DIAGNOSTIC TESTS

HANDBOOK

W9-CST-937

DIAGNOSTIC TESTS

HANDBOOK

Springhouse Corporation
Springhouse, Pennsylvania

...ord, RN, BSN, MA

...itors: Mary Chapman Gyetvan, RN, BSEd; Judith A. Schilling
...cann, RN, BSN; Helen Hahler D'Angelo, RN, MSN; Nina Poorman
Welsh, RN; Sandra Ludwig Nettina, RN, MSN

Editorial Services Manager: David Moreau

Art Director: John Hubbard

Senior Production Manager: Deborah Meiris

Some material in this book was adapted from *Diagnostics,* 2nd edition (Nurse's
Reference Library®), © 1986 by Springhouse Corporation.

Library of Congress Cataloging-in-Publication Data
Diagnostic tests handbook.

   "Material in this book adapted from Diagnostics, 2nd edition... c1986"—T.p.
verso.
   Includes bibliographies and index.
   1. Diagnosis, Laboratory—Handbooks, manuals, etc.   2. Nursing—
Handbooks, manuals, etc.   I. Springhouse Corporation.   II. Diagnostics.
[DNLM: 1. Diagnostic Tests, Routine—handbooks.   2. Diagnostic Tests,
Routine—nurses' instruction   QY 39 D5366]
RT48.5.D53 1987   616.07′5   87-10197
ISBN 0-87434-030-6 (Flex cover) and 0-87434-138-8 (Paper cover)

CONTENTS

ADVISORY BOARD, CONTRIBUTORS, AND CONSULTANTS

ADVISORY BOARD

CONTRIBUTORS

John W. Breckenridge, MD, Associate Radiologist, Abington (Pa.) Memorial Hospital

Debra C. Broadwell, RN, PhD, ET, Associate Professor of Nursing, Emory University, Atlanta

Dorothy Brooten, RN, PhD, FAAN, Chairperson, Health Care of Women and Childbearing Family Section; Director, Graduate Perinatal Nursing Program, University of Pennsylvania School of Nursing, Philadelphia

Frank Lowell Brown, CUT, Chief Urology Technician, Department of Surgery, Division of Urology, Maricopa Medical Center, Phoenix, Ariz.

Judith Byrne, BS, MT(ASCP), Affiliate Member, American Society of Clinical Pathologists

Donald C. Cannon, MD, PhD, Resident in Internal Medicine, University of Kansas School of Medicine, Wichita

Deborah L. Dairymple, RN, MSN, Assistant Professor of Nursing, Montgomery County Community College, Blue Bell, Pa.; Staff, Doylestown (Pa.) Hospital

William M. Dougherty, BS, Manager, Corporate Technical Services, SmithKline Beckman Co., Philadelphia

Patricia A. Dowen BA, COT, OT, Ophthalmic Technician, Franklin Eye Consultants, Southfield, Mich.

Barbara Boyd Egoville, RN, MSN, Former Instructor, Critical Care Nursing, Lankenau Hospital School of Nursing, Philadelphia

Jane Farrell, RN, BS, Orthopedic Nursing Specialist, Bellin Memorial Hospital. Green Bay, Wis.

John J. Fenton, PhD, DABcc, FNACB, Directory of Chemistry, Crozer-Chester Medical Center, Chester, Pa.; Associate Professor of Clinical Chemistry, West Chester University of Pennsylvania

Sr. Rebecca Fidler, MT(ASCP), PhD, Chairperson, Health Sciences, Salem (W.Va.) College

Margaret C. Fisner, MD, Assistant Professor of Pediatrics, Temple University School of Medicine, Philadelphia; Epidemiologist, St. Christopher's Hospital for Children, Philadelphia

Cynthia G. Fowler, PhD, Audiologist and Assistant Clinical Instructor, Veterans Administration Medical Center/University of California, Irvine

Katherine L. Fulton, RN, Clinical Supervisor, Gastrointestinal Unit, The Genesee Hospital, Rochester, N.Y.

Corre J. Garrett, RN, EdD, CCRN, Assistant Professor, East Carolina University School of Nursing, Greenville, N.C.

Shirley Given, HT(ASCP), Supervisor of Histology, Crozer-Chester Medical Center, Chester, Pa.

Thad C. Hagen, MD, Chief, Medical Service, Veterans Administration Medical Center, Milwaukee; Professor and Co-chairman, Department of Medicine, Medical College of Wisconsin, Milwaukee

Patrice M. Harman, RN, Staff Builders Registry, Ventura, Calif.

Annette L. Harmon, RN, MSN, CEN, Assistant Director of Nursing, Newton-Wellesley Hospital, Newton—Lower Falls, Mass.

Lenora R. Haston, RN, MSN, Assistant Executive Director for Nursing Services, Rolling Hill Hospital, Elkins Park, Pa.

Cynthia Weidman Haughey, RN, MSN, Lecturer, BSN Program, University of California—Fresno

Kathy A. Hausman, RN, MS, CNRN, Neuroscience Consultant and Program Planner, Resource Applications, Baltimore

Tobie Virginia Hittle, RN, BSN, CCRN, Head Nurse, Intensive Care Unit, The Genesee Hospital, Rochester, N.Y.

Sr. Eileen Marie Hollen, RN, BSN, CCRN, Special Care Unit Supervisor, Nazareth Hospital, Philadelphia

Richard Edward Honigman, MD, FAAP, Pediatrician, Levittown, N.Y.

Susan A. Kayes, BS, SM(ASCP), Supervisor, Microbiology Laboratory, Southwestern Vermont Medical Center, Bennington

Sr. Mary Brian Kelber, RN, SM, DNS, Associate Professor, School of Nursing, University of San Francisco

Dana Kathryn Kelly, RN, BSN, Teaching Assistant, Psychomotor Skills Laboratory, Rush University School of Nursing, Chicago

Catherine E. Kirby, RN, MSN, Nurse Consultant, Nursing Technomics of National Technomics, Inc., West Chester, Pa.

William E. Kline, MS, MT(ASCP), SBB, Director, Technical Services, St. Paul (Minn.) Red Cross

Clarke Lambe, MD, Clinical Assistant III, Department of Pathology, University of Arizona, Tucson

Laurel Kareus Lambe, MS, RD, Nutrition Consultant, Tucson, Ariz.

Dennis E. Leavelle, MD, Associate Professor and Consultant, Mayo Medical Laboratories, Department of Laboratory Medicine, Mayo Clinic, Rochester, Minn.

Cheryl Longinotti, PhD, Audiologist, Veterans Administration Westside Medical Center, Chicago

Marylou K. McHugh, RN, MSN, Academic Counselor, Department of Nursing, LaSalle University, Philadelphia

Joan C. McManus, RN, MA, Assistant Professor of Nursing, Bergen Community College, Paramus, N.J.

Claire B. Mailhot, RN, MS, Director of Operating Room Services and Assistant Director of Nursing, Stanford (Calif.) University Hospital

Elizabeth Anne Mallon, MS, MT(ASCP), Transplant Coordinator, Thomas Jefferson University Hospital, Philadelphia

Nancy L. Mauldin, RN, Nurse-Technician, St. Mary's Hospital, Galveston, Tex.

Malinda S. Mitchell, RN, MS, Associate Director of Nursing, Stanford (Calif.) University Hospital

Marilee Warner Mohr, RN, MSN, Assistant Director of Nursing, Mercy Catholic Medical Center, Misericordia Division, Philadelphia

S. Breanndan Moore, MD, DCH, FCAP, Staff Physician in Blood Bank and Transfusion Service, Mayo Clinic, Rochester, Minn.

Roger M. Morrell, MD, PhD, FACP, Chief, Neurology Service, Veterans Administration Medical Center, Allen Park, Mich.; Professor of Neurology and Microbiology/Immunology, Wayne State University School of Medicine, Detroit

Susan F. Morrow, RN, ASN, Head Nurse, Endocrinology and Neurology, Alachua General Hospital, Gainesville, Fla.

Patricia J. Noone, RN, BSN, MEd, Senior Associate Professor of Nursing, Bucks County Community College, Newtown, Pa.

Lynda Palmer, RN, BSN, Head Nurse, Respiratory and Thoracic Surgical Nursing, Toronto Western Hospital

Chan H. Park, MD, FACR, Professor and Director, Nuclear Medicine Division, Thomas Jefferson University Hospital, Philadelphia

Deborah S. Parziale, RN, MS, Assistant Professor of Nursing, Ohione College, Fremont, Calif.

Mae E. Paulfrey, RN, MN, Assistant Professor, University of San Francisco School of Nursing

Linda K. Peterson, RN, RVT, Research Clinician, Vascular Laboratory, Northwestern Memorial Hospital, Chicago

Barbara Madigan Preston, RN, MSN, Vascular Nurse Clinical Specialist and Consultant, Hospital of the University of Pennsylvania, Philadelphia

Frances W. Quinless, RN, PhD, Assistant Professor, Rutgers University College of Nursing, Newark, N.J.

Brendal Joy Randall, RN, BSN, Clinical Coordinator, Coronary Care Unit, Graduate Hospital, Philadelphia

Frank C. Riggall, MD, Associate Professor and Head, Division of Reproductive Endocrinology, University of Florida College of Medicine, Gainesville

Carolyn Robertson, RN, MSN, Diabetes Nurse Specialist, New York University School of Medicine

Suzanne G. Rotzell, RN, BSN, Staff, Intensive Care Unit, Miami Valley Hospital, Dayton, Ohio

E. Nancy Scott, RN, Staff Nurse, Nuclear Medicine Division, Thomas Jefferson University Hospital, Philadelphia

Janice Selekman, RN, MSN, DNSc, Associate Professor, Thomas Jefferson University, Philadelphia

Ellen Shipes, RN, MN, MEd, ET, Clinical Nurse Specialist, Enterostomal Therapy, Vanderbilt University Hospital, Nashville, Tenn.

Marcia S. Slaughter, RRT, Assistant Director, Respiratory Care Services, Duke University Medical Center, Durham, N.C.

Mary C. Smolenski, MSN, RNC, ARNP, Family Nurse Practitioner, University of Miami Primary Care Internal Medicine Group

Starr Shelhorse Sordelett, RN, MSN, CNS, Clinical Nurse Specialist, John Randolph Hospital, Hopewell, Va.

Harvey Spector, MD, Chief Pathologist and Director of Laboratories, Crozer-Chester Medical Center, Chester, Pa.

Arlene B. Strong, RN, MN, ANP, Cardiac Clinical Specialist, Veterans Administration Medical Center, Portland, Ore.

Basia Belza Tack, RN, MSN, Nursing Consultant, El Camino Hospital, Mountain View, Calif.; Formerly: Clinical Nurse Educator, Allergy & Infectious Diseases Nursing Service, National Institutes of Health, Bethesda, Md.

Barry L. Tonkonow, MD, Staff, Doylestown (Pa.) Hospital

Karen Dyer Vance, RN, BSN, Former Clinical Editor, Nurse's Reference Library, Springhouse Corporation, Springhouse, Pa.

Paula Brammer Vetter, RN, BSN, CCRN, Nursing Instructor, Lorain County Community College, Elyria, Ohio

Cheryl A. Walker, RN, MN, CFNP, C-ANP, MBA, Assistant Professor, School of Nursing, University of Colorado Health Science Center, Denver

Ronald J. Wapner, MD, Director, Division of Maternal and Fetal Medicine, Thomas Jefferson University Hospital, Philadelphia

Joseph B. Warren, RN, BSN, Neurosurgical Nurse Consultant, Kinetic Concepts, Inc., San Antonio, Tex.

Martin Weisberg, MD, FACOG, Assistant Professor of Obstetrics/Gynecology, Psychiatry, and Human Behavior, Jefferson Medical College, Thomas Jefferson University, Philadelphia

Charles E. Wexler, MD, Radiologist. Encino, Calif.

Beverly A. Zenk Wheat, RN, MA, Oncology Nurse Consultant, Stanford (Calif.) University Hospital

Elaine G. Whelan, RNC, MSN, MA, Associate Professor of Nursing, Bergen Community College, Paramus, N.J.

Peter Wilding, PhD, FRC, Professor and Head of Clinical Chemistry, Department of Pathology and Laboratory Medicine, Hospital of the University of Pennsylvania, Philadelphia

CONSULTANTS

Bonnie L. Anderson, MD, Radiologist, Mercy Hospital, New Orleans; formerly: Radiologist, Bowman Gray School of Nursing, Wake Forest University, Winston-Salem, N.C.

Rita S. Axelrod, MD, Assistant Professor of Medicine, Temple University School of Medicine, Philadelphia

John M. Bertoni, MD, PhD, Associate Professor of Neurology, Thomas Jefferson University, Philadelphia

Vanessa A. Fortin, RN, Day Team Leader—ICU, The Genesee Hospital, Rochester, N.Y.

Carol Ann Gramse, RN, CNA, PhD, Associate Professor of Nursing, Hunter-Bellevue School of Nursing, New York

Susan A. Kayes, BS, SM(ASCP), Supervisor, Microbiology Laboratory, Southwestern Vermont Medical Center, Bennington, Vt.

Joyce K. Keithley, RN, DNSc, Acting Chairperson, Department of OR and Surgical Nursing, Rush–Presbyterian–St. Luke's Medical Center, Chicago

Marc S. Lapayowker, MD, Chairman, Department of Radiology, Abington (Pa.) Memorial Hospital

William Levy, MD, Staff Cardiologist, Abington (Pa.) Memorial Hospital

J. Thomas Rosenthal, MD, Associate Professor, Urological Surgery, University of Pittsburgh School of Medicine

Basia Belza Tack, RN, MSN, Nursing Consultant, El Camino Hospital, Mountain View, Calif.; formerly: Clinical Nurse Educator, Allergy and Infectious Disease Nursing Service, National Institutes of Health, Bethesda, Md.

Martin Weisberg, MD, FACOG, Assistant Professor of Obstetrics/Gynecology, Psychiatry, and Human Behavior, Jefferson Medical College, Thomas Jefferson University, Philadelphia

Peter Wilding, PhD, FRC, Professor and Head of Clinical Chemistry, Department of Pathology and Laboratory Medicine, Hospital of the University of Pennsylvania, Philadelphia.

FOREWORD

More than ever before, professional responsibility for patient care is likely to involve laboratory tests and other diagnostic procedures. Such involvement may include multiple aspects of preparing for the test, assisting during its course, monitoring its effects, and modifying care based on test results.

To meet these responsibilities effectively, you need much more than just a superficial familiarity with any given test. You must have a ready source of fundamental information about the test itself: why it is useful, how it is performed, how it is likely to affect the patient, and what the test results indicate. DIAGNOSTIC TESTS HANDBOOK provides this comprehensive information in a readily accessible form.

The handbook contains 13 chapters, which include over 450 diagnostic tests. Chapters 1 through 6 present laboratory tests performed on blood, urine, other body fluids, and feces. These include hematologic chemistry and immunodiagnostic tests. Chapter 7 presents microbiological tests used in diagnosing infection. Chapter 8 presents endoscopic tests performed on a variety of body organs. Chapter 9 presents histologic and cytologic tests important in diagnosing malignancy, and cytogenetic tests important in diagnosing genetic disorders. Chapters 10 through 12 present diagnostic imaging tests—both invasive and noninvasive—including radiologic, nuclear medicine, and ultrasound tests. Chapter 13 presents such specialized tests as cardiac studies as well as other organ studies.

Each chapter begins with essential information about the category of tests included in the chapter, followed by "Patient-Teaching Guidelines." Individual test entries are easy to find within each chapter, since they are organized alphabetically. Each test entry follows a consistent format, beginning with *Purpose*, a brief summary of common indications for the test. Next, *Normal Results* summarizes values or findings generally regarded as normal. (Some numeric values listed may vary by laboratory and by method and are provided as a general guide.) The entry continues with *Abnormal Results,* which summarizes how results may deviate from normal, when appropriate, and lists the clinical conditions causing abnormalities. Next, *The Basics* includes significant information about the test: relevant physiology that supports understanding of the test, its clinical importance, contraindications, and other pertinent facts. *Procedure* explains how the test is performed, using a concise format to identify each essential step. *Special Precautions,* used when needed, draws attention to special measures important for test accuracy, patient safety, or other vital health needs. The *Patient Care Checklist* is a helpful guide to ensure that patients' needs are met before and after the test. "Before the test" always includes a reminder concerning patient teaching and evaluation of patient understanding; it itemizes the necessary physical and psychological preparation for the test, including dietary and drug restrictions. "After the test" is used, when needed, to itemize post-test care measures, such as activity or dietary restrictions, special assessment measures, health teaching, and referrals based on test results. Finally, *Interfering Factors* summarizes elements of preparation or procedure that can invalidate the test or make its interpretation difficult or unreliable. "Clinical Alerts" are used in some entries to call attention to urgent information.

When appropriate, each entry also includes helpful information on related tests as well as illustrations, graphs, and charts that isolate and emphasize useful supplementary information. A special introductory section on *Collection Techniques* summarizes recommended procedures and offers practical guidelines for obtaining and handling blood and urine samples—the two most common laboratory specimens.

A major feature of this handbook is a separate section, "Diagnostic Test Profiles for Common Disorders." This convenient chart profiles 101 of the most common and/or important medical disorders along with pertinent diagnostic tests that may be performed for each. Most helpful is the inclusion of such newer tests as magnetic resonance imaging and positron emission tomography. Expected results for each test are identified, and meaningful comments are included where appropriate.

Useful appendices follow the chapters. Normal results for laboratory tests included throughout the book are arranged alphabetically and are condensed into one handy reference chart. Similarly, charts with laboratory values are provided for therapeutic drug monitoring and toxicology. Another unique appendix features home tests, a relatively new and growing phenomenon. A representative sample of tests for glucose, pregnancy, ovulation, occult blood, and infection is included.

The DIAGNOSTIC TESTS HANDBOOK provides a clear, concise, and comprehensive presentation of information concerning current diagnostic tests. I highly recommend this volume not only to nurses, but also to all medical professionals who deal with diagnostic testing in any way. A thorough knowledge of its contents will promote your understanding of diagnostic procedures and enhance your effectiveness as a member of the health care team.

Dennis E. Leavelle, MD
Mayo Medical Laboratories
Department of Laboratory Medicine
Mayo Clinic
Rochester, Minnesota

COLLECTION TECHNIQUES: BLOOD AND URINE SAMPLES

Blood

The type of blood sample required—whole blood, plasma, or serum—depends on the nature of the test. *Whole blood*—containing all blood elements—is the sample of choice for blood gas analysis, determination of hemoglobin derivatives, and measurement of RBC constituents. In addition, most routine hematologic studies, such as complete blood count, erythrocyte sedimentation rate, reticulocyte and platelet counts, and the osmotic fragility test, require whole blood samples.

Plasma is the liquid part of whole blood, which contains all the blood proteins; *serum,* the liquid that remains after whole blood clots. Plasma and serum samples, which contain most of the physiologically and clinically significant substances found in blood, are used for most biochemical, immunologic, and coagulation studies. They also provide useful electrolyte evaluation, enzyme analysis, glucose concentration, protein determination, and bilirubin level.

Venous, arterial, and capillary blood

Venous blood represents physiologic conditions throughout the body and is relatively easy to obtain; therefore, it is used for most laboratory procedures.

Arterial blood samples are necessary for pH, PaO_2, and $PaCO_2$ determinations, and oxygen saturation studies, even though an arterial puncture increases the risks of hematoma and arterial spasm.

Capillary blood samples are most useful for studies such as hemoglobin and hematocrit determinations; blood smears; microtechniques for clinical chemistry; and platelet, RBC, and WBC counts requiring only small amounts of blood.

Quantities and containers

Sample quantities needed for diagnostic studies depend on the laboratory, available equipment, and the type of test. Some laboratories, for example, use automated analyzer systems that require a serum sample of 100 μl or less; others use manual systems that require a larger amount. The desired sample quantity determines the collection procedure, and the type and size of the container. A single venipuncture with a conventional glass or disposable plastic syringe can provide 15 ml of blood—sufficient for many hematologic, immunologic, chemical, and coagulation tests, but hardly enough for a series of tests.

To avoid multiple venipunctures when tests require a large blood sample, an evacuated tube system (Vacutainer, Corvac) with interchangeable glass tubes, optional draw capacities, and a selection of additives is used. Evacuated tubes are commercially prepared with or without additives (indicated by their color-coded stoppers), and with enough vacuum to draw a predetermined blood volume (2 to 20 ml per tube).

Microanalysis of minute amounts of capillary blood collected with micropipettes or glass capillary tubes allows numerous hematologic and routine laboratory studies on infants, children, and patients with severe burns or poor veins. Micropipettes are color-coded by sample capacity and hold 30 to 50 μl of whole blood; glass capillary tubes hold 80 to 130 μl of serum or plasma.

Venous sample

The nature of the test and the patient's age and condition determine the appropriate blood sample, collection site, and technique. Most tests require a venous sample. Although a relatively simple procedure, venipuncture must be performed carefully to avoid hemolysis or hemoconcentration of the sample, to prevent hematoma formation, and to prevent damage to the patient's veins. For these reasons and also to decrease patient discomfort, venipuncture is usually performed by laboratory technicians and nurses skilled in the technique.

Label all test tubes clearly with the patient's name and room number, doctor's name, date, and collection time.

Select a venipuncture site. The most common site is the antecubital fossa area; other sites include the wrist and the dorsum of the hand or foot. When drawing the sample at bedside, instruct the patient to lie on his back, with his head slightly elevated and his arms resting at his sides. When drawing blood from an ambulatory patient, tell him to sit in a chair, with his arm supported securely on an armrest or table.

When using an evacuated tube, attach the needle to the holder before applying the tourniquet. Apply a soft rubber tourniquet above the puncture site to prevent venous blood return and to increase venous pressure, thus making the veins more prominent and increasing the volume of blood at the puncture site. Make sure the tourniquet is snug but not tight enough to constrict arteries. Using a tourniquet for a patient with large, distended, and highly visible veins increases the risk of hematoma. If the patient's veins appear distinct, you may not need to apply a tourniquet.

Instruct the patient to make a fist several times to further enlarge the veins. Select a vein by palpation and inspection.

If you cannot feel a vein distinctly, *do not* attempt venipuncture. Working in a circular motion from the center outward, clean the puncture site with alcohol or povidone-iodine solution, and dry it with a gauze pad. If you must touch the cleansed puncture site again to relocate the vein, palpate with an antiseptically clean finger, and wipe

Safeguards for Venipuncture

● Make sure the patient is adequately supported, in case of syncope.
● When using a syringe to draw a sample, avoid injecting air into a vein by checking that the plunger is fully depressed before injection.
● If possible, avoid drawing blood from an arm or leg used for I.V. infusion of blood, dextrose, or electrolyte solutions, since this dilutes the blood sample. If you must collect blood near an I.V. site, choose a location below it.
● For easier identification of veins in patients with tortuous or sclerosed veins, or with veins damaged by repeated venipuncture, antibiotic therapy, or chemotherapy, apply warm, wet compresses 15 minutes before attempting venipuncture.
● If you are not successful after two attempts, ask another nurse to perform the venipuncture.
● When you cannot find a vein quickly, release the tourniquet temporarily, to avoid tissue necrosis and circulation problems.
● Be sure to insert the needle at the correct angle to reduce the risk of puncturing the opposite wall of the vein and causing a hematoma.
● Always release the tourniquet before withdrawing the needle, to prevent a hematoma. When drawing multiple samples, release the tourniquet within 1 minute after beginning to draw blood to prevent a hemoconcentration sample.

the area again with an alcohol swab.

Draw the skin tautly over the vein by pressing just below the puncture site with your thumb, to keep the vein from moving.

Hold the syringe or tube with the needle bevel up and the shaft parallel to the path of the vein at a 15-degree angle to the arm. Enter the vein with a single direct puncture of the skin and vein wall. If you use a syringe, venous blood will appear in the hub. Withdraw the blood slowly, gently pulling on the syringe to create steady suction until you obtain the desired amount. For an evacuated tube, when a drop of blood appears just inside the needle holder, grasp the needle holder securely and push down on the collection tube until the needle punctures the rubber stopper; blood flows into the tube automatically. When the tube is filled, remove it, and if drawing multiple samples, repeat the procedure with additional tubes.

To prevent stasis, release the tourniquet as soon as you establish adequate blood flow. If the flow is sluggish, you may want to leave the tourniquet in place longer. However, always remove the tourniquet before withdrawing the needle.

After drawing the sample, ask the patient to open his fist as soon as you collect the desired amount. Release the tourniquet. Place a gauze pad over the puncture site, then withdraw the needle slowly and gently. Apply gentle pressure to the puncture site. If the patient is alert and cooperative, tell him to hold the gauze in place for several minutes until the bleeding stops, to prevent hematoma. If the patient is not alert or cooperative, hold the pad in place, or apply a small adhesive bandage.

After collection with a syringe, remove the needle and carefully empty the sample into the appropriate test tube, without delay. To prevent foaming and possible hemolysis, *do not* eject the blood through the needle or force it out of the syringe.

Place the appropriate color-coded stoppers on the tubes. Gently invert a tube containing anticoagulant several times to mix the sample thoroughly. Examine the sample for clots or clumps; if none appears, send the sample to the laboratory. *Do not* shake the tube.

Before leaving the patient, check his condition. If a hematoma develops at the puncture site, apply warm soaks. If the patient has lingering discomfort or undue bleeding, instruct him to lie down. Watch for anxiety or signs of shock, such as hypotension and tachycardia.

Make sure the specimen is sent to the laboratory immediately.

Arterial sample

Arterial blood is rarely required for routine studies. Since arterial puncture carries risks, samples are generally collected by a doctor or a specially trained nurse from the radial, brachial, or femoral artery. Arterial blood may also be drawn from an arterial line.

Although a local anesthetic may be administered at the puncture site, this is done only when necessary because it delays the proedure and may cause an allergic reaction, and resulting vasoconstriction may prevent successful puncture.

To heparinize the syringe, first attach a 20G needle to the syringe; then, break open the ampul of heparin and draw 1 ml into the syringe. While rotating the barrel, pull the plunger back past the 7-ml mark. Hold the syringe in an upright position, and slowly force the heparin toward the hub of the syringe, as you continue to rotate the barrel. Leave enough heparin—about 0.1 ml—to fill the syringe tip.

Heparinize the needle by removing the first needle and replacing it with a 23G needle. Continue to hold the syringe upright, but tilt it slightly. Then push the plunger all the way up to eject the remaining heparin.

Perform the Allen's test (see *How to Perform the Allen's Test*) to assess circulation in the radial artery. Choose either the radial or brachial artery, whichever has the better circulation. Because complications can be more severe, arterial blood is usually collected from the femoral artery only when circulation in the brachial and radial artery is poor. *Do not* choose a site where the patient has had a vascular graft or has an atrioventricular fistula in situ.

Next, using a circular motion, clean the puncture site with a swab soaked in povidone-iodine solution. Then wipe the site with a swab soaked in alcohol to remove the povidone-iodine solution, which is sticky and may hinder palpation. Palpate the artery with the forefinger and middle finger of one hand, while holding the syringe over the puncture site with the other hand.

With the needle bevel up, puncture the skin at a 45-degree angle for the radial artery and at a 60-degree angle for the brachial artery. For a femoral arterial puncture, the needle is inserted at a 90-degree angle.

Advance the needle, but do not pull the plunger back. When you have punctured the artery, blood will pulsate into the syringe. Allow it to fill 5 to 10 ml. If the syringe does not fill immediately, you may have pushed the needle through the artery. Pull the needle back slightly, but do not pull the plunger back. If the syringe still does not fill, withdraw the needle and start over with a fresh heparinized needle. Never make more than two attempts to draw blood from one site.

After drawing the sample, remove the needle and apply firm pressure to the puncture site with a gauze pad for at least 5 minutes, to prevent hematoma (a significant risk after arterial puncture). If the patient is receiving an anticoagulant or has a bleeding disorder, apply pressure for at least 15 minutes. *Do not* ask the patient to apply pressure to the site. The patient may not apply the continuous, firm pressure that is needed.

How to Perform the Allen's Test

Before drawing blood from a radial artery, perform the Allen's test. This test tells you whether or not the patient will receive enough blood through the ulnar artery to supply his hand if occlusion of the radial artery occurs.

First, have the patient rest his arm on the mattress or bedside stand, supporting his wrist with a rolled towel. Ask him to clench his fist. Then, using your index and middle fingers, exert pressure on both the radial and ulnar arteries. Hold this position for a few seconds.

Without removing your fingers from the patient's arteries, ask the patient to unclench his fist and hold his hand in a relaxed position. The palm will be blanched, because you have impaired the normal blood flow with your fingers.

Now, release the pressure on the patient's ulnar artery. If the hand becomes flushed, indicating the rush of oxygenated blood to the hand, you can safely proceed with the radial artery puncture. If it does not, repeat the test on the other arm. If neither arm produces a positive result, use the brachial artery for arterial puncture.

Rotate the syringe to mix the heparin with the sample. If air bubbles appear, try to remove them by holding the syringe upright and tapping it lightly with your finger. If the bubbles do not disappear, hold the syringe upright and pierce a 2" x 2" gauze pad or alcohol swab with the needle (slowly forcing some of the blood out of the syringe eliminates the bubbles, and the gauze pad catches the ejected blood). After removing air bubbles, plunge the needle into a rubber stopper to seal it from the air, and transfer the sample to the iced specimen container.

Note on the laboratory slip the patient's temperature, hemoglobin count, and the type and amount of oxygen he is receiving. Send the sample to the laboratory immediately.

After releasing pressure on the puncture site and checking for bleeding, tape a bandage firmly over it. (Do not tape the entire wrist, as this may restrict circulation.)

CLINICAL ALERT: **After arterial puncture, observe carefully for signs of circulatory impairment distal to the puncture site, such as swelling, discoloration, pain, numbness, or tingling in the bandaged extremity.**

Before drawing an arterial blood sample for blood gas studies, carefully check the patient's oxygen level. If ABG levels are being measured to monitor response to withdrawal of oxygen therapy, but the patient continues to receive it, results will be misleading. For the same reason, do not draw an arterial sample immediately after suctioning or after placement on a ventilator. Wait at least 15 minutes to allow circulating blood levels to accurately reflect response to mechanical ventilation.

Capillary sample

Collection of a capillary blood sample requires skin puncture of the fingertip or earlobe of adults, or puncture of the great toe or the heel of newborns.

To facilitate collection of a capillary sample, first dilate the vessels by applying warm, moist compresses to the area for about 10 minutes. Select the puncture site, wipe it with gauze and alcohol, and dry it thoroughly with another gauze pad so the blood will well up. Avoid cold, cyanotic, or swollen sites, to ensure an adequate blood sample.

To draw a sample from the fingertip, use a lancet smaller than 2 mm, and make the puncture perpendicular to the lines of the patient's fingerprints.

After drawing the sample, wipe away the first drop of blood to reduce the chance of sample dilution with tissue fluid. For the same reason, avoid squeezing the puncture site. After collecting the sample, briefly apply pressure to the puncture site to prevent painful extravasation of blood into the subcutaneous tissues. Ask the adult patient to hold a sterile gauze pad over the puncture site until bleeding has stopped. Then apply a small adhesive bandage.

Interfering factors

Food or medications can interfere with test methods, so be sure to check the patient's diet and medication history before tests, and to schedule them after an overnight fast of 12 to 14 hours. Although the concentration of most blood constituents does not change significantly after a meal, fasting is customary, because blood collected shortly after eating often appears cloudy (turbid) from a temporary increase in triglyceride levels that can interfere with many chemical reactions. Transient, food-related lipemia usually disappears 4 to 6 hours after a meal, making such short fasts acceptable before blood collection.

Baseline studies often depend on the patient's diet. For example, valid glucose tolerance test results require an adequate daily carbohydrate intake (250 mg) for 3 days before testing. Similarly, recent protein and fat consumption influences uric acid, urea, and lipid levels.

Numerous drugs and their metabolites affect test results by pharmacologic or chemical interference. Pharmacologic interference results from temporary or permanent drug-induced physiologic change in a blood component. For example, long-term administration of such drugs as erythromycin can damage the liver and alter the results of liver function studies. Chemical interference results from a drug's physical characteristic that alters the test reaction. For example, high dosages of ascorbic acid may raise blood glucose levels. To identify such interference with test results, all unexpected changes in blood values require a meticulous review of the patient's drug and dietary history and of his clinical status.

Urine

The type of urine specimen required—random, second-voided, clean-catch midstream, first morning, fasting, or timed—depends on the patient's condition and age, and the purpose of the test. Random, second-voided, and clean-catch midstream specimens can be collected at any time; first morning, fasting, or timed specimens require collection at specific times.

To collect a *random* specimen (for such routine tests as urinalysis), the patient simply collects one voiding in a specimen container. Although this method provides quick laboratory results, the information it provides is less reliable than that from a controlled specimen.

To collect a *second-voided* specimen, the patient voids, discards the urine, and then 30 minutes later voids again into a specimen container.

To collect a *clean-catch* specimen, the patient voids first into either a bedpan or toilet, and collects a sample in midstream. Originally used mainly to test for bacteriuria and pyuria, this specimen is now replacing the random specimen because it is aseptic.

First morning and *fasting* specimens must be collected when the patient awakes. Since the *first morning* specimen is the most concentrated of the day, it is the specimen of choice for nitrate, protein, and urinary sediment analyses. For this specimen, the patient voids and discards the urine just before going to bed, then collects the first voiding of the morning. For the *fasting* specimen, which is used for glucose testing, the patient maintains an overnight fast and collects a *first morning* specimen.

The *timed* specimen determines the urinary concentration of such substances as hormones, proteins, creatinine, and electrolytes over a specified period—usually 2, 12, or 24 hours. The 24-hour collection, the most common timed specimen, provides a measure of average excretion for substances eliminated in variable amounts during the day, such as hormones. Timed specimens may also be collected after administration of a challenge dose of a chemical, to measure physiologic efficiency—for example, ingestion of glucose to test for incipient diabetes mellitus or hypoglycemia. This type of specimen is also preferred for quantitative analysis of urobilinogen, xylose, amylase, phenolsulfonphthalein dye excretion, or an Addis count.

Random and second-voided collections

For random collection, tell the ambulatory patient to urinate directly into a clean, dry specimen container. Tell the nonambulatory patient to void into a clean bedpan or urinal, to minimize bacterial or chemical contamination; then transfer about 30 ml of urine to the specimen container, and secure the cap.

For second-voided collection, instruct the patient to void and discard the urine. Then, offer him at least one glass of water, to stimulate urine production. Collect urine 30 minutes later, using the random collection technique.

Label the container with the patient's name and room number (if applicable), doctor's name, date, and collection time. Send the specimen and a completed request slip to the laboratory immediately. On the chart, record the procedure and the time the specimen was sent.

First morning and fasting collections

Unless the patient is an infant or is catheterized or unable to urinate, the following collection techniques are used for first morning and fasting specimens.

For fasting specimen collection, instruct the patient to restrict food and fluids after midnight before the test. For both collection procedures, instruct the patient to void and discard the urine before retiring for the night; then collect the first voiding of the next day in a clean, dry specimen container. (If the patient must void during the night, note it on the specimen label—for example, "Urine specimen, 2:15 a.m. to 8:00 a.m.")

Label the container with the patient's name and room number (if applicable), doctor's name, date, and collection time. Send the specimen and a completed request slip to the laboratory immediately. On the chart, record the procedure and the time the specimen was sent.

Clean-catch midstream collection

This aseptic technique for obtaining a clean-catch midstream urine specimen has recently become the more acceptable procedure for collecting a random urine specimen.

Because this method is used to collect a virtually uncontaminated specimen, explain the procedure to the patient carefully. Provide illustrations to emphasize correct collection technique, if possible.

Tell the patient first to cleanse the periurethral area (tip of the penis, or labial folds, vulva, and urethral meatus) with soap and water. Then, wipe the area three times, each time with a fresh $2'' \times 2''$ gauze pad soaked in povidone-iodine solution or, if you are using a commercial kit, with the wipes provided. Instruct the female patient to separate her labial folds with the thumb and forefinger; to wipe down one side with the first pad and discard it; to wipe the other side with the second pad and discard it; and finally, to wipe down the center over the urinary meatus with the third pad and discard it. Stress the importance of cleansing

from front to back to prevent contamination of the genital area with fecal matter. For the uncircumcised male patient, emphasize the need to retract his foreskin to effectively cleanse the meatus and to keep it retracted during voiding. Tell the female patient to straddle the bedpan or toilet to allow labial spreading. She should continue to keep her labia separated with her fingers while voiding.

Instruct the patient to begin voiding into the bedpan, urinal, or toilet, because the urinary stream washes bacteria from the urethra and urinary meatus. Then, tell the patient to void directly into the sterile container, collecting about 30 to 50 ml at the midstream portion of the voiding. The patient can then finish voiding into the bedpan, urinal, or toilet. Emphasize that the first and the last portions of the voiding are discarded.

Take the sterile container from the patient, and cap it securely. Wash your hands thoroughly to prevent cross-contamination, and tell the patient to do the same.

Label the container with the patient's name and room number, type of specimen, collection time, and suspected diagnosis, if known. If a urine culture is to be performed, note any current antibiotic therapy on the laboratory request slip. Send the container to the laboratory immediately, or place it on ice to prevent specimen deterioration and altered test results.

Timed collection

All timed specimens—2-, 12-, and 24-hour—are collected in virtually the same way. This procedure is applicable for uncatheterized adults and continent children.

Explain the procedure to the patient, and instruct him to collect all urine during the test period, to notify you after each voiding, and to avoid contaminating the specimen with toilet tissue or stool. Also, provide him with written instructions for home collection. Explain any necessary dietary, drug, or activity restrictions.

Obtain the proper preservative from the laboratory. Write down the test requirements on the nursing-care Kardex.

Label a gallon jug or commercial urine collection container with the patient's name and room number (if applicable); doctor's name; date and time the collection begins and ends; a warning "Do Not Discard"; and instructions to keep the container refrigerated. Prominently display signs indicating that a 24-hour urine collection is in progress: one at the head of the patient's bed, a second over the toilet bowl in his bathroom, and a third over the utility room bedpan hopper.

Tell the patient to void and discard the urine; then begin 24-hour collection with the next voiding. After placing the first voiding in the container, add the preservative. Add each voiding to the container immediately. If any urine is lost, restart the test, but remember the test should end at a time the laboratory is open. Just before the end of the collection period, have the patient void, and add the urine to the gallon jug.

Send the labeled container to the laboratory immediately after the collection period. On the chart, record the time urine collection ended and when the specimen was sent to the laboratory.

Special timed collections

Some tests require specimen collection at specified times—for example, the glucose tolerance test requires collection of urine at ½ hour, 1 hour, 2 hours, 3 hours, and occasionally, 4 and 5 hours after a test meal. To ensure that the patient can void at the specified times, provide water at least every hour. Other tests, including urea clearance, require only 2-hour collection periods. For these tests, give the patient at least 20 oz (600 ml) of water 30 minutes before the test, and instruct him to drink at least one full glass each hour during the test.

Pediatric urine collection

Pediatric urine collection is used to obtain a random, second-voided, first morning, fasting, or timed specimen from infants.

Position the patient on his back, with his hips externally rotated and abducted, and knees flexed. Clean the perineal area with cotton swabs, soap, and water. Rinse the area with warm water; dry it thoroughly.

For *boys*, apply the collection device over the penis and scrotum, and closely press the flaps of the collection bag against the perineum to ensure a tight fit.

For *girls*, tape the pediatric collection device to the perineum, starting at the point between the anus and the vagina and working anteriorly.

Place a diaper over the collection bag to discourage the child from tampering with it. Elevate the head of the bed to facilitate drainage.

Remove the bag immediately after collection is complete to prevent skin excoriation. Transfer the urine to a clean, dry specimen container. Label the container with the patient's name and room number (if applicable), doctor's name, date, and collection time. Send the specimen and the completed request slip to the laboratory immediately, and note the collection time on the chart.

Catheter collection

Although catheter collection increases the risk of bacterial infection in the lower genitourinary tract, it may be necessary to obtain a random, second-voided, first morning, fasting, or timed specimen in a patient who cannot void voluntarily.

Using sterile technique, the patient is catheterized. A few milliliters of urine are allowed to drain into the basin and then, depending on test requirements, 10 to 60 ml of urine are collected in a sterile plastic container. The catheter is removed, and the area is cleansed and dried.

The specimen and a completed request slip are sent to the laboratory within 10 minutes after collection, or the specimen is refrigerated. On the chart, record the procedure and the time the specimen was sent.

Collection from an indwelling catheter

You can minimize the risk of bacterial contamination by aspirating a urine specimen from a Foley catheter made of self-sealing rubber or from a collection tube with a special sampling port. However, *do not* aspirate a Silastic, silicone, or plastic catheter. This technique can provide a random, second-voided, first morning, fasting, or special timed specimen.

About 30 minutes before collecting the specimen, clamp the collection tube. (This procedure is contraindicated for patients who have just undergone genitourinary surgery.) If the collection tube has a sampling port, wipe the sampling port with an alcohol sponge, insert the needle at a 90-degree angle, and aspirate the urine into the syringe. If it does not have a port, but if the catheter is made of rubber, you can obtain the specimen from the catheter. Other types of catheters will leak after you withdraw the needle. To do this, wipe the catheter with alcohol just above the connection of the collection tube to the catheter. Insert the needle at a 45-degree angle into the rubber catheter, and withdraw the urine specimen. Never insert the needle into the shaft of the catheter since this may puncture the lumen leading to the balloon.

Be sure to unclamp the tube after collecting the specimen. Failure to do so can cause bladder distension and may predispose the patient to a bladder infection. If you cannot draw any urine, lift the tube a little, but make sure urine does not return to the bladder. Aspirate urine, and transfer the specimen to a sterile container.

If a 12-hour or 24-hour urine collection is necessary and the patient has an indwelling catheter, empty the drainage tubing into the collection bag, then empty the collection bag and put the bag into an ice-filled container at his bedside. Also, depending on the institution's policy, a clean collection bag may be attached to the indwelling catheter for this technique.

Interfering factors

A common interfering factor in urine collection, especially in timed collections, is the patient's or nurse's failure to follow the correct collection procedure. Improper specimens may result from *overcollection,* by failing to discard the last voiding before the test period; *undercollection,* by failing to include all urine voided during the test; *contamination,* by including toilet tissue or stool in the specimen; or, for procedures requiring collection at specified times or for the second-voided collection, the patient's *inability to urinate on demand.* In urine specimens collected from females, vaginal drainage—such as menses, which elevates RBCs—can alter the results of a urinalysis.

Improper collection or handling of the specimen can also produce unreliable results. For instance, failure to thoroughly clean the urethral meatus and glans before collection can contaminate a clean-catch midstream specimen. Similarly, failure to send a urine specimen to the laboratory immediately allows bacterial proliferation and thus invalidates the colony count on bacterial culture.

Obviously, foods and drugs can also affect test results by changing the composition of the urine. For example, ingestion of sugar increases urine glucose. Drugs can cause chemical or pharmacologic interference with the laboratory analysis. For example, aspirin causes false-positive results with Clinitest, and corticosteroids tend to elevate glucose levels.

1 HEMATOLOGIC TESTING

Introduction

Hematologic testing involves studying blood components as well as the actual process of hemostasis.

Red cells, also known as erythrocytes and red corpuscles, maintain a high concentration of circulatory hemoglobin. Hemoglobin—the main component of the red cell—is a conjugated protein that enables red cells to carry oxygen from the lungs to the tissues, and to carry carbon dioxide from the tissues back to the lungs, for excretion. Three major types of hemoglobin are found in normal blood: Hgb A, Hgb A_2, and Hgb F. Red cells also transport large quantities of carbon dioxide through the activity of carbonic anhydrase, a red cell enzyme. Thus, red cells help to maintain the body's acid-base balance.

Abnormal red cell production can result in anemias, characterized by an abnormally low hemoglobin concentration, red cell count, and hematocrit or polycythemia, and overproduction of red blood cells. More than 200 abnormal hemoglobins result from genetic and acquired variations.

White blood cells (leukocytes, WBCs) include neutrophils, eosinophils, basophils, monocytes, and lymphocytes. The special function of white cells, particularly neutrophils, is to protect against infection. Malignant mutation of the blood-forming tissues can cause unrestrained white-cell production (leukemia). Leukemias are classified according to the type of white-cell proliferation: lymphocytic, granulocytic, or monocytic.

Plasma cells are usually found in the lymphoid tissue, but rarely in the peripheral circulation. They produce antibodies to help fight disease. Contact with a specific antigen causes certain lymphocytes to become plasma cells and stimulates the immune activity. Plasma cells may appear in the circulation during severe infection, to reinforce immunity when insufficient antibodies are available. The presence of such cells in the blood may indicate multiple myeloma, plasma cell leukemia, scarlet fever, measles, or chicken pox.

Reticuloendothelial system (RES) cells are much less mobile than circulating white cells, but like them, RES cells remove foreign matter and endogenous debris from the blood, lymph, and interstitial spaces of the body. For example, when hemoglobin enters the blood from ruptured red cells, RES cells digest it.

Platelets, also known as thrombocytes, protect vascular surfaces and help stop bleeding. Platelet disorders stemming from abnormalities of number (thrombocytopenia and thrombocytosis) or function (thrombasthenia and thrombocytopathia) can interfere with hemostasis by impairing vascular integrity and the coagulation mechanism.

Hemostasis is the process in which the circulatory system protects itself from excessive blood loss. Vascular injury activates a complex chain of events—vasoconstriction, platelet aggregation, and coagulation—leading to clotting, which stops the bleeding without hindering blood flow through the injured vessel. Interference in the normal clotting process, whether hereditary or acquired, can result in coagulation defects and bleeding disorders, such as hypoprothrombinemia or hemophilia. (See *Collection Techniques: Blood and Urine Samples*, pp. xii to xx.)

Patient-teaching guidelines
Patient-learner objectives:
- Define the test.
- State the specific purpose of the test.
- Explain the procedure.
- Discuss test preparation, procedure, and post-test care.

Teaching content:
- Define the test in terms the patient can understand.
- Explain the specific purpose of the test.
- Describe the procedure if the patient is unfamiliar with it. If collection of a capillary blood sample is necessary, explain that this requires a small skin puncture of the fingertip or earlobe of adults, or a puncture of the great toe or heel of newborns. If a venipuncture is necessary, explain that the patient's vein will be punctured, usually by a steel needle attached to a tube or syringe, so blood can be collected for testing.
- Explain that collection of the blood sample causes some discomfort; however, the procedure is brief.
- Inform the patient that mild pressure will be applied to the puncture site following the procedure. Usually, a few minutes' pressure at most is sufficient to stop the bleeding. If the patient has a bleeding tendency, inform him that pressure may be necessary for a longer period to control bleeding.
- When appropriate, list the medications that may interfere with test results, and instruct the patient to withhold these medications for the designated period of time before the test. Accompany verbal instructions with written ones for the outpatient.

- When appropriate, inform the patient that the hematological tests are part of routine hospital screening procedures.

Evaluation:
- After the patient-teaching session is completed, evaluate whether the patient has successfully met each patient-learner objective, by obtaining necessary patient feedback. Refocus teaching as needed.

Activated partial thromboplastin time (APTT)

Purpose
- To screen for deficiencies of the clotting factors in the intrinsic pathways (except Factors VII and XIII)
- To monitor heparin therapy.

Normal results
A fibrin clot forms 25 to 36 seconds after the addition of reagent.

Abnormal results
Prolonged APTT times may indicate:
  Deficiency of certain plasma clotting factors
  Presence of heparin
  Presence of fibrin split products, fibrinolysins, or circulating anticoagulants that are antibodies to specific clotting factors.

The basics
The APTT test evaluates all the clotting factors of the intrinsic pathway—except Factors VII and XIII—by measuring the time required for formation of a fibrin clot. Since most congenital coagulation deficiencies occur in the intrinsic pathway, APTT is valuable in preoperative screening for bleeding tendencies. It is also the test of choice for monitoring heparin therapy. The partial thromboplastin time (PTT) test is similar to the APTT but is less sensitive and less commonly performed.

Heparin Neutralization Assay

This complex quantitative test is sometimes used to monitor heparin therapy. It can also help determine if prolonged thrombin time results from effective heparin therapy or from the presence of circulating anticoagulants, such as fibrin split products. To perform this test, a specimen is divided into small plasma samples. Thrombin time is determined on one sample; the other samples are added to various dilutions of protamine sulfate. After a brief incubation, equal amounts of thrombin are added to each solution and thrombin time is measured. Because protamine sulfate neutralizes heparin, reduced thrombin time in the protamine-treated samples indicates the presence of heparin.

A fibrometer is used to select the sample with the thrombin time closest to standard. Then a chart or formula is used to convert the sample's protamine concentration to units of heparin/ml, providing an accurate measurement of heparin blood levels. If none of the samples shows a reduced thrombin time, no heparin is present, indicating that the prolonged thrombin time is due to other anticoagulants, such as fibrin split products.

Procedure
Perform a venipuncture, and collect the sample in a 7-ml blue-top tube.

Patient care checklist
Before the test
☑ Explain or clarify test purpose and procedure.
☑ Evaluate patient understanding.
☑ Inform the patient who is receiving heparin therapy that this test may be repeated at regular intervals, to assess response to treatment.

Interfering factors
• Failure to use the proper anticoagulant, to fill the collection tube completely, or to mix the sample and the anticoagulant adequately may interfere with accurate determination of test results.
• Hemolysis due to rough handling of the sample or to excessive probing at the venipuncture site may alter test results.
• Failure to send the sample to the laboratory immediately or to place it on ice may cause spurious test results. (See *Heparin Neutralization Assay*.)

Bleeding time

Purpose
• To assess overall hemostatic function (platelet response to injury and functional capacity of vasoconstriction)
• To detect congenital and acquired platelet function disorders.

Normal results
Template method: 2 to 8 minutes
Modified template method: 2 to 10 minutes
Ivy method: 1 to 7 minutes
Duke method: 1 to 3 minutes

Abnormal results
Prolonged bleeding time
Associated with low platelet count in:
    Hodgkin's disease
    Acute leukemia
    Disseminated intravascular coagulation (DIC)
    Hemolytic disease of the newborn
    Schönlein-Henoch purpura
    Severe hepatic disease (cirrhosis, for example)
    Severe deficiency of Factors I, II, V, VII, VIII, IX, and XI.
Associated with normal platelet count in:

Platelet function disorders, such as thrombasthenia and thrombocytopathia.

The basics

This test measures the duration of bleeding after a standardized skin incision. Bleeding time depends on the elasticity of the blood vessel wall and on the number and functional capacity of platelets. Although this test is usually performed on patients with personal or family histories of bleeding disorders, it is also useful for preoperative screening, along with a platelet count. Bleeding time may be measured by one of four methods: Duke, Ivy, template, or modified template. The template methods are the most frequently used and the most accurate, since they standardize the incision size, making test results reproducible.

Usually, the test is not recommended for a patient whose platelet count is less than 75,000/mm³. However, some patients with altered platelet morphology may have normal bleeding times despite their low platelet counts.

Procedure

Template and modified template methods:
• Wrap the pressure cuff around the upper arm and inflate the cuff to 40 mmHg.
• Select an area on the forearm that is free of superficial veins, and cleanse it with antiseptic. Allow the skin to dry completely before making the incision.
• Apply the appropriate template lengthwise to the forearm.
• For the template method, use the lancet to make two incisions, 1 mm deep and 9 mm long. For the modified template method, use the spring-loaded blade to make two incisions, 1 mm deep and 5 mm long.
• Start the stopwatch.
• Taking care not to touch the cuts, gently blot the drops of blood with filter paper every 30 seconds, until the bleeding stops in both cuts.
• Note the amount of time it takes for each cut to stop bleeding.
• Average the bleeding time of the two cuts, and record the result.

Ivy method
• After applying the pressure cuff and preparing the test site, make three small punctures with a disposable lancet.
• Follow the same procedure as above but average the bleeding times of the three punctures, and record the result.

Duke method
• Drape the patient's shoulder with a towel. Clean the earlobe, and let the skin air-dry.
• Make a puncture wound 2 to 4 mm deep on the earlobe with a disposable lancet.
• Start the stopwatch.
• Being careful not to touch the ear, blot the site with filter paper every 30 seconds, until the bleeding stops.
• Record the bleeding time.

Special precautions

If the bleeding does not diminish after 15 minutes, discontinue the test by applying compression to the incision site.

Patient care checklist

Before the test
☑ Explain or clarify test purpose and procedure.
☑ Tell the patient that, although he may feel some discomfort from the incisions, the antiseptic, and the tightness of the blood pressure cuff, the test takes only 10 to 20 minutes.
☑ Advise the patient that the incisions will leave two small, hairline scars that should be barely visible when healed.
☑ Evaluate patient understanding.
☑ Review patient history for recent ingestion of drugs that prolong bleeding time. Check with the laboratory for special instructions if the patient has taken such drugs.

After the test
☑ In a patient with a bleeding tendency (hemophilia, for example),

maintain a pressure bandage over the incision for 24 to 48 hours to prevent further bleeding. Keep the edges of the cuts aligned to minimize scarring.

Interfering factors

Sulfonamides, thiazides, antineoplastics, anticoagulants, nonsteroidal anti-inflammatory drugs, aspirin and aspirin compounds, and some nonnarcotic analgesics may prolong bleeding times.

Capillary fragility
[Tourniquet test, Rumpel-Leede capillary fragility test, positive pressure test]

Purpose

• To assess the fragility of capillary walls
• To identify platelet deficiency (thrombocytopenia).

Normal results

A few petechiae may normally be present before the test. Fewer than 10 petechiae on the forearm 5 minutes after the test is considered normal, or negative. The test result for the presence of zero to 10 petechiae may be reported as a score of 1 +.

Abnormal results

Positive test, using the following scale:

Number of petechiae	Score
10 to 20	2 +
20 to 50	3 +
50	4 +

Occurs in conditions related to bleeding defects, such as:

Thrombocytopenia
Thrombasthenia
Purpura senilis
Scurvy
Disseminated intravascular coagulation (DIC)
Von Willebrand's disease

Vitamin K deficiency
Dysproteinemia
Polycythemia vera
Severe deficiencies of Factor VII, fibrinogen, or prothrombin.

Occurs in conditions unrelated to bleeding defects, such as:

Scarlet fever
Measles
Influenza
Chronic renal disease
Hypertension
Diabetes with coexistent vascular disease.

Sometimes appears:

Before menstruation in some healthy women, especially in those over age 40.

The basics

A nonspecific method for evaluating bleeding tendencies, the capillary fragility test (positive-pressure test) measures the capillaries' ability to remain intact under increased intracapillary pressure. In this test, a laboratory technician or other specially trained person places a blood pressure cuff around the patient's upper arm and raises the pressure to a point midway between the systolic and diastolic blood pressures, but no higher than 100 mmHg. At this pressure, blood can enter the arm and hand but cannot easily return to circulation. Pressure is maintained for 5 minutes. This temporary increase in pressure may cause rhexis bleeding of the capillaries and formation of petechiae on the arm, wrist, or hand. The number of petechiae within a given circular space is recorded as the test result.

Contraindications: a diagnosis of DIC or other bleeding disorders, or significant petechiae.

Procedure

• Select and mark a 2″ (5-cm) space on the patient's forearm. Select a site free of petechiae; otherwise, record the number of petechiae already present on the site before starting the test. To ensure accurate results, the patient's

skin temperature and the room temperature should be normal.
• Fasten the cuff around the arm, and raise the pressure to a point midway between the systolic and diastolic blood pressures.
• Maintain this pressure for 5 minutes, then release the cuff.
• Count the number of petechiae that appear in the space. Record the test results.

Patient care checklist
Before the test
☑ Explain or clarify test purpose and procedure.
☑ Evaluate patient understanding.
After the test
☑ Encourage the patient to open and close his hand a few times to hasten the return of blood to his forearm.

Interfering factors
• Decreased estrogen levels in postmenopausal women may increase capillary fragility.
• Glucocorticoids may increase capillary resistance, even in a patient with thrombocytopenia.
• A high number of pretest petechiae may be caused by allergy to certain foods or drugs.
• Repeating the test on the same arm within 1 week may lead to an error in counting the number of petechiae.

Erythrocyte sedimentation rate (ESR)

Purpose
• To monitor inflammatory or malignant disease
• To aid in detection and diagnosis of occult disease, such as tuberculosis, tissue necrosis, or connective tissue disease.

Normal results
Normal ESRs range from 0 to 20 mm/hour; rates gradually increase with age.

Abnormal results
Increased ESR may indicate:
Pregnancy
Acute or chronic inflammation
Tuberculosis
Paraproteinemias (especially multiple myeloma and Waldenström's macroglobulinemia)
Rheumatic fever
Rheumatoid arthritis
Some malignancies
Anemia.
Decreased ESR may indicate:
Polycythemia
Sickle cell anemia
Hyperviscosity
Low plasma protein.

The basics
The ESR measures the time required for erythrocytes in a whole blood sample to settle to the bottom of a vertical tube. Factors affecting ESR include red cell volume, surface area, density, aggregation, and surface charge. Plasma proteins (notably fibrinogen and globulin) encourage aggregation, thereby increasing ESR.

The ESR is a sensitive but nonspecific test that is frequently the earliest indicator of disease when other chemical or physical signs are normal. It often rises significantly in widespread inflammatory disorders due to infection or autoimmune mechanisms; such elevations may be prolonged in localized inflammation and malignancy.

Procedure
Perform a venipuncture, and collect the sample in a 7-ml lavender-top, 4.5-ml black-top, or 4.5-ml blue-top tube. (Check with the laboratory to determine its preference.)

Patient care checklist
Before the test
☑ Explain or clarify test purpose and procedure.
☑ Evaluate patient understanding.

Interfering factors
• Failure to use the proper anticoagulant in the collection tube or to mix the sample and anticoagulant adequately may interfere with accurate determination of test results.
• Hemolysis due to rough handling or excessive mixing of the sample may affect the ESR.
• Since prolonged standing decreases the ESR, send the sample to the laboratory immediately after examining it for clots or clumps (it must be tested within 2 hours).
• Prolonged tourniquet constriction may cause hemoconcentration.

Euglobulin lysis time

Purpose
• To assess systemic fibrinolysis
• To help detect abnormal fibrinolytic states.

Normal results
Normal euglobulin lysis time is at least 2 hours.

Abnormal results
Euglobulin lysis within 1 hour indicates increased plasminogen activator activity. In pathologic fibrinolysis, lysis time may be as brief as 5 to 10 minutes.

The basics
This test measures the interval between clot formation and dissolution in the euglobulin fraction of plasma. In the laboratory, a blood sample is acidified and mixed with calcium to form a clot. The time required for this clot to lyse is recorded.

Procedure
• Perform a venipuncture. Collect a 4.5-ml sample in a blue-top tube or in a chilled tube with 0.5 ml sodium oxalate.
• If a blue-top tube is used, mix the sample and anticoagulant thoroughly.

If a chilled tube containing 0.5 ml sodium oxalate is used, mix the sample and preservative adequately, pack the sample in ice, and send it to the laboratory immediately.

Patient care checklist
Before the test
☑ Explain or clarify test purpose and procedure.
☑ Evaluate patient understanding.

Interfering factors
• Prolonged tourniquet constriction, vigorous vein preparation, or excessive pumping of the fist shortens lysis time.
• Hemolysis due to excessive probing during venipuncture or to rough handling of the sample may alter test results.
• Failure to follow appropriate precautions for the type of collection tube used may hinder accurate results.
• Depressed fibrinogen levels (less than 100 mg/dl) can shorten lysis time.

Ferritin

Purpose
• To screen for iron deficiency and iron overload
• To measure iron storage
• To distinguish between iron deficiency (a condition of low iron storage) and chronic inflammation (a condition of normal storage).

Normal results
Normal serum ferritin values vary with age. According to the Mayo Medical Laboratories, serum ferritin levels range as follows:
Men: 20 to 300 ng/ml
Women: 20 to 120 ng/ml
6 months to 15 years: 7 to 140 ng/ml
2 to 5 months: 50 to 200 ng/ml
1 month: 200 to 600 ng/ml
Neonates: 25 to 200 ng/ml.

Abnormal results
Increased serum ferritin levels may indicate:
  Acute or chronic hepatic disease
  Iron overload
  Leukemia
  Acute or chronic infection or inflammation
  Hodgkin's disease
  Chronic hemolytic anemias.
Slightly increased (or normal) serum ferritin may indicate:
  Chronic renal disease.
Decreased serum ferritin levels may indicate:
  Chronic iron deficiency.

The basics
Ferritin, a major iron-storage protein found in reticuloendothelial cells, normally appears in small quantities in serum. In healthy adults, serum ferritin levels are directly related to the amount of available iron stored in the body and can be measured accurately by radioimmunoassay. Unlike many other blood studies, the serum ferritin test is not affected by moderate hemolysis of the sample or by any known drugs.

Procedure
Perform a venipuncture, and collect the sample in a 10-ml red-top tube.

Patient care checklist
Before the test
☑ Explain or clarify test purpose and procedure.
☑ Evaluate patient understanding.

Interfering factors
Recent transfusion may elevate serum ferritin levels.

Fibrinogen
[Factor I]

Purpose
To aid diagnosis of suspected bleeding disorders.

Normal results
Plasma fibrinogen levels normally range from 195 to 365 mg/dl.

Abnormal results
Decreased plasma fibrinogen levels may indicate:
  Congenital afibrinogenemia
  Hypofibrinogenemia or dysfibrinogenemia
  Disseminated intravascular coagulation (DIC)
  Fibrinolysis
  Severe hepatic disease
  Cancer of the prostate, pancreas, or lung
  Bone marrow lesions
  Recent obstetric complications
  Recent trauma.
Increased plasma fibrinogen levels may indicate:
  Cancer of the stomach, breast, or kidney
  Inflammatory disorders, such as membranoproliferative glomerulonephritis or pneumonia.

The basics
Fibrinogen (Factor I), a plasma protein originating in the liver, is not normally present in serum; it is converted to fibrin by thrombin during clotting. Since fibrin is a necessary part of a blood clot, fibrinogen deficiency can produce mild to severe bleeding disorders. When fibrinogen levels drop below 100 mg/dl, accurate interpretation of all coagulation tests involving a fibrin clot as an end point becomes most difficult.

Contraindications: active bleeding, acute infection or illness or blood transfusion within 4 weeks.

Procedure
• If the patient is receiving heparin therapy, notify the laboratory; such therapy requires the use of a different reagent.
• Perform a venipuncture, and collect the sample in a 7-ml blue-top tube.

Patient care checklist
Before the test

☑ Explain or clarify test purpose and procedure.

☑ Evaluate patient understanding.

☑ Notify physician regarding patients who are actively bleeding, have an acute infection or illness, or have received a blood transfusion within 4 weeks; these are all contraindications.

Interfering factors

• Fibrinogen levels may also be elevated postoperatively and during pregnancy (third trimester).

• Hemolysis caused by traumatic venipuncture or by rough handling of the sample may affect test results.

• Failure to fill the collection tube completely, to mix the sample and anticoagulant adequately, to send the sample to the laboratory promptly, or to place it on ice may interfere with accurate determination of test results.

• Use of heparin and oral contraceptives may interfere with the accurate determination of test results.

Fibrin split products *(FSP)* *[Fibrinogen degradation products (FDP)]*

Purpose

• To detect FSP in the circulation
• To help diagnose disseminated intravascular coagulation (DIC) and distinguish it from other coagulation disorders
• To determine the degree of fibrinolysis during coagulation.

Normal results

In a screening assay, serum contains less than 10 mcg/ml of FSP. A quantitative assay shows normal levels of less than 3 mcg/ml.

Abnormal results

Increased FSP levels may indicate:
Primary fibrinolytic states

Secondary fibrinolytic states due to DIC and subsequent fibrinolysis
Other disorders, such as alcoholic cirrhosis, postcesarean birth, pre-eclampsia, abruptio placentae, congenital heart disease, sunstroke, burns, intrauterine death, pulmonary embolus, deep-vein thrombosis (transient increase), and myocardial infarction (after 1 or 2 days).

Increased FSP levels above 100 mcg/ ml may indicate:
Active renal disease
Renal transplant rejection.

The basics

After a fibrin clot forms in response to vascular injury, the fibrinolytic system acts to prevent excessive clotting by converting plasminogen into the fibrin-dissolving enzyme plasmin. Plasmin breaks down fibrin and fibrinogen into fragments, or split products, labeled X, Y, D, and E, in order of decreasing molecular weight. These products may combine with fibrin monomers to prevent polymerization; that is, the fragments retain some anticoagulant activity. An excess of such products in circulation leads to abnormally active fibrinolysis and to coagulation disorders, such as DIC.

Procedure

• Perform a venipuncture, and draw 2 ml of blood into a plastic syringe.
• Transfer the sample to the tube provided by the laboratory, which contains a soybean trypsin inhibitor and bovine thrombin.

Special precautions

CLINICAL ALERT: **Draw the sample before administering heparin, which may cause false-positive test results.**

Patient care checklist
Before the test

☑ Explain or clarify test purpose and procedure.

☑ Evaluate patient understanding.

Interfering factors
• Pretest administration of heparin causes false-positive results.
• Fibrinolytic drugs, such as urokinase, and large doses of barbiturates increase FSP levels.
• Failure to fill the collection tube completely or to mix the sample and anticoagulant gently and adequately may interfere with the accurate determination of test results.
• Hemolysis caused by rough handling of the sample may alter test results.
• Since the blood must be incubated at 98.6° F. (37° C.) for 30 minutes before testing proceeds, send the sample to the laboratory immediately, or test results may not be accurate.

Glycosylated hemoglobin
[Total fasting hemoglobin, glycohemoglobin]

Purpose
To assess control of diabetes mellitus.

Normal results
Glycosylated hemoglobin values are reported as a percentage of the total hemoglobin within an erythrocyte. Hemoglobins A_{1a} and A_{1b} account for about 1.6% and 0.8%, respectively; $HgbA_{1c}$ accounts for approximately 5%; and total glycosylated hemoglobin accounts for 5.5% to 9%.

Abnormal results
In diabetes mellitus, hemoglobins A_{1a} and A_{1b} constitute approximately 2.5% to 3.9% of total hemoglobin; $HgbA_{1c}$ constitutes 8% to 11.9%; and total glycosylated hemoglobin, 10.9% to 15.5%.

The basics
The glycosylated hemoglobin test is a relatively new diagnostic tool for monitoring diabetes therapy. The three minor hemoglobins measured in this test—hemoglobins A_{1a}, A_{1b}, and A_{1c}—are variants of Hgb A formed by glycosylation, a nearly irreversible molecular process in which glucose becomes chemically incorporated in Hgb A. Since glycosylation occurs at a constant rate during the 120-day life span of an erythrocyte, glycosylated hemoglobin levels reflect the average blood glucose level during the preceding 2 to 3 months, and therefore can be used to evaluate the long-term effectiveness of diabetes therapy. As effective therapy brings diabetes under control, glycosylated hemoglobin levels approach the normal range. This test has several distinct advantages over traditional blood or urine glucose tests, since it requires only one venipuncture every 6 to 8 weeks and reflects diabetes control over several months. In addition, since this test measures glucose within an erythrocyte, levels are more stable than with plasma glucose, which is affected by metabolic processes within the body.

Procedure
• Perform a venipuncture, and collect the sample in a 5-ml lavender-top tube.
• Completely fill the collection tube, and invert it gently several times to mix the sample and anticoagulant adequately.

Patient care checklist
Before the test
☑ Explain or clarify test purpose and procedure. Instruct patient to maintain his prescribed medication and diet regimen.
☑ Evaluate patient understanding.
After the test
☑ Schedule patient for an appointment in 6 to 8 weeks for appropriate follow-up testing.

Interfering factors
Failure to mix the sample and anticoagulant adequately may interfere with accurate determination of test results.

Haptoglobin

Purpose
• To serve as an index of hemolysis
• To distinguish between hemoglobin and myoglobin in plasma, since haptoglobin does not bind with myoglobin
• To investigate hemolytic transfusion reactions
• To establish proof of paternity, using genetic (phenotypic) variations in haptoglobin structure.

Normal results
Normal serum haptoglobin concentrations, measured in terms of the protein's hemoglobin-binding capacity, are 38 to 270 mg/dl.

Abnormal results
Markedly increased serum haptoglobin levels may indicate:
   Acute and chronic hemolysis
   Severe hepatocellular disease
   Infectious mononucleosis
   Transfusion reactions
   Ahaptoglobinemia.
Strikingly increased serum haptoglobin levels may indicate:
   Diseases marked by chronic inflammatory reactions, such as rheumatoid arthritis
   Diseases marked by tissue destruction, such as malignant neoplasms.

The basics
Using radial immunodiffusion, this test measures serum levels of haptoglobin, a glycoprotein produced in the liver. Haptoglobin binds with free hemoglobin and prevents its accumulation in plasma, permitting clearance by reticuloendothelial cells and conserving body iron. Normally, hemoglobin circulates inside erythrocytes, but it appears in plasma when bacterial toxins, mechanical disruption (from a prosthetic heart valve, for example), or antibodies cause intravascular hemolysis.

When haptoglobin levels are inadequate to remove all hemoglobin from plasma, hemolysis is severe. After such hemolysis, low haptoglobin levels may persist for 5 to 7 days, until the liver can synthesize more of this glycoprotein.

Hepatocellular disease inhibits the synthesis of haptoglobin. In hemolytic transfusion reactions, haptoglobin levels begin falling after 6 to 8 hours and drop to 40% of pretransfusion levels after 24 hours.

Although haptoglobin is absent in 90% of neonates, levels will gradually rise to normal by age 4 months in most of these infants. In about 1% of the population—including 4% of blacks—haptoglobin is permanently absent; this disorder is known as congenital ahaptoglobinemia.

Procedure
Draw a venous blood sample into a 10- to 15-ml red-top tube.

Special precautions
If serum haptoglobin values are very low, watch for symptoms of hemolysis: chills, fever, back pain, flushing, distended neck veins, tachycardia, tachypnea, and hypotension.

Patient care checklist
Before the test
☑ Explain or clarify test purpose and procedure.
☑ Evaluate patient understanding.

Interfering factors
• Steroids and androgens can elevate haptoglobin levels and mask hemolysis in patients with inflammatory disease.
• Hemolysis caused by rough handling of the sample can interfere with accurate determination of test results.

Heinz bodies

Purpose
To help detect causes of hemolytic anemia.

Normal results
Absence of Heinz bodies is the normal (negative) test result.

Abnormal results
Positive for Heinz bodies may indicate:
    Inherited red cell deficiency
    Presence of unstable hemoglobins
    Thalassemia
    Drug-induced red cell injury
    Post-splenectomy.

The basics
Heinz bodies are particles of denatured hemoglobin that have precipitated out of the cytoplasm of red blood cells and have collected in small masses attached to cell membranes. They form as a result of drug injury to red cells, the presence of unstable hemoglobins, unbalanced globin chain synthesis due to thalassemia, or a red cell enzyme deficiency (such as glucose 6-phosphate dehydrogenase deficiency). Although Heinz bodies are rapidly removed from red cells in the spleen, they are a major factor contributing to hemolytic anemias.

Procedure
Perform a venipuncture, and collect the sample in a 7-ml lavender-top tube.

Patient care checklist
Before the test
☑ Explain or clarify test purpose and procedure.
☑ Evaluate patient understanding.
☑ Withhold medications that may interfere with test results as ordered. If they must be continued, note them on the laboratory slip.

Interfering factors
• Antimalarials, furazolidone (in infants), nitrofurantoin, phenacetin, procarbazine, and sulfonamides can cause false-positive results.
• Failure to use the appropriate anticoagulant in the collection tube, to fill the collection tube completely, to mix the sample and the anticoagulant adequately and gently, or to send the sample immediately to the laboratory may interfere with the accurate determination of test results.

Hematocrit *(HCT)*

Purpose
• To aid diagnosis of abnormal states of hydration, polycythemia, and anemia
• To aid in calculating red cell indices.

Normal results
Hematocrit values vary, depending on the patient's sex and age, type of sample and the laboratory performing the test. (See *Normal Hematocrit Levels.*)

Abnormal results
Decreased HCT levels may indicate:
    Anemia
    Hemodilution.
Increased HCT levels may indicate:
    Polycythemia
    Hemoconcentration due to blood loss.

Normal Hematocrit Levels

Age	Hematocrit level
Newborn	55% to 68%
1 Week	47% to 65%
1 Month	37% to 49%
3 Months	30% to 36%
1 Year	29% to 41%
10 Years	36% to 40%
Adult Male	42% to 54%
Adult Female	38% to 46%

The basics

HCT, a common, reliable test, may be done by itself or as part of a complete blood count. It measures the percentage by volume of packed red blood cells (RBCs) in a whole blood sample; for example, an HCT of 40% means that a 100-ml sample contains 40 ml of packed RBCs. This packing is achieved by centrifuging anticoagulated whole blood in a capillary tube, so that RBCs are tightly packed without hemolysis.

Most commonly, HCT is measured electronically, producing results 3% lower than when HCT is measured manually. (Manual measurement traps plasma in the column of packed RBCs.) Test results may be used to calculate two erythrocyte indices: mean corpuscular volume (MCV) and mean corpuscular hemoglobin concentration (MCHC).

Procedure

• Perform a finger stick, using a heparinized capillary tube with a red band on the anticoagulant end.
• Fill the capillary tube from the red-banded end to about two-thirds capacity, and seal this end with clay.
• Or, if you perform the test, place the tube in the centrifuge, with the red end pointing outward.

Patient care checklist

Before the test

☑ Explain or clarify test purpose and procedure.
☑ Evaluate patient understanding.

Interfering factors

• Failure to use the proper anticoagulant in the collection tube or to fill it appropriately may interfere with accurate determination of test results.
• Hemolysis due to rough handling of the sample may affect test results.
• Tourniquet constriction for longer than 1 minute causes hemoconcentration and typically raises HCT by 2.5% to 5%.

• Taking the blood sample from the same arm that is being used for I.V. infusion of fluids causes hemodilution.
• Failure to mix the sample and the anticoagulant adequately may hinder accurate determination of test results.
• Excessive centrifugation of the sample results in hemolysis.

Hemoglobin, total *(Hgb)*

Purpose

• To measure the severity of anemia or polycythemia and monitor response to therapy
• To supply figures for calculating mean corpuscular hemoglobin (MCH) and mean corpuscular hemoglobin concentration (MCHC).

Normal results

Hgb concentration varies, depending on the patient's age and sex, and on the type of blood sample drawn. Except for infants, values for age groups listed in the accompanying chart are based on venous blood samples. (See *Normal Hemoglobin Levels,* p. 14.)

Abnormal results

Increased Hgb levels suggest:
  Hemoconcentration from polycythemia or dehydration.
Decreased Hgb levels may indicate:
  Anemia
  Recent hemorrhage
  Fluid retention causing hemodilution.

The basics

This test measures the grams of Hgb found in a deciliter (100 ml) of whole blood. Hgb concentration correlates closely with the red blood cell (RBC) count and is affected by the Hgb-RBC ratio (MCH) and free plasma Hgb. In the laboratory, Hgb is chemically converted to pigmented compounds and is measured by spectrophotometric or colorimetric technique.

Normal Hemoglobin Levels

Age	Hemoglobin level
Newborns	17 to 22 g/dl
1 Week	15 to 20 g/dl
1 Month	11 to 15 g/dl
Children	11 to 13 g/dl
Men	14 to 18 g/dl
Men after middle age	12.4 to 14.9 g/dl
Women	12 to 16 g/dl
Women after middle age	11.7 to 13.8 g/dl

The test is usually performed as part of a complete blood count.

Procedure
• For adults and older children, perform a venipuncture, and collect the sample in a 7-ml lavender-top tube.
• For younger children and infants, collect capillary blood in a pipette.

Patient care checklist
Before the test
☑ Explain or clarify test purpose and procedure. (If the patient is an infant or young child, explain to the parents and to the child, if he is old enough to understand.)
☑ Evaluate patient and/or parent understanding.

Interfering factors
• Failure to use the proper anticoagulant in the collection tube or to mix the sample and anticoagulant adequately may interfere with accurate determination of test results.

• Hemolysis due to rough handling of the sample may adversely affect the test results.
• Prolonged tourniquet constriction may cause hemoconcentration.
• Very high white cell counts, lipemia, or red cells that are resistant to lysis will falsely elevate Hgb values.

Hemoglobin derivatives, abnormal
[Carboxyhemoglobin, methemoglobin, sulfhemoglobin]

Purpose
• To rule out abnormal hemoglobin derivatives as a cause of cyanosis or anoxia
• To monitor persons in danger of overexposure to a substance causing cyanosis or anoxia, such as carbon monoxide.

Normal results
Normally, carboxyhemoglobin concentration is 3% of total hemoglobin (up to 15% in tobacco smokers); methemoglobin concentration, less than 3%; and sulfhemoglobin concentration, undetectable.

Abnormal results
Concentrations of carboxyhemoglobin, methemoglobin and sulfhemoglobin higher than normal. (See the chart *Toxic Signs and Symptoms of Hemoglobin Derivatives*.)

The basics
This quantitative test measures the percentage of total hemoglobin-containing abnormal derivatives—primarily, carboxyhemoglobin, methemoglobin, and sulfhemoglobin—after the onset of signs of toxicity, such as cyanosis and anoxia. By changing the pH or adding a reducing substance, then analyzing the blood with a spectrophotometer, the specific form of he-

Toxic Signs and Symptoms of Hemoglobin Derivatives

Hemoglobin derivatives	Levels	Signs and symptoms
Carboxyhemoglobin	20%	Headache, mild dyspnea
	20% to 40%	Fatigue, irritability, diminished judgment, dimmed vision, nausea
	40% to 60%	Confusion, hallucinations, ataxia, collapse, coma, reddened skin and mucous membranes
	60% to 80%	Death
Methemoglobin	10% to 25%	Cyanosis
	35% to 40%	Exertional dyspnea, headache
	>60%	Lethargy, stupor
	>70%	Death
Sulfhemoglobin	10 g/dl	Cyanosis with few or no toxic symptoms

moglobin present can be determined, thus confirming the diagnosis.

When combined with certain chemicals or drugs, hemoglobins are converted into compounds that are incapable of transporting oxygen. One such compound is carboxyhemoglobin, which results when hemoglobin and carbon monoxide unite. (This compound's affinity for hemoglobin is 210 times greater than that of oxygen.) The major effect of carbon monoxide toxicity is tissue hypoxia, because carboxyhemoglobin cannot carry oxygen and also prevents the release of oxygen from as yet unaffected hemoglobin. Serious symptoms can occur in patients with chronic carbon monoxide poisoning or in children when carboxyhemoglobin levels are even lower than those seen in patients with acute carbon monoxide poisoning. Treatment with 100% oxygen or with 95% oxygen and 5% carbon dioxide can help to reverse carbon monoxide toxicity. The principal sources of carbon monoxide include tobacco smoke and exhaust from the incomplete combustion of petroleum and natural gas fuels, such as that from gasoline and diesel motors, unvented natural gas heaters, and defective gas stoves.

Another compound, sulfhemoglobin, results when hemoglobin combines with certain drugs, such as phenacetin or sulfonamides. Methemoglobin results when ferrous iron oxidizes to the ferric form. Such oxidation usually results from chemicals and drugs—such as nitrates, nitrites, sulfonamides, aniline, chlorates, or phenacetin—or from primary methemoglobinemia. Sulfhemoglobin cannot be removed by therapy and disappears only with the destruction of the affected red blood cells. Levels of each of these hemoglobin derivatives depend on the duration of exposure as well as the concentration. Treatment of toxicity and exposure limitations depend on the identification of the various hemoglobins and the levels noted.

Procedure
Perform a venipuncture, and collect the sample in a 4.5-ml blue-top tube for carboxyhemoglobin, or in a 7-ml green-top (heparinized) tube for sulfhemoglobin or methemoglobin.

Patient care checklist
Before the test
☑ Explain or clarify test purpose and procedure.
☑ Evaluate patient understanding.
☑ Have a consent form signed by the patient or a responsible family member, if the test is being performed for medicolegal purposes.

Interfering factors
Air contamination of the specimen may affect the accuracy of test results.

Hemoglobin *(Hgb)* electrophoresis

Purpose
• To measure the amount of Hgb A and to detect abnormal hemoglobins
• To aid diagnosis of thalassemias.

Normal results
In adults, Hgb A accounts for over 95% of all hemoglobins; A_2, 2% to 3%; and F, less than 1%. In neonates, Hgb F normally accounts for half the total. Hemoglobins S and C are normally absent.

Abnormal results
Hgb electrophoresis allows identification of various types of Hgb, many of which clinically may imply a hemolytic disease. (See *Variations of Hemoglobin Type and Distribution*.)

The basics
Hgb electrophoresis is probably the most useful laboratory method for separating and measuring normal and certain abnormal hemoglobins. Electrophoresis apparatus consists of an anode (+) and a cathode (−), separated by cellulose acetate, to which Hgb molecules migrate when an electrical current is passed through the medium. Different groups migrate toward the anode at different speeds, creating a series of distinctively pigmented bands in the medium, which are then compared with a normal sample.

In practice, the laboratory may change the medium (from cellulose acetate to starch gel) or its pH (from 6.2 to 8.6), to clearly separate hemoglobins and to expand the range of this test beyond those hemoglobins routinely checked: hemoglobins A, A_2, S, and C.

Procedure
Perform a venipuncture, and collect the sample in a 7-ml lavender-top tube.

Patient care checklist
Before the test
☑ Explain or clarify test purpose and procedure.
☑ Evaluate patient understanding.

Interfering factors
• A blood transfusion within the past 4 months may invalidate test results.
• Failure to use the proper anticoagulant in the collection tube, to fill the tube completely, or to mix the sample and the anticoagulant adequately may interfere with accurate determination

Variations of Hemoglobin Type and Distribution

Hemoglobin	% of Total Hemoglobin	Clinical Implications
Hgb A$_2$	4% to 5.8%	β-thalassemia minor
	Under 2%	Hgb H disease
Hgb F	2% to 5%	β-thalassemia minor
	10% to 90%	β-thalassemia major
	5% to 15%	β-δ-thalassemia minor
	5% to 35%	Heterozygous hereditary persistence of fetal hemoglobin (HPFH)
	100%	Homozygous HPFH
	15%	Homozygous Hgb S
Homozygous Hgb S	70% to 98%	Sickle cell disease
Homozygous Hgb C	90% to 98%	Hgb C disease
Heterozygous Hgb C	24% to 44%	Hemoglobin C trait

of test results.
• Hemolysis due to rough handling of the sample may hinder accurate determination of test results.

Iron and total iron-binding capacity (TIBC)

Purpose
• To estimate total iron storage
• To aid diagnosis of hemochromatosis
• To help distinguish between iron deficiency anemia and anemia of chronic disease
• To provide data for evaluating nutritional status.

Normal results
Normal serum iron and TIBC values are as follows:

Serum Iron (mcg/dl)	TIBC (mcg/dl)	Saturation (%)
Men: 70 to 150	300 to 400	20 to 50
Women: 80 to 150	300 to 450	20 to 50

Abnormal results
Decrease in serum iron level and increased TIBC suggests:
  Iron deficiency.
Decrease in serum iron level (in presence of adequate body stores) and normal or slight drop in TIBC suggests:
  Chronic inflammation, such as in rheumatoid arthritis.

Increase in serum iron level and normal TIBC suggests:
   Iron overload (may not alter serum levels until relatively late).

The basics
Iron is essential to the formation and function of hemoglobin, as well as many other heme and nonheme compounds. After iron is absorbed by the intestine, it is distributed to various body compartments for synthesis, storage, and transport. Since iron appears in the plasma, bound to a glycoprotein called transferrin, it is easily sampled and measured.

Serum iron and TIBC are of great diagnostic usefulness when performed with the serum ferritin assay, but together these tests may not accurately reflect the state of other iron compartments, such as myoglobin iron and the labile iron pool. Bone marrow or liver biopsy, and iron absorption or excretion studies may yield more information.

Procedure
Perform a venipuncture, and collect the sample in a 7-ml red-top tube.

Patient care checklist
Before the test
☑ Explain or clarify test purpose and procedure.
☑ Evaluate patient understanding.
☑ Withhold medications that may interfere with test results, as ordered. If they must be continued, note them on the laboratory slip.

Interfering factors
• Chloramphenicol and oral contraceptives can cause false-positive test results; ACTH can produce false-negative results. Iron supplements can cause false-positive serum iron values but a false-negative TIBC.
• Hemolysis due to rough handling of the sample, or failure to send the sample to the laboratory immediately may interfere with accurate determination results.

One-stage assay: Extrinsic coagulation system
[Factor II assay, Factor V assay, Factor VII assay, Factor X assay]

Purpose
• To identify a specific factor deficiency in persons with prolonged prothrombin time (PT) or activated partial thromboplastin time (APTT)
• To study patients with congenital or acquired coagulation defects
• To monitor the effects of anticoagulant therapy.

Normal results
Factor II assay: 225 to 290 u/ml
Factor V assay: 50% to 150% activity
Factor VII assay: 65% to 135% activity
Factor X assay: 45% to 155% activity.

Abnormal results
Deficiency of Factor II may indicate:
   Hepatic disease
   Vitamin K deficiency
   Hypoprothrombinemia (rare).
Deficiency of Factor V may indicate:
   Severe hepatic disease
   Disseminated intravascular clotting (DIC)
   Fibrinolysis.
Deficiency of Factor VII may indicate:
   Hepatic disease
   Vitamin K deficiency.
Deficiency of Factor X may indicate:
   DIC.

The basics
When PT and APTT are abnormal (prolonged), a one-stage assay helps detect deficiency of Factors II, V, or X. If PT is abnormal but APTT is normal, Factor VII may be deficient.

Deficiencies of all four factors may be congenital, although congenital Factor II deficiency is rare. Absence of Factor II is lethal.

The Missing Link: Factor XIII Assay

When the patient shows poor wound healing and other symptoms of a bleeding disorder, despite normal results of coagulation screening tests, a Factor XIII assay is recommended.

Factor XIII is responsible for stabilizing the fibrin clot, the final step in the clotting process. If the clot is unstable, it breaks loose, resulting in scarring and poor wound healing. Deficiency of this factor is usually transmitted as an autosomal recessive trait but may result from hepatic disease or from tumors. Clinical effects of Factor XIII deficiency include umbilical bleeding in neonates; recurrent ecchymoses, hematomas, and poor wound healing; prolonged bleeding after trauma; hemarthrosis; spontaneous abortion (rarely);

and intraovarian bleeding (more common in Factor XIII deficiency than in other bleeding disorders). Bleeding after trauma may begin immediately or may be delayed as long as 12 to 36 hours. Treatment with infusions of plasma or cryoprecipitate has improved the prognosis; some patients may even live normal lives.

Before appropriate treatment for Factor XIII deficiency can begin, diagnostic evaluation must rule out other bleeding disorders. Dysfibrinogenemia, hyperfibrinogenemia, and disseminated intravascular coagulation also cause rapid clot dissolution in this assay, but unlike Factor XIII deficiency, they also cause an abnormal fibrinogen level and thrombin time.

Procedure

Perform a venipuncture, and collect the sample in a 7-ml blue-top tube.

Special precautions

If the patient has a suspected coagulation defect, avoid excessive probing during venipuncture, do not leave the tourniquet on too long (it will cause bruising), and apply pressure to the puncture site for 5 minutes, or until the bleeding stops.

Patient care checklist

Before the test

☑ Explain or clarify test purpose and procedure.

☑ Tell the patient that a series of tests will be needed to monitor the effects of anticoagulant therapy, if appropriate.

☑ Evaluate patient understanding.

Interfering factors

• Hemolysis caused by rough handling of the sample may interfere with accurate determination of test results.

• Failure to mix the sample and anticoagulant adequately, to send the sample to the laboratory immediately, or to place it on ice may alter test results.

• Oral anticoagulant therapy may increase bleeding time by inhibiting vitamin K–dependent synthesis and activation of Factors II, VII, and X, which are formed in the liver. (See *The Missing Link: Factor XIII Assay*.)

One-stage assay: Intrinsic coagulation system
[Factor VIII assay, Factor IX assay, Factor XI assay, Factor XII assay]

Purpose

• To identify a specific factor deficiency

• To study patients with congenital or acquired coagulation defects.

Normal results

Factor VIII activity values: 55% to 145%
Factor IX activity values: 60% to 140%
Factor XI activity values: 65% to 135%
Factor XII activity values: 50% to 150%.

Abnormal results

Factor VIII deficiency may indicate:
Hemophilia A
Von Willebrand's disease
Factor VIII inhibitor
Disseminated intravascular clotting (DIC)
Fibrinolysis.

Hereditary Coagulation Defects

Deficient factor	Coagulation disorder
II	Hypoprothrombin-emia
V	Parahemophilia
VII	Factor VII deficiency
VIII	Hemophilia A (classic hemophilia), von Willebrand's disease (vascular hemophilia)
IX	Hemophilia B (Christmas disease)
X	Stuart factor deficiency
XI	Plasma thromboplastin antecedent deficiency (PTA deficiency)
XII	Hageman trait

Factor IX deficiency may indicate:
Hemophilia B
Hepatic disease
Factor IX inhibitor
Vitamin K deficiency
Coumarin therapy.
Factor XI deficiency may occur:
Transiently in neonates.
Factor XII deficiency may occur:
In nephrosis.
Transiently in neonates.

The basics

When prothrombin time (PT) is normal but activated partial thromboplastin time (APTT) is abnormal, a one-stage assay helps identify a deficiency in the intrinsic coagulation system—Factors VIII, IX, XI, or XII.

Factor VIII antigen and ristocetin cofactor tests distinguish between hemophilia A (and its carrier state) and von Willebrand's disease.

(Factors VIII and IX inhibitors occur after transfusions in patients deficient in either factor and are antibodies specific to each factor.)

Procedure

Perform a venipuncture, and collect the sample in a 7-ml blue-top tube.

Special precautions

If a coagulation defect is suspected, avoid excessive probing during venipuncture, do not leave the tourniquet on too long (it will cause bruising), and apply pressure to the puncture site for 5 minutes, or until the bleeding stops. A pressure bandage may be necessary.

Patient care checklist

Before the test
☑ Explain or clarify test purpose and procedure.
☑ Evaluate patient understanding.
☑ Withhold medications that may interfere with test results, as ordered. If they must be continued, note them on the laboratory slip.

Factor VIII–Related Antigen Test

Bleeding time tests and patient history can usually distinguish between classic hemophilia and von Willebrand's disease. But when bleeding time tests prove inconclusive and the patient has no family history of bleeding, the Factor VIII–related antigen test can provide helpful diagnostic information.

Persons with hemophilia and carriers of hemophilia demonstrate normal activity (45% to 185% of the control sample). Patients with von Willebrand's disease, however, show absent or deficient levels of Factor VIII antigen.

Interfering factors
• Hemolysis caused by rough handling of the sample may interfere with accurate determination of test results.
• Failure to mix the sample and the anticoagulant gently and adequately, to send the sample to the laboratory immediately, or to place it on ice may alter test results.
• Oral anticoagulants decrease Factor IX levels; pregnancy elevates Factor VIII. (See *Hereditary Coagulation Defects* and *Factor VIII–Related Antigen Test*.)

Osmotic fragility

Purpose
• To aid diagnosis of hereditary spherocytosis
• To confirm morphologic red cell abnormalities.

Normal results
Osmotic fragility values (percent of red blood cells hemolyzed) that have been obtained photometrically are plotted against decreasing saline tonicities, producing an S-shaped curve with a slope characteristic of the disorder. (See *Patterns of Hemolytic Response to Varying Saline Hypotonicity*, p. 22.)

Abnormal results
Low osmotic fragility (increased resistance to hemolysis) may indicate:
Thalassemia
Iron deficiency anemia
Sickle cell anemia
Other red cell disorders in which codocytes (target cells) and leptocytes are found
Post-splenectomy.
High osmotic fragility (increased tendency to hemolysis) may indicate:
Hereditary spherocytosis
Spherocytosis associated with autoimmune hemolytic anemia
Severe burns
Chemical poisoning
Erythroblastosis fetalis.

The basics
Osmotic fragility measures the resistance of red cells to hemolysis when exposed to a series of increasingly dilute saline solutions. The test is based on osmosis—movement of water across a membrane from a less concentrated solution to a more concentrated one, in a natural tendency to correct the imbalance.

The degree of hypotonicity needed to produce hemolysis varies inversely with the red cells' osmotic fragility: the closer saline tonicity is to normal physiologic values when hemolysis occurs, the more fragile the cells.

This test offers quantitative confirmation of red cell morphology and should supplement the stained cell examination.

Procedure
Perform a venipuncture, and collect the sample in a 7-ml green-top (hep-

arinized) tube, or secure a special heparinized tube for collecting defibrinated blood.

Patient care checklist
Before the test
☑ Explain or clarify test purpose and procedure.
☑ Evaluate patient understanding.

Interfering factors
The following factors may affect the accurate determination of test results:

• Failure to use the proper anticoagulant in the collection tube, to fill the tube completely, or to mix the sample and anticoagulant adequately
• Hemolysis due to rough handling of the sample
• Presence of hemolytic organisms in the sample
• Severe anemia, or other condition in which a reduced number of red cells are available for testing.
(See *Patterns of Hemolytic Response to Varying Saline Hypotonicity*.)

Patterns of Hemolytic Response to Varying Saline Hypotonicity

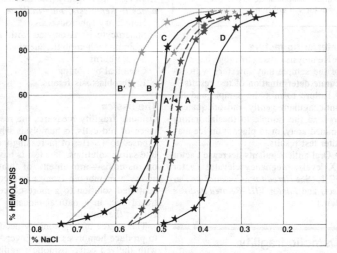

These curves show what happens when red cells are subjected to increasingly dilute (hypotonic) saline solution concentrations. Normal red cells behave as in curve A, and incubation for 24 hours (to improve test sensitivity) produces only a slight increase in their osmotic fragility (curve A′). But in hereditary spherocytosis, the cells burst easily (curve B), and even more easily upon incubation (curve B′). Acquired hemolytic anemia produces a line like curve C. Lowered osmotic fragility and, hence, increased resistance to hemolysis occur in thalassemia (curve D).

Adapted with permission from Maxwell M. Wintrobe, et al, *Clinical Hematology*, 7th ed. (Philadelphia: Lea & Febiger, 1974).

Plasminogen

Purpose
• To assess fibrinolysis
• To detect congenital and acquired fibrinolytic disorders.

Normal results
Normal plasminogen levels are 65% or greater (expressed as a percentage of normal), or 2.7 to 4.5 μ/ml (expressed as activity units).

Abnormal results
Decreased plasma plasminogen levels may indicate:
  Disseminated intravascular clotting (DIC)
  Tumors
  Preeclampsia
  Eclampsia
  Some liver diseases.

The basics
Plasminogen, the precursor molecule of plasmin, is measured to assess fibrinolysis. During fibrinolysis, plasmin dissolves fibrin clots to prevent excessive coagulation and the resulting impairment of blood flow. However, because plasmin does not circulate in active form, it cannot be measured directly; its circulating precursor, plasminogen, can be measured and provides an estimate of fibrinolysis.

Procedure
Perform a venipuncture, and collect the sample in a 7-ml blue-top tube.

Patient care checklist
Before the test
☑ Explain or clarify test purpose and procedure.
☑ Evaluate patient understanding.

Interfering factors
• Failure to collect the sample as quickly as possible may cause stasis, which can slow blood flow, causing coagulation and plasminogen activation.
• Failure to use the proper tube, to mix the sample and citrate adequately, to send the sample to the laboratory immediately, or to have it separated and frozen may alter results.
• Hemolysis caused by excessive probing during venipuncture or by rough handling of the sample may alter results.
• Prolonged tourniquet use before venipuncture may cause stasis, falsely decreasing plasminogen levels.
• Oral contraceptives may slightly increase plasminogen levels. Thrombolytic drugs, such as streptokinase or urokinase, may also decrease levels.

Platelet aggregation

Purpose
• To assess platelet aggregation
• To detect congenital and acquired platelet bleeding disorders.

Normal results
Normal aggregation occurs in 3 to 5 minutes, but findings are temperature-dependent and vary between laboratories.

Abnormal results
Reduced platelet aggregation may indicate:
  Von Willebrand's disease
  Bernard-Soulier syndrome
  Storage pool disease
  Glanzmann's thrombasthenia
  Polycythemia vera.

The basics
After vascular injury, platelets gather at the injury site and clump together to form an aggregate—a plug—that helps maintain hemostasis and promotes healing. This test is a major diagnostic tool for detecting von Willebrand's disease.

Procedure

Perform a venipuncture, and collect the sample in a 7-ml blue-top siliconized tube.

Special precautions

• If a coagulation defect is suspected, avoid excessive probing at the venipuncture site and do not leave the tourniquet on too long (it causes bruising). Apply pressure to the venipuncture site for 5 minutes, or until the bleeding stops.

• Keep the sample between 71.6° F. (22° C.) and 98.6° F. (37° C.) to prevent aggregation.

• If the patient has taken aspirin within the past 2 weeks and the test cannot be postponed, notify the laboratory. The technician will then use a different reagent to verify the presence of aspirin in the plasma. If test results are abnormal for such a sample, aspirin must be discontinued and the test repeated in 2 weeks.

Patient care checklist

Before the test

☑ Explain or clarify test purpose and procedure.

☑ Evaluate patient understanding.

☑ Provide a nonfat diet for 8 hours prior to the test, because lipemia can affect test results.

☑ Withhold aspirin and aspirin compounds for 14 days before the test. Withhold other medications that may interfere with test results for 48 hours before the test, as ordered. If these medications must be continued, note them on the laboratory slip.

Interfering factors

• Hemolysis caused by rough handling of the sample or by trauma at the venipuncture site may interfere with accurate determination of test results.

• Failure to use the proper anticoagulant or to mix the sample and anticoagulant adequately may alter test results.

• Failure to observe restrictions of diet and medications may hinder accurate

determination of test results. Platelet aggregation is inhibited by aspirin and aspirin compounds, phenylbutazone, sulfinpyrazone, phenothiazines, antihistamines, anti-inflammatory drugs, and tricyclic antidepressants.

• Since the list of medications known to alter the results of this test is long and continually growing, the patient should be as free of drugs as possible before the test.

Platelet count

Purpose

• To evaluate platelet production

• To assess effects of chemotherapy or radiation therapy on platelet production

• To aid diagnosis of thrombocytopenia and thrombocytosis

• To confirm a visual estimate of platelet number and morphology from a stained blood film.

Normal results

Normal platelet counts range from 130,000 to 370,000/mm³.

Abnormal results

Increased platelet count (thrombocytosis) may indicate:

    Hemorrhage

    Infectious disorders

    Malignancies

    Iron deficiency anemia

    Recent surgery

    Pregnancy

    Splenectomy

    Inflammatory disorder, such as collagen vascular disease

    Primary thrombocytosis

    Polycythemia vera

    Chronic myelogenous leukemia.

Decreased platelet count (thrombocytopenia) may indicate:

    Aplastic or hypoplastic bone marrow

    Infiltrative bone marrow disease, such as carcinoma, leukemia, or disseminated infection

Megakaryocytic hypoplasia
Ineffective thrombopoiesis due to folic acid or vitamin B_{12} deficiency
Pooling of platelets in an enlarged spleen
Increased platelet destruction due to drugs or immune disorders
Disseminated intravascular coagulation
Bernard-Soulier syndrome
Mechanical injury to platelets.

The basics

Platelets, or thrombocytes, are the smallest formed elements in the blood. They are vital to the formation of the hemostatic plug in vascular injury and promote coagulation by supplying phospholipids to the intrinsic thromboplastin pathway. Platelet count is one of the most important screening tests of platelet function. A platelet count that falls below 50,000 can cause spontaneous bleeding; when it drops below 5,000, fatal CNS bleeding or massive GI hemorrhage is possible.

When the platelet count is abnormal, diagnosis usually requires further studies, such as a complete blood count, bone marrow biopsy, direct antiglobulin test (direct Coombs' test), and serum protein electrophoresis.

Procedure

Perform a venipuncture, and collect the sample in a 7-ml lavender-top tube.

Patient care checklist

Before the test

☑ Explain or clarify test purpose and procedure.

☑ Evaluate patient understanding.

Interfering factors

● Failure to use the proper anticoagulant or to mix the sample and anticoagulant promptly and adequately may interfere with the accurate determination of test results.

● Hemolysis due to rough handling of the sample or to excessive probing at the venipuncture site may alter test results.

● Medications that may decrease platelet count include acetazolamide, acetohexamide, antimony, antineoplastics, brompheniramine maleate, carbamazepine, chloramphenicol, ethacrynic acid, furosemide, gold salts, hydroxychloroquine, indomethacin, isoniazid, mephenytoin, mefenamic acid, methazolamide, methimazole, methyldopa, oral diazoxide, oxyphenbutazone, penicillamine, penicillin, phenylbutazone, phenytoin, pyrimethamine, quinidine sulfate, quinine, salicylates, streptomycin, sulfonamides, thiazide and thiazide-like diuretics, and tricyclic antidepressants. Heparin causes transient, reversible thrombocytopenia.

● Platelet counts normally increase at high altitudes, with persistent cold temperature, and during strenuous exercise and excitement; the count decreases just before menstruation.

Platelet survival

Purpose

● To aid diagnosis of idiopathic thrombocytopenic purpura

● To assess platelet survival and life span.

Normal results

Normally, half the radiolabeled platelets disappear from circulation in 84 to 116 hours. The remaining radioactivity normally disappears in 8 to 10 days, which is thought to be the normal platelet life span.

Abnormal results

Diminished platelet survival time (may be as brief as 1 to 4 hours) indicates:

Idiopathic thrombocytopenic purpura
Systemic lupus erythematosus
Consumptive coagulopathy
Some cases of Hodgkin's disease and lymphosarcoma.

The basics
The platelet survival test measures the rate at which platelets are destroyed and renewed in the peripheral circulation. Platelets labeled with radioactive chromium-51 (^{51}Cr) are injected into the bloodstream. For 8 to 10 days, labeled platelets remaining in circulation are counted in serial samples of peripheral blood and are plotted to obtain a platelet survival curve. Findings are easily reproducible and closely express the life span of circulation platelets. This test provides important information for diagnosis of idiopathic thrombocytopenic purpura, a disorder marked by shortened platelet life span.

Procedure
• Perform a venipuncture, and collect the sample in a 7-ml lavender-top tube. This is performed to obtain platelets for tagging with ^{51}Cr isotope (donor platelets from a blood bag may be used instead).
• Inject the ^{51}Cr-tagged platelets into the bloodstream.
• Draw two blood samples: one at 30 minutes and another at 2 hours after the platelet injection.
• A venipuncture is performed daily for the next 8 to 10 days, and the blood samples are collected in 7-ml lavender-top tubes.

Special precautions
If the patient has a suspected coagulation defect, avoid excessive probing during venipuncture, do not leave the tourniquet on too long (it will cause bruising), and be sure to apply pressure to the venipuncture site for 5 minutes, or until the bleeding stops.

Patient care checklist
Before the test
☑ Explain or clarify test purpose and procedure.
☑ Evaluate patient understanding.

Interfering factors
Presence of antiplatelet antibodies after multiple transfusions, platelet transfusion, or repeated pregnancies may interfere with accurate determination of test results by shortening platelet survival time.

Prothrombin consumption time *(PCT)*

Purpose
To detect deficiencies of platelets or clotting factors essential to thromboplastin formation (Factors VIII, IX, XI, and XII).

Normal results
Prothrombin consumption is normally complete after 20 seconds.

Abnormal results
Increased PCT may indicate:
   Hemolysis
   Contamination of the blood sample with tissue thromboplastin.
Decreased PCT (excessive prothrombin in the serum) may indicate:
   Deficiency in some or all of the stage I clotting factors (Factors VIII, IX, XI, and XII)
   Platelet abnormalities.

The basics
Using a serum sample, this test measures the rate and the amount of prothrombin activation in the clotting process. In normal coagulation, the thromboplastin formed in the intrinsic coagulation pathway converts most plasma prothrombin into thrombin, leaving little or no prothrombin in normal serum. Consequently, the presence of prothrombin in serum indicates a deficiency of platelets or of the clotting factors that generate thromboplastin. Such deficiencies allow only a small amount of prothrombin to be converted to thrombin, shortening the PCT. Decreased PCT suggests that one or more of the stage I clotting factors is at 10% or less of its normal concentration.

Patients with abnormal results require factor assays, platelet studies, and further tests of thromboplastin function (activated partial thromboplastin time, for example) to confirm diagnosis.

Procedure
Perform a venipuncture, and collect the sample in a 7-ml red-top tube.

Patient care checklist
Before the test
☑ Explain or clarify test purpose and procedure.
☑ Evaluate patient understanding.

Interfering factors
• Traumatic venipuncture, hemolysis caused by rough handling of the sample, or failure to send the sample to the laboratory immediately or to place it on ice may interfere with accurate determination of test results.
• Anticoagulant therapy may alter test results.

Prothrombin time
[Pro time, PT]

Purpose
• To evaluate the extrinsic coagulation system
• To monitor response to oral anticoagulant therapy.

Normal results
Normally, PT values range from 9.6 to 11.8 seconds in males, and from 9.5 to 11.3 seconds in females. However, values vary, depending on the source of tissue thromboplastin and the type of sensing devices used to measure clot formation.

Abnormal results
Increased PT may indicate:
Deficiencies in fibrinogen, prothrombin, or Factors V, VII, or X

(Specific assays can pinpoint such deficiencies.)
Vitamin K deficiency
Hepatic disease
Ongoing oral anticoagulant therapy.

The basics
PT indirectly measures prothrombin and is an excellent screening procedure for overall evaluation of extrinsic coagulation Factors V, VII, and X, and of prothrombin and fibrinogen. Prothrombin time is the test of choice for monitoring oral anticoagulant therapy. In a patient receiving oral anticoagulants, PT is usually maintained between one and a half and two times the normal control value. Prolonged PT that exceeds two and a half times the control value is commonly associated with abnormal bleeding.

Although test results are frequently reported as a percentage of normal activity, compared with a curve of the clotting rate of normal diluted plasma, this method is inaccurate, because dilution of the sample affects the coagulation mechanism. The most reliable and accurate method reports both the patient's and the control clotting times in seconds.

Procedure
Perform a venipuncture, and collect the sample in a 7-ml blue-top tube.

Special precautions
Send the sample to the laboratory promptly. If transport is delayed more than 4 hours, and the sample is kept at room temperature, Factor V may deteriorate, prolonging the PT; however, if the sample is refrigerated, Factor VII may be activated, shortening the PT.

Patient care checklist
Before the test
☑ Explain or clarify test purpose and procedure.
☑ Evaluate patient understanding.

☑ Tell the patient that the test will be performed daily when therapy begins and will be repeated at longer intervals when medication levels stabilize, if the test is performed to monitor effects of anticoagulants.

Interfering factors
• Hemolysis caused by excessive probing during venipuncture or by rough handling of the sample may interfere with accurate determination of test results.
• Failure to mix the sample and anticoagulant adequately or to send the sample to the laboratory promptly may alter test results.
• Fibrin or fibrin split products in the sample, or plasma fibrinogen levels less than 100 mg/dl can prolong PT.
• Falsely prolonged results may occur if the collection tube is not filled to capacity with blood, since then the amount of anticoagulant would be excessive for the blood sample.
• Prolonged PT can also result from the use of adrenocorticotrophic hormone (ACTH), alcohol (large quantities), anabolic steroids, cholestyramine resin, heparin I.V. (within 5 hours of sample collection), indomethacin, mefenamic acid, para-aminosalicylic acid, methimazole, oxyphenbutazone, phenylbutazone, phenytoin, propylthiouracil, quinidine, quinine, thyroid hormones, and vitamin A.
• Shortened PT can result from the use of antihistamines, chloral hydrate, corticosteroids, digitalis, diuretics, glutethimide, griseofulvin, progestinestrogen combinations, pyrazinamide, vitamin K, and xanthines (caffeine, theophylline).
• Prolonged or shortened PT results can follow ingestion of antibiotics, barbiturates, hydroxyzine, sulfonamides, salicylates (more than 1 g/day prolongs PT), mineral oil, or clofibrate.

Red blood cell (RBC) count
[Erythrocyte count]

Purpose
• To supply figures for computing erythrocyte indices, which reveal RBC size and hemoglobin content
• To support other hematologic tests in diagnosis of anemia and polycythemia.

Normal results
Normal RBC values vary, depending on age, sex, sample, and geographic location. In adult males, red cell counts range from 4.5 to 6.2 million/μl of venous blood; in adult females, 4.2 to 5.4 million/μl of venous blood; in children, 4.6 to 4.8 million/μl of venous blood. In full-term infants, values range from 4.4 to 5.8 million/μl of capillary blood at birth; fall to 3 to 3.8 million/μl at age 2 months and increase slowly thereafter. Values are generally higher in persons living at high altitudes.

Abnormal results
Increased RBC count may indicate:
   Primary or secondary polycythemia
   Dehydration.
Decreased RBC count may indicate:
   Anemia
   Fluid overload
   Recent hemorrhage.

The basics
This test reports the number of RBCs found in a microliter (cubic millimeter) of whole blood and is included in the complete blood count. (See *Complete Blood Count.*) The RBC count itself provides no qualitative information regarding the size, shape, or concentration of hemoglobin within the corpuscles but may be used to calculate two erythrocyte indices: mean corpuscular volume (MCV) and mean corpuscular hemoglobin (MCH).

Complete Blood Count (CBC)

This often requested test gives a fairly complete picture of all the blood's formed elements. The CBC generally is composed of two sections: direct measurement of cellular components, including hemoglobin and erythrocyte indices, and differentiation of white blood cells, with an assessment of WBC, RBC, and platelet morphology. The following tests are usually included: hemoglobin concentration, hematocrit, red and white counts, differential white cell count, and stained red cell examination. Besides pointing the way toward further definitive studies, CBC data have proven extremely valuable in themselves.

CBC data can detect anemias, determine their severity, and compare the status of specific blood elements. Thus, the CBC is especially useful for evaluating conditions in which hematocrit does not parallel the red cell count. Normally, as the red cell count rises, so does hematocrit. However, in patients with microcytic or macrocytic anemia, this natural correlation does not hold true. For example, the patient with iron deficiency anemia has undersized red cells that cause his hemocrit to decrease, even though his red cell count may be reported as nearly normal. Conversely, the patient with pernicious anemia has many oversized red cells that cause his hematocrit to be higher than his red cell count.

The stained red cell examination often accompanies the white cell differential as part of the CBC. After the differential, the same stained slide is evaluated for RBC distribution and morphology, including changes in cell contents, color, size, and shape, providing additional information for detecting leukemia, anemia, and thalassemia. Variations in size and shape are reported as occasional, slight, moderate, marked, or very marked; structural variations are reported as the number of immature or nucleated RBCs/100 WBCs, noting cell inclusions.

Further tests, such as stained cell examination, hematocrit, hemoglobin, red cell indices, and white cell studies, are needed to confirm diagnosis.

Procedure

For adults and older children, draw venous blood into a 7-ml lavender-top tube. For younger children, collect capillary blood in a pipette or Microtainer.

Patient care checklist

Before the test

☑ Explain or clarify test purpose and procedure. (If the patient is an infant or young child, explain to the parents and to the child, if he is old enough to understand.)

☑ Evaluate patient and/or parent understanding.

Interfering factors

The following factors may interfere with accurate determination of test results:

• Failure to use the proper anticoagulant in the collection tube and to mix the sample and anticoagulant adequately

• Hemolysis due to rough handling of the sample

• Hemoconcentration due to prolonged tourniquet constriction

• Hemodilution caused by drawing the sample from the same arm that is being used for I.V. infusion of fluids

• High white cell count, which falsely elevates red cell count in semiautomated and automated counters

• Diseases that cause RBCs to agglutinate or form rouleaux, which falsely decreases red cell count.

Red cell indices
[Erythrocyte indices, Mean corpuscular volume (MCV), Mean corpuscular hemoglobin (MCH), Mean corpuscular hemoglobin concentration (MCHC)]

Purpose
To aid diagnosis and classification of anemias.

Normal results
The range of normal red cell indices is as follows:
MCV: 84 to 99 μ^3/red cell
MCH: 26 to 32 pg/red cell
MCHC: 30% to 36%.

Abnormal results
Increased MCV values may indicate:
Macrocytic anemias caused by megaloblastic anemias
Inherited disorders of DNA synthesis
Reticulocytosis
Deficiency of folic acid or vitamin B_{12}.
Increased MCH values may indicate:
Macrocytic anemia.
Increased MCHC values may indicate:
Spherocytosis.
Decreased MCV and MCHC values may indicate:

Microcytic, hypochromic anemias caused by iron deficiency anemia
Pyridoxine-responsive anemia
Thalassemia.
Decreased MCH values may indicate:
Microcytic anemia (see *Comparative Red Cell Indices in Anemias*).

The basics
Using the results of the RBC count, hematocrit, and total hemoglobin tests, the red cell indices provide important information about the size, hemoglobin concentration, and hemoglobin weight of an average red cell.

MCV, the ratio of hematocrit (packed cell volume) to the RBC count, expresses the average size of the erythrocytes and indicates whether they are undersized (microcytic), oversized (macrocytic), or normal (normocytic). MCH, the hemoglobin-RBC ratio, gives the weight of hemoglobin in an average red cell. MCHC, the ratio of hemoglobin weight to hematocrit, defines the concentration of hemoglobin in 100 ml of packed red cells. It helps distinguish normally colored (normochromic) red cells from paler (hypochromic) red cells.

Procedure
Perform a venipuncture, and collect the sample in a 7-ml lavender-top tube.

Comparative Red Cell Indices in Anemias

	Normal values (Normocytic, normochromic)	Iron deficiency anemia (Microcytic, hypochromic)	Pernicious anemia (Macrocytic, normochromic)
MCV	84 to 99μ^3	60 to 80μ^3	95 to 150μ^3
MCH	26 to 32 pg	5 to 25 pg	33 to 53 pg
MCHC	30% to 36%	20% to 30%	33% to 38%

Patient care checklist
Before the test
☑ Explain or clarify test purpose and procedure.
☑ Evaluate patient understanding.

Interfering factors
The following factors may interfere with accurate determination of test results:
• Failure to use the proper anticoagulant in the collection tube or to mix adequately the sample and anticoagulant
• Hemolysis due to rough handling of the sample
• Hemoconcentration due to prolonged tourniquet constriction
• High white cell count, which falsely elevates red cell count in semiautomated and automated cell counters and invalidates MCV and MCH results
• Diseases that cause RBCs to agglutinate or form rouleaux falsely decrease red cell count and invalidate test results.

Reticulocyte count

Purpose
• To aid in distinguishing between hypo- and hyperproliferative anemias
• To help assess blood loss, bone marrow response to anemia, and therapy for anemia.

Normal results
Reticulocytes account for 0.5% to 2% of the total RBC count. In infants, the percentage is normally higher, ranging from 3.2% at birth to 0.7% at age 12 weeks.

Abnormal results
Above-normal reticulocyte count:
Indicates a bone marrow response to anemia caused by hemolysis or blood loss
May occur after therapy for iron deficiency anemia or pernicious anemia.

Below-normal reticulocyte count occurs in:
Hypoplastic anemia
Pernicious anemia.

The basics
Reticulocytes are nonnucleated, immature red blood cells (RBCs) that remain in the peripheral blood for 24 to 48 hours while maturing. Generally larger than mature RBCs, they contain ribosomes, a centriole, particles of Golgi vesicles, and mitochondria that produce hemoglobin.

In this test, reticulocytes in a whole blood sample are counted and expressed as a percentage of the total red cell count. The reticulocyte count is useful in evaluating anemia and is an index of effective erythropoiesis and bone marrow response to anemia.

When following a patient with an abnormal reticulocyte count, look for trends in repeated tests or very gross changes in the numerical value, since the error rate for one test is very high.

Because the manual method for reticulocyte counting is imprecise, values may be reported as being below normal, normal, or above normal.

Procedure
Perform a venipuncture, and collect the sample in a 7-ml lavender-top tube.

Patient care checklist
Before the test
☑ Explain or clarify test purpose and procedure.
☑ Evaluate patient understanding. (If the patient is an infant or young child, explain to the parents and to the child if he is old enough to understand.)
☑ Withhold medications that may interfere with test results, as ordered. If they must be continued, note them on the laboratory slip.

Interfering factors
• False-negative test results can be caused by azathioprine, chloramphenicol, dactinomycin, and methotrexate.

False-positive results can be caused by adrenocorticotrophic hormone (ACTH), antimalarials, antipyretics, furazolidone (in infants), and levodopa. Sulfonamides can cause false-negative or false-positive results.

• Failure to use the proper anticoagulant in the collection tube or to mix the sample and anticoagulant adequately may interfere with accurate determination of the reticulocyte count.

• Prolonged tourniquet constriction may influence accurate determination of test results.

• Hemolysis due to rough handling of the sample may affect test results.

Sickle cell test
[Hemoglobin S test, Hgb S]

Purpose
To identify sickle cell disease and sickle cell trait.

Normal results
Negative for Hgb S.

Abnormal results
Positive for Hgb S indicates:
   Presence of sickle cells.

The basics
Sickle cells are severely deformed erythrocytes. The sickling phenomenon results from a hemoglobinopathy—most commonly, the polymerization of Hgb S, in the presence of low pH, low oxygen tension, elevated osmolarity, and elevated temperature, to form elongated structures (tactoids) that deform red cells. Reversing these conditions depolymerizes Hgb S and allows the red cells to resume their normal shape. However, repeated sickling leads to permanent red cell deformity. Hgb S is found almost exclusively in blacks; 0.2% of the blacks born in the United States have sickle cell anemia.

Persons with sickle cell disease (who have homozygous Hgb S) usually show abundant spontaneously sickled red cells on a peripheral blood smear. Persons with sickle cell trait (who have heterozygous Hgb S) or those who are doubly heterozygous may have normal red cells that can be easily changed to sickled forms by lowering oxygen tension.

Because sickle cell anemia is inherited, serious risks occur. When both parents have it, childbearing—if possible at all—is dangerous for the mother, and all offspring will have the disease. When only one parent has sickle cell anemia, all offspring will be carriers of the disease.

Although this test is useful as a rapid screening procedure, it may produce

Fetal Sickle Cell Test

When both parents of a developing fetus are suspected carriers of sickle cell trait, a reliable test is now available that can detect whether the fetus has the sickle cell trait or the disease. This test, developed in 1979 at the University of California at San Francisco, was the first diagnostic tool resulting from recombinant DNA research. Many major medical centers throughout the United States currently perform the test. In addition, any doctor can request the fetal sickle cell test if he suspects that both parents are carriers. He need only mail the appropriate samples to the nearest location.

The test requires a venous blood sample from both parents and an amniotic fluid sample. Diagnosis is based on analysis of the genes and the DNA in the fetal cells, and on the DNA in parental leukocytes. About 1 week is required to complete the test, which can generally be performed between the 14th and 18th weeks of pregnancy. This provides a sufficient opportunity for the couple to seek genetic counseling.

Sickle Cell Trait

This relatively benign condition results from heterozygous inheritance of the abnormal hemoglobin S–producing gene. Like sickle cell anemia, this condition is most common in blacks.

In persons with sickle cell trait, 20% to 40% of the total hemoglobin is hemoglobin S; the rest is normal. Such persons, called carriers, usually have no symptoms. They have normal hemoglobin and hematocrit values and can expect a normal life span. Nevertheless, they must avoid situations that provoke hypoxia, which occasionally causes a sickling crisis similar to that in sickle cell anemia.

Genetic counseling is essential for sickle cell carriers. Every child of two sickle cell carriers has a 25% chance of inheriting sickle cell anemia and a 50% chance of being a carrier.

false-positive and false-negative results. Consequently, an Hgb electrophoresis should be performed if the presence of Hgb S is strongly suspected. An Hgb electrophoresis is also needed to distinguish between homozygous and heterozygous forms.

Procedure

Perform a venipuncture, and collect the sample in a 7-ml lavender-top tube.

Patient care checklist

Before the test

☑ Explain or clarify test purpose and procedure.

☑ Evaluate patient understanding.

Interfering factors

• Hgb concentration under 10%, elevated Hgb F levels in infants under age 6 months, and blood transfusion within the past 3 months may produce false-negative test results.

• Failure to use the proper anticoag-

ulant in the collection tube, to fill the tube completely, or to mix the sample and the anticoagulant adequately may interfere with accurate determination of test results.

• Hemolysis due to rough handling of the sample may affect test results.

(See *Fetal Sickle Cell Test* and *Sickle Cell Trait*.)

Thrombin time
[*Thrombin clotting time*]

Purpose

• To detect fibrinogen deficiency or defect

• To aid diagnosis of disseminated intravascular coagulation (DIC) and hepatic disease

• To monitor the effectiveness of treatment with heparin, streptokinase, or urokinase.

Normal results

Normal thrombin times range from 10 to 15 seconds. Test results are usually reported with a normal control value.

Abnormal results

Thrombin time > 1.3 times the control may indicate:

Effective heparin therapy

Hepatic disease

DIC

Hypofibrinogenemia or dysfibrinogenemia.

The basics

The thrombin time test measures how quickly a clot forms when a standard amount of bovine thrombin is added to a platelet-poor plasma sample from the patient and to a normal plasma control sample. Since thrombin rapidly converts fibrinogen to a fibrin clot, this test allows a quick but imprecise estimation of plasma fibrinogen levels, which are a function of clotting time.

Patients with prolonged thrombin times require quantitation of fibrinogen levels; in suspected DIC, the test for fibrin split products is also necessary.

Procedure
Perform a venipuncture, and collect the sample in a 7-ml blue-top tube.

Patient care checklist
Before the test
☑ Explain or clarify test purpose and procedure.
☑ Evaluate patient understanding.

Interfering factors
• Hemolysis caused by excessive probing during venipuncture or by rough handling of the sample may alter test results.
• Failure to use the proper anticoagulant in the collection tube, to mix the sample and the anticoagulant adequately, to send the sample to the laboratory immediately, or to place it on ice may interfere with the accurate determination of test results.
• Administration of heparin may prolong clotting time. (See *Antithrombin III Test*.)

Antithrombin III Test

This test helps detect the cause of impaired coagulation, especially hypercoagulation. Antithrombin III (AT III) inactivates thrombin and inhibits coagulation. Normally, a balance between AT III and thrombin creates hemostasis, whereas AT III deficiency increases coagulation.

The normal value exceeds 50% of the control value. Decreased AT III levels can indicate disseminated intravascular coagulation (DIC) or thromboembolic, hypercoagulation, or hepatic disorders. Slightly decreased levels can result from use of oral contraceptives. Elevated levels can result from kidney transplant and use of oral anticoagulants or anabolic steroids.

Unstable hemoglobins

Purpose
To detect and/or confirm the presence of unstable hemoglobins.

Normal results
Heat stability test—negative (this result means that no unstable hemoglobins appear in the sample.)
Isopropanol solubility test—stable.

Abnormal results
A positive heat stability or unstable solubility test, especially with hemolysis, strongly suggests the presence of unstable hemoglobins.

The basics
Unstable hemoglobins are rare congenital red cell defects caused by amino acid substitutions in the normally stable structure of hemoglobin. These abnormal replacements produce a molecule that spontaneously denatures into clumps and aggregations called Heinz bodies, which separate from the red cell cytoplasm and accumulate at the cell membrane. Although Heinz bodies are usually removed efficiently by the spleen or liver, they may cause mild to severe hemolysis.

Unstable hemoglobins are best detected by precipitation tests (heat stability or isopropanol solubility) performed in the laboratory. Although a hemoglobin electrophoresis and the Heinz body test can demonstrate certain unstable hemoglobins, these tests do not always confirm the presence of such hemoglobins. Globin chain analysis identifies them more reliably, but because this procedure is time-consuming and technically complex, it is not performed routinely.

Procedure
Perform a venipuncture, and collect the sample in a 7-ml lavender-top tube.

Clinical Signs of Unstable Hemoglobins

More than 60 varieties of unstable hemoglobins exist, each named after the city in which it was discovered. Their effects vary according to their number, severity of instability, the condition of the spleen, and the oxygen-binding abilities of the unstable hemoglobin. Common indications of unstable hemoglobins include pallor, jaundice, splenomegaly, and, with severely unstable hemoglobins, cyanosis, pigmenturia, and hemoglobinuria. Thalassemia often causes similar clinical effects, but the molecular bases of the two diseases differ greatly.

Patient care checklist
Before the test
☑ Explain or clarify test purpose and procedure.
☑ Evaluate patient understanding.
☑ Withhold medications that may interfere with test results, as ordered. If they must be continued, note them on the laboratory slip.

Interfering factors
• Antimalarials, furazolidone (in infants), nitrofurantoin, phenacetin, procarbazine, and sulfonamides can induce Heinz body formation, resulting in a positive or unstable test.
• High levels of Hgb F may cause a false-positive isopropanol test.
• Failure to use the proper anticoagulant in the collection tube, to fill the tube completely, or to mix the sample and the anticoagulant adequately may interfere with accurate determination of test results.
• Hemolysis due to rough handling of the sample or hemoconcentration due to prolonged tourniquet constriction may influence test results.
(See *Clinical Signs of Unstable Hemoglobins.*)

White blood cell *(WBC)* count
[Leukocyte count]

Purpose
• To determine infection or inflammation
• To determine the need for further tests, such as the WBC differential or bone marrow biopsy
• To monitor response to chemotherapy or radiation therapy.

Normal results
The WBC count ranges from 4,100 to 10,900/μl.

Abnormal results
Increased WBC count (leukocytosis) may suggest:
  Infection or inflammation, such as an abscess, meningitis, appendicitis, or tonsillitis
  Leukemia
  Tissue necrosis due to burns, myocardial infarction, or gangrene.
Decreased WBC count (leukopenia) may suggest:
  Bone marrow depression, possibly due to a viral infection or to toxic reactions, such as those following treatment with antineoplastics, ingestion of mercury or other heavy metals, or exposure to benzene or arsenicals
  Influenza
  Typhoid fever
  Measles
  Infectious hepatitis
  Mononucleosis
  Rubella.

The basics
Part of the complete blood count, the WBC count reports the number of white cells found in a microliter (cubic millimeter) of whole blood. On any given day, WBC counts may vary by as much as 2,000 WBC/μl. Such variation can be the result of strenuous

exercise, stress, or digestion. The WBC count may rise or fall significantly in certain diseases, but is diagnostically useful only when interpreted in light of the white cell differential and of the patient's current clinical status. Patients with severe leukopenia may have little or no resistance to infection and, therefore, may require reverse isolation.

Procedure

Perform a venipuncture, and collect the sample in a 7-ml lavender-top tube.

Patient care checklist

Before the test

☑ Explain or clarify test purpose and procedure.

☑ Advise patient to avoid strenuous exercise for 24 hours before the test and to avoid ingesting a heavy meal before the test.

☑ Tell the patient that the test will be repeated to monitor his progress, if he is being treated for an infection.

☑ Evaluate patient understanding.

Interfering factors

• Hemolysis caused by rough handling of the sample may interfere with accurate determination of test results.

• Exercise, stress, or digestion raises the WBC count, thus yielding inaccurate results.

• Some drugs, including most antineoplastic agents; anti-infectives, such as metronidazole and flucytosine; anticonvulsants, such as phenytoin derivatives; thyroid hormone antagonists; and nonsteroidal antiinflammatories, such as indomethacin, lower the WBC count, altering results.

White blood cell differential

Purpose

• To evaluate the body's capacity to resist and overcome infection

• To detect and identify various types of leukemia

• To determine the stage and severity of an infection

• To detect allergic reactions and parasitic infections and to assess their severity (eosinophil count).

Normal results

Normal values for the five types of white blood cells (WBCs) that are classified in the differential—neutrophils, eosinophils, basophils, lymphocytes, and monocytes—are given for adults and children in the accompanying chart. (See *White Blood Cell Count Differential.*) For an accurate diagnosis, differential test results must always be interpreted in relation to the total WBC count.

Abnormal results

Evidence of a wide range of diseases and other conditions is revealed by abnormal differential patterns, as shown in the chart. (See *Influence of Disease on Blood Cell Count,* p. 38.)

The basics

Because the WBC differential evaluates the distribution and morphology of white cells, it provides more specific information about a patient's immune system than the WBC count. In the differential test, the laboratory classifies 100 or more white cells in a stained film of peripheral blood according to two major types of leukocytes—granulocytes (neutrophils, eosinophils, and basophils) and nongranulocytes (lymphocytes and monocytes)—and determines the percentage of each type. The differential count is the relative number of each type of white cell in the blood. By multiplying the percentage value of each type by the total WBC count, the investigator obtains the absolute number of each type of white cell. Although little is known about the func-

White Blood Cell Count Differential

| Cells | FOR ADULTS | | FOR CHILDREN (Age 6 to 18) | |
	Value	Absolute value	Relative value Boys	Girls
Neutrophils	47.6% to 76.8%	1,950 to 8,400/μl	38.5% to 71.5%	41.9% to 76.5%
Lymphocytes	16.2% to 43%	660 to 4,600/μl	19.4% to 51.4%	16.3% to 46.7%
Monocytes	0.6% to 9.6%	24 to 960/μl	1.1% to 11.6%	0.9% to 9.9%
Eosinophils	0.3% to 7%	12 to 760/μl	1% to 8.1%	0.8% to 8.3%
Basophils	0.3% to 2%	12 to 200/μl	0.25% to 1.3%	0.3% to 1.4%

Interpreting the Differential

To make an accurate diagnosis, the examiner must consider both relative and absolute values of the differential. Considered alone, relative results may point to one disease while masking the true pathology that would be revealed by considering the results of the white cell count. For example, consider a patient whose white blood cell (WBC) count is 6,000/μl and whose differential shows 30% neutrophils and 70% lymphocytes. His relative lymphocyte count would seem to be quite high (lymphocytosis), but when this figure is multiplied by his white cell count—6,000 × 70% = 4,200 lymphocytes/μl—it is well within the normal range.

This patient's neutrophil count, however, is low (30%), and when this is multiplied by the white cell count—6,000 × 30% = 1,800 neutrophils/μl—the result is a low absolute number.

This low result indicates decreased neutrophil production, which may mean depressed bone marrow.

tion of eosinophils in the blood, abnormally high levels of them are associated with various allergic diseases and reactions to parasites. In such cases, an eosinophil count is sometimes ordered as a follow-up to the white cell differential. This test is also appropriate if the differential WBC count shows a depressed eosinophil level. (See *Thorn [ACTH] Test,* p. 39.)

Procedure

Perform a venipuncture, and collect the sample in a 7-ml lavender-top tube.

Patient care checklist
Before the test
☑ Explain or clarify test purpose and procedure.
☑ Evaluate patient understanding.

Influence of Disease on Blood Cell Count

Cell type	How affected
Neutrophils	**Increased by:** • Infections: osteomyelitis, otitis media, salpingitis, septicemia, gonorrhea, endocarditis, smallpox, chickenpox, herpes, Rocky Mountain spotted fever • Ischemic necrosis due to myocardial infarction, burns, carcinoma • Metabolic disorders: diabetic acidosis, eclampsia, uremia, thyrotoxicosis • Stress response due to acute hemorrhage, surgery, excessive exercise, emotional distress, third trimester of pregnancy, childbirth • Inflammatory disease: rheumatic fever, rheumatoid arthritis, acute gout, vasculitis and myositis **Decreased by:** • Bone marrow depression due to radiation or cytotoxic drugs • Infections: typhoid, tularemia, brucellosis, hepatitis, influenza, measles, mumps, rubella, infectious mononucleosis • Hypersplenism: hepatic disease and storage diseases • Collagen vascular disease, such as systemic lupus erythematosus • Deficiency of folic acid or vitamin B_{12}
Eosinophils	**Increased by:** • Allergic disorders: asthma, hay fever, food or drug sensitivity, serum sickness, angioneurotic edema • Parasitic infections: trichinosis, hookworm, roundworm, amebiasis • Skin diseases: eczema, pemphigus, psoriasis, dermatitis, herpes • Neoplastic diseases: chronic myelocytic leukemia, Hodgkin's disease, metastases and necrosis of solid tumors • Miscellaneous: collagen vascular disease, adrenocortical hypofunction, ulcerative colitis, polyarteritis nodosa, postsplenectomy, pernicious anemia, scarlet fever, excessive exercise **Decreased by:** • Stress response due to trauma, shock, burns, surgery, mental distress • Cushing's syndrome
Basophils	**Increased by:** • Chronic myelocytic leukemia, polycythemia vera, some chronic hemolytic anemias, Hodgkin's disease, systemic mastocytosis, myxedema, ulcerative colitis, chronic hypersensitivity states, nephrosis **Decreased by:** • Hyperthyroidism, ovulation, pregnancy, stress

(continued)

Influence of Disease on Blood Cell Count *(continued)*

Cell type	How affected
Lymphocytes	**Increased by:** • Infections: pertussis, brucellosis, syphilis, tuberculosis, hepatitis, infectious mononucleosis, mumps, German measles, cytomegalovirus • Other: thyrotoxicosis, hypoadrenalism, ulcerative colitis, immune diseases, lymphocytic leukemia **Decreased by:** • Severe debilitating illness, such as congestive heart failure, renal failure, advanced tuberculosis • Defective lymphatic circulation, high levels of adrenal corticosteroids, immunodeficiency due to immunosuppressives
Monocytes	**Increased by:** • Infections: subacute bacterial endocarditis, tuberculosis, hepatitis, malaria, Rocky Mountain spotted fever • Collagen vascular disease: systemic lupus erythematosus, rheumatoid arthritis, polyarteritis nodosa • Carcinomas, monocytic leukemia, lymphomas

Thorn (ACTH) Test

This test evaluates adrenal cortex function by determining the effect of adrenocorticotrophic hormone (ACTH) on the eosinophil count. It is useful as an aid in the diagnosis of Addison's disease and helps distinguish functional hypopituitarism from organic disease of the adrenal cortex.

Food and fluids are restricted for 12 hours before the test. Then, a baseline eosinophil count is done. Next, 25 mg of ACTH is administered intramuscularly to stimulate the adrenal cortex. A second eosinophil count is done 4 hours after the ACTH is given. If the adrenal cortex is functioning normally, the second eosinophil count will show a decrease of 50% or more from the baseline count. If adrenal cortex insufficiency is present, the second eosinophil count will be decreased by less than 20%.

Interfering factors
• Hemolysis caused by rough handling of the sample may affect test results.
• Failure to use the proper anticoagulant, to fill the collection tube completely, or to mix the sample and anticoagulant adequately may influence accurate determination of test results.
• Many drugs influence the eosinophil count: methysergide and desipramine increase or decrease eosinophil count; indomethacin or procainamide decrease the eosinophil count; anticonvulsants, capreomycin, cephalosporins, D-penicillamine, gold compounds, isoniazid, nalidixic acid, novobiocin, para-aminosalicylic acid, paromomycin, penicillins, phenothiazines, rifampin, streptomycin, sulfonamides, and tetracyclines increase the eosinophil count by provoking an allergic reaction. (See *Leukocyte Alkaline Phosphatase Stain*, p. 40.)

Leukocyte Alkaline Phosphatase Stain

Levels of leukocyte alkaline phosphatase (LAP), an enzyme found in neutrophils, may be altered by infection, stress, chronic inflammatory diseases, Hodgkin's disease, and hematologic disorders. Most of these conditions elevate LAP levels; only a few, notably chronic myelogenous leukemia (CML), depress them. Thus, this test is most often used to differentiate CML from other disorders that produce an elevated white blood cell count.

To perform this test, a blood sample is obtained by venipuncture or finger stick. The venous blood sample is collected in a 7-ml green-top tube and transported immediately to the laboratory. Normally, values for LAP fall in the range of 40 to 100, depending upon the laboratory's standards.

Depressed LAP values typically indicate CML; however, low values may also occur in paroxysmal nocturnal hemoglobinuria, aplastic anemia, and infectious mononucleosis. Elevated values may indicate Hodgkin's disease, polycythemia vera, or a neutrophilic leukemoid reaction—a response to conditions such as infection, chronic inflammation, or pregnancy.

After a diagnosis of CML, the LAP stain may also be used to help detect onset of the blastic phase of the disease, when LAP levels typically rise. However, LAP levels also increase toward normal in response to therapy; because of this, test results must be correlated with the patient's condition.

Whole blood clotting time and clot retraction time
[Lee-White coagulation time, coagulation time, venous clotting time]

Purpose
• To assess the intrinsic system of blood coagulation
• To monitor effectiveness of heparin therapy, although less reliable than the activated partial thromboplastin time (APTT).

Normal results
Whole blood clotting time: 5 to 15 minutes
Clot retraction time: Normal if after 1 hour, the clot becomes firm and retracted from the sides of the tube, occupying about half the original blood volume (most of the serum has been expressed from the clot). Approximately 50% retraction is normal.

Abnormal results
Increased whole blood clotting time may indicate:
Severe deficiency of coagulation factors (except Factors VII and XIII)
Presence of anticoagulants.
Slow or incomplete clot retraction may indicate:
Thrombocytopenia
Thrombasthenia (produces reduced retraction and a soft clot)
Hyperfibrinogenemia (abnormal clot retraction)
Anemia (abnormal clot retraction)
Secondary fibrinolysis (clot appears soft and ill-defined)
Disseminated intravascular coagulation (clot appears soft and ill-defined).

The basics
Whole blood clotting time measures the interval required for fresh whole blood to clot in vitro at 98.6° F. (37° C.) and grossly evaluates the intrinsic clotting mechanism. Developed in 1939, this test is nonspecific for any

coagulation factor, time-consuming, difficult to standardize, subject to technical error, and unreliable as a screening test. Abnormal clotting time necessitates further tests, including prothrombin time, APTT, and specific factor assays. Other tests, such as the APTT, are more useful. Using the same whole blood sample, the clot retraction study measures the time needed for the platelet and fibrinogen network to contract into a firm clot. Successful retraction is based on the number and activity of platelets, fibrinogen and other intrinsic factor levels, and hematocrit. (See *Using the Hemochron*.)

Procedure
• Perform a venipuncture, using the two-syringe technique. Draw 3 ml of blood with a plastic syringe; disconnect the syringe from the needle and discard it (to minimize contamination of the sample with tissue thromboplastin).
• Attach a new syringe, and start a stopwatch as soon as blood enters the new syringe.
• Apply pressure to the puncture site after withdrawing the needle, and instruct the patient to continue this pressure until the bleeding stops.
• Remove the needle from the syringe, and immediately transfer 1-ml portions of the sample into three 12 x 75 mm plain glass tubes set in a water bath at 98.6° F. (37° C.).
• Take the last tube filled and tilt it gently every 30 seconds until a clot

Using the Hemochron

To prevent complications (such as hemorrhage) from an extremely prolonged clotting time, a fast, precise way to monitor a patient's whole blood clotting time is needed. The Hemochron Portable Blood Coagulation Timing System, shown at right, usually provides clotting time measurements within 10 minutes of specimen collection.

Because the Hemochron has no water bath or heating block, it is easy to operate. The patient can be monitored at his bedside, which eliminates laboratory delays and specimen mix ups. The Hemochron runs on either battery or outlet power.

To use the Hemochron system, first perform venipuncture. Collect the specimen in a specially prepared test tube provided by the manufacturer. Then, place the tube in the Hemochron's incubated test well. When clotting has been detected, a tone sounds and the results appear on the Hemochron's display screen.

When monitoring a patient receiving heparin therapy, use the Hemochron to:

• detect any initial sensitivity or resistance to the heparin
• detect any variation in heparin potency
• evaluate the rate of heparin consumption
• assess for heparin rebound.

Note: Consider using the Hemochron to monitor a patient undergoing hemodialysis. By doing so, you protect him against overheparinization and still prevent clotting in the artificial kidney.

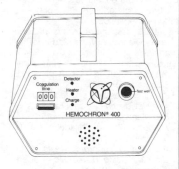

forms; next, do the same with the second tube filled and finally with the first.

• Stop the watch when clotting has occurred in all three tubes, and record the time elapsed as the whole blood clotting time.

• Observe the three samples at hourly intervals for signs of clot retraction. Record retraction as complete when the clot has separated from the sides and bottom of the tube.

Special precautions

• If a coagulation defect is suspected, avoid excessive probing during venipuncture, do not leave the tourniquet on too long (it will cause bruising), and apply pressure to the venipuncture site for 5 minutes, or until the bleeding stops.

• Since the inside surface of the collection tube affects clot retraction, use only plain glass tubes.

Patient care checklist

Before the test

☑ Explain or clarify test purpose and procedure.

☑ Evaluate patient understanding.

Interfering factors

• Failure to record the sample collection time, to maintain the sample at 98.6° F. (37° C.), or to fill the collection tubes to the proper level may affect accuracy of test results.

• Hemolysis due to poor venipuncture technique or rough handling of the sample may affect test results.

• Contamination of the sample with tissue thromboplastin may interfere with accuracy of test results.

• Use of a plastic or silicone-coated collection tube, instead of glass, prolongs clotting time.

• Depressed fibrinogen levels (less than 100 mg/dl) prolong clotting time.

• Anticoagulants increase clotting time.

Selected References

Beck, William S., ed. *Hematology,* 3rd ed. Cambridge, Mass.: MIT Press, 1981.

Brown, Barbara A. *Hematology: Principles and Procedures,* 3rd ed. Philadelphia: Lea & Febiger, 1980.

Diagnostics, 2nd ed. Nurse's Reference Library. Springhouse, Pa.: Springhouse Corp., 1986.

Diseases, 2nd ed. Nurse's Reference Library. Springhouse, Pa.: Springhouse Corp., 1987.

Fischbach, Frances. *A Manual of Laboratory Diagnostic Tests,* 2nd ed. Philadelphia: J.B. Lippincott Co., 1984.

Guyton, Arthur C. *Textbook of Medical Physiology,* 6th ed. Philadelphia: W.B. Saunders Co., 1981.

Henry, John Bernard, ed. *Todd-Sanford-Davidsohn Clinical Diagnosis and Management by Laboratory Methods,* 17th ed. Philadelphia: W.B. Saunders Co., 1984.

Lamb, Jane O. *Laboratory Tests for Clinical Nursing.* Bowie, Md.: Robert J. Brady Co., 1984.

Miale, John B. *Laboratory Medicine:*

Hematology, 6th ed. St. Louis: C.V. Mosby Co., 1982.

Nursing87 Drug Handbook. Springhouse, Pa.: Springhouse Corp., 1987.

Petersdorf, Robert G., and Adams, Raymond D., eds. *Harrison's Principles of Internal Medicine,* 10th ed. New York: McGraw-Hill Book Co., 1983.

Price, Sylvia, and Wilson, Lorraine. *Pathophysiology: Clinical Concepts of Disease Processes,* 2nd ed. New York: McGraw-Hill Book Co., 1982.

Ravel, Richard A. *Clinical Laboratory Medicine,* 4th ed. Chicago: Year Book Medical Pubs., 1984.

Selkurt, Ewald E. *Basic Physiology for the Health Sciences,* 2nd ed. Boston: Little, Brown & Co., 1981.

Tilkian, Sarko M., et al. *Clinical Implications of Laboratory Tests,* 3rd ed. St. Louis: C.V. Mosby Co., 1983.

Widmann, Frances K. *Clinical Interpretation of Laboratory Tests,* 9th ed. Philadelphia: F.A. Davis Co., 1983.

Wintrobe, Maxwell M., et al. *Clinical Hematology,* 8th ed. Philadelphia: Lea & Febiger, 1981.

2 BLOOD CHEMISTRY TESTING

Introduction

Blood chemistry testing identifies numerous chemical substances found in the body.

Analysis of these substances provides valuable clues to the functioning of the major body systems. Analysis of blood gases and electrolytes, for example, helps evaluate the respiratory and metabolic states of the body. Serum levels of enzymes can also give valuable information. When tissue cells are damaged by disease or some other defect, they release enzymes specific to that area into the bloodstream, where they can be readily detected. For example, leakage from dying cells is the source of elevated serum enzymes in myocardial infarction, infectious hepatitis, and other disease states. Although serum levels of any one enzyme may not identify its tissue of origin, comparing serum levels of several enzymes may give important diagnostic information, since individual enzymes are present in different tissues in different ratios. Such an analysis may reveal the extent of pathology and monitor the progress of healing. Some enzymes—creatine phosphokinase and lactic dehydrogenase, for instance—occur in multiple forms (isoenzymes) that differ in molecular details while retaining their basic identity. Certain organs or tissues contain greater or lesser amounts of one isoenzyme than another; therefore, testing for isoenzymes sometimes provides better sensitivity or specificity than measuring an entire enzyme group.

Hormones are powerful, complex chemicals, normally produced by the endocrine system and transported through the bloodstream to stimulate or inhibit the metabolic activity of target glands or organs to maintain homeostasis. A change in the circulating blood level of any one hormone eventually changes the secretion of others. Consequently, the circulating blood levels of hormones have enormous diagnostic significance, and numerous tests have been devised to detect and evaluate abnormal secretion. Hormonal blood tests are subject to such variables as drug effects, stress, nutritional status, or diurnal rhythms in hormone secretion, which necessitate careful collection scheduling.

Lipids must combine with plasma proteins into a lipid-protein molecular complex called lipoproteins for transportation through the body. Lipoprotein phenotyping—classifying patients by the pattern of their lipoprotein levels—is an important procedure for diagnosing and treating hyper- and hypolipoproteinemias. Lipoprotein determinations are also useful in evaluating the risk of coronary artery disease (CAD).

Tests for blood glucose measure the capacity for conversion of carbohydrates by insulin. These tests are used to identify hypo- or hyperglycemic states.

Serum proteins have diagnostic significance because of their various and vital functions: binding and detoxifying drugs and other potentially toxic substances; synthesizing antibodies, enzymes, and hormones; sustaining the physical stability of the blood; maintaining acid-base balance; and serving as a reserve source of nutrition for tissues. The major serum proteins are albumin and the globulins (alpha$_1$, alpha$_2$, beta, and gamma).

Bile pigments are waste products of heme degradation, initiated by the breakdown of erythrocytes at the end of their life cycle. Although bile pigments have no known function, abnormalities in their overall transformation have considerable significance in the diagnosis of hepatobiliary disease and in conditions marked by excessive hemolysis.

Vitamins and trace elements—organic and inorganic nutrients, respectively—are indispensable to normal metabolism and proper nutrition. Today, a far greater danger than trace element deficiency is toxic excess—through industrial exposure to poten-tially toxic levels of trace elements. Fortunately, sophisticated diagnostic techniques have been developed to detect minute concentrations of trace elements in serum. Equally sensitive tests are available to investigate vitamin toxicity or deficiency. (See *Automatic Test Series: SMA 12/60 and SMAC.*) (Also see *Collection Techniques: Blood and Urine Samples,* pp. xii to xx.)

Patient-teaching guidelines
Patient-learner objectives:
• Define the test.
• State the specific purpose of the test.
• Explain the procedure.
• Discuss test preparation, procedure, and post-test care.
Teaching content:
• Explain the purpose of the test.
• Describe the procedure if the patient is unfamiliar with it. If a venipuncture is necessary, explain that the patient's vein will be punctured, usually by a steel needle attached to a tube or sy-

---

Automatic Test Series: SMA 12/60 and SMAC

Many laboratories now use automated electronic systems, such as the sequential multiple analyzer (SMA) 12/60 and the sequential multiple analyzer with computer (SMAC), in chemistry, blood banking, and serologic and bacteriologic procedures. These systems perform blood studies rapidly, economically, and comprehensively. They can detect unsuspected abnormalities and indicate the need for additional tests.

• The SMA 12/60 can make 12 determinations on 60 serum specimens in 1 hour. It can determine glucose, cholesterol, albumin, and total protein levels (nutritional status); bilirubin levels (liver function); blood urea nitrogen (BUN) and uric acid levels (kidney function); serum glutamic-oxaloacetic acid (SGOT) and lactate dehydrogenase (LDH) enzyme levels (tissue injury); alkaline phosphatase (bone tissue injury); and calcium and phosphate levels (parathyroid function).

• The SMAC can perform 20 to 40 biochemical determinations on 120 serum specimens in 1 hour. It can analyze selected blood components singly or in combination, as well as provide an entire test profile on each specimen. This system also automatically reports special cardiac, renal, hepatic, lipid, bone, enzyme, and electrolyte profiles. With SMAC, tests performed on a 450-μl sample include cholesterol, triglycerides, glucose, BUN, calcium, phosphorus, sodium, potassium, chloride, carbon dioxide, total protein, total bilirubin, albumin, creatinine, gamma glutamyl transferase, SGOT, serum glutamic-pyruvic transaminase, LDH, uric acid, acid and alkaline phosphatase, and iron levels.

ringe, so that blood can be collected for testing.

• Explain that collection of the blood sample causes some discomfort; however, the procedure is brief.

• Inform the patient that mild pressure will be applied to the puncture site following the procedure, usually for a few minutes.

• Identify any dietary or medication restrictions necessary before the test. List items to be avoided, and give a definite time period. Explain that these steps are necessary to provide accurate test results. Verbal instructions should be accompanied by written instructions for outpatients.

• If hormonal tests are ordered, explain that physical or emotional stress may influence test results. To decrease this possibility, instruct the patient to limit physical activity for 10 to 12 hours before the test, and encourage the patient to relax and remain recumbent for 30 minutes before the test.

• When appropriate, inform the patient that the blood chemistry tests are part of routine hospital screening procedures.

Evaluation:
After the patient-teaching session has been completed, evaluate whether or not the patient has satisfactorily met each patient-learner objective by obtaining necessary patient feedback. Refocus teaching as needed.

Acid phosphatase

Purpose
• To detect prostatic cancer
• To monitor response to therapy for prostatic cancer.

Normal results
Serum values for total acid phosphatase depend on the method and range from 0 to 1.1 Bodansky units/ml; 1 to 4 King-Armstrong units/ml; 0.13 to 0.63 Bessey-Lowery-Brock (BLB) units/ml.

Abnormal results
Markedly increased acid phosphatase levels:
  A tumor that has spread beyond the prostatic capsule.
Moderately increased acid phosphatase levels:
  Prostatic infarction
  Paget's disease
  Gaucher's disease
  Other conditions, such as multiple myeloma.
Declining high acid phosphatase levels:
  Successful treatment of prostatic cancer.

The basics
Acid phosphatase, a group of phosphatase enzymes most active at a pH of about 5.0, appears primarily in the prostate gland and semen, and to a lesser extent, in the liver, spleen, red blood cells, bone marrow, and platelets. Prostatic and erythrocytic enzymes are this group's two major isoenzymes, which can be separated in the laboratory; the prostatic isoenzyme is more specific for prostatic cancer. The more widespread the tumor, the more likely it is to produce high serum acid phosphatase levels.

Procedure
Perform a venipuncture, and collect the sample in a 7-ml, red-top tube.

Patient care checklist
Before the test
☑ Explain or clarify test purpose and procedure.
☑ Evaluate patient understanding.
☑ Withhold medications that may interfere with test results as ordered. If they must be continued, note them on the laboratory slip.

Interfering factors
• Fluorides and phosphates can cause false-negative test results; clofibrate can cause false-positive results.
• Prostate massage, catheterization, or rectal examination within 48 hours

of the test may interfere with test results.

• Hemolysis due to rough handling of the sample or improper sample storage may interfere with test results. Acid phosphatase levels drop by 50% within 1 hour if the sample remains at room temperature without the addition of a preservative or if it is not packed in ice.

ACTH
[Adrenocorticotropic hormone, corticotropin]

Purpose
• To facilitate differential diagnosis of primary and secondary adrenal hypofunction
• To aid in differential diagnosis of adrenal hyperfunction (Cushing's syndrome).

Normal results
Reference values are not yet firmly established. The Mayo Clinic sets baseline values at less than 120 pg/ml, but these values may vary, depending on the laboratory.

Abnormal results
Increased plasma ACTH levels:
   Primary adrenal hypofunction (Addison's disease)
   Pituitary adenoma
   Stress (physical or emotional).
Decreased or low-normal plasma ACTH levels:
   Adrenocortical hyperfunction due to adrenocortical tumor or hyperplasia
   Secondary adrenal hypofunction resulting from pituitary or hypothalamic dysfunction.

The basics
This test measures the plasma levels of ACTH by radioimmunoassay. ACTH, a hormone released by the anterior pituitary, stimulates the adrenal cortex to secrete cortisol and, to a lesser degree, androgens and aldosterone. ACTH levels vary diurnally, peaking between 6 a.m. and 8 a.m. and ebbing between 6 p.m. and 11 p.m.

Through a negative feedback mechanism, plasma cortisol levels control ACTH secretion—for example, high cortisol levels suppress ACTH secretion. Emotional and physical stress (pain, surgery, insulin-induced hypoglycemia) stimulate secretion and can override the effects of plasma cortisol levels.

In primary adrenal hypofunction (Addison's disease), the pituitary gland attempts to compensate for the unresponsiveness of the target organ by releasing excessive ACTH.

In Cushing's disease, pituitary dysfunction (due to adenoma) causes continuous hypersecretion of ACTH and, consequently, continuously elevated plasma cortisol levels, without diurnal variations.

In adrenal hyperfunction due to adrenocortical tumor or hyperplasia, ACTH levels are low-normal (or undetectable) because the high plasma cortisol levels suppress ACTH secretion through negative feedback.

In secondary adrenal hypofunction, pituitary or hypothalamic dysfunction causes decreased output of ACTH.

ACTH suppression or stimulation testing is usually necessary to confirm the diagnosis. The instability and unavailability of plasma ACTH greatly limit its diagnostic significance and reliability.

Procedure
• For a patient with suspected adrenal hypofunction, perform the venipuncture for a baseline level between 6 a.m. and 8 a.m. (peak secretion).
• For a patient with suspected Cushing's syndrome, perform the venipuncture between 6 p.m. and 11 p.m. (low secretion).
• Collect the sample in a plastic tube, since ACTH may adsorb to glass, or in a green-top (heparinized) tube.
• Pack the sample in ice, and send it

to the laboratory immediately. The collection technique may vary, depending on the laboratory.

Patient care checklist
Before the test
☑ Explain or clarify test purpose, preparation, and procedure.
☑ Evaluate patient understanding.
☑ Restrict the patient's physical activity for 10 to 12 hours before the test.
☑ Withhold medications that may interfere with test results as ordered for 48 hours or longer before the test. If medications must be continued, note them on the laboratory slip.
☑ Give the patient a low-carbohydrate diet for 2 days before the test (if required by the laboratory).

Interfering factors
• Failure to observe restrictions of diet or physical activity may interfere with accurate determination of the test results.
• ACTH levels are depressed by corticosteroids, including cortisone and its analogues, and by drugs that increase endogenous cortisol secretion (estrogens, calcium gluconate, amphetamines, spironolactone, and ethanol). Lithium carbonate decreases cortisol levels and may interfere with ACTH secretion.
• ACTH levels are also affected by the menstrual cycle and pregnancy.
• A radioactive scan performed within 1 week before the test may influence test results.
• Failure to transfer the sample to the laboratory immediately or to pack the sample in ice may affect accurate determination of test results.

Aldosterone

Purpose
To aid in diagnosis of primary and secondary aldosteronism, adrenal hyperplasia, hypoaldosteronism, and salt-losing syndrome.

Normal results
Serum aldosterone levels (in a standing, nonpregnant patient) range from 1 to 21 ng/dl. Specifically, a normal serum aldosterone level for an adult male or female who has been supine for at least 2 hours is 7.4 ± 4.2 ng/dl; for an adult male or female who has been standing for at least 2 hours, 13.2 ± 8.9 ng/dl.

Abnormal results
Increased serum aldosterone levels:
Primary aldosteronism (Conn's syndrome) resulting from adrenocortical adenoma or carcinoma, or bilateral adrenal hyperplasia
Secondary aldosteronism resulting from renovascular hypertension, congestive heart failure, cirrhosis of the liver, nephrotic syndrome, idiopathic cyclic edema, or the third trimester of pregnancy.
Decreased serum aldosterone levels:
Primary hypoaldosteronism
Salt-losing syndrome
Toxemia of pregnancy
Addison's disease.

The basics
Aldosterone, the principal mineralocorticoid secreted by the adrenal cortex, regulates ion transport across cell membranes in the renal tubules to promote reabsorption of sodium and chloride in exchange for potassium and hydrogen ions. Consequently, aldosterone helps to maintain blood pressure and blood volume, and to regulate fluid and electrolyte balance.

Aldosterone secretion is controlled primarily by the renin-angiotensin system and by the circulating concentration of potassium. Thus, high serum potassium levels elicit secretion of aldosterone through a potent feedback system; similarly, hyponatremia, hypovolemia, and other disorders that provoke the release of renin stimulate aldosterone secretion. This test identifies aldosteronism and, when supported by plasma renin levels, distinguishes between the primary and secondary forms of this disorder.

Procedure
• While the patient is still supine after a night's rest, perform a venipuncture.
• Collect the sample in a 7-ml, red-top collection tube, and send it to the laboratory.
• To evaluate the effect of postural change, draw another sample while the patient is standing 4 hours later, after the patient has been up and about.
• Collect the second sample in a 7-ml, red-top collection tube, and send it to the laboratory.
• Record on the laboratory slip whether the patient was supine or standing during the venipuncture.
• If the patient is a premenopausal female, specify the phase of her menstrual cycle on the laboratory slip, since aldosterone levels may fluctuate during the menstrual cycle.

Patient care checklist
Before the test
☑ Explain or clarify test purpose, preparation, and procedure.
☑ Evaluate patient understanding.
☑ Keep the patient on a low-carbohydrate, normal-sodium (135 mEq or 3 g/day) diet for at least 2 weeks or, preferably, for 30 days before the test.
☑ Inform the patient that the laboratory requires at least 10 days to complete the multistage analysis.
☑ Withhold medications, as ordered: diuretics, antihypertensives, steroids, cyclic progestational agents, and estrogens—for at least 2 weeks or, preferably, for 30 days before the test; all renin inhibitors (such as propranolol)—for 1 week before the test. If medications must be continued, note them on the laboratory slip.
☑ Instruct the patient to avoid licorice for at least 2 weeks before the test. (It produces an aldosterone-like effect.)

Interfering factors
• Hemolysis due to rough handling of the sample may interfere with accurate determination of test results.
• Failure to observe restrictions of diet, medications, or posture may interfere with accurate determination of test results. Some antihypertensives—methyldopa, for example—promote sodium and water retention, and therefore may reduce aldosterone levels. Diuretics promote sodium excretion and may raise aldosterone levels. Some corticosteroids—fludrocortisone, for example—mimic mineralocorticoid activity and therefore may lower aldosterone levels.
• A radioactive scan performed within 1 week before the test may influence test results.

Alkaline phosphatase

Purpose
• To detect and identify skeletal diseases, primarily those characterized by marked osteoblastic activity
• To detect focal hepatic lesions causing biliary obstruction, such as tumors or abscesses
• To assess response to vitamin D in the treatment of deficiency-induced rickets.

Normal results
The normal range of serum alkaline phosphatase varies with the laboratory method used. Total alkaline phosphatase levels, when measured by chemical inhibition, range from 90 to 239 units/liter for males; for females under age 45, the range is 76 to 196 units/liter; for women over age 45, the range widens from 87 to 250 units/liter, for unknown reasons. Since alkaline phosphatase concentrations rise during active bone formation in growth, infants, children, and adolescents normally have levels that may be three times as

high as those of adults. Pregnancy also causes a physiologic rise in alkaline phosphatase levels.

When the Bodansky method is used, normal range is from 1.5 to 4 Bodansky units/dl; for the King-Armstrong method, normal adult values range from 4 to 13.5 King-Armstrong units/dl.

Abnormal results

Markedly increased alkaline phosphatase levels:

Severe biliary obstruction by gallstones, malignant or infectious infiltrations, or fibrosis
Paget's disease
Bone metastasis
Hyperparathyroidism.

Moderately increased alkaline phosphatase levels:

Cirrhosis of liver
Mononucleosis
Viral hepatitis
Osteomalacia
Deficiency-induced rickets.

Decreased alkaline phosphatase levels:

Hypophosphatasia
Protein deficiency
Magnesium deficiency.

The basics

This test measures serum levels of alkaline phosphatase, an enzyme that is most active at about pH 9.0. Alkaline phosphatase influences bone calcification and lipid and metabolite transport. Total serum levels reflect the combined activity of several alkaline phosphatase isoenzymes.

The alkaline phosphatase test is particularly sensitive to mild biliary obstruction and is a primary indicator of space-occupying hepatic lesions. However, since both skeletal and hepatic diseases can raise alkaline phosphatase levels, its most specific clinical application is in the diagnosis of metabolic bone disease; additional liver function studies are usually required to identify hepatobiliary disorders.

Alkaline Phosphatase Isoenzymes

Separation of alkaline phosphatase isoenzymes in the laboratory, using heat inactivation, electrophoresis, or chemical means, is sometimes used in place of serum gamma glutamyl transferase, leucine aminopeptidase, or 5'-nucleotidase tests to differentiate hepatic and skeletal diseases. Sixteen molecularly distinct isoenzyme fractions have been identified electrophoretically in human serum, stimulating continuing controversy about the origins, proportions, and methods of isoenzyme determination. Although the number and concentration of alkaline phosphatase isoenzymes in total serum levels vary with the laboratory separation method used, the five isoenzymes of greatest clinical significance originate in the liver (including kidney and bile fractions), bone (may also include bile fraction), intestine, and placenta.

On electrophoresis, the liver isoenzyme usually measures from 20 to 130 units/liter; the bone isoenzyme, from 20 to 120 units/liter; and the intestinal fraction—which occurs almost exclusively in individuals with blood group B or O and is markedly elevated 8 hours after a fatty meal—from undetectable to 18 units/liter. The placental isoenzyme first appears in the second trimester of pregnancy, accounts for roughly half of all alkaline phosphatase during the third trimester, and drops to normal levels the 1st month postpartum. Another isoenzyme, Regan, resembles the placental isoenzyme and appears in a small percentage of patients with cancer; it may be used as a tumor marker.

Procedure

Perform a venipuncture, and collect the sample in a 7-ml, red-top tube.

Patient care checklist

Before the test

☑ Explain or clarify test purpose, preparation, and procedure.

☑ Evaluate patient understanding.

☑ Restrict food and fluids for 10 to 12 hours before the test, since fat intake stimulates intestinal alkaline phosphatase secretion.

Interfering factors

• Recent ingestion of vitamin D may increase levels of alkaline phosphatase, because of the effect of vitamin D on osteoblastic activity.

• Recent infusion of albumin prepared from placental venous blood causes extreme increases in serum alkaline phosphatase levels.

• Drugs that influence liver function or cause cholestasis, such as barbiturates, chlorpropamide, oral contraceptives, isoniazid, methyldopa, phenothiazine, phenytoin, and rifampin, can mildly elevate alkaline phosphatase levels; halothane sensitivity may increase levels drastically. Clofibrate decreases alkaline phosphatase levels.

• Healing long bone fractures, age (infants, children, adolescents, and women over 45), and pregnancy (third trimester) can produce physiologic elevations of alkaline phosphatase levels.

• Hemolysis due to rough handling of the sample or a delay of more than 8 hours in sending the sample to the laboratory may interfere with accurate determination of alkaline phosphatase levels. (See *Alkaline Phosphatase Isoenzymes,* p. 49.)

Amino acid screening

Purpose

To screen for inborn errors of amino acid metabolism.

Normal results

Chromatography shows a normal plasma amino acid pattern.

Abnormal results

Abnormal plasma amino acid pattern:

Congenital enzymatic deficiency.

(Also see *Chromatographic Identification of Amino Acid Disorders,* pp. 214 and 215.)

The basics

This test is a qualitative but effective screen for inborn errors of amino acid metabolism. Thin-layer chromatography is the method used, since it can profile many amino acids simultaneously.

Amino acids are the chief components of all proteins and polypeptides. The body contains at least 20 amino acids; 10 are considered "essential"—that is, the body does not form them, so they must be acquired through the diet. Certain congenital enzymatic deficiencies interfere with normal metabolism of one or more amino acids and cause accumulation or deficiency of these amino acids. Excessive accumulation of amino acids typically produces overflow aminoacidurias. Congenital abnormalities of the amino acid transport system in the kidneys produce a second group of disorders called renal aminoacidurias. The plasma amino acid pattern is normal in renal aminoacidurias and abnormal in overflow aminoacidurias. Comparisons of blood and urine chromatography can help distinguish between the two types of aminoacidurias.

Procedure

Perform a heel-stick, and collect 0.1 ml of blood in a heparinized capillary tube.

Patient care checklist

Before the test

☑ Explain or clarify test purpose, preparation, and procedure to the parents of an infant.

☑ Evaluate understanding.
☑ Restrict food and fluid for 4 hours before the test.

Interfering factors
Failure to observe restrictions of diet may influence amino acid levels.

Ammonia

Purpose
• To help monitor the progression of severe hepatic disease and the effectiveness of therapy
• To recognize impending or established hepatic coma.

Normal results
Plasma ammonia levels are less than 50 mcg/dl.

Abnormal results
Increased plasma ammonia levels characteristically occur in:
   Hepatic coma.
also occur in:
   Reye's syndrome
   Severe congestive heart failure
   Gastrointestinal hemorrhage
   Erythroblastosis fetalis.

The basics
This test measures plasma levels of ammonia, a nonprotein nitrogen compound that helps maintain acid-base balance. Most ammonia is absorbed from the intestinal tract, where it is produced by bacterial action on protein; a smaller amount of ammonia is produced in the kidneys. Normally, the body uses the nitrogen fraction of ammonia to rebuild amino acids; then it converts the ammonia to urea in the liver, for excretion by the kidneys. In diseases such as cirrhosis of the liver, however, ammonia can bypass the liver and accumulate in the blood; therefore, plasma ammonia levels may help indicate the severity of hepatocellular damage.

Procedure
• Notify the laboratory before performing the venipuncture, so that preliminary preparations can begin before you send the sample.
• Perform a venipuncture, and collect the sample in a 10-ml, green-top (heparinized) tube.
• Pack the sample in ice and send it to the laboratory immediately. (Do not use a chilled container.)

Patient care checklist
Before the test
☑ Explain or clarify test purpose, preparation, and procedure to the patient or family member if patient is comatose.
☑ Evaluate understanding.
☑ Instruct the patient to fast overnight.
After the test
☑ Before removing pressure from the venipuncture site, make certain that bleeding has stopped. Hepatic disease can prolong bleeding time.
☑ If plasma ammonia levels are high, assess the patient for impending or established hepatic coma.

Interfering factors
• Acetazolamide, thiazides, ammonium salts, or furosemide can raise ammonia levels, as can hyperalimentation or a portacaval shunt. Lactulose, neomycin, and kanamycin depress ammonia levels.
• Hemolysis caused by rough handling of the sample may alter test results.

Amylase

Purpose
• To diagnose acute pancreatitis
• To distinguish between acute pancreatitis and other causes of abdominal pain that require immediate surgery
• To evaluate possible pancreatic injury caused by abdominal trauma or surgery.

Normal results
Serum levels range from 60 to 180 Somogyi units/dl.

Abnormal results
Markedly increased serum amylase levels:
Acute pancreatitis (4 to 12 hours after onset).
Moderately increased serum amylase levels:
Obstruction of common bile duct, pancreatic duct, or ampulla of Vater
Pancreatic injury from perforated peptic ulcer
Pancreatic cancer
Acute salivary gland disease.
Decreased serum amylase levels:
Chronic pancreatitis
Pancreatic cancer
Cirrhosis
Hepatitis
Toxemia of pregnancy.

The basics
Amylase, synthesized primarily in the pancreas and the salivary glands, is secreted into the gastrointestinal tract. This enzyme helps digest starch and glycogen in the mouth, stomach, and intestine. In cases of suspected acute pancreatic disease, measurement of serum or urine amylase is the most important laboratory test. Highest serum amylase levels occur 4 to 8 hours after onset of acute pancreatitis, then drop to normal in 48 to 72 hours. Determination of urine levels should follow normal serum amylase results, to rule out pancreatitis.

An amylase fractionation test helps determine the source of the amylase and aids in selection of additional tests. More than 20 methods of measuring serum amylase exist, with different ranges of normal values. Unfortunately, test values cannot always be converted to a standard measurement. The classic saccharogenic method described here reports serum amylase in Somogyi units/dl.

Procedure
Perform a venipuncture, and collect the sample in a 7-ml, red-top tube.

Special precautions
If the patient has severe abdominal pain, draw the sample before diagnostic or therapeutic intervention. For accurate results, it is important to obtain an early sample.

Patient care checklist
Before the test
☑ Explain or clarify test purpose and procedure.
☑ Restrict alcohol before the test, as ordered.
☑ Evaluate patient understanding.
☑ Withhold medications that may elevate amylase level, as ordered. If they must be continued, note them on the laboratory slip.

Interfering factors
• The following conditions may produce false-positive test results:
—ingestion of ethyl alcohol in large amounts; certain drugs, such as aminosalicylic acid, asparaginase, azathioprine, corticosteroids, cyproheptadine, narcotic analgesics, oral contraceptives, rifampin, sulfasalazine, or thiazide and loop diuretics
—recent peripancreatic surgery, perforated ulcer or intestine, or abscess
—spasm of the sphincter of Oddi or, rarely, macroamylasemia, a benign condition that does not cause symptoms
—coughing, sneezing, or talking near an open collection tube (saliva contains amylase).
• Hemolysis due to rough handling of the sample may alter test results.

Androstenedione

Purpose
To aid in determining the cause of gonadal dysfunction, menstrual or meno-

pausal irregularities, and premature sexual development.

Normal results

Females: premenopausal—0.6 to 3 ng/ml; postmenopausal—0.3 to 8 ng/ml.

Males: 0.9 to 1.7 ng/ml.

Abnormal results

Increased androstenedione levels:
Stein-Leventhal syndrome
Cushing's syndrome
Ovarian, testicular, or adrenocortical tumors
Ectopic ACTH-producing tumors
Late-onset congenital adrenal hyperplasia
Ovarian stromal hyperplasia.

Decreased androstenedione levels:
Hypogonadism.

The basics

This test helps identify the causes of various disorders related to altered estrogen levels. Androstenedione, secreted by the adrenal cortex and the gonads, is converted to estrone (an estrogen of relatively low biologic activity) by adipose tissue and the liver. In premenopausal women, the amount of estrogen derived from androstenedione is relatively small compared with the amount of the potent estrogen, estradiol, secreted by the ovaries. Usually, estrogen derived from androstenedione does not interfere with gonadotropin feedback during the menstrual cycle. But in such conditions as obesity, increased adrenal production of androstenedione or increased conversion of androstenedione to estrone may interfere with normal feedback, causing menstrual irregularities.

In children and postmenopausal women, estrone is a major source of estrogen. Increased androstenedione production or increased conversion to estrone may induce premature sexual development in children and renewed ovarian stimulation, endometriosis, bleeding, and polycystic ovaries in postmenopausal women. In men, overproduction of androstenedione may cause feminizing signs, such as gynecomastia.

Procedure

• Perform a venipuncture, and collect a serum sample in a 10-ml, red-top tube. (Collect a plasma sample in a green-top tube.)
• If a plasma sample is taken but cannot be sent to the laboratory immediately, refrigerate it or place it on ice.
• Record the patient's age, sex, and (if appropriate) phase of menstrual cycle on the laboratory slip.

Patient care checklist

Before the test
☑ Explain or clarify test purpose, preparation, and procedure.
☑ Evaluate patient understanding.
☑ When appropriate, have the test performed 1 week before or after the patient's menstrual period.
☑ Inform the patient that the test may have to be repeated.
☑ Withhold medications that may interfere with test results, as ordered. If they must be continued, note them on the laboratory slip.

Interfering factors

• Hemolysis due to rough handling of the sample may affect test results.
• Ingestion of steroids or pituitary hormones may alter test results.

Angiotensin-converting enzyme *(ACE)*

Purpose

• To aid in diagnosis of sarcoidosis, especially pulmonary sarcoidosis
• To monitor response to therapy in sarcoidosis
• To help confirm Gaucher's disease or leprosy.

Normal results
In the colorimetric assay, values for serum ACE range from 18 to 67 units/ liter for patients over age 20. (Patients under age 20 have variable ACE levels and are not usually tested.)

Abnormal results
Increased ACE levels:
  Sarcoidosis
  Gaucher's disease
  Leprosy.
Declining ACE levels:
  Response to prednisone
  Therapy for sarcoidosis.

The basics
ACE is found in high concentrations in lung capillaries and in lesser concentrations in blood vessels and kidney tissue. Its primary function is to help regulate arterial pressure by converting angiotensin I to angiotensin II, a powerful vasoconstrictor. This test measures serum levels of ACE. Despite ACE's role in blood pressure regulation, this test is of little use in diagnosing hypertension. Instead, it is primarily used to diagnose sarcoidosis because of the high correlation between elevated serum ACE levels and this disease. Presumably, elevated serum levels reflect macrophage activity. Results must be correlated with the patient's clinical condition.

Procedure
• Perform a venipuncture and collect the sample in a 7-ml, red-top tube. (A green-top tube may be required, depending on the laboratory method used.)
• Note the patient's age on the laboratory slip.
• Send the sample to the laboratory immediately, or freeze the sample and place it on dry ice until the test can be performed.

Patient care checklist
Before the test
☑ Explain or clarify test purpose, preparation, and procedure.
☑ Evaluate patient understanding.
☑ Restrict food and fluid for 12 hours before the test.
☑ Question doctor about postponing test if patient is under age 20.

Interfering factors
• Use of a lavender-top collection tube or other EDTA contamination can decrease ACE levels.
• Hemolysis due to rough handling of the sample may interfere with accurate determination of ACE levels.
• Failure to fast before the test may cause significant lipemia of the sample, which may interfere with accurate test measurement.
• Failure to send the sample to the laboratory immediately or to freeze it and place it on dry ice may cause enzyme degradation and yield artificially low ACE levels.

Anion gap

Purpose
• To distinguish types of metabolic acidosis
• To monitor renal function and I.V. hyperalimentation.

Normal results
Values range from 8 to 14 mEq/liter.

Abnormal results
Increased anion gap
occurs with metabolic acidosis, as in:
  Renal failure
  Ketoacidosis caused by starvation, diabetes mellitus, or alcohol
  Lactic acidosis
  Toxic ingestion, including ingestion of salicylates, methanol, ethylene glycol (antifreeze), or paraldehyde.
Decreased anion gap
rarely occurs with:
  Hypermagnesemia
  Multiple myeloma
  Waldenström's macroglobulinemia.

The basics

The anion gap reflects serum anion-cation balance and helps distinguish types of metabolic acidosis without expensive, time-consuming measurement of all serum electrolytes. This test uses serum levels of routinely measured electrolytes—sodium (Na^+), chloride (Cl^-), and bicarbonate (HCO_3^-)—for a quick calculation based on a simple physical principle: Total concentrations of cations and anions are normally equal, thereby maintaining electrical neutrality in serum. Since sodium accounts for more than 90% of circulating cations, whereas chloride and bicarbonate together account for 85% of the counterbalancing anions, the gap between measured cation and anion levels represents those anions not routinely measured (sulfates, phosphates, organic acids such as ketone bodies and lactic acid, and proteins).

An increased anion gap indicates an increase in one or more of these unmeasured anions, which may occur with acidoses characterized by excessive organic or inorganic acids, such as lactic acidosis or ketoacidosis. A normal anion gap does not rule out metabolic acidosis. When acidosis results from loss of bicarbonate in the urine or other body fluids, renal reabsorption of sodium promotes retention of chloride, and the anion gap remains unchanged. Thus, metabolic acidosis resulting from excessive chloride levels is known as a normal anion gap acidosis.

A normal anion gap occurs in hyperchloremic acidoses, renal tubular acidosis, and severe bicarbonate-wasting conditions, such as biliary or pancreatic fistulas and poorly functioning ileal loops.

Because the anion gap only determines total anion-cation balance, it does not necessarily reflect abnormal values for individual electrolytes. Further investigation and diagnostic tests are usually necessary to determine the specific cause of metabolic acidosis.

Procedure

Perform a venipuncture, and collect the sample in a 10- to 15-ml, red-top tube.

Patient care checklist

Before the test

☑ Explain or clarify test purpose and procedure.

☑ Evaluate patient understanding.

Interfering factors

• Diuretics, lithium, chlorpropamide, and vasopressin suppress serum sodium, possibly decreasing the anion gap; corticosteroids and antihypertensives elevate serum sodium and may increase the anion gap.

• Salicylates, paraldehyde, methicillin, dimercaprol, ammonium chloride, acetazolamide, ethylene glycol, and methyl alcohol decrease serum bicarbonate, possibly increasing the anion gap; ACTH, cortisone, mercurial or chlorthiazide diuretics, and excessive ingestion of alkalis or licorice elevate serum bicarbonate and may decrease the anion gap.

• Ammonium chloride, cholestyramine, boric acid, oxyphenbutazone, phenylbutazone, and excessive I.V. infusion of sodium chloride may elevate serum chloride and possibly decrease the anion gap.

• Thiazides, furosemide, ethacrynic acid, bicarbonates, or prolonged I.V. infusion of 5% dextrose in water can lower serum chloride and may increase the anion gap.

• Iodine absorption from wounds packed with povidone-iodine, or excessive use of magnesium-containing antacids (especially by patients with renal failure) may cause a spuriously low anion gap.

• Hemolysis due to rough handling of the sample may interfere with accurate determination of test results.

Antidiuretic hormone
(ADH)
[Vasopressin]

Purpose
To aid in the differential diagnosis of pituitary diabetes insipidus, nephrogenic diabetes insipidus (congenital or familial), and syndrome of inappropriate antidiuretic hormone (SIADH).

Normal results
Values range from 1 to 5 pg/ml.

Abnormal results
Decreased or absent serum ADH levels:
Pituitary diabetes insipidus resulting from a neurohypophyseal or hypothalamic tumor, viral infection, metastatic disease, sarcoidosis, tuberculosis, Hand-Schüller-Christian disease, syphilis, neurosurgical procedures, or head trauma.

Increased serum ADH levels:
SIADH, possibly as a result of bronchogenic carcinoma, acute porphyria, hypothyroidism, Addison's disease, cirrhosis of the liver, infectious hepatitis, severe hemorrhage, or circulatory shock.

The basics
ADH is produced by the hypothalamus and released from storage sites in the posterior pituitary on neural stimulation. The primary function of ADH is to promote water reabsorption in response to increased osmolality (water deficiency with high concentration of sodium and solutes). In response to decreased osmolality (water excess), reduced secretion of ADH allows increased excretion of water to maintain fluid balance. In an interlocking feedback mechanism with aldosterone, ADH helps regulate sodium, potassium, and fluid balance. It also stimulates vascular smooth-muscle contraction, causing an increase in arterial blood pressure.

The laboratory requires at least 5 days to complete analysis for this relatively rare test. It may be ordered as part of dehydration or hypertonic saline infusion testing, which determines the body's response to states of hyperosmolality.

Normal ADH levels, in the presence of typical clinical features of diabetes insipidus (such as polydipsia, polyuria, and hypotonic urine), may indicate the nephrogenic form of the disease, marked by renal tubular resistance to ADH. Levels may be elevated, however, if the pituitary attempts to compensate for renal resistance.

Procedure
Perform a venipuncture, and collect the sample in a red-top, plastic collection tube.

Patient care checklist
Before the test
☑ Explain or clarify test purpose, preparation, and procedure.
☑ Evaluate patient understanding.
☑ Restrict food and fluid and limit physical activity for 10 to 12 hours before the test.
☑ Encourage the patient to relax and remain recumbent for 30 minutes before the test.
☑ Withhold medications that may interfere with test results, as ordered. If they must be continued, note them on the laboratory slip.

Interfering factors
• Failure to observe restrictions of diet, medications, or activity may hinder accurate determination of test results. Morphine, anesthetics, estrogens, oxytocin, chlorpropamide, vincristine, carbamazepine, cyclophosphamide, and chlorothiazide elevate ADH levels, as do stress, pain, and positive-pressure ventilation. Alcohol and negative-pressure ventilation inhibit ADH secretion.

• A radioactive scan performed within 1 week before the test may influence the results, since serum ADH level is determined by radioimmunoassay.

• Failure to immediately send the sample to the laboratory, where serum must be separated from the clot within 10 minutes, may affect test results.

• Use of a glass syringe or collection tube causes the fragile ADH to undergo degradation.

Arginine test
[Growth hormone stimulation test]

Purpose
• To aid in diagnosis of pituitary tumors
• To confirm plasma growth hormone (hGH) deficiency in infants and children with low baseline levels.

Normal results
Arginine should raise hGH levels to more than 10 ng/ml in men, 15 ng/ml in women, and 48 ng/ml in children. Such an increase may appear in the first sample, drawn 30 minutes after arginine infusion is discontinued, or in the samples drawn 60 and 90 minutes afterward.

Abnormal results
Increased fasting hGH levels and elevated levels during sleep:
Rule out hGH deficiency.
Failure of hGH levels to rise after arginine infusion:
Decreased anterior pituitary hGH reserve. In children, this deficiency causes dwarfism; in adults, it can indicate panhypopituitarism.

The basics
This test measures hGH levels after I.V. administration of arginine, an amino acid that normally stimulates hGH secretion, and is commonly used to identify pituitary dysfunction in infants and children with growth retardation and to confirm hGH deficiency. This test may be performed concomitantly with an insulin tolerance test or after administration of other hGH stimulants, such as glucagon, vasopressin, and L-dopa.

When hGH levels fail to reach 10 ng/ml, retesting is required at the same time of day as the original test.

Procedure
• Between 6 a.m. and 8 a.m., draw 6 ml of venous blood (basal sample) into a 10- to 15-ml, red-top collection tube.
• Start an I.V. infusion of arginine (0.5 g/kg body weight) in normal saline solution, and continue for 30 minutes. Use of an indwelling venous catheter avoids repeated venipunctures and minimizes stress and anxiety.
• Discontinue I.V. infusion, then draw a total of three 6-ml samples at 30-minute intervals.
• Collect each sample in a 10- to 15-ml, red-top collection tube, and label it appropriately. Be sure to specify collection time.

Patient care checklist
Before the test
☑ Explain or clarify test purpose, preparation, and procedure to the patient and/or parents.
☑ Evaluate patient and/or parent understanding.
☑ Restrict food and fluid and limit physical activity for 10 to 12 hours before the test.
☑ Inform the patient and/or parents that the test takes at least 2 hours to perform; results are available in 2 days.
☑ Withhold medications that may interfere with test results, as ordered. If they must be continued, note them on the laboratory slip.
☑ Instruct the patient to remain relaxed and recumbent for at least 90 minutes before the test.

Interfering factors
• Failure to observe restrictions of diet, medications, and physical activity may affect test results.
• A radioactive scan performed within 1 week before the test may affect results.
• Hemolysis due to rough handling of the sample may affect test results.
• Failure to send each sample to the laboratory immediately may affect test results, since hGH has a half-life of 20 to 25 minutes.

Arterial blood gas analysis
[ABG analysis]

Purpose
• To evaluate the efficiency of pulmonary gas exchange
• To assess integrity of the ventilatory control system
• To determine the acid-base level of the blood
• To monitor respiratory therapy.

Normal results
PaO_2: 75 to 100 mm Hg
$PaCO_2$: 35 to 45 mm Hg
pH: 7.35 to 7.42
O_2Ct: 15% to 23%
O_2Sat: 94% to 100%
HCO_3^-: 22 to 26 mEq/liter

Abnormal results
(See *Clarifying Blood Oxygen Disorders; Acid-Base Disorders;* and *Abnormal ABG Values,* p. 60.)

The basics
Partial pressure exerted by the small amount of oxygen dissolved in arterial blood (PaO_2) indicates how much oxygen the lungs are delivering to the blood.

Clarifying Blood Oxygen Disorders

Status and ABG finding	Possible causes
Impaired respiratory functioning PaO_2—low O_2Ct—low O_2Sat—low $PaCO_2$—high	• Respiratory muscle weakness or paralysis such as with myasthenia gravis • Respiratory center inhibition such as from head injury, brain tumor, or drug abuse • Airway obstruction as from mucous plugs or a tumor • Bronchiole obstruction caused by asthma, emphysema • Abnormal ventilation perfusion ratio such as from near drowning
Insufficient oxygen from inspired air PaO_2—low O_2Ct—low O_2Sat—low $PaCO_2$—may be normal	• Pneumothorax • Arteriovenous shunt that permits blood to bypass the lungs • Impaired diffusion between alveoli and blood, such as from interstitial fibrosis
Impaired oxygen hemoglobin capability PaO_2—normal O_2Ct—low O_2Sat—normal $PaCO_2$—may be normal	• Severe anemia • Decreased blood volume • Reduced hemoglobin oxygen-carrying capacity

Acid-Base Disorders

Disorders and ABG findings	Possible causes
Respiratory acidosis (excess CO_2 retention) pH < 7.35 HCO_3^- > 26 mEq/liter (if compensating) $Paco_2$ > 45 mm Hg	• Central nervous system depression from drugs, injury, or disease • Asphyxia • Hypoventilation due to pulmonary, cardiac, musculoskeletal, or neuromuscular disease
Respiratory alkalosis (excess CO_2 excretion) pH > 7.42 HCO_3^- < 22 mEq/liter (if compensating) $Paco_2$ < 35 mm Hg	• Hyperventilation due to anxiety, pain, or improper ventilator settings • Respiratory stimulation by drugs, disease, hypoxia, fever, or high room temperature • Gram-negative bacteremia
Metabolic acidosis (HCO_3^- loss, acid retention) pH < 7.35 HCO_3^- < 22 mEq/liter $Paco_2$ < 35 mm Hg (if compensating)	• HCO_3^- depletion due to renal disease, diarrhea, or small-bowel fistulas • Excessive production of organic acids due to hepatic disease; endocrine disorders, including diabetes mellitus; hypoxia; shock; or drug intoxication • Inadequate excretion of acids due to renal disease
Metabolic alkalosis (HCO_3^- retention, acid loss) pH > 7.42 HCO_3^- > 26 mEq/liter $Paco_2$ > 45 mm Hg (if compensating)	• Loss of hydrochloric acid from prolonged vomiting, gastric suctioning • Loss of potassium from increased renal excretion (as in diuretic therapy), steroid overdose • Excessive alkali ingestion

Partial pressure exerted by carbon dioxide dissolved in arterial blood ($Paco_2$) indicates how efficiently the lungs eliminate carbon dioxide.

Hydrogen ion concentration (pH) indicates the acid-base level of the blood; acidity indicates hydrogen ion excess; alkalinity, hydrogen ion deficit.

Oxygen content (O_2Ct) measures the volume of oxygen combined with hemoglobin in arterial blood. This value is used infrequently.

Oxygen saturation (O_2Sat) is the percentage of hemoglobin carrying oxygen. Hemoglobin carries most oxygen in the blood.

The amount of bicarbonate or alkaline substance dissolved in blood (HCO_3-) is primarily influenced by metabolic changes; HCO_3- is under renal control.

Procedure

Perform an arterial puncture. (See "Arterial sample," p. xiv.)

Special precautions

• If the patient has recently had an intermittent positive-pressure breathing treatment, wait at least 20 minutes before drawing arterial blood, because such treatment alters blood gas values.

Abnormal ABG Values

Pao₂

Value less than 50 mm Hg indicates hypoxia. Pao₂ between 0 and 80 mm Hg may or may not indicate hypoxia, depending on age of patient and oxygen concentration being given. A newborn has a Pao₂ between 40 and 60 mm Hg. After age 60, Pao₂ may fall below 80 mm Hg without hypoxia.

Paco₂

Value above 45 mm Hg indicates hypoventilation (hypercapnia). Value below 35 mm Hg indicates hyperventilation (hypocapnia). Paco₂ level may also indicate respiratory (lung-regulated) acid-base imbalance. If patient's pH shows an imbalance, Paco₂ above 45 mm Hg indicates respiratory acidosis; Paco₂ below 35 mm Hg indicates respiratory alkalosis.

pH

Value greater than 7.45 indicates alkalosis. Value less than 7.35 indicates acidosis.

O₂ Sat

If Pao₂ is between 60 and 95 mm Hg, O₂ Sat should remain above 85%. Sharply decreased values usually indicate drop in Pao₂ below 50 mm Hg.

HCO₃ –

Value greater than 26 mEq/liter indicates metabolic (kidney-regulated) alkalosis. Value less than 22 mEq/liter indicates metabolic acidosis.

• If the patient is receiving oxygen therapy, find out whether the order for ABG measurements specifies that these be obtained on room air or on oxygen therapy. If the order indicates room air, discontinue oxygen therapy for 15 to 20 minutes before drawing the sample.

Before sending the sample to the laboratory, include the following information on the requisition slip:

• Indicate whether the patient was breathing room air or receiving oxygen therapy when the sample was drawn. If he was receiving oxygen therapy, give the flow rate.

• If the patient is on a ventilator, note the fraction of inspired oxygen and tidal volume.

• Record the patient's rectal temperature and respiratory rate.

Patient care checklist

Before the test

☑ Explain or clarify test purpose, preparation, and procedure.

☑ Instruct the patient to breathe normally during the test, and warn him that he may experience a brief cramping or throbbing pain at the puncture site.

☑ Evaluate patient understanding.

After the test

☑ After applying pressure to the puncture site, tape a gauze pad firmly over it. (If the puncture site is on the arm, do not tape the entire circumference; this may restrict circulation.)

CLINICAL ALERT: **Monitor vital signs, and observe for signs of circulatory impairment, such as swelling, discoloration, pain, numbness, or tingling in the bandaged arm or leg. Assess for bleeding from the puncture site.**

Interfering factors

• Exposing the sample to air affects Pao₂ and Paco₂ levels and interferes with accurate determination of results.

• Failure to heparinize the syringe, to place the sample correctly in an iced bag, or to send the sample to the laboratory immediately adversely affects the test results.

• Venous blood in the sample may lower PaO_2 and elevate $PaCO_2$.

• Bicarbonate, ethacrynic acid, hydrocortisone, metolazone, prednisone, and thiazides may elevate $PaCO_2$ levels. Acetazolamide, methicillin, nitrofurantoin, and tetracycline may decrease $PaCO_2$ levels.

Bilirubin

Purpose
• To evaluate liver function
• To aid in differential diagnosis of jaundice and to monitor the progression of this disorder
• To aid in diagnosis of biliary obstruction and hemolytic anemia
• To determine whether a newborn requires an exchange transfusion or phototherapy because of dangerously high unconjugated bilirubin levels.

Normal results
In an adult, indirect serum bilirubin measures 1.1 mg/dl or less; direct serum bilirubin, less than 0.5 mg/dl. Total serum bilirubin in the newborn measures 1 to 12 mg/dl.

Abnormal results
Increased indirect serum bilirubin levels:
  Hepatic damage
  Hemolytic anemia
  Congenital enzyme deficiencies, such as Gilbert's disease and Crigler-Najjar syndrome.
Increased direct serum bilirubin levels:
  Biliary obstruction.
Increased direct and indirect serum bilirubin levels:
  Continued hemolysis
  Continued biliary obstruction with resulting hepatic damage.

The basics
This test measures serum levels of bilirubin, the predominant pigment in bile. Bilirubin is the major product of hemoglobin catabolism. After being formed in the reticuloendothelial cells, bilirubin is bound to albumin and is transported to the liver, where it is conjugated with glucuronide. The resulting compound—bilirubin diglucuronide—is then excreted in bile.

Effective conjugation and excretion of bilirubin depends on a properly functioning hepatobiliary system and a normal red blood cell turnover rate. Therefore, measurement of unconjugated (indirect), or prehepatic, bilirubin and conjugated (direct), or posthepatic, bilirubin can help evaluate hepatobiliary and erythropoietic functions. Serum bilirubin measurements are especially significant in the newborn, since elevated unconjugated bilirubin can accumulate in the brain and cause irreparable tissue damage.

Therefore, in newborn infants, total bilirubin levels that reach or exceed 20 mg/dl indicate the need for exchange transfusion. With hepatic damage, the parenchymal cells can no longer conjugate bilirubin with glucuronide. Consequently, indirect bilirubin reenters the bloodstream. With hemolysis, excessive indirect bilirubin overwhelms the liver's conjugating mechanism. With biliary obstruction, direct bilirubin, blocked from its normal pathway from the liver into the biliary tree, overflows into the bloodstream.

Procedure
• If the patient is an adult, perform a venipuncture, and collect the sample in a 10- to 15-ml, red-top tube.
• If the patient is an infant, perform a heel stick, and fill the microcapillary tube to the designated level with blood.

Special precautions
Protect the sample from strong sunlight and ultraviolet light, since bili-

rubin breaks down when exposed to light.

Patient care checklist
Before the test

☑ Explain or clarify test purpose, preparation, and procedure to the patient or parents of infants.

☑ Evaluate patient and/or parent understanding.

☑ Restrict solid food for at least 4 hours before the test. (Fasting is not necessary for a newborn.)

Interfering factors

• Novobiocin raises bilirubin levels.

• Exposure of the sample to direct sunlight or ultraviolet light may depress bilirubin levels.

• Hemolysis due to rough handling of the sample may alter test results.

Blood urea nitrogen (BUN)

Purpose

• To evaluate renal function and aid in diagnosis of renal disease

• To aid in assessment of hydration.

Normal results

BUN values normally range from 8 to 20 mg/dl.

Abnormal results

Increased BUN levels:
  Renal disease
  Reduced renal blood flow, as in dehydration
  Urinary tract obstruction
  Increased protein catabolism, as in burns.
Decreased BUN levels:
  Severe hepatic damage
  Malnutrition
  Overhydration.

The basics

This test measures the nitrogen fraction of urea, the chief end product of protein metabolism. Formed in the liver from ammonia and excreted by the kidneys, urea constitutes 40% to 50% of the blood's nonprotein nitrogen. The BUN level reflects protein intake and renal excretory capacity, but is a less reliable indicator of uremia than the serum creatinine level.

Procedure

Perform a venipuncture, and collect the sample in a 10- to 15-ml, red-top tube.

Patient care checklist
Before the test

☑ Explain or clarify test purpose and procedure.

☑ Evaluate patient understanding.

Interfering factors

• Chloramphenicol can depress BUN levels.

• Nephrotoxic drugs, such as aminoglycosides, amphotericin B, and methicillin, can elevate BUN levels.

• Hemolysis caused by rough handling of the sample may affect test results.

Calcitonin
[Thyrocalcitonin]

Purpose

To aid in diagnosis of thyroid medullary carcinoma or ectopic calcitonin-producing tumors (rare).

Normal results

Basal serum calcitonin levels ≤ 0.155 ng/ml in males; ≤ 0.105 ng/ml in females. Values after provocative testing with 4-hour calcium infusion are:
  males: 0.265 ng/ml
  females: 0.120 ng/ml.
Values after provocative testing with pentagastrin infusion are:
  males: 0.210 ng/ml
  females: 0.105 ng/ml.
Detection limit of assay is 0.030 ng/ml.

Abnormal results

Increased plasma calcitonin levels usually indicate:
Medullary carcinoma of the thyroid (in the absence of hypocalcemia).
occasionally occur with:
Oat cell carcinoma of the lung
Breast carcinoma.

The basics

This radioimmunoassay measures plasma levels of calcitonin, a hormone secreted by the thyroid gland in response to rising serum calcium levels. The exact role of calcitonin in normal human physiology has not been fully defined. However, calcitonin is known to inhibit bone resorption by osteoclasts and osteocytes, and to increase calcium excretion by the kidneys; thereby, calcitonin acts as an antagonist to parathyroid hormone and lowers serum calcium levels. The usual clinical indication for this test is suspected medullary carcinoma of the thyroid, which causes hypersecretion of calcitonin (without associated hypocalcemia). Equivocal results require provocative testing with I.V. pentagastrin or calcium to rule out disease. (See *Calcitonin Stimulation Testing*.)

Procedure

Draw venous blood into a 10-ml, green-top (heparinized) tube.

Patient care checklist

Before the test
☑ Explain or clarify test purpose, preparation, and procedure.
☑ Evaluate patient understanding.
☑ Restrict food and fluid overnight before the test.
☑ Inform the patient that the laboratory requires several days to complete the analysis.

Interfering factors

• Failure to observe an overnight fast before the test may interfere with accurate determination of test results.

Calcitonin Stimulation Testing

Stimulation testing is often necessary in patients with medullary thyroid carcinoma when baseline calcitonin levels fail to rise high enough to confirm diagnosis. The most common test is a 4-hour I.V. calcium infusion (15 mg/kg) to provoke calcitonin secretion. Samples are taken just before the infusion and at 3 and 4 hours afterward. After the infusion, calcitonin levels rise rapidly in patients with medullary thyroid carcinoma.

Another test involves I.V. infusion of pentagastrin 0.5 mcg/kg over 5 to 10 seconds. A blood sample is drawn just before the I.V. infusion, and at 90 seconds, 5 minutes, and 10 minutes postinfusion. In patients with medullary thyroid carcinoma, calcitonin levels rise markedly over the baseline reading. This test is now being used in some centers.

• Hemolysis due to rough handling of the sample may interfere with accurate determination of test results.

Calcium

Purpose

To aid in diagnosis of neuromuscular, skeletal, and endocrine disorders; dysrhythmias; blood-clotting deficiencies; and acid-base imbalance.

Normal results

Levels range from 8.9 to 10.1 mg/dl (atomic absorption), or from 4.5 to 5.5 mEq/liter. In children, serum calcium levels are higher than in adults. Calcium levels can rise as high as 12 mg/dl or 6 mEq/liter during phases of rapid bone growth.

Abnormal results
Increased serum calcium levels (hypercalcemia):
  Hyperparathyroidism
  Parathyroid tumors
  Paget's disease of the bone
  Multiple myeloma
  Metastatic carcinoma
  Multiple fractures
  Prolonged immobilization
  Inadequate calcium secretion, as in adrenal insufficiency and renal disease
  Excessive calcium ingestion
  Overuse of antacids, such as calcium carbonate.
Decreased serum calcium levels (hypocalcemia):
  Hypoparathyroidism
  Total parathyroidectomy
  Malabsorption
  Cushing's syndrome
  Renal failure
  Acute pancreatitis
  Peritonitis.

The basics
This test measures serum levels of calcium, a predominantly extracellular cation that helps regulate and promote neuromuscular and enzyme activity, skeletal development, and blood coagulation. The body absorbs calcium from the gastrointestinal tract, provided sufficient vitamin D is present, and excretes it in the urine and feces. Over 98% of the body's calcium is found in the bones and teeth. However, calcium can shift in and out of these structures. For example, when calcium concentrations in the blood fall below normal, calcium ions can move out of the bones and teeth to help restore blood levels.

Parathyroid hormone, vitamin D, and to a lesser extent calcitonin and adrenal steroids control calcium blood levels. Calcium and phosphorus are closely related, usually reacting together to form insoluble calcium phosphate. To prevent formation of a precipitate in the blood, calcium levels vary inversely with phosphorus; as serum calcium levels rise, phosphorus levels should decrease through renal excretion. Since the body excretes calcium daily, regular ingestion of calcium in food (at least 1 g/day) is necessary for normal calcium balance.

Procedure
Perform a venipuncture, and collect the sample in a 10- to 15-ml, red-top tube.

Special precautions
CLINICAL ALERT: **Observe the patient with hypercalcemia for deep bone pain, flank pain due to renal calculi, and muscle hypotonicity. Hypercalcemic crisis begins with nausea, vomiting, and dehydration, leading to stupor and coma, and can end in cardiac arrest. In a patient with hypocalcemia, be alert for circumoral and peripheral numbness and tingling, muscle twitching, Chvostek's sign (facial muscle spasm), tetany, muscle cramping, Trousseau's sign (carpopedal spasm), seizure activity, and dysrhythmias.**

Patient care checklist
Before the test
☑ Explain or clarify test purpose and procedure.
☑ Evaluate patient understanding.

Interfering factors
• Excessive ingestion of vitamin D or its derivatives (dihydrotachysterol, calcitriol) and the use of androgens, calciferol-activated calcium salts, progestins-estrogens, and thiazides can elevate serum calcium levels.
• Chronic use of laxatives, excessive transfusions of citrated blood, and administration of acetazolamide, corticosteroids, and mithramycin can suppress calcium levels.

Carbon dioxide content, total *(CO₂)*

Purpose
To help evaluate acid-base balance.

Normal results
Total CO_2 content levels range from 22 to 34 mEq/liter.

Abnormal results
Increased CO_2 content may occur:
in metabolic alkalosis, such as in:
Severe vomiting
Continuous gastric drainage.
in respiratory acidosis, as in:
Hypoventilation from emphysema or pneumonia.
Also may occur in:
Primary aldosteronism
Cushing's syndrome.
Decreased CO_2 content may occur:
in metabolic acidosis, as in:
Diabetic acidosis
Renal tubular acidosis
Severe diarrhea
Intestinal drainage.
in respiratory alkalosis, as in:
Hyperventilation.

The basics
CO_2 is present in small amounts in the air, and in the body as an end product of food metabolism. When the pressure of CO_2 in the red cells exceeds 40 mm Hg, CO_2 spills out of the cells and dissolves in plasma. There, it may combine with water (H_2O) to form carbonic acid (H_2CO_3), which, in turn, can dissociate into hydrogen ($H+$) and bicarbonate ions (HCO_3-). This test measures the total concentration of all such forms of CO_2 in serum, plasma, or whole blood samples. Since about 90% of CO_2 in serum is in the form of bicarbonate, this test closely assesses bicarbonate levels. Total CO_2 content reflects the adequacy of gas exchange in the lungs and the efficiency of the carbonic acid–bicarbonate buffer system, which maintains acid-base balance and normal pH. Consequently, this test is commonly ordered for patients with respiratory insufficiency and is usually included in any assessment of electrolyte balance. For maximum clinical significance, test results must be considered with both pH and arterial blood gas values.

Procedure
• Perform a venipuncture. Since CO_2 content is usually measured along with electrolytes, a 10- to 15-ml, red-top tube may be used. When this test is performed alone, a green-top (heparinized) tube is appropriate.
• Completely fill the tube to prevent diffusion of CO_2 into the vacuum.

Patient care checklist
Before the test
☑ Explain or clarify test purpose and procedure.
☑ Evaluate patient understanding.

Interfering factors
• CO_2 levels rise with administration of excessive adrenocorticotropic hormone, cortisone, or thiazide diuretics, or with excessive ingestion of alkalis or licorice.
• CO_2 levels decrease with administration of salicylates, paraldehyde, methicillin, dimercaprol, ammonium chloride, acetazolamide, and accidental ingestion of ethylene glycol or methyl alcohol.

Catecholamines

Purpose
• To rule out adrenal medullary or extraadrenal pheochromocytoma in patients with hypertension
• To help identify neuroblastoma, ganglioneuroblastoma, and ganglioneuroma

• To distinguish between adrenal medullary tumors and other catecholamine-producing tumors, through fractional analysis.

• To aid in diagnosis of autonomic nervous system dysfunction, such as idiopathic orthostatic hypotension.

Normal results

In fractional analysis, catecholamine levels range as follows:

supine: epinephrine, undetectable to 110 pg/ml; norepinephrine, 70 to 750 pg/ml; dopamine, undetectable to 30 pg/ml

standing: epinephrine, undetectable to 140 pg/ml; norepinephrine, 200 to 1,700 pg/ml; dopamine, undetectable to 30 pg/ml.

Abnormal results

Increased catecholamine levels:

Pheochromocytoma
Neuroblastoma
Ganglioneuroblastoma
Ganglioneuroma
Thyroid disorders
Hypoglycemia
Cardiac disease
Shock resulting from hemorrhage, endotoxins, or anaphylaxis
Electroshock therapy.

The basics

This test has significant clinical importance in patients with hypertension and signs of adrenal medullary tumor, and in patients with neural tumors that affect endocrine function. Elevated plasma catecholamine levels necessitate supportive confirmation by urinalysis that shows catecholamine degradation products, such as vanillylmandelic acid and metanephrine.

Major catecholamines include the hormones epinephrine, norepinephrine, and dopamine, which are produced almost exclusively in the brain, sympathetic nerve endings, and adrenal medulla. When secreted into the bloodstream, adrenal medullary cat-

echolamines prepare the body for the fight-or-flight reaction to stress.

Since many factors influence catecholamine secretion, diurnal variations are common; for example, plasma levels may fluctuate in response to temperature, stress, postural change, diet, smoking, and many drugs.

In the patient with normal or low baseline catecholamine levels, failure to show increased catecholamine levels in the sample taken after standing suggests autonomic nervous system dysfunction. No known dysfunction is associated with insufficiency of the adrenal medulla.

Fractional analysis helps identify the specific abnormality that is producing elevated catecholamine levels. For example, adrenal medullary tumors secrete epinephrine; ganglioneuromas, ganglioblastomas, and neuroblastomas secrete norepinephrine. The laboratory requires at least one week to complete analysis of plasma catecholamines.

Procedure

• Perform a venipuncture between 6 a.m. and 8 a.m.

• Collect the sample in a 10-ml, chilled tube containing EDTA (sodium metabisulfite solution), which can be obtained from the Mayo laboratory on request.

• Then have the patient stand for 10 minutes, and draw a second sample into another tube, exactly like the first. If a heparin lock is used, it may be necessary to discard the first 1 or 2 ml of blood.

• Check with the laboratory for the preferred procedure.

Special precautions

• After collecting each sample, roll the tube slowly between your palms to distribute the EDTA without agitating the blood.

• Then, pack the tube in crushed ice, to minimize deactivation of catecholamines, and send it to the laboratory immediately.

• Indicate on the laboratory slip whether the patient was supine or standing, and the time the sample was drawn.

Patient care checklist
Before the test
☑ Explain and clarify test purpose, preparation, and procedure. Stress the need to follow pretest instructions strictly since the action of catecholamines is so transitory.
☑ Evaluate patient understanding.
☑ Restrict patient use of self-prescribed medications (especially cold or hay fever remedies that may contain sympathomimetics) for 2 weeks before the test.
☑ Advise the patient to exclude from his diet amine-rich foods and beverages (such as bananas, avocados, cheese, coffee, tea, cocoa, beer, and Chianti) for 48 hours before the test.
☑ Instruct the patient to abstain from smoking for 24 hours before the test.
☑ Restrict food and fluid for 10 to 12 hours before the test.
☑ As ordered, withhold medications that may interfere with the test in the hospitalized patient.
☑ Make sure an indwelling venous catheter (heparin lock) is inserted as ordered 24 hours before the test.
☑ Encourage the patient to relax and remain recumbent and warm for 45 to 60 minutes before the test.

Interfering factors
• Failure to observe pretest restrictions may interfere with accurate determination of test results.
• Epinephrine, levodopa, amphetamines, phenothiazines (chlorpromazine), sympathomimetics, decongestants, and tricyclic antidepressants raise plasma catecholamine levels. Reserpine lowers plasma catecholamine levels.
• A radioactive scan performed within 1 week before the test may influence results, since plasma catecholamine levels are determined by radioimmunoassay.

Ceruloplasmin

Purpose
To aid in diagnosis of Wilson's disease, Menkes' kinky hair syndrome, and copper deficiency.

Normal results
Serum ceruloplasmin levels range from 22.9 to 43.1 mg/dl.

Abnormal results
Decreased serum ceruloplasmin levels:
  Wilson's disease
  Menkes' kinky hair syndrome
  Nephrotic syndrome
  Hypocupremia caused by total parenteral nutrition.
Increased serum ceruloplasmin levels:
  Some hepatic diseases
  Some infections.

The basics
This test measures serum levels of ceruloplasmin, an $alpha_2$-globulin that binds about 95% of serum copper (little copper exists in a free state), usually in the liver. Because ceruloplasmin catalyzes oxidation of ferrous compounds to ferric ions, it is thought to regulate iron uptake by transferrin, making iron available to reticulocytes for heme synthesis. Although decreased levels usually indicate Wilson's disease, this is confirmed by Kayser-Fleischer rings (copper deposits in the corneas that form green-gold rings) or liver biopsy results that show 250 mcg of copper/g of dry weight.

Procedure
Perform a venipuncture, and collect the sample in a 7-ml, red-top tube.

Patient care checklist
Before the test
☑ Explain or clarify test purpose and procedure.
☑ Evaluate patient understanding.

Interfering factors
Estrogen, methadone, and phenytoin may elevate serum ceruloplasmin levels.

Chloride

Purpose
To detect acid-base imbalance (acidosis and alkalosis) and to aid in evaluation of fluid status and extracellular cation-anion balance.

Normal results
Serum chloride levels range from 100 to 108 mEq/liter.

Abnormal results
Increased serum chloride levels (hyperchloremia):
   Severe dehydration
   Complete renal shutdown
   Head injury producing neurogenic hyperventilation
   Primary aldosteronism.
Decreased serum chloride levels (hypochloremia):
   Prolonged vomiting
   Gastric suctioning
   Intestinal fistula
   Chronic renal failure
   Addison's disease
   Congestive heart failure (dilutional hypochloremia)
   Edema (dilutional hypochloremia).

The basics
This test, a quantitative analysis, measures serum levels of chloride, the major extracellular fluid anion. Interacting with sodium, chloride helps maintain the osmotic pressure of blood and therefore helps regulate blood volume and arterial pressure. Chloride levels relate inversely to those of bicarbonate and thus reflect acid-base balance. Excessive loss of gastric juices or of other secretions containing chloride may cause hypochloremic metabolic alkalosis; excessive chloride retention or ingestion may lead to hyperchloremic metabolic acidosis.

Serum concentrations of this electrolyte are regulated by aldosterone secondarily to regulation of sodium. Chloride is absorbed from the intestines and is excreted primarily by the kidneys. Low chloride levels are usually associated with low sodium and potassium levels.

Procedure
Perform a venipuncture, and collect the sample in a 10- to 15-ml, red-top tube.

Special precautions
CLINICAL ALERT: **Observe a patient with hypochloremia for hypertonicity of muscles, tetany, and depressed respirations. In a patient with hyperchloremia, be alert for signs of developing stupor, rapid deep breathing, and weakness that may lead to coma.**

Patient care checklist
Before the test
☑ Explain and clarify test purpose and procedure.
☑ Evaluate patient understanding.

Interfering factors
• Elevated serum chloride levels may result from administration of ammonium chloride, cholestyramine, boric acid, oxyphenbutazone, phenylbutazone, or excessive I.V. infusion of sodium chloride.
• Serum chloride levels are decreased by thiazides, furosemide, ethacrynic acid, bicarbonates, or prolonged I.V. infusion of dextrose 5% in water.
• Hemolysis due to rough handling of the sample may interfere with accurate determination of test results.

Cholesterol, total

Purpose
• To assess the risk of coronary artery disease (CAD)

- To evaluate fat metabolism
- To aid in diagnosis of nephrotic syndrome, pancreatitis, hepatic disease, and hypo- and hyperthyroidism.

Normal results

Total cholesterol concentrations vary with age and sex, and may range from 120 mg/dl to 330 mg/dl.

Abnormal results

Increased serum cholesterol levels (hypercholesterolemia):
   Risk of CAD
   Incipient hepatitis
   Lipid disorders
   Bile duct blockage
   Nephrotic syndrome
   Obstructive jaundice
   Pancreatitis
   Hypothyroidism.

Decreased serum cholesterol levels (hypocholesterolemia):
   Malnutrition
   Cellular necrosis of the liver
   Hyperthyroidism.

The basics

This test, the quantitative analysis of serum cholesterol, measures the circulating levels of free cholesterol and cholesterol esters. Total cholesterol is the only cholesterol routinely measured. Cholesterol, a structural component in cell membranes and plasma lipoproteins, is both absorbed from the diet and synthesized in the liver and other body tissues. It is then metabolized to steroid hormones, glucocorticoids, and bile acids. A diet high in saturated fat raises cholesterol levels by stimulating absorption of lipids, including cholesterol, from the intestine; a low-saturated-fat diet lowers them. High serum cholesterol levels may be associated with an increased risk of CAD.

Procedure

Perform a venipuncture, and collect the sample in a 7-ml red-top tube.

Patient care checklist

Before the test
☑ Explain or clarify test purpose, preparation, and procedure.
☑ Evaluate patient understanding.
☑ Restrict food and fluid overnight before the test.
☑ Advise the patient to abstain from alcohol for 24 hours before the test.
☑ Withhold medications that may interfere with test results, as ordered. If they must be continued, note them on the laboratory slip.

Interfering factors

- Cholesterol levels are lowered by cholestyramine, clofibrate, colestipol, dextrothyroxine, haloperidol, neomycin, niacin, and chlortetracycline. Levels are raised by epinephrine, chlorpromazine, trifluoperazine, oral contraceptives, and trimethadione. Androgens may have a variable effect on cholesterol levels.
- Failure to follow dietary restrictions may interfere with test results.
- Failure to send the sample to the laboratory immediately may interfere with test results, since cholesterol is not stable at room temperature.

Cholinesterase

Purpose

- To evaluate, preoperatively or before electroconvulsive therapy, the patient's potential response to succinylcholine, which is hydrolyzed by cholinesterase
- To identify atypical forms of pseudocholinesterase to detect those patients who may have reactions to muscle relaxants
- To assess overexposure to insecticides containing organophosphate compounds
- To assess liver function and aid diagnosis of liver disease (a rare purpose).

Normal results

Pseudocholinesterase levels range from 8 to 18 units/ml (when determined by kinetic colorimetric technique).

Abnormal results

Severely decreased pseudocholinesterase levels:
  Congenital deficiency
  Organophosphate insecticide poisoning.
Decreased pseudocholinesterase levels:
  Acute infections
  Chronic malnutrition
  Anemia
  Myocardial infarction
  Obstructive jaundice
  Metastasis.
Variably decreased pseudocholinesterase levels:
  Hepatitis
  Cirrhosis.

The basics

The cholinesterase test measures the amounts of two similar enzymes that hydrolyze acetylcholine: pseudocholinesterase (also known as PCHE, or serum cholinesterase) and acetylcholinesterase (or true cholinesterase). Acetylcholinesterase inactivates acetylcholine at nerve junctions and helps transmit impulses across nerve endings to muscle fibers. Pseudocholinesterase has no known function; however, its measurement is significant, because certain chemicals that inactivate acetylcholinesterase also affect pseudocholinesterase.

Two groups of anticholinesterase chemicals—organophosphates and muscle relaxants—are important. Organophosphates, which are used by the military as nerve gases and are common ingredients in many insecticides, inactivate acetylcholinesterase directly. Muscle relaxants (such as succinylcholine), which interfere with acetylcholine-mediated transmission across nerve endings, are normally destroyed by pseudocholinesterase.

When poisoning by an organophosphate (such as parathion) is suspected, either cholinesterase may be measured. For technical reasons, pseudocholinesterase is generally tested (although this analysis is less sensitive than the one for acetylcholinesterase).

In "muscle relaxant poisoning," prolonged apnea develops not from the drug itself, but because the patient lacks adequate pseudocholinesterase, which normally inactivates the muscle relaxant. In this case, measurement of pseudocholinesterase is required.

Procedure

• Perform a venipuncture, and collect the sample in a 7-ml, red-top tube.
• If the sample cannot be sent to the laboratory within 6 hours after being drawn, refrigerate it.

Special precautions

Pseudocholinesterase levels near zero necessitate emergency treatment.

Patient care checklist

Before the test
☑ Explain or clarify test purpose, preparation, and procedure.
☑ Evaluate patient understanding.
☑ Withhold substances that may interfere with test results, as ordered. If they must be continued, note on the laboratory slip.

Interfering factors

• Hemolysis due to rough handling of the sample may interfere with accurate determination of test results.
• Pregnancy or recent surgery may hinder accurate determination of test results.
• Serum cholinesterase levels can be falsely depressed by cyclophosphamide, echothiophate iodide, MAO inhibitors, succinylcholine, neostigmine, quinine, quinidine, chloroquine, caffeine, theophylline, epinephrine, ether, barbiturates, atropine, morphine, codeine, phenothiazines, vitamin K, and folic acid.

Chromium

Purpose
To detect chromium toxicity.

Normal results
Serum chromium values range from 0.30 to 0.85 ng/ml.

Abnormal results
Significant increases in serum chromium levels:
  Chromium toxicity.

The basics
Chromium, a trace element found in most body tissues, aids in the transport of amino acids to the liver and heart cells and appears to enhance the effects of insulin in glucose utilization. The effect of impaired chromium metabolism on diabetes mellitus is under investigation. Chromium toxicity can result from industrial overexposure to the metal, such as in the tanning, electroplating, and steelmaking industries. High chromium levels are normal at birth but steadily decrease with age. Chromium toxicity causes dermatitis, and liver and kidney impairment. (See

Industrial Exposure to Chromium VI.)

Procedure
Perform a venipuncture, and collect the sample in a metal-free collection tube. Laboratories provide special kits for this test on request.

Patient care checklist
Before the test
☑ Explain or clarify test purpose and procedure.
☑ Evaluate patient understanding.

Interfering factors
• Recently performed diagnostic tests in which radioactive hexavalent chromium was used may interfere with accurate determination of test results.
• Failure to use a metal-free collection tube may interfere with accurate determination of test results.
• Hemolysis due to rough handling of the sample may interfere with accurate determination of test results.

Cortisol

Purpose
To aid in the diagnosis of Cushing's

Industrial Exposure to Chromium VI

Approximately 175,000 industrial workers risk toxic exposure to chromium VI, the most toxic form of chromium. Such overexposure can result from inhalation or skin contact in the following industries and occupations:

• Abrasives manufacturing

• Cement manufacturing

• Diesel locomotive repair

• Electroplating

• Explosives manufacturing

• Furniture polishing

• Fur processing

• Glassmaking

• Jewelrymaking

• Metal cleaning

• Oil drilling

• Photography

• Textile dyeing

• Wood preservative manufacturing

disease, Cushing's syndrome, Addison's disease, and secondary adrenal insufficiency.

Normal results

Plasma cortisol levels range from 7 to 28 mcg/dl in the morning, and from 2 to 18 mcg/dl in the afternoon. (The afternoon level is usually half the morning level.)

Abnormal results

Increased plasma cortisol levels:
  Adrenocortical hyperfunction in Cushing's disease, Cushing's syndrome.
Decreased cortisol levels:
  Primary adrenal hypofunction (Addison's disease)
  Secondary adrenal insufficiency, such as hypophysectomy, postpartum pituitary necrosis, craniopharyngioma, or chromophobe adenoma.

The basics

Cortisol—the principal glucocorticoid secreted by the adrenal cortex, primarily in response to adrenocorticotropic hormone (ACTH) stimulation—helps metabolize nutrients, mediate physiologic stress, and regulate the immune system. Production of this hormone is influenced by physical or emotional stress, which activates ACTH. Thus, intense heat or cold, infection, trauma, exercise, obesity, and debilitating disease influence cortisol secretion. Cortisol secretion normally follows a diurnal pattern: levels rise during the early morning hours and peak around 8 a.m., then decline to very low levels in the evening and during the early phase of sleep. However, in most patients with Cushing's syndrome, the adrenal cortex tends to secrete independently of any natural rhythm. Thus, absence of diurnal variation in cortisol secretion is a significant finding in almost all patients with Cushing's syndrome; in these patients, little difference in values, if any, is found between morning samples and those taken in the afternoon. Diurnal variations may also be absent in otherwise healthy persons who are under considerable emotional or physical stress.

This test is usually ordered for patients with signs of adrenal dysfunction, but dynamic tests, suppression test for hyperfunction, and stimulation tests for hypofunction are generally required for confirmation of diagnosis.

Procedure

• Between 6 a.m. and 8 a.m., perform a venipuncture.
• Collect the sample in a green-top tube.
• Label appropriately, including the collection time, and send it to the laboratory immediately.
• For diurnal variation testing, draw another sample between 4 p.m. and 6 p.m.
• Collect it in a green-top tube, label appropriately (including the collection time) and send it to the laboratory immediately.

Patient care checklist

Before the test
☑ Explain or clarify test purpose, preparation, and procedure.
☑ Evaluate patient understanding.
☑ Instruct the patient to maintain a normal salt intake (2 to 3 g/day) for 3 days before the test.
☑ Restrict food and fluid and limit physical activity for 10 to 12 hours before the test.
☑ Withhold medications that may interfere with test results, as ordered, for 48 hours before the test. If medication is necessary, note this on the laboratory slip.
☑ Encourage the patient to relax and remain recumbent for 30 minutes before the test.

Interfering factors

• Failure to observe restrictions of diet, medications, or physical activity may interfere with accurate determination of test results. Plasma cortisol levels are falsely elevated by estrogens (during pregnancy or use of oral contraceptives), which increase plasma proteins that bind with cortisol. Obesity, stress, or severe hepatic or renal disease may also increase these levels. Plasma cortisol levels may be decreased by androgens and phenytoin, which decrease cortisol-binding proteins.

• A radioactive scan performed within 1 week before the test may influence the results.

• Hemolysis due to rough handling of the sample may interfere with accurate determination of test results.

Creatine

Purpose
To aid in diagnosis of muscular diseases, including muscular dystrophies.

Normal results
Serum creatine values in males normally range from 0.2 to 0.6 mg/dl; in females, from 0.6 to 1 mg/dl.

Abnormal results
Greatly increased serum creatine levels:
Follow necrosis or atrophy of skeletal muscle, as in trauma, amyotrophic lateral sclerosis, dermatomyositis, and progressive muscular dystrophies.
Increased serum creatine levels:
Hyperthyroidism
Pregnancy
Excessive dietary intake of protein.

The basics
Creatine, an end product of protein metabolism, is formed in the liver, kidneys, small intestinal mucosa, and pancreas, and is distributed to muscle tissues, where it combines with phosphate to form phosphocreatine—a high-energy compound. In the anaerobic stage of muscle contraction, some creatine enters the bloodstream, nor-

mally in an amount proportional to the body's muscle mass. However, muscular diseases may greatly increase the amount of creatine released into the blood.

Procedure
Perform a venipuncture, and collect the sample in a 10- to 15-ml, red-top tube.

Patient care checklist
Before the test
☑ Explain or clarify test purpose, preparation, and procedure.
☑ Evaluate patient understanding.
☑ Restrict foods, fluids, and exercise for approximately 12 hours before the test.

Interfering factors
• Testosterone therapy increases creatine synthesis by the liver and can therefore elevate serum creatine levels.
• Hemolysis caused by rough handling of the sample may alter test results.

Creatine phosphokinase
(CPK)
[Creatine kinase (CK)]

Purpose
• To detect and diagnose acute myocardial infarction (MI) and reinfarction (CPK-MB primarily used)
• To evaluate possible causes of chest pain and to monitor the severity of myocardial ischemia after cardiac surgery, cardiac catheterization, or cardioversion (CPK-MB primarily used)
• To detect skeletal muscle disorders that are not neurogenic in origin, such as Duchenne muscular dystrophy (total CPK primarily used), and early dermatomyositis.

Normal results
Total CPK values determined by ultraviolet or kinetic measurement range

from 23 to 99 units/liter for men, and from 15 to 57 units/liter for women. CPK levels may be significantly higher in very muscular people. Infants up to age 1 have levels two to four times higher than adult levels, possibly reflecting birth trauma and striated muscle development. Normal ranges for isoenzyme levels are as follows: CPK-BB, undetectable; CPK-MB, undetectable to 7 IU/liter; CPK-MM, 5 to 70 IU/liter.

Abnormal results
Detectable CPK-BB isoenzyme:
  Brain tissue injury
  Certain widespread malignant tumors
  Severe shock
  Renal failure.
CPK-MB isoenzyme greater than 5% of total CPK (or more than 10 IU/ liter):
  MI
  Cardiac surgery—in acute MI and following cardiac surgery, CPK-MB begins to rise in 2 to 4 hours, peaks in 12 to 24 hours, and usually returns to normal in 24 to 48 hours; persistent elevations or increasing levels indicate ongoing myocardial damage.
Mild increase in CPK-MB isoenzyme:
  Muscular dystrophies
  Polymyositis
  Severe myoglobinuria.
Increased CPK-MM isoenzyme:
  Trauma to skeletal muscle, such as surgery and I.M. injections
  Dermatomyositis and muscular dystrophy
  Hypothyroidism
  Muscular activity due to agitation as in acute psychotic episode.
Increased total CPK levels:
  Severe hypokalemia
  Carbon monoxide poisoning
  Malignant hyperthermia
  Postconvulsions
  Alcoholic cardiomyopathy.
occasionally in:
  Pulmonary or cerebral infarction.

The basics
CPK is an enzyme that catalyzes the creatine-creatinine metabolic pathway in muscle cells and brain tissue. Because of its intimate role in energy production, CPK reflects normal tissue catabolism; an increase above normal serum levels indicates trauma to cells with high CPK content. CPK may be separated into three isoenzymes with distinct molecular structures: CPK-BB, CPK-MB, and CPK-MM. CPK-BB is found primarily in brain tissue; CPK-MB, in cardiac muscle (a small amount also appears in skeletal muscle); and CPK-MM, in skeletal muscle. CPK-MM constitutes over 99% of total CPK normally present in serum.

An assay of total serum CPK was once widely used to detect acute MI, but elevated serum CPK levels caused by skeletal muscle damage reduce the test's specificity for this disorder. Fractionation and measurement of CPK isoenzymes is rapidly replacing use of total CPK to accurately localize the site of increased tissue destruction.

Procedure
Perform a venipuncture, and collect the sample in a 7-ml, red-top tube.

Special precautions
• Draw the sample before or within 1 hour of giving I.M. injections, as muscle trauma raises total CPK levels.
• Obtain the sample on schedule. Note on the laboratory slip the time the sample was drawn and the hours elapsed since onset of chest pain.

Patient care checklist
Before the test
☑ Explain or clarify test purpose, preparation, and procedure.
☑ Evaluate patient understanding.
☑ Instruct the patient to avoid exercise for 24 hours before the test if he is being evaluated for skeletal muscle disorders.
☑ Withhold alcohol and interfering medications, as ordered. If medica-

tions must be continued, note them on the laboratory slip.

Interfering factors
• Hemolysis due to rough handling of the sample may affect CPK levels.
• Failure to send the sample to the laboratory immediately or to refrigerate the serum if testing will be delayed for more than 2 hours may hinder accurate determination of CPK levels.
• Failure to draw the samples at the scheduled time, missing peak levels, may interfere with accurate determination of test results.
• Halothane and succinylcholine, alcohol, lithium, and large doses of aminocaproic acid reportedly cause elevated CPK levels. Intramuscular injections, cardioversion, invasive diagnostic procedures, surgery, trauma, recent vigorous exercise or muscle massage, and severe coughing also increase total CPK levels.

Creatinine

Purpose
• To assess renal glomerular filtration
• To screen for renal damage.

Normal results
Serum creatinine concentrations in males normally range from 0.8 to 1.2 mg/dl; in females, from 0.6 to 0.9 mg/dl.

Abnormal results
Increased serum creatinine levels:
  Renal disease that has seriously damaged 50% or more of the nephrons
  Gigantism
  Acromegaly.

The basics
This test provides a more sensitive measure of renal damage than blood urea nitrogen levels, because renal impairment is virtually the only cause of creatinine elevation. Creatinine is a nonprotein end product of creatine metabolism. Similar to creatine, creatinine appears in serum in amounts proportional to the body's muscle mass; unlike creatine, it is easily excreted by the kidneys, with minimal or no tubular reabsorption. Creatinine levels, therefore, are directly related to the glomerular filtration rate. Since creatinine levels normally remain constant, elevated levels usually indicate diminished renal function.

Procedure
Perform a venipuncture, and collect the sample in a 10- to 15-ml, red-top tube.

Patient care checklist
Before the test
☑ Explain or clarify test purpose, preparation, and procedure.
☑ Evaluate patient understanding.
☑ Restrict foods and fluids for about 8 hours before the test.

Interfering factors
• Ascorbic acid, barbiturates, and diuretics may raise serum creatinine levels.
• Sulfobromophthalein or phenolsulfonphthalein given within the previous 24 hours can elevate creatinine levels if the test is based on the Jaffé reaction.
• Patients with exceptionally large muscle masses, such as athletes, may have above-average creatinine levels, even in the presence of normal renal function.

Dexamethasone suppression test *(DST)*

Purpose
• To measure increased cortisol activity
• To diagnose and etiologically differentiate Cushing's syndrome
• To investigate neuroendocrine abnormalities in affective disorders and

to help diagnose and manage depression.

Normal results
Overnight-screening DST (single dose):
Plasma cortisol: 8 a.m.—less than 5 μg/dl.
Low-dose or high-dose DST:
Plasma cortisol: less than 5 μg/dl
Urinary free cortisol: less than 20 μg/24 hours, or more than a 50% reduction from baseline level.

Abnormal results
Nonsuppression, or "escape" of cortisol, with urine or plasma cortisol levels greater than 50% of normal levels following dexamethasone administration occurs with:
Diurnal rhythm
Cushing's syndrome
Hyperthyroidism
Affective disorders
Severe stress.

The basics
The most important and most abundant steroid produced by the adrenal cortex is cortisol, a glucocorticoid whose release is stimulated by adrenocorticotropic hormone (ACTH) from the pituitary gland via a negative feedback mechanism. Cortisol also exhibits a diurnal pattern of production, with the highest levels occurring between 6 a.m. and 10 a.m. and the lowest between 4 p.m. and midnight. Activation of this hypothalamic-pituitary-adrenocortical (HPA) axis, with concurrent increased cortisol production, also occurs during periods of heightened emotional stress (such as excitement or fear), as well as in some psychiatric conditions. HPA axis function may be evaluated by measurement of cortisol levels.

Dexamethasone is a potent synthetic glucocorticoid with properties similar to those of cortisol. When given orally in low doses, dexamethasone will usually cause reduced adrenal stimulation by inhibiting ACTH secretion. This will result in lowered (or suppressed) plasma and urine cortisol levels.

The DST is used to diagnose Cushing's syndrome. This syndrome results in increased secretion of cortisol, which may be from pituitary ACTH hypersecretion (Cushing's disease), an autonomous adrenal tumor hypersecreting cortisol, or ectopic or paraneoplastic ACTH hypersecretion. The combination of the low-dose and the high-dose DST allows differentiation of hyperplastic from neoplastic causes of Cushing's syndrome. Low-dose nonsuppression plus high-dose suppression indicate bilateral adrenal hyperplasia; low-dose nonsuppression plus high-dose nonsuppression indicate adrenal tumor or carcinoma, or an ectopic ACTH-secreting tumor.

The DST is also being used increasingly to assist in the identification and diagnosis of affective diseases in psychiatry, particularly melancholia (endogenous depression), and as a predictor of treatment response. Research results are not yet conclusive, but it is generally agreed that approximately 45% of these patients fail to suppress, or "escape" from suppression more rapidly than the normal population. Failure to suppress plasma cortisol following administration of dexamethasone has been suggested for use as a biological marker for endogenous depression in adult and possibly in adolescent psychiatric patients, in identification of patients with major depression, and in work with autistic children and adolescents.

Procedure
(Not fully standardized; may vary depending on test purpose and physician preference.)
Overnight-screening DST (single dose):
Day 1
• Administer 0.5 to 2.0 mg dexamethasone (or dosage according to body weight at 5 μg/kg) orally at 11 p.m., as ordered.

Day 2
• Perform a venipuncture and collect the sample in a red-top tube between 8 a.m. and 9 a.m.

Low-dose DST:
Day 1
• Collect a baseline 24-hour urine specimen (urine free cortisol test) with creatinine content, using a collection container with preservative added.

Days 2 and 3
• Administer 0.5 mg dexamethasone (or dosage according to weight at 5 μg/kg/6 hours) orally every 6 hours for 2 days, as ordered.
• Collect a 24-hour urine specimen for urinary free cortisol with creatinine content, using a collection container with preservative added.
• Perform a venipuncture and collect the sample in a red-top tube for plasma cortisol at 8 a.m. and 4 p.m. If a third sample is required, it should be drawn at 11 p.m.

Day 4
• Occasionally, an 8 a.m. plasma cortisol sample will be ordered, using the same procedure. (If suppression fails to occur, the high-dose DST will be performed.)

High-dose DST:
Day 1
• Collect a baseline 24-hour urine specimen (urinary free cortisol test) with creatinine content, using a collection container with preservative added. (This procedure may be omitted if this is a continuation of the low-dose DST.)

Days 2 and 3
• Administer 2.0 mg dexamethasone orally every 6 hours for 2 days, as ordered.
• Collect a 24-hour urine specimen for urinary free cortisol with creatinine content, using a collection container with preservative added.
• Perform a venipuncture and collect the sample in a red-top tube for plasma cortisol at 8 a.m. and 4 p.m. If a third sample is required, it should be drawn at 11 p.m.

Day 4
• Occasionally, an 8 a.m. plasma cortisol sample will be ordered, using the same procedure.

Special precautions

• If urine is collected, keep it refrigerated or on ice during the collection period.
• Be certain blood samples for plasma cortisol levels are drawn at the exact times they are ordered.
• Administer oral dexamethasone at the exact time it is ordered. Milk or antacid may be ordered to prevent gastric irritation.
• If urine samples are ordered, be sure no interfering drugs are given to the patient during testing time. Consult with the physician, as needed.

Patient care checklist
Before the test
☑ Explain or clarify test purpose, preparation, and procedure.
☑ Evaluate patient understanding.
☑ Restrict food and fluids, except water, for 10 to 12 hours before the test.
☑ Try to minimize patient anxiety and stress, since they can interfere with accurate testing; if undue emotional or physical stress (such as fever or infection) arises, report it to the physician.
☑ Check patient history for preexisting medical conditions that interfere with the hypothalamic-pituitary axis.
☑ Check patient history to be sure interfering drugs were withheld, as ordered, for 2 weeks.
☑ Explain that, if nonsuppression occurs with the low dexamethasone dose, a second test may be ordered using a higher dose of dexamethasone.
☑ If ordered, administer a hypnotic for sleep.

Interfering factors
• Caffeine (equivalent to 4 to 5 cups of coffee) may cause false-positive results.

• Obesity may cause failure to suppress with the overnight-screening DST.

• Medical conditions that may interfere with the accuracy of test results by increasing cortisol levels include major physical illnesses, hyperthyroidism, trauma, increased temperature, temporal lobe disease, gastrointestinal disturbances (nausea), pregnancy, diabetes mellitus, dehydration, malnutrition, anorexia nervosa, alcohol use, acute alcohol withdrawal, or electroconvulsive therapy.

• ACTH, cortisone, estrogens, hydrocortisone, oral contraceptives, ethanol, lithium, or methadone taken in the 2 weeks prior to testing plasma cortisol levels may cause an increase in test levels; phenytoin and androgens may decrease plasma cortisol levels.

• Salicylates, acetaminophen, morphine, barbiturates, reserpine, furosemide, thiazides, paraldehyde, monoamine oxidase inhibitors, spironolactone, cloxacillin, or licorice taken during collection of urine for free cortisol may interfere with test results.

• ACTH or oral contraceptives taken in the 2 weeks prior to testing urinary free cortisol may cause an increase in test levels.

Erythrocyte total porphyrins
[Erythropoietic porphyrins]

Purpose
• To aid in diagnosis of congenital or acquired erythropoietic porphyrias
• To help confirm diagnosis of disorders affecting red blood cell activity.

Normal results
Total porphyrin levels range from 16 to 60 mg/dl of packed red blood cells. Protoporphyrin levels range from 16 to 60 mg/dl; coproporphyrins and uroporphyrins each have levels below 2 mg/dl.

Abnormal results
Increased protoporphyrin levels:
  Erythropoietic protoporphyria
  Infection
  Increased erythropoiesis
  Thalassemia
  Sideroblastic anemia
  Iron deficiency anemia
  Lead poisoning.
Increased coproporphyrin levels:
  Congenital erythropoietic porphyria
  Erythropoietic protoporphyria or coproporphyria
  Sideroblastic anemia.
Increased uroporphyrin levels:
  Congenital erythropoietic porphyria
  Erythropoietic protoporphyria.

The basics
This test measures total erythrocyte porphyrins—mostly protoporphyrin, but also coproporphyrin and uroporphyrin. Porphyrins are pigments that are present in all protoplasm and have a significant role in energy storage and use. Protoporphyrin, coproporphyrin, and uroporphyrin are produced during heme biosynthesis. Small amounts of these porphyrins or their precursors normally appear in blood, urine, and feces. Production and excretion of porphyrins or their precursors increase in porphyrias, which are separated into erythropoietic and hepatic types. This test detects erythropoietic porphyrias.

After an initial screening test for total porphyrins, quantitative fluorometric analysis can identify specific porphyrins and suggest specific disorders.

Procedure
• Perform a venipuncture and collect the sample in a 5-ml or larger green-top tube.
• Label the sample, place it on ice, and send it to the laboratory.

Patient care checklist
Before the test
☑ Explain or clarify test purpose, preparation, and procedure.
☑ Evaluate patient understanding.

☑ Restrict food and fluids (water is permitted) for 12 to 14 hours before the sample is drawn.

Interfering factors
Hemolysis or failure to observe dietary restrictions may alter test results.

Estrogens

Purpose
• To determine sexual maturation and fertility
• To aid in diagnosis of gonadal dysfunction: precocious or delayed puberty, menstrual disorders (especially amenorrhea), or infertility
• To determine fetal well-being
• To aid in diagnosis of tumors known to secrete estrogen.

Normal results
Serum estrogen levels for premenopausal females vary widely during the menstrual cycle:

1 to 10 days: 24 to 68 pg/ml
11 to 20 days: 50 to 186 pg/ml
21 to 30 days: 73 to 149 pg/ml.

Serum estrogen levels in males range from 12 to 34 pg/ml. In girls age 6 and older, levels rise gradually to adult female values. In menopause, serum estrogen decreases to a constant low level. In children under age 6, the normal range of serum estrogen is 3 to 10 pg/ml.

Abnormal results
Decreased estrogen levels:
Primary hypogonadism, or ovarian failure, as in Turner's syndrome or ovarian agenesis
Secondary hypogonadism, as in hypopituitarism.
Increased estrogen levels:
Estrogen-producing tumors
Precocious puberty
Cirrhosis
Congenital adrenal hyperplasia.

The basics
Estrogens (and progesterone) are secreted by the ovaries under the influence of the pituitary gonadotropins, follicle-stimulating hormone (FSH), and luteinizing hormone (LH). Estrogens—in particular, estradiol, which is the most potent estrogen—interact with the hypothalamic-pituitary axis through both negative and positive feedback mechanisms. Slowly rising or sustained high levels inhibit secretion of FSH and LH (negative feedback), but a rapid rise in estrogen that occurs just before ovulation seems to stimulate LH secretion (positive feedback).

Estrogens are responsible for the development of secondary female sexual characteristics and for normal menstruation. These hormones are secreted by ovarian follicular cells during the first half of the menstrual cycle, and by the corpus luteum during the luteal phase and during pregnancy.

This radioimmunoassay measures serum levels of estradiol, estrone, and estriol—the only estrogens that appear in serum in measurable amounts—and has diagnostic significance in evaluating female gonadal dysfunction. Tests of hypothalamic-pituitary function may be required to confirm diagnosis. (See *Estriol: Clue to Fetal Well-Being,* p. 80.)

Procedure
Procedure may vary slightly, depending on choice of plasma or serum assay.
• Perform a venipuncture, and collect the sample in a 10-ml, red-top tube.
• If the patient is premenopausal, indicate the phase of her menstrual cycle on the laboratory slip.

Patient care checklist
Before the test
☑ Explain or clarify test purpose, preparation, and procedure.
☑ Advise patient that the test may be repeated during the various phases of the menstrual cycle.

Estriol: Clue to Fetal Well-Being

Estriol represents about 90% of the estrogen produced during pregnancy after 20 weeks' gestation. The placenta converts fetal adrenal precursors into estriol, which is then conjugated by the maternal liver and excreted in maternal urine. Because estriol production depends on the fetus and placenta, levels serve as an index of fetal well-being and placental adequacy.

Disagreement exists as to the merits of measuring total plasma estriol, plasma unconjugated estriol (about 10% to 15% of total plasma estriol), and urine estriol. However, plasma estriol has several advantages over urine estriol—samples do not have to be collected at specific times and are less affected by medications. Of the plasma samples, unconjugated estriol appears to be preferred, because the sample is easier to analyze in the laboratory. Despite these differences, all three types of samples are commonly used to assess placental function and fetal well-being.

☑ Evaluate patient understanding.
☑ Withhold medications that may interfere with test results, as ordered. If these medications must be continued, note them on the laboratory slip.

Interfering factors
• Pregnancy and pretest use of estrogens (oral contraceptives) can increase serum estrogen levels. Clomiphene, an estrogen antagonist, can decrease serum estrogen levels. Ingestion of steroids or pituitary-based hormones can alter test results. For example, dexamethasone may suppress adrenal androgen secretion.
• Hemolysis caused by rough handling of the sample may interfere with accurate determination of test results.

Fasting plasma glucose
[Fasting blood sugar]

Purpose
• To screen for diabetes mellitus
• To monitor drug or dietary therapy in patients with diabetes mellitus.

Normal results
Range for fasting plasma glucose varies according to the laboratory procedure. Generally, normal values after a 12- to 14-hour fast are 70 to 100 mg of "true glucose"/100 ml of blood when measured by the glucose oxidase and hexokinase methods.

Abnormal results
Increased fasting plasma glucose levels:
with values of 140 mg/100 ml obtained on two or more occasions:
   Confirms diabetes mellitus.
may also occur with:
   Pancreatitis
   Recent acute illness, such as myocardial infarction
   Cushing's syndrome
   Acromegaly
   Pheochromocytoma
   Hyperlipoproteinemia (especially Type III, IV, or V)
   Chronic hepatic disease
   Nephrotic syndrome
   Brain tumor
   Sepsis
   Dumping syndrome
   Eclampsia
   Anoxia
   Convulsive disorders.
Decreased fasting plasma glucose levels:
   Hyperinsulinism
   Insulinoma
   von Gierke's disease
   Functional or reactive hypoglycemia
   Myxedema
   Adrenal insufficiency
   Congenital adrenal hyperplasia

Hypopituitarism
Malabsorption syndrome
Hepatic insufficiency (possibly).

The basics

Commonly used to screen for diabetes mellitus, the fasting plasma glucose test measures plasma glucose levels following a 12- to 14-hour fast; however, borderline or transient elevated levels require the 2-hour postprandial plasma glucose test or the oral glucose tolerance test to confirm diagnosis.

In the fasting state, plasma glucose levels decrease, stimulating release of the hormone glucagon. Glucagon then acts to raise plasma glucose by accelerating glycogenolysis, stimulating glyconeogenesis, and inhibiting glycogen synthesis. Normally, secretion of insulin checks this rise in glucose levels. In diabetes, however, absence or deficiency of insulin allows persistently high glucose levels.

Procedure

• Perform a venipuncture, and collect the sample in a 5-ml, gray-top tube.
• Send the sample to the laboratory immediately.
• If transport is delayed, refrigerate the sample.
• Specify on the laboratory slip the time when the patient last ate, the sample collection time, and the time the last pretest insulin or oral hypoglycemic dose (if applicable) was given.

Patient care checklist

Before the test

☑ Explain or clarify test purpose, preparation, and procedure

☑ Evaluate patient understanding.

☑ Restrict food and fluid for 12 to 14 hours before the test.

☑ Withhold medications that may affect test results, as ordered. If these must be continued, note them on the laboratory slip.

CLINICAL ALERT: **Alert the patient to symptoms of hypoglycemia (weakness, restlessness, nervousness, hunger, and sweating), and tell him to report such symptoms immediately.**

After the test

☑ Provide a balanced meal or snack.

Interfering factors

• False-positive findings may be caused by acetaminophen when the glucose oxidase/hexokinase method is used. Other drugs known to elevate plasma glucose levels are chlorthalidone, thiazide diuretics, furosemide, triamterene, oral contraceptives (estrogen-progestogen combination), benzodiazepines, phenytoin, phenothiazines, lithium, epinephrine, arginine, phenolphthalein, dextrothyroxine, diazoxide, large doses of nicotinic acid, corticosteroids, and recent I.V. glucose infusions. Ethacrynic acid may also cause hyperglycemia, but large doses can produce hypoglycemia in patients with uremia.

• Decreased plasma glucose levels may be caused by beta-adrenergic blockers, ethanol, clofibrate, insulin, oral hypoglycemic agents, and monoamine oxidase inhibitors.

• Failure to observe dietary restrictions may elevate plasma glucose levels.

• Recent illness, infection, or pregnancy can elevate plasma glucose levels; strenuous exercise can depress them.

• Glycolysis due to failure to refrigerate the sample or to send it to the laboratory immediately can result in false-negative results. (Also see *Home Tests*, pp. 685 to 687.)

Folic acid
[Pteroylglutamic acid, folacin folate]

Purpose

• To aid in differential diagnosis of megaloblastic anemia, which may result from deficiency of folic acid or vitamin B_{12}

• To assess folate stores in pregnancy.

Normal results

Serum folic acid values range from 2 to 14 ng/ml.

Abnormal results

Decreased serum folic acid levels:

Anemia (especially megaloblastic anemia)

Leukopenia

Thrombocytopenia

Hypermetabolic states, such as hyperthyroidism

Inadequate dietary intake

Chronic alcoholism

Small-bowel malabsorption syndrome

Pregnancy.

Increased serum folic acid levels (more than 20 ng/ml):

Excessive dietary intake of folic acid or folic acid supplements.

The basics

This test is often performed concomitantly with serum vitamin B_{12} determinations. Like vitamin B_{12}, folic acid is a water-soluble vitamin that influences hematopoiesis, DNA synthesis, and overall body growth. Because the body stores only small amounts of folic acid (mostly in the liver), inadequate dietary intake causes a deficiency, especially during pregnancy, when the metabolic demand for folic acid rises. Because of folic acid's vital role in hematopoiesis, the usual indication for this test is a suspected hematologic abnormality. Levels less than 2 ng/ml may indicate such abnormalities. The Schilling test is often performed to rule out vitamin B_{12} deficiency, which also causes megaloblastic anemia (pernicious anemia). This vitamin is nontoxic in humans, even when taken in large doses.

Procedure

Perform a venipuncture, and collect the sample in a 7-ml, red-top tube.

Patient care checklist

Before the test

☑ Explain or clarify test purpose, preparation, and procedure.

☑ Evaluate patient understanding.

☑ Restrict food and fluid overnight before the test.

Interfering factors

• Alcohol and phenytoin interfere with folic acid absorption and lower serum folic acid. Pyrimethamine can induce folate deficiency and low folic acid levels.

• Hemolysis caused by rough handling of the sample may alter test results.

Follicle-stimulating hormone
(FSH)

Purpose

• To aid in the diagnosis of infertility and disorders of menstruation, such as amenorrhea

• To aid in the diagnosis of precocious puberty in girls (before age 9) and in boys (before age 10)

• To aid in the differential diagnosis of hypogonadism.

Normal results

Values vary greatly, depending on the patient's age, stage of sexual development, and—for a female—phase of her menstrual cycle. For menstruating females, approximate values are as follows:

follicular phase: 5 to 20 mIU/ml

midcycle peak: 15 to 30 mIU/ml

luteal phase: 5 to 15 mIU/ml.

Approximate values for adult males are 5 to 20 mIU/ml; for menopausal women, 50 to 100 mIU/ml.

Abnormal results

Increased FSH levels occur in:

Turner's syndrome (primary hypogonadism)

Stein-Leventhal syndrome (polycystic ovary syndrome)

Congenital absence of the gonads

Precocious puberty (idiopathic or with central nervous system lesions)

Early-stage acromegaly

Destruction of the testes (from mumps orchitis or X-ray exposure)

Testicular failure

Seminoma.

Decreased FSH levels occur in:
Anorexia nervosa
Panhypopituitarism
Hypothalamic lesions.

The basics

This test of gonadal function, performed more often on females than on males, measures plasma FSH levels by radioimmunoassay and is usually vital to infertility studies. Decreased FSH levels may cause male or female infertility: aspermatogenesis in males and anovulation in females. However, its overall diagnostic significance often depends on the results of related hormone tests (for luteinizing hormone, estrogen, or progesterone, for example). Secreted by the anterior pituitary, FSH stimulates gonadal activity in both sexes. In females, FSH spurs development of primary ovarian follicles into graafian follicles for ovulation. Secretion fluctuates rhythmically during the menstrual cycle, peaking at ovulation. In males, continuous secretion of FSH (and testosterone) stimulates and maintains spermatogenesis. Plasma levels fluctuate widely in females, and to obtain a true baseline level, daily testing for 3 to 5 days may be necessary, or multiple samples can be drawn on the same day. The laboratory requires at least 3 days to complete the analysis.

Procedure

• Perform a venipuncture, preferably between 6 a.m. and 8 a.m., using a 7-ml, red-top collection tube.

• If the patient is a female, indicate the phase of her menstrual cycle on the laboratory slip. If she is menopausal, note this on the laboratory slip.

Patient care checklist

Before the test

☑ Explain or clarify test purpose, preparation, and procedure.

☑ Evaluate patient understanding.

☑ Withhold medications that may interfere with test results, as ordered. If they must be continued, note them on the laboratory slip.

☑ Encourage the patient to relax and remain recumbent for 30 minutes before the test.

Interfering factors

• Failure to observe restriction of medications may hinder accurate determination of test results. Ovarian steroid hormones, such as estrogen or progesterone, and related compounds may, through negative feedback, inhibit the flow of releasing hormones from the hypothalamus and pituitary; phenothiazines (such as chlorpromazine) may exert a similar effect.

• A radioactive scan performed within 1 week before the test may affect results.

• Hemolysis due to rough handling of the sample may interfere with accurate determination of test results.

Free thyroxine and free triiodothyronine
[FT₄ and FT₃]

Purpose

• To measure the metabolically active form of the thyroid hormones

• To aid in diagnosis of hyper- or hypothyroidism when thyroxine-binding globulin (TBG) levels are abnormal.

Normal results

Range for FT_4 is from 0.8 to 3.3 ng/dl; for FT_3, from 0.2 to 0.6 ng/dl. Values vary, depending on the laboratory.

Abnormal results

Increased FT₄ and FT₃ levels:
Hyperthyroidism.

Increased FT$_3$ levels with low or normal FT$_4$ levels:
   T$_3$ toxicosis (a distinct form of hyperthyroidism).
Decreased FT$_4$ levels:
   Hypothyroidism (except in patients receiving T$_3$ replacement therapy).

The basics
These tests, often done simultaneously, measure serum levels of FT$_4$ and FT$_3$, the minute portions of T$_4$ and T$_3$ not bound to TBG and other serum proteins. As the active components of T$_4$ and T$_3$, these unbound hormones enter target cells and are responsible for the thyroid's effects on cellular metabolism. Since levels of circulating FT$_4$ and FT$_3$ are regulated by a feedback mechanism that compensates for changes in binding protein concentrations by adjusting total hormone levels, measurement of free hormone levels is the best indicator of thyroid function. Disagreement exists as to whether FT$_4$ or FT$_3$ is the better indicator; therefore, laboratories commonly measure both. The disadvantages of these tests include a cumbersome and difficult laboratory method, inaccessibility, and cost. The laboratory requires several days to complete the analysis. This test may be useful in the 5% of patients in whom the standard T$_3$ or T$_4$ tests fail to produce diagnostic results. Serial tests may be performed. Patients on thyroid therapy may have varying levels of FT$_4$ and FT$_3$, depending on the preparation used and the time of sample collection; however, thyroid medications should not be withheld.

Procedure
Draw venous blood into a 7-ml, red-top tube.

Patient care checklist
Before the test
☑ Explain or clarify test purpose and procedure.
☑ Evaluate patient understanding.

Interfering factors
Except for hemolysis due to rough handling of the sample, this test is virtually free of interfering factors.

Galactose-1-phosphate uridyl transferase

Purpose
• To screen infants for galactosemia.
• To detect heterozygous carriers of galactosemia.

Normal results
The qualitative test is negative (fluorescence is strong 1 and 2 hours after the test begins). The range for the quantitative test is 18.5 to 28.5 kU/mol of hemoglobin. Check the normal range for your laboratory if a different method is used.

Abnormal results
A positive test (no fluorescence) may indicate:
   Transferase deficiency.
Results less than 5 kU/mol of hemoglobin indicate:
   Galactosemia.
Results between 5 and 18.5 kU/mol may indicate:
   A carrier state.

The basics
This enzyme helps convert galactose to glucose during lactose metabolism. Deficiency of these enzymes causes galactosemia, an autosomal-recessive disorder marked by elevated serum galactose and decreased serum glucose. Unless detected and treated soon after birth, galactosemia can impair eye, brain, and liver development, causing irreversible cataracts, mental retardation, and cirrhosis.

A deficiency of galactose-1-phosphate uridyl transferase causes the most common and severe form of galactosemia. Both qualitative and quantitative tests are widely used to detect it. The qualitative method, a simple screening test performed at birth, is required in some hospitals for all neonates. If positive, a follow-up quantitative test should be performed as soon as possible.

Prenatal testing of amniotic fluid can also detect transferase deficiency. However, such testing is rarely performed because neonatal screening can detect the deficiency in time to prevent irreversible damage.

Procedure
• For a qualitative (screening) test, collect cord blood or blood from a heel stick on special filter paper, saturating all three circles.
• For a quantitative test, perform a venipuncture and collect a 4-ml sample in a green-top or lavender-top tube, depending on the laboratory method used.
• Indicate the patient's age on the laboratory slip.
• Send the collection tube to the laboratory on wet ice.

Patient care checklist
Before the test
☑ Explain or clarify test purpose and procedure to an adult patient or parents of a neonate.
☑ Evaluate understanding.
☑ Review the patient's history for a recent exchange transfusion. Note it on the laboratory slip or postpone the test, as ordered.
After the test
☑ If test results indicate galactosemia, provide nutritional counseling for the parents and a galactose- and lactose-free diet for their infant. A soybean or meat-based formula may be substituted for milk.
☑ If one or both partners in a couple are carriers, stress the importance of having a screening test performed on their infant at birth.

Interfering factors
• Failure to use the proper tube or to send the sample on wet ice may cause a false-positive result, because heat inactivates the transferase.
• A total exchange transfusion causes a transient false-negative result, because normal transfused blood contains the transferase.
• Hemolysis caused by rough handling of the sample may alter test results.

Gamma glutamyl transferase *(GGT)* *[Gamma glutamyl transpeptidase]*

Purpose
• To provide information about hepatobiliary diseases, to assess liver function, and to detect alcohol ingestion
• To distinguish between skeletal disease and hepatic disease when serum alkaline phosphatase is elevated. (A normal GGT level suggests such elevation stems from skeletal disease.)

Normal results
Serum GGT values vary with the assay method used (colorimetric or kinetic method). In females under age 45, normal levels range from 5 to 27 units/liter; in females over age 45 and in males, levels range from 6 to 37 units/liter.

Abnormal results
Sharpest increases in GGT levels:
    Obstructive jaundice
    Hepatic metastasis.
Increase in GGT levels:
    Any acute hepatic disease
    Acute pancreatitis
    Renal disease
    Prostatic metastasis
    Postoperative status
    Alcohol ingestion.
Possible increases in GGT levels:
    Epilepsy
    Brain tumor
    Acute MI; occur 5 to 10 days after.

The basics

This test, which measures serum GGT levels, is a somewhat more sensitive indicator of hepatic necrosis than serum glutamic-oxaloacetic transaminase, and is as sensitive as or more sensitive than alkaline phosphatase, since GGT is not elevated in bone growth or pregnancy. However, the test is nonspecific, providing little data about the type of hepatic disease. GGT is particularly sensitive to the effects of alcohol in the liver, and levels may be elevated after moderate alcohol intake and in chronic alcoholism, even without clinical evidence of hepatic injury.

Procedure

Perform a venipuncture, and collect the sample in a 7-ml, red-top tube.

Patient care checklist

Before the test

☑ Explain or clarify test purpose, preparation, and procedure.

☑ Evaluate patient understanding.

☑ Restrict food and fluid, especially alcohol, for 12 hours before the test if required by the laboratory.

Interfering factors

• Clofibrate and oral contraceptives decrease serum GGT levels. Aminoglycosides, barbiturates, and phenytoin produce elevated values.

• Moderate intake of alcohol causes increased serum GGT levels that may persist for at least 60 hours.

• Hemolysis due to rough handling of the sample may interfere with accurate determination of serum GGT levels.

Gastrin

Purpose

• To confirm diagnosis of gastrinoma, the gastrin-secreting tumor in Zollinger-Ellison syndrome

• To aid in differential diagnosis of gastric and duodenal ulcers and pernicious anemia.

Normal results

Serum gastrin levels are less than 300 pg/ml.

Abnormal results

Strikingly high serum gastrin (over 1,000 pg/ml) levels:

Confirm Zollinger-Ellison syndrome.

Increased serum gastrin levels:

Duodenal ulcer (less than 1% of patients)

Achlorhydria

Extensive stomach carcinoma.

The basics

Gastrin is a hormone produced and stored primarily by specialized G cells in the antrum of the stomach and, to a lesser degree, by the islets of Langerhans, in the pancreas. The main function of gastrin is to aid in digestion of food by triggering gastric acid secretion in the parietal area of the stomach in response to food (especially proteins), vagal stimulation, or decreased stomach acidity. Through a stong negative feedback control mechanism, acid in the gastric antrum inhibits gastrin release in response to all stimuli. However, the concomitant findings of very low gastric juice pH and a very high serum gastrin level indicate autonomous hormone secretion not governed by a negative feedback mechanism.

Procedure

Perform a venipuncture, and collect the sample in a 10- to 15-ml, red-top tube.

Patient care checklist

Before the test

☑ Explain or clarify test purpose, preparation, and procedure.

☑ Evaluate patient understanding.

☑ Restrict food and fluid (water is permitted) for 12 hours before the test.

☑ Advise the patient to abstain from alcohol for at least 24 hours before the test.

☑ Withhold medications that may interfere with test results, especially anticholinergics or insulin, as ordered. If they must be continued, note on the laboratory slip.

☑ Encourage the patient to relax and to remain recumbent for at least 30 minutes before the test.

Interfering factors

• Failure to observe restrictions of diet, medications, or physical activity may interfere with accurate determination of test results.

• Gastrin secretion is increased by amino acids (especially glycine), calcium carbonate, acetylcholine, calcium chloride, and ethanol; gastrin secretion is decreased by anticholinergics (atropine), hydrochloric acid, or secretin (a strongly basic polypeptide).

• Insulin-induced hypoglycemia increases gastrin secretion.

• Hemolysis caused by rough handling of the sample may interfere with accurate determination of test results.

• Failure to send the sample to the laboratory immediately may cause destruction of serum gastrin by proteolytic enzymes. (See *Gastrin Stimulation Tests*.)

Glucagon

Purpose

To aid in diagnosis of glucagonoma (alpha-cell tumor) and hypoglycemia due to chronic pancreatitis or idiopathic glucagon deficiency.

Normal results

Fasting glucagon levels are normally less than 250 pg/ml.

Abnormal results

Markedly increased fasting glucagon levels:

Glucagonoma (values may range from 900 to 7,800 pg/ml).

Increased glucagon levels:

Gastrin Stimulation Tests

Since some patients with duodenal or gastric ulcers have normal fasting levels of gastrin, provocative testing is necessary to identify such patients; a protein-rich test meal serves this purpose. In a patient with duodenal or gastric ulcers, gastrin levels increase markedly after such a meal, while these levels rise only moderately in a healthy person.

Provocative testing is also necessary to distinguish a patient with duodenal or gastric ulcers from one suspected of having Zollinger-Ellison syndrome, since both may show similar baseline gastrin levels. One effective test involves I.V. infusion of calcium gluconate in a dosage of 5 mg/kg of body weight over 3 hours. After the infusion, 10 ml of venous blood is drawn and sent to the laboratory. Gastrin levels double, rising to about 500 pg/ml, in a patient with Zollinger-Ellison syndrome; a patient with duodenal or gastric ulcers shows only a moderate rise or no change at all.

A third indication for provocative testing is an abnormally—but not strikingly—high fasting serum gastrin level. This is possible in both Zollinger-Ellison syndrome and in patients with pernicious anemia. To distinguish between the two, hydrochloric acid may be infused into the stomach through a nasogastric tube. Such an infusion causes a sharp drop in gastrin levels in patients with pernicious anemia but not in patients with Zollinger-Ellison syndrome.

Diabetes mellitus
Acute pancreatitis
Pheochromocytoma.
Decreased glucagon levels:
Idiopathic glucagon deficiency
Hypoglycemia due to chronic pancreatitis.

The basics

Glucagon, a hormone secreted by the alpha cells of the islets of Langerhans in the pancreas, acts primarily on the liver to promote glucose production and control glucose storage. Glucagon is secreted in response to hypoglycemia; secretion is inhibited by the other pancreatic hormones, insulin and somatostatin. Normally, the coordinated release of glucagon, insulin, and somatostatin ensures an adequate and constant fuel supply while maintaining blood glucose levels within relatively stable limits. Glucagon is usually measured concomitantly with serum glucose and insulin, since glucose and insulin levels influence glucagon secretion. With abnormally low glucagon levels, stimulation or suppression tests may be necessary to confirm the diagnosis.

Procedure

• Perform a venipuncture, and collect a blood sample in a chilled 10-ml, lavender-top tube.
• Place the sample on ice and send it to the laboratory immediately.

Patient care checklist

Before the test
☑ Explain or clarify test purpose, preparation, and procedure.
☑ Evaluate patient understanding.
☑ Restrict food and fluid for 10 to 12 hours before the test.
☑ Withhold medications that may interfere with test results, as ordered. If they must be continued, note them on the laboratory slip.
☑ Encourage the patient to relax and to remain recumbent for 30 minutes before the test.

Interfering factors

• Prolonged fasting, undue stress, or use of catecholamines or insulin before the collection of blood samples may elevate glucagon levels.
• Hemolysis caused by rough handling of the sample may interfere with accurate determination of test results.
• Failure to pack the sample in ice and send it to the laboratory immediately may affect test results.

Glucose-6-phosphate dehydrogenase (G-6-PD)

Purpose

• To detect hemolytic anemia caused by G-6-PD deficiency
• To aid in differential diagnosis of hemolytic anemia.

Normal results

Serum values of G-6-PD vary with the method used; for example, with the fluorescent spot-screening test, values are simply reported as normal or abnormal.

Abnormal results

Screening tests detect (but do not confirm):
G-6-PD deficiency.

The basics

This test, which measures serum G-6-PD levels, detects deficiency of this enzyme. Such deficiency is a hereditary, sex-linked condition carried on the female X chromosome (with clinical disease found mostly in males) that produces hemolytic anemia. About 10% of all black males in the United States inherit mild G-6-PD deficiencies; certain peoples of Mediterranean origin inherit severe deficiencies. In some whites, fava beans may produce hemolytic episodes. Although deficiency of G-6-PD provides partial immunity to falciparum malaria, it precipitates an adverse reaction to antimalarials.

Procedure
• Perform a venipuncture, and collect the sample in a 7-ml, lavender-top tube.
• Completely fill the collection tube, and invert it gently several times to mix the sample and the anticoagulant adequately.

Patient care checklist
Before the test
☑ Explain or clarify test purpose and procedure.
☑ Evaluate patient understanding.

Interfering factors
• Performing the test after a hemolytic episode or a blood transfusion can cause false-negative results.
• Failure to use a collection tube containing the proper anticoagulant or to mix the sample and anticoagulant adequately may hinder accurate determination of test results.
• Hemolysis caused by rough handling of the sample may affect test results.
• The following substances decrease G-6-PD enzyme activity and precipitate hemolytic episodes: aspirin, sulfonamides, nitrofurantoin, vitamin K derivatives, primaquine, and fava beans.

Growth hormone
[Human growth hormone (hGH), somatotrophic hormone (STH)]

Purpose
• To aid in differential diagnosis of dwarfism, since retarded growth in children can result from pituitary or thyroid hypofunction
• To confirm diagnosis of acromegaly and gigantism

• To aid in diagnosis of pituitary or hypothalamic tumors
• To help evaluate hGH therapy.

Normal results
hGH levels for men range from undetectable to 5 ng/ml; for women, from undetectable to 10 ng/ml. Higher values in women are due to estrogen effects. Children generally have higher hGH levels; nevertheless, they may range from undetectable to 16 ng/ml.

Abnormal results
Increased hGH levels:
associated with gigantism or acromegaly:
    Pituitary tumor
    Hypothalamic tumor.
not associated with gigantism or acromegaly:
    Diabetes mellitus (sometimes).
Decreased hGH levels:
possibly associated with dwarfism:
    Pituitary infarction
    Pituitary adenoma
    Pituitary metastatic disease.

The basics
hGH, a protein secreted by the anterior pituitary, is the primary regulator of human growth. Secretion of hGH appears to be regulated by the hypothalamus by means of a growth hormone–releasing factor and a growth hormone release–inhibiting factor (somatostatin). Secretion of hGH is diurnal and varies with such factors as exercise, sleep, stress, and nutritional status. Altered hGH levels are common in patients with pituitary dysfunction. Increased hGH levels cause gigantism in children and acromegaly in adults and adolescents. Dwarfism may be due to low hGH levels, although only 15% of all cases of growth failure relate to endocrine dysfunction.

This test, a quantitative analysis of plasma hGH levels, is usually performed as part of an anterior pituitary stimulation or suppression test. Such testing is crucial, since clinical manifestations of an hGH deficiency can rarely be reversed by therapy.

Procedure
Between 6 a.m. and 8 a.m. on 2 consecutive days, or as ordered, draw at least 7 ml of venous blood into a 10-ml, red-top collection tube.

Patient care checklist
Before the test
☑ Explain or clarify test purpose, preparation, and procedure to the patient or his parents.
☑ Evaluate understanding.
☑ Restrict food and fluid and limit physical activity for 10 to 12 hours before the test.
☑ Withhold medications that may interfere with test results, as ordered. If they must be continued, note on the laboratory slip.
☑ Encourage the patient to relax and remain recumbent for 30 minutes before the test.

Interfering factors
• Failure to follow restrictions of diet, medications, or physical activity may alter test results.
• Amphetamines, arginine, beta-blocking agents (propranolol), bromocriptine, dopamine, estrogens, glucagon, histamine, insulin, levodopa, methyldopa, and nicotinic acid raise hGH secretion. Phenothiazines (chlorpromazine) and corticosteroids reduce hGH secretion.
• A radioactive scan performed within 1 week before the test may affect results, since plasma hGH levels are determined by radioimmunoassay.
• Hemolysis due to rough handling of the sample may interfere with accurate determination of test results.
• Failure to send the sample to the laboratory immediately may affect test results, since hGH has a half-life of only 20 to 25 minutes.

Growth hormone suppression test
[Glucose loading]

Purpose
• To assess elevated baseline growth hormone (hGH) levels
• To confirm diagnosis of gigantism in children and acromegaly in adults.

Normal results
Glucose suppresses hGH to levels ranging from undetectable to 3 ng/ml in 30 minutes to 2 hours. In children, rebound stimulation may occur after 2 to 5 hours.

Abnormal results
Failure to suppress hGH levels in response to glucose loading:
Confirms acromegaly or gigantism.

The basics
This test evaluates excessive baseline levels of hGH from the anterior pituitary by measuring the secretory response to a loading dose of glucose. Normally, hGH raises plasma glucose and fatty acid concentrations; in response, insulin secretion increases to counteract these effects. Consequently, a glucose load should suppress hGH secretion.

Procedure
• Between 6 a.m. and 8 a.m., draw 6 ml of venous blood (basal sample) into a 10- to 15-ml, red-top collection tube.
• Administer 100 g of glucose solution P.O. To prevent nausea, advise the patient to drink the glucose slowly.
• After 1 to 2 hours, draw another 6 ml of venous blood into a second 10- to 15-ml, red-top collection tube.
• Label the tubes appropriately, and send each tube to the laboratory immediately.

Patient care checklist
Before the test

☑ Explain or clarify test purpose, preparation, and procedure.

☑ Evaluate patient understanding.

☑ Restrict food and fluid intake, and limit physical activity for 10 to 12 hours before the test.

☑ Warn the patient that he may experience nausea after drinking the glucose.

☑ Withhold medications that may interfere with test results, as ordered. If they must be continued, note on the laboratory slip.

☑ Encourage the patient to relax and remain recumbent for 30 minutes before the test.

Interfering factors
• Failure to observe restrictions of diet, medications, and physical activity may interfere with accurate determination of test results.

• Amphetamines, arginine, beta-blocking agents (propranolol), bromocriptine, dopamine, estrogens, glucagon, histamine, insulin, levodopa, methyldopa, and nicotinic acid increase hGH secretion.

• Phenothiazines (chlorpromazine) and corticosteroids reduce hGH secretion.

• Radioactive scans performed within 1 week before the test may affect results, since hGH levels are determined by radioimmunoassay.

• Hemolysis due to rough handling of the sample may interfere with accurate determination of test results.

• Failure to send each sample to the laboratory immediately may affect test results, since hGH has a half-life of only 20 to 25 minutes.

Hexosaminidase A and B

Purpose
• To confirm or rule out Tay-Sachs disease in neonates
• To screen for Tay-Sachs carriers

• To establish prenatal diagnosis of hexosaminidase A deficiency.

Normal results
Total serum levels of hexosaminidase range from 5 to 12.9 units/liter, with hexosaminidase A accounting for 55% to 76% of the total.

Abnormal results
Absence of hexosaminidase A:
   Tay-Sachs disease.
Absence of hexosaminidase A and hexosaminidase B:
   Sandhoff's disease.

The basics
Hexosaminidase is a group of enzymes necessary for the metabolism of gangliosides—water-soluble glycolipids found primarily in brain tissue. Deficiency of hexosaminidase A (one of the two hexosaminidase isoenzymes) causes Tay-Sachs disease. In this autosomal-recessive disorder, GM_2 ganglioside accumulates in brain tissue, resulting in progressive destruction and demyelination of central nervous system cells and, usually, death before age 5. The disorder strikes persons of Ashkenazic Jewish ancestry about 100 times more often than the general population. Sandhoff's disease, an uncommon, virulent variant of Tay-Sachs disease, produces more rapid deterioration. It results from total hexosaminidase (both A and B) deficiency, and is uncommon and not prevalent in any ethnic group. Hexosaminidase deficiency can also be identified by testing cultured skin fibroblasts. However, because this procedure is costly and technically complex, analysis of blood or of amniotic fluid is the prevalent method.

Procedure
• Perform a venipuncture, collect cord blood, or assist with amniocentesis, as appropriate.
• Collect the sample in a 7-ml, red-top tube.

• When testing a neonate, check with the laboratory concerning its preferred method for collecting serum samples from the patient. Obtain the sample from the neonates's arm, neck, or umbilical cord, as appropriate.

Patient care checklist
Before the test
☑ Explain or clarify test purpose, preparation, and procedure to the adult patient or parents of neonate.
☑ Evaluate understanding.
☑ Inform the Ashkenazic Jewish couple being tested that they both must carry the defective gene to transmit Tay-Sachs disease to their offspring.
After the test
☑ If both partners in a couple are carriers of Tay-Sachs disease, refer them for genetic counseling. Stress the importance of having amniocentesis performed as early as possible during pregnancy.
☑ If only one partner is a carrier, reassure the couple that there is no risk of their offspring inheriting the disease, since both parents must be carriers for transmission of Tay-Sachs disease to occur.

Interfering factors
Hemolysis caused by rough handling of the sample may interfere with accurate determination of test results.

Human chorionic gonadotropin (hCG)

Purpose
• To detect early pregnancy
• To determine adequacy of hormonal production in high-risk pregnancies (for example, habitual abortion)
• To aid in diagnosis of trophoblastic tumors, such as hydatidiform moles or choriocarcinoma, and of tumors that ectopically secrete hCG
• To monitor treatment for induction of ovulation and conception.

Normal results
Values for hCG are less than 3 mIU/ml. During pregnancy, hCG levels are quite variable and depend partially on the number of days after the last normal menstrual period. (See *Rate of hCG Production at Different Stages of Pregnancy.*)

Abnormal results
Very high hCG beta-subunit levels indicate:
   Multiple pregnancy.
Increased hCG beta-subunit levels usually indicate:
   Pregnancy.
may also occur in:
   Hydatidiform mole
   Trophoblastic neoplasms of the placenta
   Gastric, pancreatic, and ovarian adenocarcinoma.
Slightly increased hCG levels indicate:
   Ectopic pregnancy
   Pregnancy of less than 9 days.

The basics
hCG is a glycoprotein hormone produced by the trophoblastic cells of the placenta. If conception occurs, a specific assay for hCG—commonly called the beta-subunit assay—may detect this hormone in the blood 9 days after ovulation. This interval coincides with the implantation of the fertilized ovum into the uterine wall. Although the precise function of hCG is still unclear, it appears that hCG, with progesterone, maintains the corpus luteum during early pregnancy.

   Production of hCG increases steadily during the first trimester, peaking around the 10th week of gestation. Levels then fall to less than 10% of first trimester peak levels during the remainder of the pregnancy. At approximately 2 weeks after delivery, the hormone may no longer be detectable.

   Beta-subunit levels cannot differentiate between pregnancy and tumor recurrence, because these levels are high in both conditions.

Rate of hCG Production at Different Stages of Pregnancy

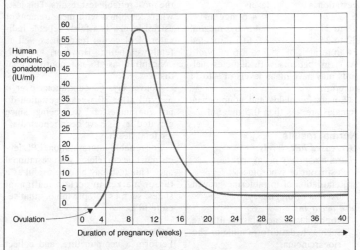

Production of human chorionic gonadotropin (hCG) increases steadily during the first trimester, peaking around the 10th week of gestation. Levels then fall to less than 10% of first trimester levels during the remainder of the pregnancy.

Adapted with permission from Arthur C. Guyton, *Textbook of Medical Physiology* (Philadelphia: W.B. Saunders Co., 1981), p.1026.

Procedure
Perform a venipuncture, and collect the sample in a 7-ml, red-top tube.

Patient care checklist
Before the test
☑ Explain or clarify test purpose and procedure.
☑ Evaluate patient understanding.

Interfering factors
• Heparin anticoagulants or EDTA depress plasma hCG levels and may interfere with accurate determination of test results. (Check with the laboratory to be sure whether the test is to be performed on plasma or serum.)
• Hemolysis due to rough handling of the sample may affect test results.

Human placental lactogen
(hPL)
[Human chorionic somatomammotropin (hCS)]

Purpose
• To assess placental function
• To aid in diagnosis of hydatidiform mole and choriocarcinoma. However, human chorionic gonadotropin levels are more diagnostic in these conditions.
• To aid in diagnosis and monitor treatment of nontrophoblastic tumors that ectopically secrete hPL.

Normal results

For pregnant females, values are as follows:

Weeks of gestation	Normal hPL levels
5 to 27	< 4.6 mcg/ml
28 to 31	2.4 to 6.1 mcg/ml
32 to 35	3.7 to 7.7 mcg/ml
36 to term	5 to 8.6 mcg/ml

At term, patients with diabetes mellitus may have mean levels of 9 to 11 mcg/ml.

Levels for males and nonpregnant females are less than 0.5 mcg/ml.

Normal results

Decreased hPL levels:
characteristically occur with:
   Postmaturity syndrome
   Retardation of intrauterine growth
   Toxemia of pregnancy.
also occur in:
   Trophoblastic neoplastic disease, such as hydatidiform mole or choriocarcinoma.
Increased hPL levels:
suggest large placenta, as in:
   Diabetes mellitus
   Multiple pregnancy
   Rh isoimmunization.
also occur in:
   Bronchogenic carcinoma
   Hepatoma
   Lymphoma
   Pheochromocytoma.

The basics

hPL, a hormone secreted by placental trophoblasts, displays lactogenic and somatotropic (growth hormone) properties in the pregnant female. Secretion is autonomous, beginning about the 5th week of gestation and declining rapidly after delivery. According to some evidence, this hormone may not be essential for a successful pregnancy.

This radioimmunoassay measures plasma hPL levels, which are roughly proportional to placental mass, as evidenced by higher levels in a multiple pregnancy. Such assays may be required in high-risk pregnancies or in suspected placental tissue dysfunction. Since values vary widely during the last half of pregnancy, serial determinations over several days provide the most reliable test results. This test, when combined with measurement of estriol levels, is a fairly reliable indicator of placental function as well as fetal well-being. However, low hPL concentrations do not confirm fetal distress.

Conversely, concentrations over 4 mcg/ml after 30 weeks' gestation do not guarantee fetal well-being, since elevated levels have been reported after fetal death.

For reliable interpretation, hPL levels must be correlated with gestational age. This test may also be useful as a tumor marker in certain malignant states, such as ectopic tumors that secrete hPL.

Procedure

Perform a venipuncture, and collect the sample in a 7-ml, red-top tube.

Patient care checklist

Before the test
☑ Explain or clarify test purpose and procedure.
☑ Evaluate patient understanding.
☑ Inform the pregnant patient that this test may be repeated during her pregnancy.

Interfering factors

Hemolysis caused by rough handling of the sample may interfere with accurate determination of test results.

Hydroxybutyric dehydrogenase *(HBD)* *[Alpha-hydroxybutyric dehydrogenase]*

Purpose

● To aid in diagnosis of myocardial infarction (MI) when lactic dehydrogenase (LDH) isoenzyme assay is unavailable

• To monitor cardiac isoenzyme activity after LDH_1 is proven to be elevated

• To detect MI after other enzyme levels drop to normal (HBD remains elevated longer)

• To aid in differentiating between cardiac and hepatic cellular damage when total LDH is elevated (LDH/HBD ratio is commonly used).

Normal results

Serum HBD values range from 114 to 290 units/ml. Ratio of serum LDH to HBD normally varies from 1.2:1 to 1.6:1.

Abnormal results

Increased HBD levels:

MI (levels peak 72 hours after onset of chest pains and remain elevated for 2 weeks)

Acute hepatocellular damage

Artifact blood sample hemolysis

Hemolytic or megaloblastic anemia.

The basics

HBD is actually total LDH that is tested using a hydroxybutyric acid substrate instead of lactic or pyruvic acid. With this substrate, the electrophoretically fast-moving LDH_1 and LDH_2 (cardiac) isoenzymes exhibit more activity than the slow-moving LDH_5 (liver) fraction, so that HBD activity roughly parallels LDH_1 and LDH_2 activity. Measurement of serum HBD is sometimes used as a substitute for LDH isoenzyme fractionation because this analysis is easier to perform and less expensive than LDH electrophoresis.

Although HBD concentration predominately reflects LDH_1 and LDH_2 activity, it may also show LDH_5 activity, if enough of this isoenzyme is present (as it is in some forms of hepatic disease). In MI, the LDH/HBD ratio is decreased due to greater activity of LDH_1 and LDH_2. However, HBD is not consistently reliable in distinguishing between myocardial and hepatocellular damage, and is less popular than it used to be.

Acute hepatitis increases the LDH/HBD ratio, since HBD levels are less sensitive to hepatocellular damage than LDH levels, which increase moderately.

Procedure

Perform a venipuncture, and collect the sample in a 7-ml, red-top tube.

Special precautions

For patients with MI, draw blood at the same time each morning.

Patient care checklist

Before the test

☑ Explain or clarify test purpose and procedure.

☑ Evaluate patient understanding.

☑ Tell the patient suspected of having an MI that the test will be repeated on subsequent mornings to monitor his progress.

Interfering factors

• Failure to draw the sample on schedule, missing peak levels, may interfere with accurate determination of values.

• If the sample is not sent to the laboratory promptly or is not refrigerated, test results may be affected.

• Cardioversion or extensive surgery can elevate HBD levels.

• Hemolysis caused by rough handling of the sample may affect test results.

Insulin

Purpose

• To aid in diagnosis of hypoglycemia resulting from tumor or hyperplasia of pancreatic islet cells, glucocorticoid deficiency, or severe hepatic disease

• To aid in diagnosis of diabetes mellitus and insulin-resistant states.

Normal results

Serum insulin levels range from undetectable to 25 μU/ml.

Abnormal results

Insulin levels are interpreted in light of the prevailing glucose concentration. A normal insulin level may be inappropriate for the glucose results. High insulin and low glucose levels after a significant fast suggest an insulinoma. In insulin-resistant diabetic states, insulin levels are elevated; in non-insulin-resistant diabetes, they are low.

The basics

This radioimmunoassay is a quantitative analysis of serum insulin levels, which are always measured concomitantly with glucose levels, since glucose is the primary stimulus for insulin release from pancreatic islet cells. It helps evaluate patients suspected of having hyperinsulinemia due to pancreatic tumor or hyperplasia. Prolonged fasting or stimulation testing may be required to confirm diagnosis of an insulinoma.

Insulin, a hormone secreted by beta cells of the islets of Langerhans, regulates the metabolism and transport or mobilization of carbohydrates, amino acids, and lipids. Stimulated by increased plasma levels of glucose, insulin secretion reaches peak levels after meals, when metabolism and food storage are greatest. An insufficient level of insulin or resistance to its effects is the primary abnormality in diabetes mellitus.

Procedure

• Perform a venipuncture, and collect one sample for insulin level in a 7-ml, red-top tube.
• Collect another sample, for glucose, in a gray-top tube.
• Pack the sample for insulin in ice, and send it, along with the glucose sample, to the laboratory immediately.

Special precautions

CLINICAL ALERT: **In the patient with an insulinoma, this test may precipitate dangerously severe hypoglycemia. Keep glucose I.V. (50%) available to combat possible hypoglycemia.**

Connecting Peptide

Connecting peptide (C-peptide) is a biologically inactive peptide chain formed during the proteolytic conversion of proinsulin to insulin in the pancreatic beta cells. It has no insulin effect, either biologically or immunologically. This is important, because circulating insulin is measured by immunologic assay. As insulin is released into the bloodstream, the C-peptide chain splits off from the hormone. Except in patients with islet cell tumors and, possibly, in obese patients, serum C-peptide levels generally parallel those of insulin: normal values range between 0.9 and 4.2 ng/ml.

A C-peptide assay may help to:
• Determine the cause of hypoglycemia by distinguishing between endogenous hyperinsulinism and insulinoma (elevated C-peptide levels) and surreptitious insulin injection (decreased C-peptide levels).
• Determine beta cell function in patients with diabetes mellitus. Absence of C-peptide indicates no beta cell function; presence indicates residual beta cell function.
• Indirectly measure insulin secretion in the presence of circulating insulin antibodies, which interfere with insulin assays but not with C-peptide assays.
• Detect residual tissue (some C-peptide present) after total pancreatectomy for carcinoma.
• Indicate the remission phase (some C-peptide present) of diabetes mellitus.

Patient care checklist
Before the test

☑ Explain or clarify test purpose, preparation, and procedure.

☑ Evaluate patient understanding.

☑ Restrict food and fluid for 10 to 12 hours before the test. (Questionable results may make it necessary to repeat the test or, commonly, to perform a glucose tolerance test simultaneously, which requires that the patient drink glucose solution.)

☑ Withhold medications that may interfere with test results, as ordered. If they must be continued, note them on the laboratory slip.

☑ Encourage the patient to relax and remain recumbent for 30 minutes before the test.

Interfering factors

• Failure to observe restrictions of diet and activity may affect test results.

• Use of adrenocorticotropic hormone, steroids (including oral contraceptives), thyroid hormones, or epinephrine increases insulin requirements by exerting a hyperglycemic effect, thereby raising serum insulin levels.

• Use of insulin by non-insulin-dependent patients suppresses endogenous insulin secretion, lowering levels. (See *Connecting Peptide*.)

• In patients with insulin-dependent diabetes mellitus, high levels of insulin antibodies may interfere with the test.

• Failure to pack the insulin sample in ice and send it to the laboratory promptly, or hemolysis caused by rough handling of the sample, may hinder accurate determination of test results.

Insulin tolerance test

Purpose

• To aid in diagnosis of human growth hormone (hGH) or adrenocorticotropic hormone (ACTH) deficiency

• To identify pituitary dysfunction

• To aid in differential diagnosis of primary and secondary adrenal hypofunction.

Normal results

Blood glucose falls to 50% of the fasting level 20 to 30 minutes after insulin administration. This stimulates a 10 to 20 ng/dl increase over baseline values in both human chorionic gonadotropin (hCG) and ACTH, with peak levels occurring 60 to 90 minutes after insulin administration.

Abnormal results
Failure of stimulation of a blunted response:
  Hypothalamic-pituitary-adrenal axis dysfunction.
hGH levels increased less than 10 ng/ dl above basal suggest:
  hGH deficiency.
ACTH levels increased less than 10 ng/dl above basal suggest:
  Adrenal insufficiency.

The basics

This test measures serum levels of hGH and ACTH after administration of a loading dose of insulin. It is more reliable than direct measurement of hGH and ACTH, because healthy persons often have undetectable fasting levels of these hormones. Insulin-induced hypoglycemia stimulates hGH and ACTH secretion in persons with an intact hypothalamic-pituitary-adrenal axis. Failure of stimulation indicates anterior pituitary or adrenal hypofunction, and helps confirm an hGH or ACTH insufficiency. However, definitive diagnosis of hGH deficiency requires a supplementary stimulation test, such as the arginine test. Additional testing is necessary to determine the site of the abnormality.

The metyrapone or ACTH stimulation test confirms adrenal insufficiency and determines whether insufficiency is primary or secondary.

Because the insulin tolerance test stimulates an adrenergic response, it is not recommended for patients with cardiovascular or cerebrovascular disorders, epilepsy, or low basal plasma cortisol levels.

Procedure

• Between 6 a.m. and 8 a.m., collect three 5-ml samples of venous blood for basal levels—one in a gray-top tube (for blood glucose) and two in green-top tubes (for hGH and ACTH).
• Then, administer an I.V. bolus of U-100 regular insulin (0.15 unit/kg, or as ordered) over a 1- to 2-minute period.
• Draw additional blood samples 15, 30, 45, 60, 90, and 120 minutes after administration of insulin. Use an indwelling venous catheter to avoid repeated venipunctures. At each interval, collect three samples: one in a gray-top tube and two in green-top tubes.
• Label the tubes appropriately, including the collection time, and send them to the laboratory immediately.

Special precautions

CLINICAL ALERT: Have concentrated glucose solution readily available in case of severe hypoglycemic reaction to insulin. To minimize the possibility of such a reaction, use highly purified pork or human insulin.

Patient care checklist

Before the test

☑ Explain or clarify test purpose, preparation, and procedure.
☑ Evaluate patient understanding.
☑ Withhold food and restrict physical activity for 10 to 12 hours before the test.
☑ Warn the patient that he may experience an increased heart rate, diaphoresis, hunger, and anxiety after administration of the insulin. Reassure him that these symptoms are transient, but that if they become severe, the test will be discontinued.
☑ Inform the patient that the test takes about 2 hours, and that results are usually available in 2 days.

☑ Encourage the patient to relax and remain recumbent for 90 minutes before the test.
☑ Withhold medications that may interfere with test results, as ordered. If they must be continued, note them on the laboratory slip.

Interfering factors

• Failure to follow restrictions of diet, physical activity, and medications may prevent reliable test results.
• Steroids such as progestogen, estrogen, and pituitary-based drugs elevate hGH levels; glucocorticoids and beta blockers depress hGH levels.
• Glucocorticoids, estrogens, calcium gluconate, amphetamines, methamphetamines, spironolactone, and ethanol depress ACTH levels.
• Hemolysis caused by rough handling of the sample may affect test results.

Isocitrate dehydrogenase (ICD)

Purpose

• To aid in diagnosis of acute hepatocellular damage
• To detect early viral hepatitis and infectious mononucleosis
• To distinguish between hepatic disease and myocardial infarction (MI) when serum glutamic-oxaloacetic transaminase (SGOT) is elevated.

Normal results

Serum ICD values range from 1.2 to 7 units/liter at 86° F. (30° C.), as measured by continuous monitoring. Neonates may have serum levels four times as high as normal adult values for the first 2 weeks after birth.

Abnormal results

Markedly increased serum ICD levels (10 to 40 times normal):
    Acute viral hepatitis.
Moderately increased levels:
    Hepatic metastases

Moderate or severe passive hepatic
congestion
Active cirrhosis
Biliary tract inflammation
Neonatal biliary duct atresia
Drug-induced hepatic injury
Infectious mononucleosis.

The basics

ICD, an enzyme involved in the Krebs
cycle, appears primarily in the liver in
a stable, electrophoretically fast-moving form, and in the heart in a heat-
labile form that quickly loses its activity when released into serum. It is
also present in skeletal muscles, platelets, red blood cells, and the placenta.
This test, which measures total ICD
levels in a serum sample, is as sensitive
as but more specific for hepatic disease than measurement of SGOT: ICD
levels generally rise in acute hepatocellular damage but remain normal in
acute MI.

ICD levels increase as early as the
incubation period in acute viral hepatitis
and return to normal during the 3rd week
of illness, unless the infection becomes
chronic. Since ICD offers no advantages
over serum glutamic-pyruvic transaminase (SGPT), it is rarely ordered, and
no clinical significance has been associated with isoenzyme fractionation.

Procedure

Perform a venipuncture, and collect
the sample in a 7-ml red-top tube.

Patient care checklist

Before the test

☑ Explain or clarify test purpose and
procedure.

☑ Evaluate patient understanding.

Interfering factors

• Alcohol, aminosalicylic acid, isoniazid, methotrexate, and phenylbutazone increase ICD levels due to their
effect on liver cells.

• Hemolysis due to rough handling of
the sample may interfere with accurate
determination of ICD levels.

Lactic acid and pyruvic acid
[Lactate and pyruvate]

Purpose

• To assess tissue oxidation
• To help determine the cause of lactic
acidosis.

Normal results

Blood lactate values range from 0.93
to 1.65 mEq/liter; pyruvate levels,
from 0.08 to 0.16 mEq/liter. The lac-
tate-pyruvate ratio is less than 10:1.

Abnormal results

Increased blood lactate levels:

Strenuous muscle exercise
Shock
Hemorrhage
Septicemia
Myocardial infarction
Pulmonary embolism
Cardiac arrest
Diabetes mellitus
Leukemias
Lymphomas
Hepatic disease
Renal failure
Enzymatic defects, such as glyco-
gen storage disease
Ingestion of large doses of acet-
aminophen and ethanol
I.V. infusion of epinephrine, glu-
cagon, fructose, and sorbitol.

The basics

Lactic acid, present in blood as lactate
ion, is derived primarily from muscle
cells and erythrocytes. It is an intermediate product of carbohydrate metabolism and is normally metabolized
by the liver. Blood lactate concentration depends on the rate of production
and on the rate of metabolism.

Lactate is the reduction product of
pyruvate, a by-product of carbohydrate
metabolism. Together these compounds form a reversible reaction that
is regulated by oxygen supply. When
oxygen levels are deficient, pyruvate

converts to lactate; when they are adequate, lactate converts to pyruvate. When the hepatic system fails to metabolize lactate sufficiently, or when excess pyruvate converts to lactate due to tissue hypoxia and circulatory collapse, lactic acidosis (lactate levels more than 2 mEq/liter, with a pH lower than 7.37) may result. Measurement of blood lactate levels is recommended for all patients with symptoms of lactic acidosis, such as Kussmaul's respiration.

Although arterial or venous blood can be used for lactate analysis, a venous sample is more convenient to obtain. However, unless the patient rests for 1 hour before the test, venous blood may yield higher values than arterial blood. Comparison of pyruvate and lactate levels reliably mirrors tissue oxidation, but measurement of pyruvate is technically difficult and infrequently performed.

Procedure
• Perform a venipuncture, and collect the sample in a 5-ml, gray-top tube.
• Place the sample container in an ice-filled cup, and send it to the laboratory immediately.

Patient care checklist
Before the test
☑ Explain or clarify test purpose, preparation, and procedure to the patient, even though he is likely to be comatose or extremely lethargic.
☑ Restrict food and fluid overnight before the test.
☑ Advise the patient to rest for at least 1 hour before the test.
☑ Tell the patient not to clench his fist during the venipuncture.

Interfering factors
• Failure to adhere to restrictions of diet and activity may interfere with accurate determination of test results.
• Failure to pack the sample in ice and to transport it to the laboratory immediately may elevate blood lactate levels.

• Venostasis related to a clenched fist during venipuncture may raise blood lactate levels.

Lactic dehydrogenase
(LDH)

Purpose
• To aid in differential diagnosis of myocardial infarction (MI), pulmonary infarction, anemias, and hepatic disease.
• To support creatine phosphokinase (CPK) isoenzyme test results in diagnosing MI, or to provide diagnosis when CPK-MB samples are drawn too late to display elevation.
• To monitor patient response to some forms of chemotherapy.

Normal results
Total LDH levels range from 48 to 115 IU/liter. Distribution is as follows:
   LDH_1: 18.1% to 29% of total
   LDH_2: 29.4% to 37.5% of total
   LDH_3: 18.8% to 26% of total
   LDH_4: 9.2% to 16.5% of total
   LDH_5: 5.3% to 13.4% of total.

Abnormal results
(See *Diagnostic LDH Isoenzyme Variations in Disease*.)

The basics
Because LDH is present in almost all body tissues, cellular damage causes an elevation of total serum LDH, thus limiting the diagnostic usefulness of LDH. However, five tissue-specific isoenzymes can be identified and measured, using heat inactivation or electrophoresis: two of these isoenzymes, LDH_1 and LDH_2, appear primarily in the heart, red blood cells (RBCs), and kidneys; LDH_3, primarily in the lungs; and LDH_4 and LDH_5, in the liver and the skeletal muscles.

The specificity of LDH isoenzymes and their distribution pattern are useful in diagnosing hepatic, pulmonary, and erythrocytic damage. But their

Diagnostic LDH Isoenzyme Variations in Disease

Diseases	LDH$_1$	LDH$_2$	LDH$_3$	LDH$_4$	LDH$_5$
Cardiovascular					
Myocardial infarction	Diagnostic	Diagnostic			
Myocardial infarction with hepatic congestion	Diagnostic	Diagnostic			Diagnostic
Rheumatic carditis	Diagnostic	Diagnostic			
Myocarditis	Diagnostic	Diagnostic			
Congestive heart failure (decompensated)					Diagnostic
Shock	Diagnostic	Diagnostic	Diagnostic	Diagnostic	Diagnostic
Angina pectoris	Normal	Normal			
Pulmonary					
Pulmonary embolism	Normal	Normal			
Pulmonary infarction			Diagnostic		
Hematologic					
Pernicious anemia	Diagnostic	Diagnostic			
Hemolytic anemia	Diagnostic	Diagnostic			
Sickle cell anemia	Diagnostic	Diagnostic			
Hepatobiliary					
Hepatitis					Diagnostic
Active cirrhosis					Diagnostic
Hepatic congestion					Diagnostic

Normal ■   Diagnostic ▨   Not diagnostic □

Adapted with permission from information from Helena Laboratories, 1513 Lindberg Dr., Beaumont, Tex.

widest clinical application (with other cardiac enzyme tests) is in diagnosing acute MI. LDH isoenzyme assay is also useful when CPK has not been measured within 24 hours of an acute MI. The myocardial LDH level rises later than CPK (12 to 48 hours after infarction begins), peaks in 2 to 5 days, and drops to normal in 7 to 10 days, if tissue necrosis does not persist.

Specifically, in acute MI, the concentration of LDH_1 is greater than LDH_2 within 12 to 48 hours after onset of symptoms. This reversal of normal isoenzyme patterns is typical of myocardial damage and is referred to as "flipped LDH."

Procedure
• Perform a venipuncture, and collect the sample in a 7-ml, red-top tube.
• Draw the samples on schedule to avoid missing peak levels, and mark the collection time on the laboratory slip.

Patient care checklist
Before the test
☑ Explain or clarify test purpose and procedure.
☑ Evaluate patient understanding.
☑ Tell the patient suspected of having MI that the test will be repeated on the next two mornings to monitor progressive changes.

Interfering factors
• Hemolysis due to rough handling of the sample may affect accurate determination of LDH levels, since RBCs contain LDH_1.
• For diagnosis of acute MI, failure to draw the sample on schedule may interfere with test results.
• Failure to send the sample to the laboratory immediately, or to keep the sample at room temperature, may influence determination of LDH isoenzyme patterns.
• Recent surgery or pregnancy can cause elevated LDH levels. Chronic hemolysis, caused by prosthetic heart valves, may also increase LDH levels.

Leucine aminopeptidase
(LAP)
[Amino acid arylamidase]

Purpose
• To aid in differentiating hepatic disease from skeletal disease when LAP is elevated from an unknown cause
• To help distinguish between congenital biliary atresia and neonatal hepatitis.

Normal results
LAP levels should be less than 50 units/liter or, in Goldberg-Rutenberg units, 80 to 200 units/ml for males and 75 to 185 units/ml for females.

Abnormal results
Increased LAP levels:
Obstructive jaundice, such as from liver metastases, common bile duct calculus, cancer of the head of the pancreas
Hepatitis
Cirrhosis
Pancreatitis
Biliary atresia (more than 500 units/liter)
Neonatal hepatitis (less than 500 units/liter).

The basics
LAP is a proteolytic enzyme found in all body tissues but concentrated in several isoenzyme forms in the liver, pancreas, and small intestine. LAP levels tend to parallel those of alkaline phosphatase in hepatic disease and normal pregnancy; but unlike alkaline phosphatase, LAP remains normal in skeletal disease. Despite its relative hepatobiliary specificity, this test—which measures serum LAP levels—is not commonly performed. In the past, it has been used to diagnose pancreatic cancer, but has proven unreliable for this purpose. Recent research suggests that LAP isoenzyme determination may be beneficial in evalu-

ating neonatal jaundice. Two zones of electrophoretic activity suggest biliary atresia, while in neonatal hepatitis, only a single isoenzyme is detected by fractionation.

Procedure
Perform a venipuncture and collect the sample in a 7-ml, red-top tube.

Patient care checklist
Before the test
☑ Explain or clarify test purpose and procedure to the patient or to parents.
☑ Evaluate understanding.
☑ Restrict food and fluids, only if required by individual laboratory (procedures vary).

Interfering factors
• Estrogens, progesterone, pregnancy, and oral contraceptives can cause elevated LAP levels.
• Hemolysis due to rough handling of the sample may hinder accurate determination of test results.

Lipase

Purpose
To aid in diagnosis of acute pancreatitis.

Normal results
Serum levels range from 32 to 80 units/liter.

Abnormal results
Increased lipase levels:
  Acute pancreatitis
  Pancreatic duct obstruction
  Perforated peptic ulcer with chemical pancreatitis
  High intestinal obstruction
  Pancreatic cancer
  Renal disease with impaired excretion.

The basics
Lipase is produced in the pancreas and secreted into the duodenum, where it converts triglycerides and other fats into fatty acids and glycerol. Destruction of pancreatic cells, which occurs in acute pancreatitis, releases large amounts of lipase into the blood. Levels commonly remain elevated for up to 14 days. This test is most useful in diagnosing acute pancreatitis when performed with a serum or urine amylase test.

Procedure
Perform a venipuncture, and collect the sample in a 7-ml, red-top tube.

Patient care checklist
Before the test
☑ Explain or clarify test purpose, preparation, and procedure.
☑ Evaluate patient understanding.
☑ Restrict food and fluid intake overnight before the test.
☑ Withhold medications that may interfere with test results, as ordered. If they must be continued, note them on the laboratory slip.

Interfering factors
• Cholinergics, codeine, meperidine, and morphine cause spasm of the sphincter of Oddi, producing false-positive results.
• Hemolysis due to rough handling of the sample may interfere with accurate determination of test results.

Lipoprotein-cholesterol fractionation

Purpose
To assess the risk of coronary artery disease (CAD).

Normal results
Since normal cholesterol values vary according to age, sex, geographic region, and ethnic group, check the laboratory for the normal values in your hospital. An alternate method—measuring cholesterol and triglyceride levels, separating out high-density

lipoprotein (HDL) by selective precipitation, and using these values to calculate low-density lipoprotein (LDL)—provides HDL-cholesterol levels that range from 29 to 77 mg/100 ml and LDL-cholesterol levels that range from 62 to 185 mg/100 ml.

Abnormal results

Increased LDL levels indicate:
   Increased risk of CAD.
Increased HDL levels generally reflect a healthy state, but can indicate:
   Chronic hepatitis
   Early primary biliary cirrhosis
   Alcohol consumption.
Sharp increases in alpha-2-HDL levels may signal:
   CAD.

The basics
Cholesterol fractionation tests isolate

Apolipoproteins and CAD

Although measurement of apolipoproteins—the protein fractions of lipoprotein molecules—is primarily a research procedure, mounting evidence suggests that it may have important clinical applications as well. Because apolipoprotein levels can be directly measured in serum, they may more accurately indicate an individual's risk of coronary artery disease (CAD) than high-density lipoprotein (HDL) or low-density lipoprotein (LDL) levels, which must be indirectly measured.

Currently, eight apolipoproteins have been identified. Of these, apolipoprotein A (ApoA)—the major protein component of HDL—and apolipoprotein B (ApoB)—the major protein component of LDL—are the most clinically significant. Reduced ApoA levels (below 140 mg/dl) occur in ischemic heart disease, while elevated ApoB levels (above 135 mg/dl) occur in hyperlipemia, angina pectoris, and myocardial infarction.

---

and measure the cholesterol in serum—LDL and HDL—by ultracentrifugation or electrophoresis. The cholesterol in LDL and HDL fractions is significant, since the Framingham Heart Study has shown that cholesterol in HDL is inversely related to the incidence of CAD—the higher the HDL level, the lower the incidence of CAD; conversely, the higher the LDL level, the higher the incidence of CAD.

Procedure
• Perform a venipuncture, and collect the sample in a 7-ml, red-top tube.
• Send the sample to the laboratory immediately. If the sample cannot be transported immediately, it should be refrigerated but not frozen.

Patient care checklist
Before the test
☑ Explain or clarify test purpose, preparation, and procedure.
☑ Evaluate patient understanding.
☑ Instruct the patient to maintain a normal diet for 2 weeks before the test.
☑ Advise the patient to abstain from alcohol for 24 hours before the test.
☑ Tell the patient to restrict food and fluid intake and to avoid exercise for 12 to 14 hours before the test.
☑ Withhold medications that may interfere with test results, as ordered. If they must be continued, note them on the laboratory slip.

Interfering factors
• Values are lowered by antilipemic medications, such as clofibrate, cholestyramine, colestipol, dextrothyroxine, niacin, probucol, and gemfibrozil.
• Oral contraceptives, disulfiram, alcohol, miconazole, and high doses of phenothiazines may increase values.
• Estrogens usually increase but may decrease values.
• Failure to send the sample to the laboratory immediately may allow spontaneous redistribution of the lipoproteins and alter test results.
• Collecting the sample in a heparin-

ized tube may produce false elevation of values through activation of the enzyme lipase, which, in turn, causes the release of fatty acids from triglycerides.

• Presence of bilirubin, hemoglobin, salicylates, iodine, vitamins A and D, and some other substances may affect accurate determination of values. Some procedures (for example, Abell-Kendall) are less susceptible to interference than others.

• Concurrent illness, especially if accompanied by fever, recent surgery, or myocardial infarction, may interfere with accurate determination of test results. (Also see *Apolipoproteins and CAD*.)

Lipoprotein phenotyping

Purpose
To determine classification of hyper- or hypolipoproteinemia.

Normal results
Normal electrophoretic pattern.

Abnormal results
The types of familial hyperlipoproteinemias are identified by their characteristic electrophoretic patterns.
A heavy chylomicron bond with faint beta and pre-beta bands:
  Type I.
Heavy beta and negligible pre-beta bands:
  Type II-A.
Heavy beta and pre-beta bands:
  Type II-B.
Two beta bands that merge:
  Type III.
Heavy pre-beta band:
  Type IV.
Chylomicron and pre-beta bands that are most distinct:
  Type V.
  (See *Familial Hyperlipoproteinemias,* pp. 106-107; and *Hyperlipoproteinemias: Electrophoretic Patterns on Paper,* p. 108.)

The basics
Lipoprotein phenotyping is a useful screening test for younger patients with a family history of coronary artery disease that suggests a need for early preventive therapy (primarily dietary adjustments). In lipoprotein phenotyping, ultracentrifugation and electrophoresis of a blood sample determine lipoprotein levels. The lipoproteins are separated into four bands: chylomicrons, pre-beta, beta, and alpha. Their density varies, depending on their relative percentages of triglyceride and protein: chylomicrons, which are very light lipid aggregates, consist of 85% to 95% triglycerides, 5% to 10% phospholipids, 3% to 5% cholesterol, and 1% to 2% protein; very-low-density (prebeta) lipoproteins (VLDL) consist of 64% to 80% triglycerides, 7% to 14% phospholipids, 7% to 14% cholesterol, and 2% to 13% protein; low-density (beta) lipoproteins (LDL) consist of 7% to 10% triglycerides, 20% to 30% phospholipids, 35% to 45% cholesterol, and 15% to 38% protein; and high-density (alpha) lipoproteins (HDL) consist of about 1% to 7% triglycerides, 28% to 30% phospholipids, 17% to 20% cholesterol, and 49% to 50% protein.

For transportation through the blood, most lipids must combine with water-soluble proteins (apoproteins) to form lipoproteins. Several types of lipoproteins normally exist in the body, but in certain familial disorders, the blood levels of these types change. Classification of patients by the pattern of their lipoprotein levels identifies hyperlipoproteinemias and hypolipoproteinemias.

The hyperlipoproteinemias break down into six types: I, II-a, II-b, III, IV, and V. Types II-a, II-b, and IV are relatively common. In contrast, all hypolipoproteinemias are rare, and include hypobetalipoproteinemia, abetalipoproteinemia (Bassen-Kornzweig syndrome) and alpha-lipoprotein deficiency (Tangier disease).

Familial Hyperlipoproteinemias

Type	Causes and incidence	Clinical signs	Laboratory findings
I	• Deficient lipoprotein lipase, resulting in increased chylomicrons • May be induced by alcoholism • Incidence: rare	• Eruptive xanthomas • Lipemia retinalis • Abdominal pain	• Increased chylomicron, total cholesterol, and triglyceride levels • Normal or slightly increased very-low-density lipoprotein (VLDL) levels • Normal or decreased low-density lipoprotein (LDL) and high-density lipoprotein (HDL) levels • Cholesterol-triglyceride ratio under 0.2
IIa	• Deficient cell receptor, resulting in increased LDL and excessive cholesterol synthesis • May be induced by hypothyroidism • Incidence: common	• Premature coronary artery disease (CAD) • Arcus cornea • Xanthelasma • Tendinous and tuberous xanthomas	• Increased LDL • Normal VLDL • Cholesterol-triglyceride ratio over 2.0
IIb	• Deficient cell receptor resulting in increased LDL and excessive cholesterol synthesis • May be induced by dysgammaglobulinemia, hypothyroidism, uncontrolled diabetes mellitus, and nephrotic syndrome • Incidence: common	• Premature CAD • Obesity • Possible xanthelasmas	• Increased LDL, VLDL, total cholesterol, and triglycerides
III	• Unknown cause, resulting in deficient VLDL-to-LDL conversion • May be induced by hypothyroidism, uncontrolled diabetes mellitus, and paraproteinemia • Incidence: rare	• Premature CAD • Arcus cornea • Eruptive tuberous xanthomas	• Increased total cholesterol, VLDL, and triglycerides • Normal or decreased LDL • Cholesterol-triglyceride ratio of VLDL over 0.4 • Broad beta band observed on electrophoresis

(continued)

Familial Hyperlipoproteinemias (continued)

Type	Causes and incidence	Clinical signs	Laboratory findings
IV	• Unknown cause, resulting in decreased levels of lipoprotein lipase • May be induced by uncontrolled diabetes mellitus, alcoholism, pregnancy, steroid or estrogen therapy, dysgammaglobulinemia, and hyperthyroidism • Incidence: common	• Possible premature CAD • Obesity • Hypertension • Peripheral neuropathy	• Increased VLDL and triglycerides • Normal LDL • Cholesterol-triglyceride ratio of VLDL under 0.25
V	• Unknown cause, resulting in defective triglyceride clearance • May be induced by alcoholism, dysgammaglobulinemia, uncontrolled diabetes mellitus, nephrotic syndrome, pancreatitis, and steroid therapy • Incidence: rare	• Premature CAD • Abdominal pain • Lipemia retinalis • Eruptive xanthomas • Hepatosplenomegaly	• Increased VLDL, total cholesterol, and triglycerides • Chylomicrons present • Cholesterol-triglyceride ratio under 0.6

Procedure

• Perform a venipuncture, and collect the sample in a 7-ml, lavender-top tube.
• Fill the collection tube completely, and invert it gently several times to mix the sample and the anticoagulant.

Special precautions

When drawing multiple samples, collect the sample for lipoprotein phenotyping first, since venous obstruction for 2 minutes can affect test results.

Patient care checklist

Before the test

☑ Explain or clarify test purpose, preparation, and procedure.
☑ Evaluate patient understanding.
☑ Advise the patient to abstain from alcohol for 24 hours before the test.
☑ Tell the patient to eat a low-fat meal the night before the test.

☑ Instruct the patient to restrict food and fluid intake after midnight the night before the test.
☑ Withhold antilipemics, such as cholestyramine, for about 2 weeks before the test, as ordered.
☑ Notify the laboratory if the patient is hospitalized for any other condition that might alter lipoprotein metabolism, such as diabetes mellitus, nephrosis, or hypothyroidism.

Interfering factors

• Hemolysis due to rough handling of the sample may affect accurate determination of test results.
• Failure to observe diet and alcohol restrictions or recent use of antilipemics (which lower lipid levels) may interfere with accurate determination of values.
• Administration of heparin (which

Hyperlipoproteinemias: Electrophoretic Patterns on Paper

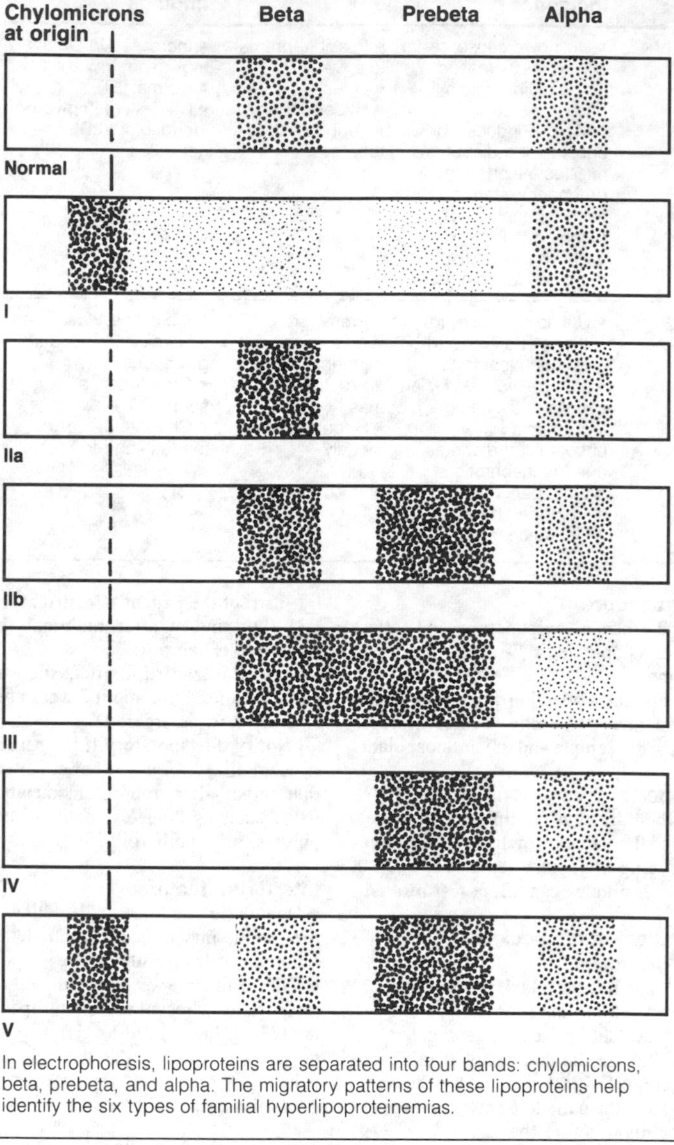

Chylomicrons at origin	Beta	Prebeta	Alpha

Normal

I

IIa

IIb

III

IV

V

In electrophoresis, lipoproteins are separated into four bands: chylomicrons, beta, prebeta, and alpha. The migratory patterns of these lipoproteins help identify the six types of familial hyperlipoproteinemias.

activates the enzyme lipase, producing fatty acids from triglycerides) or collection of the sample in a heparinized tube may falsely elevate values.

Long-acting thyroid stimulator *(LATS)*

Purpose
To confirm diagnosis of Graves' disease. (This test is not done routinely to diagnose thyroid disorders.)

Normal results
LATS does not appear in serum.

Abnormal results
LATS in serum:
  Graves' disease.

The basics
In this test, the McKenzie mouse bioassay method is used to determine whether a patient's serum contains LATS, an abnormal immunoglobulin (called 75 IgG) that mimics the action of thyroid-stimulating hormone (TSH), although its effects are more prolonged. LATS stimulates the thyroid gland to produce and secrete thyroid hormones in excessive amounts. Thus, through the normal negative feedback mechanism, it inhibits TSH secretion. LATS is found in about 80% of patients with Graves' disease, whether or not overt signs of hyperthyroidism are present. It is also found in a neonate whose mother has Graves' disease, as LATS crosses the placenta. Some authorities believe that the thyroid gland hyperplasia seen in Graves' disease may be due to LATS or other circulating antibodies. Some consider the clinical significance of this test questionable.

Procedure
Draw venous blood into a 5-ml, red-top tube.

Patient care checklist
Before the test
☑ Explain or clarify test purpose and procedure to the patient or parents of a neonate.
☑ Evaluate understanding.
☑ Note on the laboratory slip if the patient had an ^{131}I radioactive scan within 48 hours before the test.

Interfering factors
• Radioactive iodine in the serum may affect test results.
• Hemolysis due to rough handling of the sample may interfere with accurate determination of test results.

Luteinizing hormone *(LH)* *[Interstitial cell-stimulating hormone (ICSH)]*

Purpose
• To detect ovulation
• To assess male or female infertility
• To evaluate amenorrhea
• To monitor therapy designed to induce ovulation.

Normal results
Adult males: 5 to 20 mIU/ml
Postmenopausal females: 50 to 100 mIU/ml
Adult females: Values vary, depending on the phase of the patient's menstrual cycle—follicular phase: 5 to 15 mIU/ml; midcycle (ovulation): 30 to 60 mIU/ml; luteal phase: 5 to 15 mIU/ml
Children: 4 to 20 mIU/ml.

Abnormal results
For females:
Absence of a midcycle peak in LH secretion:
  Anovulation.
Decreased or low-normal LH levels:
  Hypogonadotropism.

Increased LH levels:
  Congenital absence of ovaries
  Stein-Leventhal syndrome
  Turner's syndrome
  Early-stage acromegaly.
For males:
Decreased LH levels:
  Gonadal dysfunction of hypothalamic or pituitary origin.
Increased LH levels:
  Testicular failure
  Destruction or congenital absence of testes.

The basics

This test, usually ordered for anovulation and infertility studies and performed most often on females, is a quantitative analysis of plasma LH levels. For accurate diagnosis, results must be evaluated in light of findings obtained from related hormone tests—follicle-stimulating hormone (FSH), estrogen, and testosterone tests, for example. LH is a glycoprotein secreted by the anterior pituitary. In females, cyclic LH secretion (with FSH) causes ovulation and transforms the ovarian follicle into the corpus luteum, which, in turn, secretes progesterone. In males, continuous LH secretion stimulates the cells of the testes to release testosterone, which (with FSH) stimulates and maintains spermatogenesis.

Procedure

• Perform a venipuncture, and collect the sample in a 7-ml, red-top tube.
• If the patient is a female, indicate the phase of her menstrual cycle on the laboratory slip. If the patient is menopausal, note this on the laboratory slip.

Patient care checklist

Before the test
☑ Explain or clarify test purpose, preparation, and procedure.
☑ Evaluate patient understanding.
☑ Inform the patient that the laboratory requires at least 3 days to complete the analysis.

☑ Withhold medications that may interfere with test results, as ordered, for 48 hours before the test. If they must be continued, note them on the laboratory slip.

Interfering factors

• Failure to observe medication restrictions may interfere with accurate determination of test results. Steroids (including estrogens, progesterone, and testosterone) may decrease plasma LH levels.
• A radioactive scan performed within 1 week before the test may influence test results, since plasma LH levels are determined by radioimmunoassay.
• Hemolysis due to rough handling of the sample may interfere with accurate determination of test results.

Magnesium

Purpose

• To evaluate electrolyte status
• To assess neuromuscular or renal function.

Normal results

Serum magnesium levels range from 1.7 to 2.1 mg/dl (atomic absorption) or from 1.5 to 2.5 mEq/liter.

Abnormal results

Increased serum magnesium levels:
  Renal failure
  Addison's disease.
Decreased levels:
  Chronic alcoholism
  Malabsorption syndrome
  Diarrhea
  Faulty absorption following bowel resection
  Prolonged bowel or gastric aspiration
  Acute pancreatitis
  Primary aldosteronism
  Severe burns
  Hypercalcemic conditions (including hyperparathyroidism)
  Certain diuretic therapies.

The basics

This test measures serum levels of magnesium, the most abundant intracellular cation after potassium. Vital to neuromuscular function, this often-overlooked electrolyte helps regulate intracellular metabolism, activates many essential enzymes, and affects the metabolism of nucleic acids and proteins. Magnesium also helps transport sodium and potassium across cell membranes and, through its effect on the secretion of parathyroid hormone, influences intracellular calcium levels. Most magnesium is found in bone and in intracellular fluid; a small amount is found in extracellular fluid. Magnesium is absorbed by the small intestine and is excreted in the urine and feces.

Special precautions

• Handle the sample gently to prevent hemolysis. (NOTE: This is especially important with this test, since 75% of the blood's magnesium is present in red blood cells.)

CLINICAL ALERT: **In suspected or confirmed hypermagnesemia, observe the patient for lethargy; flushing; diaphoresis; decreased blood pressure; slow, weak pulse; diminished deep-tendon reflexes; muscle weakness; and slow, shallow respirations.**

CLINICAL ALERT: **In suspected or confirmed hypomagnesemia, watch for leg and foot cramps, hyperactive deep-tendon reflexes, cardiac dysrhythmias, muscle weakness, seizures, twitching, tetany, and tremors.**

Patient care checklist

Before the test

☑ Explain or clarify test purpose, preparation, and procedure.

☑ Evaluate patient understanding.

☑ Restrict the patient's use of magnesium salts (such as Milk of Magnesia or epsom salts) for at least 3 days before the test.

Interfering factors

• Excessive use of antacids or cathartics and excessive infusion of magnesium sulfate raise magnesium levels.

• Prolonged I.V. infusions without magnesium suppress magnesium levels. Excessive use of diuretics, including thiazides and ethacrynic acid, decreases levels by increasing magnesium excretion in the urine.

• I.V. administration of calcium gluconate may falsely decrease serum magnesium levels if measured by the Titan yellow method.

• Hemolysis due to rough handling of the sample causes falsely elevated serum magnesium levels.

Manganese

Purpose

To detect manganese toxicity.

Normal results

Serum manganese values range from 0.4 to 0.85 ng/ml.

Abnormal results

Significantly increased serum manganese levels:

Manganese toxicity.

The basics

Manganese, a trace element, is found throughout the body but concentrates mainly in the pituitary, pineal, and lactating mammary glands, as well as in the liver and bones. Although the function of this element in humans is only partially understood, manganese is known to activate several enzymes—including cholinesterase and arginase—that are essential to metabolism. Because of poor intestinal absorption, the body retains only a fraction of the manganese supplied by foods such as unrefined cereals, green leafy vegetables, and nuts. However, manganese deficiency has not been linked to human disease. Industrial workers exposed to potentially dangerous levels of manganese may require testing for toxicity. Such toxicity can follow inhalation of manganese dust or fumes—a constant hazard in the steel and dry-cell battery industries—or ingestion of contaminated water. Toxicity requires prompt medical attention, since it can lead to central nervous system deterioration.

Procedure
Perform a venipuncture, and collect the sample in a metal-free collection tube. Laboratories will supply a special kit for this test on request.

Patient care checklist
Before the test
☑ Explain or clarify test purpose and procedure.
☑ Evaluate patient understanding.

Interfering factors
• High dietary intake of calcium and phosphorus can interfere with intestinal absorption of manganese and subsequently decrease serum levels.
• Serum manganese levels are influenced by estrogen, which increases levels, and by glucocorticoids, which alter its distribution in the body.
• Failure to use a metal-free collection tube can interfere with accurate determination of test results.
• Hemolysis caused by rough handling of the sample may alter test results.

Myoglobin

Purpose
• To estimate damage caused by myocardial infarction (MI) or skeletal muscle injury
• To predict exacerbation of polymyositis, a degenerative muscle disease.

Normal results
Serum myoglobin levels range from 30 to 90 ng/ml.

Abnormal results
Increased serum myoglobin levels:
  MI
  Skeletal muscle injury
  Polymyositis
  Dermatomyositis
  Systemic lupus erythematosus
  Shock
  Severe renal failure.

The basics
This test measures serum levels of myoglobin, an oxygen-binding muscle protein similar to hemoglobin. Myoglobin is normally found in skeletal and cardiac muscle, but is released into the blood after muscle injury. Thus, serum myoglobin levels help estimate the severity of muscle damage. However, because myoglobin levels do not indicate the site of injury, they are commonly used to confirm other studies, such as total creatine phosphokinase (CPK) or the myocardial-specific isoenzyme CPK-MB. Test results must also be correlated with the patient's signs and symptoms.

Procedure
Perform a venipuncture and collect the sample in a 10-ml, red-top tube.

Special precautions
• Do not collect a blood sample from a patient who has recently had an angina attack or undergone cardioversion.
• Collect a blood sample 4 to 8 hours after the onset of an acute MI, when myoglobin levels peak.

Patient care checklist
Before the test
☑ Explain or clarify test purpose and procedure.
☑ Evaluate patient understanding.

Interfering factors
• Recent cardioversion or angina attacks may increase myoglobin levels.
• Performing this test immediately after onset of an acute MI produces mis-

leading results, since myoglobin levels do not peak for 4 to 8 hours.

• A radioactive scan performed within 1 week before the test may affect results.

Neonatal thyroid-stimulating hormone
[Neonatal TSH, neonatal thyrotropin]

Purpose
To confirm diagnosis of congenital hypothyroidism.

Normal results
At age 1 to 2 days, TSH levels are normally 25 to 30 $\mu IU/ml$. Thereafter, levels are normally less than 25 $\mu IU/ml$.

Abnormal results
Neonatal TSH levels must be interpreted in light of thyroxine (T_4) concentrations.

Increased TSH and decreased T_4 indicate:

Primary congenital hypothyroidism.

Decreased TSH and decreased T_4 may be present in:

Secondary congenital hypothyroidism (pituitary or hypothalamic dysfunction).

Normal TSH and decreased T_4 may indicate:

Hypothyroidism due to a congenital defect in thyroxine-binding globulin (TBG)

Transient congenital hypothyroidism due to prematurity or prenatal hypoxia.

The basics
This radioimmunoassay confirms congenital hypothyroidism after an initial screening test detects low T_4 levels. Normally, TSH levels surge soon after birth, triggering a rise in thyroid hormone, which is essential for neurologic development. However, in primary congenital hypothyroidism, the thyroid gland does not respond to TSH stimulation, resulting in diminished thyroid hormone levels and elevated TSH levels. Early detection and treatment of congenital hypothyroidism is critical to prevent mental retardation and cretinism.

Procedure
For a filter paper sample:

• Assemble the necessary equipment and wash your hands thoroughly.

• Wipe the infant's heel with an alcohol or povidone-iodine swab, then dry it thoroughly with a gauze pad.

• Perform a heel stick.

• Squeezing the infant's heel gently, fill the circles on the filter paper with blood. Make sure the blood saturates the paper.

• Gently apply pressure with a gauze pad to ensure hemostasis at the puncture site.

• Allow the filter paper to dry, label it appropriately, and send it to the laboratory.

For a serum sample:

• Perform a venipuncture and collect the sample in a 5-ml, red-top tube.

• Label the sample and send it to the laboratory immediately.

Patient care checklist
Before the test

☑ Explain or clarify test purpose and procedure to the infant's parents. Emphasize the test's importance in detecting the disorder early, so that prompt therapy can prevent irreversible brain damage.

☑ Evaluate parents' understanding.

Interfering factors
• Corticosteroids, triiodothyronine (T_3), and T_4 lower TSH levels; lithium carbonate, potassium iodide, excessive topical resorcinol, and TSH injection raise TSH levels.

• Failure to let a filter paper sample dry completely may alter test results.

• Rough handling of a serum sample may cause hemolysis and may interfere with accurate testing.

5'-nucleotidase (5'NT)

Purpose
• To distinguish between hepatobiliary and skeletal disease when the source of elevated alkaline phosphatase levels is uncertain
• To help differentiate biliary obstruction from acute hepatocellular damage
• To detect hepatic metastasis in the absence of jaundice.

Normal results
Serum 5'NT values for adults range from 2 to 17 units/liter; values for children may be lower.

Abnormal results
Highest increases in 5'NT:
  Common bile duct obstruction due to calculi
  Hepatic tumors causing severe cholestasis.
Slight-to-moderate increases:
  Acute hepatocellular damage
  Cirrhosis.

The basics
The enzyme 5'NT is formed almost entirely in the hepatobiliary tract. Although serum 5'NT, alkaline phosphatase, and leucine aminopeptidase (LAP) levels rise in hepatic metastases, hepatocarcinoma, and biliary tract obstruction, only 5'NT remains normal in skeletal disease and pregnancy, and so is more specific for hepatic dysfunction than alkaline phosphatase or LAP. This test, which measures serum 5'NT levels, is technically more difficult than the alkaline phosphatase assay and has not been widely used as a liver function study, although some authorities consider 5'NT more sensitive than alkaline phosphatase to cholangitis, biliary cirrhosis, and malignant infiltrations of

the liver. However, 5'NT is used most often to determine whether alkaline phosphatase elevation originates from skeletal or hepatic disease.

Procedure
Perform a venipuncture, and collect the sample in a 7-ml red-top tube.

Patient care checklist
Before the test
☑ Explain or clarify test purpose and procedure.
☑ Evaluate patient understanding.

Interfering factors
• Hemolysis due to rough handling of the sample may interfere with accurate determination of serum levels.
• Ingestion of cholestatic drugs, such as phenothiazines, morphine, meperidine, and codeine, elevates 5'NT levels.

Oral glucose tolerance test (OGTT)

Purpose
• To confirm diabetes mellitus in selected patients
• To aid in diagnosis of hypoglycemia and malabsorption syndrome.

Normal results
Plasma glucose levels peak at 160 to 180 mg/100 ml within 30 minutes to 1 hour after administration of an oral glucose test dose and return to fasting levels or lower within 2 to 3 hours. Urine glucose tests remain negative throughout.

Abnormal results
Sustained elevated plasma glucose levels during at least two OGTTs:
  Help confirm diabetes mellitus. Many other diseases may cause abnormal glucose tolerance curves. (See *Glucose Tolerance Curves.*)

The basics

The OGTT, the most sensitive method of evaluating borderline cases of diabetes mellitus in selected patients, measures carbohydrate metabolism after ingestion of a challenge dose of glucose. The body absorbs this dose rapidly, causing plasma glucose levels to rise and peak within 30 minutes to 1 hour. The pancreas responds by secreting more insulin, causing glucose levels to return to normal after 2 to 3 hours. During this period, plasma and urine glucose levels are monitored to assess insulin secretion and the body's ability to metabolize glucose. Occasionally, levels are monitored an additional 2 to 3 hours to aid in diagnosis of hypoglycemia and malabsorption syndrome. Such extended testing is contraindicated when insulinoma is strongly suspected, because prolonged fasting in such a patient can lead to fainting and coma. In a patient with mild or diet-controlled diabetes, fasting plasma glucose levels may be within normal range; however, insufficient secretion of insulin after ingestion of carbohydrates causes plasma glucose to rise sharply and return to normal slowly. This decreased tolerance for glucose helps confirm mild diabetes. The oral glucose tolerance test is not necessary in patients with fasting glucose values above 140 mg/100 ml or postprandial plasma glucose above 200 mg/100 ml. Because of several limitations, the trend in laboratory testing is away from the OGTT and toward the fasting glucose tolerance test for diagnosing diabetes mellitus.

Procedure

• Between 7 a.m. and 9 a.m., perform a venipuncture to obtain a fasting blood sample. Draw this sample into a 7-ml, gray-top tube.
• Collect a urine specimen at the same time if your institution includes this as part of the test.
• After collecting these samples, administer the test load of oral glucose, and record the time of ingestion. Encourage the patient to drink the entire glucose solution within 5 minutes.
• Draw blood samples 30 minutes, 1 hour, 2 hours, and 3 hours after giving the loading dose, using 7-ml, gray-top tubes.
• Collect urine specimens at the same intervals.

Glucose Tolerance Curves

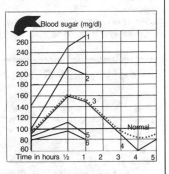

An oral glucose tolerance test measures both blood and urine sugar levels. As shown above, various diseases produce abnormal glucose tolerance curves: (1) diabetes mellitus, myasthenia gravis, brain injury, Cushing's syndrome, acromegaly (early), and hemochromatosis; (2) alimentary glycosuria and glucose infusions; (3) the dotted line indicates the normal curve while the adjoining line (4) shows that persons with insulin shock, spontaneous hypoglycemia, and hypoadrenalism have normal glucose tolerance until 2 hours after ingestion of the sugar load, but then have marked hypoglycemia; (5) pituitary deficiency and myxedema; (6) anorexia nervosa, panhypopituitarism, hyperinsulinism, and Addison's disease.

Adapted from John Bauer, et al, *Clinical Laboratory Methods*, 8th ed. (St. Louis: C.V. Mosby Co., 1974).

• Tell the patient to lie down if he feels faint from the numerous venipunctures. Encourage him to drink water throughout the test, to promote adequate urine excretion.

Special precautions
• Send blood and urine samples to the laboratory immediately, or refrigerate them. Specify when the patient last ate, and the blood and urine sample collection times. As appropriate, record the time the patient received his last pretest insulin or oral hypoglycemic dose.

CLINICAL ALERT: **If the patient develops severe hypoglycemia, notify the physician. Draw a blood sample, record the time on the laboratory slip, and discontinue the test. Have the patient drink a glass of orange juice with sugar added, or administer glucose I.V. to reverse the reaction.**

Patient care checklist
Before the test
☑ Explain or clarify test purpose, preparation, and procedure.
☑ Evaluate patient understanding.
☑ Advise the patient to abstain from smoking, coffee, alcohol, and strenuous exercise for 8 hours before or during the test.

Supplementary Glucose Tolerance Tests

Although the oral glucose tolerance test (OGTT) is the most effective test for detecting diabetes, two other glucose tolerance tests are sometimes used as research tools to sensitize or confirm OGTT findings.

The I.V. glucose tolerance test (IVGTT) measures blood glucose after the patient receives an intravenous infusion of 50% glucose over 3 or 4 minutes. Blood samples are then drawn at ½-, 1-, 2-, and 3-hour intervals. After an immediate glucose peak of 300 to 400 mg/dl (accompanied by glycosuria), the normal glucose curve falls steadily, reaching fasting levels within 1 to 1¼ hours. Failure to achieve fasting glucose levels within 2 to 3 hours generally confirms diabetes. A similarly delayed return to fasting glucose levels may result from fever, stress, old age, inactivity, carbohydrate deprivation, neoplasms, cirrhosis, and steroid-producing endocrine diseases. Nevertheless, the IVGTT has the following distinct advantages over the OGTT:
• Gastrointestinal hormones causing insulin secretion will not affect IVGTT glucose tolerance curves.

• Patients afflicted with intestinal absorption syndromes will not present abnormal curves.
• The IVGTT provides an alternative to flat OGTT curves resulting from hypopituitarism, hypoparathyroidism, or Addison's disease.
• This test avoids the inconvenience to the patient of the unpalatable oral glucose load.

The cortisone glucose tolerance test (CGTT) is occasionally used for patients with borderline carbohydrate-tolerance deficiencies and for those with strong familial predisposition to diabetes who produce a normal OGTT curve. Following a 3-day high-carbohydrate diet, oral cortisone acetate is administered 8½ and 2 hours before the standard OGTT. (Cortisone promotes glyconeogenesis and may accentuate carbohydrate intolerance in latent or mild diabetes.) Although this test is used primarily for research, values rising approximately 20 mg/dl above those of the standard OGTT after 2 hours demonstrate probable diabetes in some persons with only minimally decreased carbohydrate intolerance.

☑ Inform the patient that the test usually takes 3 hours but can last as long as 6 hours.

☑ Withhold medications that may interfere with test results, as ordered. If they must be continued, note them on the laboratory slip.

☑ Alert the patient to the symptoms of hypoglycemia—weakness, restlessness, nervousness, hunger, and sweating—and tell him to report any such symptoms immediately.

After the test

☑ Provide a balanced meal or snack; observe the patient for a hypoglycemic reaction.

Interfering factors

• Elevated plasma glucose levels may result from chlorthalidone, thiazide diuretics, furosemide, triamterene, oral contraceptives (estrogen-progestogen combination), benzodiazepines, phenytoin, phenothiazines, lithium, epinephrine, phenolphthalein, caffeine, arginine, dextrothyroxine, diazoxide, large doses of nicotinic acid, corticosteroids, and recent glucose I.V. infusions.

• Depressed glucose levels may be caused by ingestion of beta-adrenergic blockers, amphetamines, ethanol, clofibrate, insulin, oral hypoglycemics, and monoamine oxidase inhibitors.

• Failure to adhere to dietary and exercise restrictions may interfere with accurate determination of test results.

• Carbohydrate deprivation before the test can produce a diabetic response (abnormal increase in plasma glucose, with a delayed decrease), because the pancreas is unaccustomed to responding to a high-carbohydrate load.

• Recent infection, fever, pregnancy, or acute illness, such as myocardial infarction, may elevate glucose levels.

• Persons over age 50 tend toward decreasing carbohydrate tolerance, which causes an increase in glucose tolerance, to upper limits of about 1 mg/100 ml for every year over age 50.

(See *Supplementary Glucose Tolerance Tests.*)

Oral lactose tolerance test

Purpose

To detect lactose intolerance.

Normal results

Plasma glucose levels rise more than 20 mg/dl over fasting levels within 15 to 60 minutes after ingestion of the lactose loading dose. Stool sample analysis shows normal pH (7 to 8) and low glucose content (less than 1 + on a glucose-indicating dipstick).

Abnormal results

A rise in plasma glucose of less than 20 mg/dl indicates lactose intolerance, as does stool acidity (pH of 5.5 or less) and high glucose content (greater than 1 + on the dipstick).

The basics

This test measures plasma glucose levels after ingestion of a challenge dose of lactose. It is used to screen for lactose intolerance due to lactase deficiency. Lactose, a disaccharide, is found in milk and other dairy products. The intestinal enzyme lactase splits lactose into the monosaccharides glucose and galactose, for absorption by the intestinal epithelium. Absence or deficiency of lactase causes undigested lactose to remain in the intestinal lumen, producing such symptoms as abdominal cramps and watery diarrhea. True congenital lactase deficiency is rare. Usually, lactose intolerance is acquired, as lactase levels generally fall with age. Small-bowel biopsy with lactase assay may be done to confirm lactose intolerance.

Procedure

• After the patient has fasted for 8 hours, perform a venipuncture and

collect a blood sample in a 7-ml, gray-top tube.
• Then, administer the test load of lactose—for an adult, 50 g of lactose dissolved in 400 ml of water; for a child, 50 g per square meter of body surface area. Record the time of ingestion.
• Draw a blood sample 30, 60, and 120 minutes after giving the loading dose, using 7-ml, gray-top tubes.
• Collect a stool sample 5 hours after the loading dose, if ordered.

Special precautions
• Send blood and stool samples to the laboratory immediately, or refrigerate them if transport is delayed. Specify the time of collection on the laboratory slips.
• Watch for symptoms of lactose intolerance—abdominal cramps, nausea, bloating, flatulence, and watery diarrhea—caused by the loading dose.

Patient care checklist
Before the test
☑ Explain or clarify test purpose, preparation, and procedure.
☑ Evaluate patient understanding.
☑ Inform the patient that the entire procedure may take 2 hours.
☑ Restrict food and fluid intake, and tell the patient to avoid strenuous activity for 8 hours before the test.
☑ Withhold medications that may interfere with test results, as ordered. If they must be continued, note on laboratory slip.

Interfering factors
• Drugs that affect plasma glucose levels—such as thiazide diuretics, oral contraceptives, benzodiazepines, propranolol, and insulin—may alter test results.
• Delayed emptying of stomach contents can cause depressed glucose levels.
• Failure to follow diet and exercise restrictions may alter test results.
• Glycolysis may cause false-negative results.

Ornithine carbamoyltransferase (OCT)

Purpose
• To detect minimal hepatocellular damage in such disorders as chronic viral hepatitis or drug-induced hepatic dysfunction
• To confirm that abnormal values in other serum enzyme tests result from hepatic disease.

Normal results
Serum OCT levels range from undetectable to 500 Sigma units/ml, by colorimetric measurement.

Abnormal results
Marked increases in OCT levels:
   Acute viral hepatitis.
Moderate increases:
   Cholecystitis
   Cirrhosis
   Obstructive jaundice
   Metastatic carcinoma.
increases also occur from:
   Hepatotoxicity resulting from drugs or alcoholism.
increases rarely occur from:
   Extensive intestinal infarction.

The basics
OCT, an enzyme involved in urea metabolism, is found almost exclusively in the liver; small amounts are also found in the intestine. This test is one of the most sensitive indicators of acute hepatocellular dysfunction. Since only trace amounts of OCT occur normally in serum, any increase is clinically significant. Although serum OCT reveals hepatocellular damage with greater sensitivity than tests such as serum glutamic-oxaloacetic transaminase and serum glutamic-pyruvic transaminase, the test is not commonly performed—despite recent technologic advances that make possible routine laboratory measurement of OCT. Even

when an ultra-high-sensitivity analysis is required, gamma glutamyl transferase or bile acid assay is more likely to be ordered.

Procedure
Perform a venipuncture, and collect the sample in a 7-ml red-top tube.

Patient care checklist
Before the test
☑ Explain or clarify test purpose and procedure.
☑ Evaluate patient understanding.

Interfering factors
Hemolysis due to rough handling of the sample may interfere with accurate determination of OCT levels.

Parathyroid hormone *(PTH)* *[Parathormone]*

Purpose
To aid in the differential diagnosis of parathyroid disorders.

Normal results
Serum PTH levels vary, depending on the laboratory, and must be interpreted in association with serum calcium levels. Typical values are as follows:
Intact PTH: 210 to 310 pg/ml
N-terminal fraction: 230 to 630 pg/ml
C-terminal fraction: 410 to 1,760 pg/ml.

Abnormal results
(See *Clinical Implications of Abnormal Parathyroid Secretion*, p. 120.)

The basics
PTH, a polypeptide secreted by the parathyroid glands, regulates plasma concentration of calcium and phosphorus. Normally, PTH release is regulated by a negative feedback mechanism involving serum calcium.

Normal or elevated circulating calcium (especially the ionized form) inhibits PTH release; a decrease in calcium ions stimulates PTH release. The overall effect of PTH is to raise plasma levels of calcium while lowering phosphorus levels by stimulating osteoclasts and osteocytes to mobilize both calcium and phosphorus from bone; by acting on renal tubular cells to promote calcium reabsorption and phosphorus excretion (phosphaturia); and (with biologic vitamin D) by promoting intestinal absorption of calcium.

Circulating PTH exists in three distinct molecular forms: the intact PTH molecule, which originates in the parathyroids, and two smaller circulating forms—N-terminal fragments and C-terminal fragments—that are cleaved from the intact molecule by the kidneys, liver, and, to a lesser extent for the C-fragment, the parathyroids. Currently, two radioimmunoassays are available to detect PTH and the N- and C-terminal fragments. Both tests can be used to confirm diagnosis of hyperparathyroidism and hypoparathyroidism; each test has other specific applications as well. The C-terminal PTH assay is more useful in diagnosing chronic disturbances in PTH metabolism, such as secondary and tertiary hyperparathyroidism; it also better differentiates ectopic from primary hyperparathyroidism. The assay for intact PTH and the N-terminal fragment (both forms are measured concomitantly) more accurately reflects acute changes in PTH metabolism, and thus is useful in monitoring a patient's response to PTH therapy. An inappropriate excess or deficiency of PTH has clinical and diagnostic consequences directly related to the effects of PTH on bone and on the renal tubules, and to its interaction with ionized calcium and biologically active vitamin D. Consequently, measuring serum calcium, phosphorus, and creatine levels with serum PTH is useful in identifying states of pathologic parathyroid function. Suppres-

Clinical Implications of Abnormal Parathyroid Secretion

Conditions	Causes	Parathyroid hormone levels	Calcium (ionized) levels
Primary hyperparathyroidism	• Parathyroid adenoma or carcinoma • Parathyroid hyperplasia	● High	● to ◐ (High to Low)
Secondary hyperparathyroidism	• Chronic renal disease • Severe vitamin D deficiency • Calcium malabsorption • Pregnancy and lactation	● High	○ Low
Tertiary hyperparathyroidism	• Progressive secondary hyperparathyroidism leading to autonomous hyperparathyroidism	● High	● to ◐ (High to Low)
Hypoparathyroidism	• Usually, accidental removal of the parathyroid glands during surgery • Occasionally, in association with autoimmune disease	○ Low	○ Low
Malignant tumors	• Squamous cell carcinoma of the lung • Renal, pancreatic, or ovarian carcinoma	● to ◐ (High to Low)	● High

KEY High ● Normal ◐ Low ○

---

sion or stimulation tests may be of confirming value.

Procedure
Draw 3 ml of venous blood into two separate 7-ml, red-top tubes.

Patient care checklist
Before the test
☑ Explain or clarify test purpose, preparation, and procedure.
☑ Evaluate patient understanding.
☑ Restrict food and fluid intake overnight before the test.

Interfering factors
• Failure to observe an overnight fast may interfere with the accurate determination of test results.
• Hemolysis due to rough handling of the sample may interfere with accurate determination of test results.

Phenylalanine screening
[Guthrie screening test]

Purpose
To screen infants for phenylketonuria (PKU).

Normal results
Negative test indicates normal phenylalanine levels, which are less than 2 mg/dl.

Abnormal results
Positive serum phenylalanine screening indicates:
   Possibility of PKU.
also occurs with:
   Hepatic disease
   Galactosemia
   Delayed development of certain enzyme systems.

The basics
This test is a screening method used to detect elevated serum phenylalanine, an indication of possible PKU. Phenylalanine is a naturally occurring amino acid essential to growth and nitrogen balance. At birth, an infant with PKU usually has normal phenylalanine levels, but after milk or formula feeding begins (both contain phenylalanine), levels gradually rise due to a deficiency of the liver enzyme that converts phenylalanine to tyrosine. The serum phenylalanine screening test detects abnormal phenylalanine levels through the growth rate of *Bacillus subtilis,* an organism that needs phenylalanine to thrive. To ensure accurate results, the test must be performed after 3 full days (preferably 4 days) of milk or formula feeding. Diagnosis of PKU requires exact serum phenylalanine measurement and urine testing. (See *Confirming PKU.*)

Procedure
• Perform a heel stick, and collect three drops of blood—one in each circle—on the filter paper.
• Note the infant's name, birth date, and date of first milk or formula feeding on the laboratory slip.
• Send the sample to the laboratory immediately.

Patient care checklist
Before the test
☑ Explain or clarify test purpose and procedure to parents. Inform them that this test is required in many states.
☑ Evaluate understanding.
After the test
☑ Reassure the parents of a child who may have PKU that, although this disease is a common cause of congenital mental deficiency, early detection and continuous treatment with a low-phenylalanine diet can prevent permanent mental retardation.

Interfering factors
Performing the test before the infant has received at least 3 full days of milk or formula feeding yields a false-negative finding.

Confirming PKU

After the Guthrie screening test detects the possible presence of phenylketonuria (PKU), serum phenylalanine and tyrosine levels are measured to confirm diagnosis. Phenylalanine hydroxylase is the enzyme that converts phenylalanine to tyrosine. If this enzyme is absent, increasing phenylalanine levels and falling tyrosine levels indicate PKU. Samples are obtained by venipuncture (femoral or external jugular) and measured by fluorometry. Elevated serum phenylalanine (more than 4 mg/dl) and decreased tyrosine (less than 0.6 mg/dl)—with urinary excretion of phenylpyruvic acid—confirm diagnosis of PKU.

Phosphates

Purpose
• To aid in diagnosis of renal disorders and acid-base imbalance
• To detect endocrine, skeletal, and calcium disorders.

Normal results
Serum phosphate levels range from 2.5 to 4.5 mg/dl (atomic absorption), or

from 1.8 to 2.6 mEq/liter. Children have higher serum phosphate levels than adults. Phosphate levels can rise as high as 7 mg/dl or 4.1 mEq/liter during periods of increased bone growth.

Abnormal results
Values should be interpreted in light of serum calcium results.
Decreased serum phosphate levels (hypophosphatemia):
  Malnutrition
  Malabsorption syndrome
  Hyperparathyroidism
  Renal tubular acidosis
  Treatment of diabetic acidosis.
Increased serum phosphate levels (hyperphosphatemia):
  Skeletal disease
  Healing fractures
  Hypoparathyroidism
  Acromegaly
  Diabetic acidosis
  High intestinal obstruction
  Renal failure.

The basics
This test measures serum levels of phosphates, the dominant cellular anions. Phosphates help store and utilize body energy and help regulate calcium levels, carbohydrate and lipid metabolism, and acid-base balance. Phosphates are essential to bone formation; about 85% of the body's phosphates are found in bone. The intestine absorbs a considerable amount of phosphates from dietary sources, but adequate levels of vitamin D are necessary for their absorption. The kidneys excrete phosphates and serve as a regulatory mechanism. Since calcium and phosphate interact in a reciprocal relationship, urinary excretion of phosphates increases or decreases in inverse proportion to serum calcium levels. Abnormal concentrations of phosphates result more often from improper excretion than from abnormal ingestion or absorption from dietary sources.In children, hypophosphatemia can suppress normal growth. Hy-

perphosphatemia is rarely clinically significant; however, if prolonged, it can alter bone metabolism by causing abnormal calcium phosphate deposits.

Since serum phosphate values alone are of limited use diagnostically (only a few rare conditions directly affect phosphate metabolism), they should be interpreted in light of serum calcium results.

Procedure
Perform a venipuncture, and collect the sample in a 10- to 15-ml, red-top tube.

Patient care checklist
Before the test
☑ Explain or clarify test purpose and procedure.
☑ Evaluate patient understanding.

Interfering factors
• Excessive vitamin D intake or drug therapy with anabolic steroids and androgens may elevate serum phosphorus levels.
• Improper handling of the sample, resulting in hemolysis, falsely increases serum phosphate levels.
• Suppressed phosphate levels may result from excessive phosphate excretion due to prolonged vomiting and diarrhea, vitamin D deficiency (which interferes with phosphate absorption), extended I.V. infusion of dextrose 5% in water, ingestion of phosphate-binding antacids, and drug therapy with acetazolamide, insulin, and epinephrine.

Phospholipids

Purpose
• To aid in the evaluation of fat metabolism
• To aid in diagnosis of hypothyroidism, diabetes mellitus, nephrotic syndrome, chronic pancreatitis, obstructive jaundice, and hypolipoproteinemia.

Normal results

Phospholipid levels range from 180 to 320 mg/dl. Although males usually have higher levels than females, values in pregnant females exceed those of males.

Abnormal results

Increased phospholipid levels:
Hypothyroidism
Diabetes mellitus
Nephrotic syndrome
Chronic pancreatitis
Obstructive jaundice.
Decreased phospholipid levels:
Primary hypolipoproteinemia.

The basics

Phospholipid assay was formerly an important test because of the lack of more specific tests and the relative unreliability of other lipid assays. Today, however, this quantitative analysis of phospholipid levels adds minimal information to that provided by cholesterol levels. In human plasma, the main phospholipids are lecithins, cephalins, and sphingomyelins.

Procedure

Perform a venipuncture, and collect the sample in a 10- to 15-ml, red-top tube.

Patient care checklist

Before the test
☑ Explain or clarify test purpose, preparation, and procedure.
☑ Evaluate patient understanding.
☑ Advise the patient to abstain from ingestion of alcohol for 24 hours before the test.
☑ Restrict food and fluid intake from midnight before the test.
☑ Withhold medications that may interfere with test results, as ordered. If they must be continued, note them on the laboratory slip.

Interfering factors

• Clofibrate and other antilipemics may lower phospholipid levels; estrogens, epinephrine, and some phenothiazines, such as chlorpromazine, increase levels.
• Failure to follow dietary restrictions may interfere with accurate determination of test results.
• Failure to send the sample to the laboratory immediately may affect test results.

Potassium

Purpose

• To evaluate clinical signs of potassium excess (hyperkalemia) or potassium depletion (hypokalemia)
• To monitor renal function, acid-base balance, and glucose metabolism
• To evaluate neuromuscular and endocrine disorders
• To detect the origin of dysrhythmias.

Normal results

Serum potassium levels range from 3.8 to 5.5 mEq/liter.

Abnormal results

Increased serum potassium levels (hyperkalemia):
Burns
Crushing injuries
Diabetic ketoacidosis
Myocardial infarction
Renal failure
Addison's disease.
Decreased serum potassium levels (hypokalemia):
Aldosteronism
Cushing's syndrome
Loss of body fluids
Excessive licorice ingestion.

The basics

This test, a quantitative analysis, measures serum levels of potassium, the major intracellular cation. Plasma potassium levels may be measured by some laboratories. Results of plasma potassium are slightly lower than those of serum potassium. Small amounts of potassium may also be found in extracellular fluid.

Vital to homeostasis, potassium maintains cellular osmotic equilibrium and helps regulate muscle activity (it is essential in maintaining electrical conduction within the cardiac and skeletal muscles). Potassium also helps regulate enzyme activity and acid-base balance, and influences kidney function.

Potassium levels are affected by variations in the secretion of adrenal steroid hormones, and by fluctuations in pH, serum glucose levels, and serum sodium levels. A reciprocal relationship appears to exist between potassium and sodium; a substantial intake of one element causes a corresponding decrease in the other. Although it readily conserves sodium, the body has no efficient method for conserving potassium. Even in potassium depletion, the kidneys continue to excrete potassium; therefore, potassium deficiency can develop rapidly and is quite common. Although serum values and clinical symptoms can indicate a potassium imbalance, an EKG provides the definitive diagnosis.

Procedure
Perform a venipuncture, and collect the sample in a 10- to 15-ml red-top tube.

Special precautions
• Draw the sample immediately after applying the tourniquet, since a delay may elevate the potassium level by allowing leakage of intracellular potassium into the serum.
CLINICAL ALERT: **Observe a patient with hypokalemia for decreased reflexes; rapid, weak, irregular pulse; mental confusion; hypotension; anorexia; muscle weakness; and paresthesia. EKG shows a flattened T wave, depressed ST segment, and elevated U wave. In severe cases, ventricular fibrillation, respiratory paralysis, and cardiac arrest can develop.**

CLINICAL ALERT: **Observe a patient with hyperkalemia for weakness, malaise, nausea, diarrhea, colicky pain, muscle irritability progressing to flaccid paralysis, oliguria, and bradycardia. EKG reveals a prolonged PR interval; wide QRS complex; tall, tented T wave; and depressed ST segment.**

Patient care checklist
Before the test
☑ Explain or clarify test purpose and procedure.
☑ Evaluate patient understanding.

Interfering factors
• Excessive or rapid potassium infusion, spironolactone or penicillin G potassium therapy, or renal toxicity from administration of amphotericin B, methicillin, or tetracycline elevates serum potassium levels.
• Insulin and glucose administration, diuretic therapy (especially with thiazides, but not with triamterene, amiloride, or spironolactone), or I.V. infusions without potassium suppress serum potassium levels.
• Excessive hemolysis of the sample or delay in drawing blood following the application of a tourniquet elevates potassium levels.

Progesterone

Purpose
• To assess corpus luteum function as part of infertility studies
• To evaluate placental function during pregnancy
• To aid in confirming ovulation. Test results support basal body temperature readings.

Normal results
Values during menstruation:
   Follicular phase: less than 150 ng/100 ml
   Luteal phase: about 300 ng/100 ml (rises daily during periovulation)

Midluteal phase: 2,000 ng/100 ml.
Values during pregnancy:
First trimester: 1,500 to 5,000 ng/ 100 ml
Second and third trimesters: 8,000 to 20,000 ng/100 ml.

Abnormal results
Increased plasma progesterone levels:
Ovulation
Luteinizing tumors
Ovarian cysts
Adrenocortical hyperplasias and tumors producing progesterone.
Decreased plasma progesterone levels:
Amenorrhea, such as from gonadal dysfunction or panhypopituitarism
Toxemia of pregnancy
Threatened abortion
Fetal death.

The basics
Progesterone, an ovarian steroid hormone secreted by the corpus luteum, causes thickening and secretory development of the endometrium in preparation for implantation of the fertilized ovum. Progesterone levels, therefore, peak during the midluteal phase of the menstrual cycle. Progesterone may prolong the surge of luteinizing hormone after ovulation. If implantation does not occur, progesterone (and estrogen) levels drop sharply and menstruation begins about 2 days later. During pregnancy, the placenta releases about 10 times the normal monthly amount of progesterone to maintain the pregnancy. Progesterone causes thickening of the endometrium, which contains large amounts of stored nutrients for the developing ovum. Progesterone also prevents abortion by decreasing uterine contractions and, with estrogen, prepares the breasts for lactation. This radioimmunoassay provides reliable information about corpus luteum function in fertility studies or placental function in pregnancy. Serial deter-

minations are recommended. Although plasma levels provide accurate information, progesterone can also be monitored by measuring urine pregnanediol, a catabolite of progesterone.

Procedure
• Perform a venipuncture, and collect the sample in a 7-ml, green-top (heparinized) tube.
• Completely fill the collection tube, then invert it gently at least 10 times to mix the sample and anticoagulant adequately.
• Indicate the date of the patient's last menstrual period and the phase of her cycle on the laboratory slip. If the patient is pregnant, also indicate the month of gestation.

Patient care checklist
Before the test
☑ Explain or clarify test purpose and procedure.
☑ Evaluate patient understanding.
☑ Inform the patient that the test may be repeated at specific times coinciding with phases of her menstrual cycle, or with each prenatal visit.

Interfering factors
• Hemolysis caused by rough handling of the sample may affect test results.
• Progesterone or estrogen therapy may interfere with accurate determination of test results.

Prolactin
[Lactogenic hormone, lactogen]

Purpose
• To facilitate diagnosis of pituitary dysfunction, possibly due to pituitary adenoma
• To aid in the diagnosis of hypothalamic dysfunction regardless of the cause
• To evaluate secondary amenorrhea and/or galactorrhea.

Normal results
Normal prolactin values range from undetectable to 23 ng/dl in nonlactating females.

Abnormal results
Increased prolactin levels:
characteristically occur with:
  Pituitary adenoma (100 to 300 ng/ml).
may occur with:
  Hypothyroidism
  Acromegaly
  Some hypothalamic disorders.
may also be idiopathic, as in:
  Anovulatory infertility.
Decreased prolactin levels:
  Postpartum pituitary infarction (Sheehan's syndrome)
  Empty-sella syndrome.

The basics
Similar in molecular structure and biologic activity to growth hormone (hGH), prolactin is a polypeptide hormone secreted by the anterior pituitary. It is essential for the development of the mammary glands for lactation during pregnancy, and for stimulating and maintaining lactation postpartum. Prolactin is secreted in males and nonpregnant females, but its function is unknown. Like hGH, prolactin acts directly on tissues, and its levels rise in response to sleep and to physical or emotional stress. This radioimmunoassay is a quantitative analysis of serum prolactin levels, which normally rise ten- to twentyfold during pregnancy, corresponding to concomitant elevations in human placental lactogen levels. After delivery, prolactin secretion falls to basal levels in mothers who do not breast-feed. However, prolactin secretion increases during breast-feeding, apparently as a result of a stimulus triggered by suckling that curtails the release of prolactin-inhibiting factor by the hypothalamus. This, in turn, allows transient elevations in prolactin secretion by the pituitary. With Sheehan's syndrome, there is a failure of lactation due to decreased prolactin levels. This test is considered useful in patients suspected of having pituitary tumors, which are known to secrete prolactin in excessive amounts. Amenorrhea or galactorrhea is usually present.

Procedure
• Perform a venipuncture at least 2 hours after the patient wakes; samples drawn earlier are likely to show sleep-induced peak levels.
• Collect the sample in a 7-ml, red-top tube.

Patient care checklist
Before the test
☑ Explain or clarify test purpose, preparation, and procedure.
☑ Evaluate patient understanding.
☑ Encourage the patient to relax for about half an hour before the test.
☑ Inform the patient that the laboratory requires at least 4 days to complete the analysis.
☑ Withhold medications that may interfere with test results, as ordered. If they must be continued, note them on the laboratory slip.

Interfering factors
• Failure to take into account physiologic variations related to sleep or stress may invalidate test results.
• Pretest use of ethanol, haloperidol, morphine, methyldopa, estrogens, phenothiazines (such as chlorpromazine), amphetamines, and reserpine—all of which raise prolactin levels—may interfere with accurate determination of test results.
• Pretest use of apomorphine, ergot alkaloids, and levodopa—which lower prolactin levels—may also affect correct determination of test results.
• A radioactive scan performed within 1 week before the test, or recent surgery, may interfere with test results.
• Hemolysis due to rough handling of the sample may interfere with accurate determination of test results.

Protein electrophoresis

Purpose
To aid in diagnosis of hepatic disease, protein deficiency, blood dyscrasias, renal disorders, and gastrointestinal and neoplastic diseases.

Normal results
Total serum protein: 6.6 to 7.9 g/dl (100%)
Albumin: 3.3 to 4.5 g/dl (53%)
Alpha$_1$ globulin: 0.1 to 0.4 g/dl (14%)

Clinical Implications of Abnormal Protein Levels

Abnormal levels of albumin or globulin are characteristic in many pathologic states, such as those listed below.

Total proteins	Albumin	Globulins
Increased levels		
• Dehydration • Vomiting, diarrhea • Diabetic acidosis • Fulminating and chronic infections • Multiple myeloma • Monocytic leukemia • Chronic inflammatory disease (such as rheumatoid arthritis or early-stage Laennec's cirrhosis)	• Multiple myeloma only	• Chronic syphilis • Tuberculosis • Subacute bacterial endocarditis • Multiple myeloma • Collagen diseases • Systemic lupus erythematosus • Rheumatoid arthritis • Diabetes mellitus • Hodgkin's disease
Decreased levels		
• Malnutrition • Gastrointestinal disease • Blood dyscrasias • Essential hypertension • Hodgkin's disease • Uncontrolled diabetes mellitus • Malabsorption • Hepatic dysfunction • Toxemia of pregnancy • Nephroses • Surgical and traumatic shock • Severe burns • Hemorrhage • Hyperthyroidism • Benzene and carbon tetrachloride poisoning • Congestive heart failure	• Malnutrition • Nephritis/nephrosis • Diarrhea • Plasma loss from burns • Hepatic disease • Hodgkin's disease • Hypogammaglobulinemia • Peptic ulcer • Acute cholecystitis • Sarcoidosis • Collagen diseases • Systemic lupus erythematosus • Rheumatoid arthritis • Essential hypertension • Metastatic carcinoma • Hyperthyroidism	• Levels are variable in neoplastic and renal diseases, hepatic dysfunction, and blood dyscrasias.

Serum Proteins and Their Electrophoretic Values in Disease States

In electrophoresis, blood serum is placed on specially treated paper exposed to an electric current. According to their molecular size, shape, and electric charge, albumin and globulins in the serum migrate to form five homogeneous bands that indicate the relative proportions of each protein fraction. As these graphs show, variations in the proportions of these serum proteins can be plotted, making electrophoresis a valuable diagnostic tool.

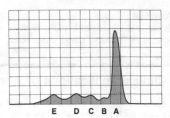

(1) Normal serum pattern

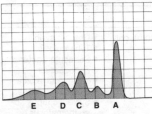

(2) Myocardial infarction causes a relative increase in alpha$_1$ and alpha$_2$ globulins.

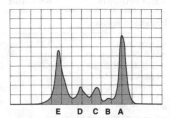

(3) An apparent decrease in albumin and, more importantly, a sharp rise in gamma globulins indicate multiple myeloma.

KEY:
A: Albumin
B: Alpha$_1$ globulin
C: Alpha$_2$ globulin

D: Beta globulin
E: Gamma globulin

Alpha$_2$ globulin: 0.5 to 1 g/dl (14%)
Beta globulin: 0.7 to 1.2 g/dl (12%)
Gamma globulin: 0.5 to 1.6 g/dl (20%).

Abnormal results
(See *Clinical Implications of Abnormal Protein Levels,* p. 127, and *Serum Proteins and Their Electrophoretic Values in Disease States.*)

The basics
This test measures serum albumin and globulins, the major blood proteins, in an electric field by separating the proteins according to their size, shape, and electric charge at pH 8.6. Because

each protein fraction moves at a different rate, this movement separates the fractions into recognizable and measurable patterns. Albumin maintains oncotic pressure (preventing leakage of capillary plasma) and transports substances that are insoluble in water alone, such as bilirubin, fatty acids, hormones, and drugs. Four types of globulins exist—alpha$_1$, alpha$_2$, beta, and gamma. The first three types act primarily as carrier proteins that transport lipids, hormones, and metals through the blood. The fourth type, gamma globulin, is an important component in the body's immune system. Electrophoresis is the most current method for measuring serum proteins. However, determinations of total protein and albumin/globulin ratio are still commonly performed. When the relative percentage of each component protein fraction is multiplied by the total protein concentration, the proportions can be converted into absolute values. Regardless of test method, however, a single protein fraction is rarely significant by itself. This test must be performed on a serum sample to avoid measuring the fibrinogen fraction.

Procedure

Perform a venipuncture, and collect the sample in a 7-ml, red-top tube.

Patient care checklist
Before the test
☑ Explain or clarify test purpose and procedure.
☑ Evaluate patient understanding.
☑ Withhold medications that may interfere with test results, as ordered. If they must be continued, note them on the laboratory slip.

Alpha₁-Antitrypsin Test

Using immunoelectrophoresis, this test measures fasting serum levels of alpha₁-antitrypsin (AAT), a major component of the alpha₁-globulin. AAT is believed to inhibit release of protease into body fluids by dying cells. Congenital absence or deficiency of AAT increases susceptibility to emphysema. As a result, the serum AAT test provides a useful screening tool for high-risk patients. Such patients must be instructed to refrain from smoking, since irritants in tobacco stimulate leukocytes in the lungs to release protease.

In addition to identifying congenital AAT deficiency, the AAT test is a nonspecific method of detecting inflammation, severe infection, and necrosis.

Interfering factors
• Pretest administration of a contrast dye (such as sulfobromophthalein) falsely elevates total protein test results. Pregnancy and the use of cytotoxic agents may lower serum albumin.
• Use of plasma instead of serum alters test results.
(See *Alpha₁-Antitrypsin Test.*)

Pyruvate kinase *(PK)*

Purpose
• To differentiate PK-deficient hemolytic anemia from other congenital hemolytic anemias—for example, glucose-6-phosphate dehydrogenase (G-6-PD) deficiency—or from acquired hemolytic anemia (when patient history or laboratory tests fail to indicate a genetic red cell defect)
• To detect PK deficiency in asymptomatic, heterozygous inheritance.

Normal results
In a routine (ultraviolet) assay, serum PK levels range from 2 to 8.8 units/g of hemoglobin; in the low-substrate assay, 0.9 to 3.9 units/g of hemoglobin.

Abnormal results
Decreased serum PK levels:
Confirm PK deficiency.

The basics
The erythrocyte enzyme PK takes part in the anaerobic metabolism of glucose. Abnormally low PK levels, revealed by erythrocyte enzyme assay using a serum sample, are inherited as an autosomal recessive trait and may result in a nonspherocytic red cell membrane defect associated with congenital hemolytic anemia. Although PK deficiency is uncommon, it is the most prevalent congenital nonspherocytic hemolytic anemia, after G-6-PD deficiency.

Procedure

• Perform a venipuncture, and collect the sample in a 7-ml, lavender-top tube.

• Completely fill the collection tube, and invert it gently several times to mix the sample and the anticoagulant.

Patient care checklist

Before the test

☑ Explain or clarify test purpose and procedure.

☑ Evaluate patient understanding.

☑ Review patient history for recent blood transfusion; note on the laboratory slip.

Interfering factors

• Failure to use a collection tube with the proper anticoagulant, or to adequately mix the sample and anticoagulant, may interfere with accurate determination of test results.

• Hemolysis caused by rough handling of the sample may affect test results.

• Since PK levels in white blood cells (WBCs) remain normal in hemolytic anemia, the laboratory removes WBCs from the sample to prevent false results.

• Failure to notify the laboratory of recent blood transfusions may interfere with accurate determination of serum PK levels.

Rapid ACTH test
[Cosyntropin test]

Purpose

To aid in identification of primary and secondary adrenal hypofunction.

Normal results

Plasma cortisol levels rise 7 or more mcg/dl above the baseline value, to a peak of 18 or more mcg/dl 60 minutes after the cosyntropin injection. Generally, a doubling of the baseline value indicates a normal response.

Abnormal results

Cortisol levels remain low:

Primary adrenal hypofunction (Addison's disease).

The basics

The rapid ACTH test is gradually replacing the 8-hour ACTH stimulation test as the most effective diagnostic tool for evaluating adrenal hypofunction (insufficiency). Using cosyntropin, a synthetic analogue of the biologically active part of ACTH, the rapid ACTH test provides faster results and causes fewer allergic reactions than the 8-hour test, which uses natural ACTH from animal sources. This test requires prior determination of baseline plasma cortisol levels to evaluate the effect of cosyntropin administration on cortisol secretion. An unequivocally high morning cortisol level rules out adrenal hypofunction and makes further testing unnecessary. Although cortisol levels remain low in patients with primary adrenal hypofunction, if test results show subnormal increases in plasma cortisol levels, prolonged stimulation of the adrenal cortex may be required to differentiate between primary and secondary adrenal hypofunction.

Procedure

• Draw 5 ml of blood for a baseline value. Collect the sample in a 5-ml, green-top (heparinized) tube.

• Label this sample "pre-injection" and send it to the laboratory.

• Inject 250 mcg (0.25 mg) of cosyntropin I.V. (preferably) or I.M. (I.V. administration affords more accurate determinations, since ineffective absorption following I.M. administration may cause wide variations in response.) Direct I.V. injection should take 2 minutes.

• Draw another 5 ml of blood 30 and

60 minutes following the cosyntropin injection. Collect the samples in 5-ml green-top (heparinized) tubes.
• Label the samples "30 minutes postinjection" and "60 minutes postinjection" and send them to the laboratory. Also include the actual collection times on the laboratory slip.

Patient care checklist
Before the test
☑ Explain or clarify test purpose, preparation, and procedure.
☑ Evaluate patient understanding.
☑ Restrict food and fluid for 10 to 12 hours before the test, if required by the specific laboratory.
☑ Encourage the patient to relax and remain recumbent for 30 minutes prior to the test.
☑ Withhold medications that may interfere with test results, as ordered. If they must be continued, note them on the laboratory slip.
After the test
☑ Observe the patient for signs of an allergic reaction to cosyntropin (rare), such as hives and itching, or tachycardia.

Interfering factors
• Failure to observe restrictions of diet, medications, and physical activity may hinder accurate determination of test results. Drugs that increase plasma cortisol levels—including estrogens (which increase plasma cortisol-binding proteins) and amphetamines—may interfere with test results. Smoking and obesity may also increase plasma cortisol levels. Lithium carbonate decreases plasma cortisol levels.
• A radioactive scan performed within 1 week before the test may influence test results, since plasma cortisol levels are determined by radioimmunoassay.
• Hemolysis due to rough handling of the sample may interfere with accurate determination of test results.

Renin activity
[Plasma renin activity (PRA)]

Purpose
• To screen for renal origin of hypertension
• To help plan the best treatment of essential hypertension, a genetic disease often aggravated by excess sodium intake
• To help identify hypertension linked to unilateral (sometimes bilateral) renovascular disease by renal vein catheterization
• To help identify primary aldosteronism (Conn's syndrome) resulting from aldosterone-secreting adrenal adenoma
• To confirm primary aldosteronism (sodium-depleted plasma renin test).

Normal results
Sodium-depleted, upright, peripheral vein: For ages 20 to 39, the range is from 2.9 to 24 ng/ml/hour; mean, 10.8 ng/ml/hour. For age 40 and over, the range is from 2.9 to 10.8 ng/ml/hour; mean, 5.9 ng/ml/hour.
Sodium-replete, upright, peripheral vein: For ages 20 to 39, the range is from 0.1 to 4.3 ng/ml/hour; mean, 1.9 ng/ml/hour. For age 40 and over, the range is from 0.1 to 3 ng/ml/hour; mean, 1 ng/ml/hour.
In renal vein catheterization, the renal venous renin ratio (the renin level in the renal vein compared with the level in the inferior vena cava) is less than 1.5:1.
Levels of plasma renin activity and of aldosterone decrease with advancing age.

Abnormal results
Increased renin levels:
    Essential hypertension (uncommon)
    Malignant hypertension
    Renovascular hypertension
    Cirrhosis

Hypokalemia
Hypovolemia due to hemorrhage
Renin-producing renal tumors
Addison's disease
Chronic renal failure
Transplantation rejection.

Decreased renin levels:
may indicate hypervolemia due to:
High-sodium diet
Salt-retaining steroids
Primary aldosteronism
Cushing's syndrome
Licorice-ingestion syndrome
Essential hypertension.

High serum and urine aldosterone levels, with low plasma renin activity, help identify primary aldosteronism; in the sodium-depleted renin test, low plasma renin confirms this and differentiates it from secondary aldosteronism (characterized by increased renin).

The basics

Renin secretion is the first stage of the renin-angiotensin-aldosterone cycle that controls the body's sodium-po-

---

Saralasin Test

In this test, saralasin, an angiotensin II antagonist, is rapidly infused I.V. while the patient's blood pressure response is monitored. This relatively new test is positive for renin-dependent hypertension if diastolic pressure drops by 7 to 10 mm Hg (or more), or by more than 8%.

To enhance test results, the physician may prepare the patient by restricting sodium intake and ordering a diuretic to cause moderate sodium depletion. However, the value of this measure is controversial.

Caution: The patient may experience a sharp blood pressure increase after the infusion ends. Closely monitor blood pressure during and after the infusion.

---

tassium balance, fluid volume, and blood pressure. Renin is released by the juxtaglomerular cells of the kidneys into the renal veins in response to sodium depletion and blood loss. It catalyzes the conversion of angiotensinogen, an alpha$_2$-globulin plasma protein, to angiotensin I, which in turn is converted by hydrolysis into angiotensin II, a vasoconstrictor that stimulates aldosterone production in the adrenal cortex. When present in excessive amounts, angiotensin II causes renal hypertension. The PRA test is a screening procedure for renovascular hypertension but does not unequivocally confirm it. When supplemented by other special tests, the PRA can help establish the cause of hypertension. For instance, sampling blood obtained from both renal veins by renal vein catheterization and analyzing the renal venous renin ratio can identify renovascular disorders. Some experts believe that essential hypertension with low, normal, and high renin levels should be treated differently, and the PRA test can categorize the disease for appropriate therapy. Plasma renin activity is measured by radioimmunoassay of a peripheral or renal blood sample. Results are expressed as the rate of angiotensin I formation per unit of time. Patient preparation is crucial and may take up to 1 month.

Special precautions

• Since renin is very unstable, the sample must be drawn into a chilled syringe and collection tube, placed on ice, and sent to the laboratory immediately.

• Completely fill the collection tube, and invert it gently several times to mix the sample and the anticoagulant.

Procedure

Peripheral vein sample:
Perform a venipuncture, and collect the sample in a 7-ml, lavender-top tube.

Renal vein catheterization:
A catheter is advanced to the kidneys

through the femoral vein, under fluoroscopic control, and samples are obtained from both renal veins and the vena cava.

Patient care checklist

Before the test

☑ Explain or clarify test purpose, preparation, and procedure.

☑ Evaluate patient understanding.

☑ Discontinue medications that may interfere with test results for 2 to 4 weeks before the test, as ordered.

☑ Advise the patient to maintain a normal sodium diet (3 g/day) for 2 to 4 weeks before the test.

☑ For the sodium-depleted renin test, give the patient furosemide (or, if he has angina or cerebrovascular insufficiency, chlorthiazide) and instruct him to follow a low-sodium diet for 3 days before the test.

☑ If a recumbent sample is ordered, have the patient remain in bed the morning of the test until a sample is obtained.

☑ If an upright sample is ordered, have the patient stand or sit upright for 2 hours before the test.

☑ If renal catheterization is ordered, ask the patient to sign an informed consent form; inform the patient that the procedure will be done in the X-ray department and that a local anesthetic will be given.

After the test

☑ After renal vein catheterization, apply pressure to the catheterization site for 10 to 20 minutes to prevent extravasation.

☑ Monitor vital signs, and check the catheterization site every 30 minutes for 2 hours, then every hour for 4 hours, to ensure that the bleeding has stopped.

☑ Check the distal pulse for signs of thrombus formation and arterial occlusion (cyanosis, loss of pulse, coolness of skin).

Interfering factors

• Failure to use the proper anticoagulant in the collection tube, to fill it completely, or to mix the sample and the anticoagulant adequately may influence renin levels. (EDTA helps preserve angiotensin I; heparin does not.)

• Failure to chill the collection tube and syringe, or failure to chill and send the sample to the laboratory immediately promotes breakdown of renin.

• Renin levels may be affected by failure to observe diet restrictions and by improper patient positioning during tests.

• Levels are increased by salt intake, diuretic therapy, oral contraceptives, severe blood loss, antihypertensives, vasodilators, licorice, and pregnancy.

• Salt-retaining steroid therapy and antidiuretic therapy decrease levels. (Also see *Saralasin Test.*)

Screening test for congenital hypothyroidism

Purpose

To screen neonates for congenital hypothyroidism.

Normal results

Immediately after birth, neonatal thyroxine (T_4) levels are considerably higher than normal adult levels. By the end of the 1st week, however, T_4 values decrease markedly:

Age (days)	Normal T_4 level
1 to 5	≤ 4.9 mcg/dl
6 to 8	≤ 4.0 mcg/dl
9 to 11	≤ 3.5 mcg/dl
12 to 120	≤ 3.0 mcg/dl.

Abnormal results

Decreased serum T_4 levels in the neonate require thyroid-stimulating hormone (TSH) testing for clarification of the diagnosis.

Decreased T_4 levels accompanied by increased TSH levels (more than 25 µIU/ml):

Primary congenital hypothyroidism.

with decreased TSH levels:
Secondary congenital hypothyroidism (strongly suspected).

The basics

This test measures serum T_4 levels in the neonate to detect congenital hypothyroidism. Characterized by low or absent levels of T_4, congenital hypothyroidism affects roughly 1 in 5,000 neonates, occurring in girls three times more often than in boys. This disorder can result from thyroid dysgenesis or hypoplasia, congenital goiter, or maternal use of thyroid inhibitors during pregnancy. If untreated, it can lead to irreversible brain damage by age 3 months. Because clinical signs are few, in the past, most cases of congenital hypothyroidism went undetected until cretinism became apparent or death followed respiratory distress. Recently, however, radioimmunoassays for T_4 and TSH have been used effectively to screen neonates for congenital hypothyroidism. This test is now mandatory in some states. A complete thyroid workup—including serum triiodothyronine (T_3), thyroxine-binding globulin (TBG), and free T_4 levels—is necessary for unequivocal diagnosis of congenital hypothyroidism before treatment begins.

Procedure

• After assembling the necessary equipment and washing your hands thoroughly, wipe the infant's heel with an alcohol or povidone-iodine swab. Then dry it thoroughly with a gauze pad.
• Perform a heel stick. Squeezing the heel gently, fill the circles on the filter paper with blood. Make sure the blood saturates the paper.
• Apply gentle pressure with a gauze pad to ensure hemostasis at the puncture site.
• When the filter paper is dry, label it appropriately and send it to the laboratory.

Patient care checklist

Before the test
☑ Explain or clarify test purpose and procedure to parents. Explain that, although hypothyroidism is uncommon in infants, the screening test detects the disorder early, before irreversible brain damage occurs. Parents should also be informed that the test will be performed before the infant is discharged from the hospital, and again 4 to 6 weeks later.
☑ Evaluate parents understanding.

After the test
☑ If results of the screening test indicate congenital hypothyroidism, tell the parents that additional testing is necessary to determine the cause of the disorder.
☑ If diagnosis is confirmed, inform the parents that replacement therapy can restore normal thyroid gland function. Also tell them that such therapy is lifelong and that the dosage will increase until adult requirement is reached.
☑ If the sample is not processed in the hospital laboratory, be sure parents are notified when the test results are available.

Interfering factors

• Failure to allow the filter paper to dry completely can alter test results.
• Failure to follow special directions for obtaining the sample can alter test results.

Serum glutamic-oxaloacetic transaminase
(SGOT)
[Aspartate aminotransferase, aspartate transaminase]

Purpose

• To detect recent myocardial infarction (MI), together with creatine phosphokinase and lactic dehydrogenase

• To aid in detection and differential diagnosis of acute hepatic disease
• To monitor patient progress and prognosis in cardiac and hepatic diseases.

Normal results

SGOT levels range from 8 to 20 units/liter. Normal values for infants are as high as four times those of adults.

Abnormal results

Very high SGOT levels (more than 20 times normal):
  Acute viral hepatitis
  Severe skeletal muscle trauma
  Extensive surgery
  Drug-induced hepatic injury
  Severe passive liver congestion.

High SGOT levels (10 to 20 times normal):
  Severe MI
  Severe infectious mononucleosis
  Alcoholic cirrhosis
  Prodromal or resolving stages of above conditions causing very high levels.

Moderately high to high levels (5 to 10 times normal):
  Duchenne muscular dystrophy
  Dermatomyositis
  Chronic hepatitis
  Prodromal or resolving stages of conditions causing high levels.

Slightly to moderately high levels (2 to 5 times normal):
  Hemolytic anemia
  Metastatic hepatic tumors
  Acute pancreatitis
  Pulmonary emboli
  Delirium tremens
  Fatty liver
  Biliary obstruction (after the first few days)
  Any preceding condition (at some past time).
  (See *SGOT Elevations in Myocardial Infarction and Hepatic Disease*.)

The basics

SGOT is an enzyme found primarily in the cells of the liver, heart, skeletal muscles, kidneys, pancreas, and to a lesser extent, in red blood cells. It is released into serum in proportion to cellular damage. SGOT levels may be transiently and minimally elevated early in the disease process, and extremely elevated during the most acute phase. Depending on when during the course of the disease the initial sample was drawn, SGOT levels can rise—indicating increasing disease severity and tissue damage—or fall—indicating disease resolution and tissue repair. Thus, the relative change in SGOT values serves as a reliable monitoring mechanism.

SGOT Elevations in Myocardial Infarction and Hepatic Disease

In acute myocardial infarction (MI), serum glutamic-oxaloacetic transaminase (SGOT) levels rise 6 to 10 hours after onset of chest pain, peak in 24 to 48 hours, and—if the infarct does not extend or another MI does not occur—drop to normal in 4 or 5 days. The degree of elevation is roughly proportional to the number of damaged cells, and to the interval between the beginning of the infarction and the time the sample is drawn. Values 15 to 20 times normal indicate extensive myocardial damage and a guarded prognosis. Variable increases occur in congestive heart failure and shock, due to hypoxia and hepatic congestion.

In hepatic disease, SGOT levels usually rise within 4 to 8 hours of onset of acute disease, peak in 24 to 48 hours, and drop to normal in 4 to 8 days or longer, depending on the disease. Subsequent elevations generally indicate a relapse. Serum levels commonly rise before symptoms (such as jaundice) appear.

Although a high correlation exists between MI and elevated SGOT, this test is sometimes considered superfluous for diagnosing MI because of its relatively low organ specificity; it does not enable differentiation between acute MI and the effects of hepatic congestion due to heart failure.

Procedure
Perform a venipuncture and collect the sample in a 7-ml, red-top tube.

Special precautions
To avoid missing peak SGOT levels, draw serum samples at the same time each day.

Patient care checklist
Before the test
☑ Explain or clarify test purpose, preparation, and procedure.
☑ Advise the patient that the test usually requires three venipunctures, one at admission and one each day for the next 2 days.
☑ Evaluate patient understanding.
☑ Withhold medications that may interfere with test results, as ordered. If they must be continued, note them on the laboratory slip.

Interfering factors
• Chlorpropamide; opiates; methyldopa; erythromycin; sulfonamides; pyridoxine; dicumarol; antitubercular agents; large doses of acetaminophen, salicylates, and vitamin A; and many other drugs known to affect the liver cause elevated SGOT levels.
• Strenuous exercise and muscle trauma caused by I.M. injections also raise SGOT levels.
• Hemolysis due to rough handling of the sample may hinder accurate determination of SGOT levels.
• Failure to draw the sample as scheduled, missing peak SGOT levels, may interfere with accurate determination of test results.

Serum glutamic-pyruvic transaminase (SGPT)
[Alanine aminotransferase, alanine transaminase]

Purpose
• To help detect and evaluate treatment of acute hepatic disease—especially hepatitis, and cirrhosis without jaundice
• To help distinguish between myocardial and hepatic tissue damage (used with serum glutamic-oxaloacetic transaminase)
• To assess hepatotoxicity of some drugs.

Normal results
Serum SGPT levels in men range from 10 to 32 units/liter; in women, from 9 to 24 units/liter. The normal range for infants is twice that of adults.

Abnormal results
Very high SGPT levels (up to 50 times normal):
Viral or severe drug-induced hepatitis
Other hepatic disease with extensive necrosis.
Moderately high to high SGPT levels:
Infectious mononucleosis
Chronic hepatitis
Intrahepatic cholestasis
Cholecystitis
Early or improving viral hepatitis
Severe hepatic congestion due to heart failure.
Slightly to moderately high SGPT levels:
Active cirrhosis
Drug-induced alcoholic hepatitis
Other conditions causing acute hepatocellular injury.
Marginal SGPT elevations:
occasionally occur in:
Acute myocardial infarction.

The basics

SGPT is an enzyme necessary for tissue energy production. It primarily appears in hepatocellular cytoplasm, with lesser amounts in the kidneys, heart, and skeletal muscles, and is a relatively specific indicator of acute hepatocellular damage. When such damage occurs, SGPT is released from the cytoplasm into the bloodstream, often before jaundice appears, resulting in abnormally high serum levels that may not return to normal for days or weeks.

Procedure

Perform a venipuncture, and collect the sample in a 7-ml, red-top tube.

Patient care checklist

Before the test

☑ Explain or clarify test purpose, preparation, and procedure.

☑ Evaluate patient understanding.

☑ Withhold medications that interfere with test results, as ordered. If they must be continued, note them on the laboratory slip.

Interfering factors

• Many medications produce hepatic injury by competitively interfering with cellular metabolism. Falsely elevated SGPT levels can follow use of barbiturates, griseofulvin, isoniazid, nitrofurantoin, methyldopa, phenothiazines, phenytoin, salicylates, tetracycline, chlorpromazine, para-aminosalicylic acid, and other drugs that affect the liver. Narcotic analgesics (morphine, codeine, meperidine) may also falsely elevate SGPT levels by increasing intrabiliary pressure.

• Ingestion of lead or exposure to carbon tetrachloride causes direct injury to hepatic cells and sharp elevations of SGPT.

• Hemolysis caused by rough handling of the sample may interfere with accurate determination of SGPT levels.

Sodium

Purpose

To evaluate fluid-electrolyte and acid-base balance, and related neuromuscular, renal, and adrenal functions.

Normal results

Serum sodium levels range from 135 to 145 mEq/liter.

Abnormal results

Sodium imbalance can result from a loss or gain of sodium, or from a change in water volume. Remember, serum sodium results must be interpreted in light of the patient's state of hydration. (See *Water Imbalances,* p. 138.)

Increased serum sodium levels (hypernatremia):

   Inadequate water intake

   Excessive sodium intake

   Water loss in excess of sodium, as in diabetes insipidus, impaired renal function, prolonged hyperventilation, severe vomiting (occasionally), severe diarrhea (occasionally)

   Sodium retention, as in aldosteronism.

Decreased serum sodium levels (hyponatremia):

   Inadequate sodium intake

   Excessive sodium loss due to profuse sweating, gastrointestinal suctioning, diuretic therapy, diarrhea, vomiting, adrenal insufficiency, burns, chronic renal insufficiency with acidosis.

The basics

This test measures serum levels of sodium, the major extracellular cation. Sodium affects body water distribution, maintains osmotic pressure of extracellular fluid, and helps promote neuromuscular function; it also helps maintain acid-base balance and influences chloride and potassium levels. Sodium is absorbed by the intestines

Water Imbalances

Causes	Signs and symptoms	Laboratory findings
Hypervolemia (Water and electrolyte retention resulting in increased extracellular fluid volume)		
• Increased water intake • Decreased water output due to renal disease • Congestive heart failure • Excessive ingestion or infusion of sodium chloride • Long-term administration of adrenocortical hormones • Excessive infusion of isotonic solutions	• Increased... —blood pressure —pulse rate —body weight —respiratory rate • Bounding peripheral pulses • Moist pulmonary rales • Moist mucous membranes • Moist respiratory secretions • Edema • Weakness • Convulsions and coma due to swelling of brain cells	• Decreased... —red cell count —hemoglobin concentration —packed cell volume —serum sodium concentration (dilutional decrease) —urine specific gravity
Hypovolemia (Decreased extracellular fluid volume due to loss of water and electrolytes)		
• Decreased water intake • Fluid loss due to diarrhea, fever, vomiting • Systemic infection • Impaired renal concentrating ability • Fistulous drainage • Severe burns • Hidden fluid in body cavities	• Increased... —pulse rate —respiratory rate • Decreased... —blood pressure —body weight • Weak and thready peripheral pulses • Thick, slurred speech • Thirst • Oliguria (diminished urine output compared with fluid intake) • Anuria • Dry skin	• Increased... —red cell count —hemoglobin concentration —packed cell volume —serum sodium concentration —urine specific gravity

and is excreted primarily by the kidneys; a small amount is lost through the skin. Since extracellular sodium concentration helps the kidneys to regulate body water (decreased sodium levels promote water excretion and increased levels promote retention), serum levels of sodium are evaluated in relation to the amount of water in the body. For example, a sodium deficit (hyponatremia) refers to a decreased level of sodium in relation to the body's water level. The body normally regulates this sodium-water balance through aldosterone, which inhibits sodium excretion and promotes its resorption (with water) by the renal tubules, to maintain balance.

Low sodium levels stimulate aldosterone secretion; elevated sodium levels depress aldosterone secretion. Urine sodium determinations are frequently more sensitive to early changes in sodium balance and should always be evaluated simultaneously with serum sodium findings.

Procedure
Perform a venipuncture, and collect the sample in a 10- to 15-ml, red-top tube.

Special precautions
CLINICAL ALERT: **In a patient with hypernatremia and associated loss of water, observe for signs of thirst, restlessness, dry and sticky mucous membranes, flushed skin, oliguria, and diminished reflexes. However, if increased total body sodium causes water retention, observe for hypertension, dyspnea, and edema.**
CLINICAL ALERT: **In a patient with hyponatremia, watch for apprehension, lassitude, headache, decreased skin turgor, abdominal cramps, and tremors that may progress to convulsions.**

Patient care checklist
Before the test
☑ Explain or clarify test purpose and procedure.
☑ Evaluate understanding.

Interfering factors
• Most diuretics suppress serum sodium levels by promoting sodium excretion; lithium, chlorpropamide, and vasopressin suppress levels by inhibiting water excretion.
• Corticosteroids elevate serum sodium levels by promoting sodium retention. Antihypertensives, such as methyldopa, hydralazine, and reserpine, may cause sodium and water retention.
• Hemolysis due to rough handling of the sample may interfere with accurate determination of test results.

Testosterone

Purpose
• To facilitate differential diagnosis of male sexual precocity (before age 10). True precocious puberty must be distinguished from pseudoprecocious puberty.
• To aid in differential diagnosis of hypogonadism. Primary hypogonadism must be distinguished from secondary hypogonadism.
• To evaluate male infertility or other sexual dysfunction.
• To evaluate hirsutism and virilization in females.

Normal results
Males: 300 to 1,200 ng/dl
Females: 30 to 95 ng/dl
Prepubertal children: In males, less than 100 ng/dl; in females, less than 40 ng/dl.
Testosterone values vary slightly among laboratories.

Abnormal results
Increased testosterone levels:
   True sexual precocity in prepubertal males
   Pseudoprecocious puberty in prepubertal males due to testicular tumor
   Congenital adrenal hyperplasia
   Adrenal tumor (benign or malignant)
   Hyperthyroidism
   Incipient puberty
   Ovarian tumors (possibly)
   Polycystic ovary syndrome (possibly).
Decreased testosterone levels:
   Primary hypogonadism, as in Klinefelter's syndrome
   Secondary hypogonadism, resulting from hypothalamic-pituitary dysfunction
   Orchiectomy
   Testicular cancer
   Prostatic cancer
   Delayed male puberty

Cirrhosis of the liver
Estrogen therapy.

The basics

The principal androgen secreted by the interstitial cells of the testes (Leydig's cells), testosterone induces puberty in the male and maintains male secondary sexual characteristics. Prepubertal levels of testosterone are low. Increased testosterone secretion during puberty stimulates growth of the seminiferous tubules and the production of sperm; it also contributes to the enlargement of external genitalia, accessory sex organs (such as prostate glands), and voluntary muscles, and to the growth of facial, pubic, and axillary hair. Testosterone production begins to increase at the onset of puberty, under the influence of luteinizing hormone from the anterior pituitary, and continues to rise during adulthood. Testosterone inhibits gonadotropin secretion by a negative feedback mechanism similar to that of ovarian hormones in females. Production begins to taper off at about age 40, eventually dropping to approximately one-fifth the peak level by age 80. In females, the adrenal glands and the ovaries secrete small amounts of testosterone.

Procedure

• Perform a venipuncture, and collect the sample in a 7-ml, red-top tube. Use a green-top (heparinized) tube if plasma is to be collected.
• Indicate the patient's age, sex, and history of hormone therapy on the laboratory slip.

Patient care checklist

Before the test
☑ Explain or clarify test purpose and procedure.
☑ Evaluate patient understanding.

Interfering factors

• Exogenous sources of estrogens or androgens can interfere with test results. Estrogens decrease free testosterone levels by increasing sex hormone–binding globulin (SHBG), which binds testosterone; androgens can elevate these levels. Both thyroid and growth hormones decrease SHBG and increase free testosterone. Other pituitary-based hormones may also influence test results.
• Hemolysis due to rough handling of the sample may affect test results.

Thyroid-stimulating hormone (TSH)
[Thyrotropin]

Purpose

• To distinguish between primary and secondary hypothyroidism
• To confirm or rule out primary hypothyroidism
• To monitor drug therapy in patients with primary hypothyroidism.

Normal results

Values for adults and children range from undetectable to 15 µIU/ml.

Abnormal results

Increased serum TSH—levels that exceed 20 µIU/ml:
Primary hypothyroidism
Endemic goiter.
Slightly increased levels:
Euthyroid patients with thyroid cancer.
Decreased or undetectable serum TSH levels:
Secondary hypothyroidism (occasionally)
Hyperthyroidism (Graves' disease)
Thyroiditis.
Note: Decreased levels may be normal.

The basics

TSH is secreted by the anterior pituitary after stimulation by thyrotropin-releasing hormone (TRH) from the hypothalamus. TSH stimulates an increase in the size, number, and secretory activity of thyroid cells; heightens iodine pump activity (active transport of iodine across basal cell membrane), often raising the ratio of intracellular to extracellular iodine as much as 350:1; and stimulates the release of triiodothyronine (T_3) and thyroxine (T_4). This test measures serum TSH levels by radioimmunoassay. It is a reliable test for primary hypothyroidism and helps determine whether hypothyroidism results from thyroid gland failure or from pituitary or hypothalamic dysfunction. Normal serum TSH levels rule out primary hypothyroidism because absence of thyroid hormone in the serum stimulates pituitary hypersecretion of TSH through negative feedback. With some laboratory techniques, this test may not distinguish between low-normal and subnormal levels, especially in secondary hypothyroidism. (There is no inadequate secretion of TSH or TRH.) Hyperthyroidism (Graves' disease) and thyroiditis are both marked by hypersecretion of thyroid hormones, which suppresses TSH release. Provocative testing with TRH is necessary to confirm diagnosis. (See *TRH Challenge Test*.)

Procedure
• Between 6 a.m. and 8 a.m., perform a venipuncture. (Some authorities consider diurnal variation insignificant.)
• Collect the sample in a 5-ml, red-top tube.

Patient care checklist
Before the test
☑ Explain or clarify test purpose, preparation, and procedure.
☑ Inform the patient that the laboratory requires at least 2 days to complete the analysis.
☑ Evaluate patient understanding.
☑ Withhold medications that may interfere with test results, as ordered. If they must be continued, note them on the laboratory slip.
☑ Encourage the patient to relax and remain recumbent for 30 minutes before the test.

Interfering factors
• Failure to observe restrictions of medications may cause spurious test results. Aspirin, corticosteroids, T_3, and heparin lower TSH levels; lithium carbonate and potassium iodide raise them.
• A radioactive scan performed within 1 week before the test may influence test results.

TRH Challenge Test

This test, which evaluates thyroid function and is the first direct test of pituitary reserve, is a reliable diagnostic tool in thyrotoxicosis (Graves' disease). The challenge test requires an injection of thyrotropin-releasing hormone (TRH), normally released by the hypothalamus.

The procedure for this test may vary greatly as to dosage and route of administration. One commonly accepted procedure is the following: After a venipuncture is performed to obtain a baseline thyroid-stimulating hormone (TSH) reading, synthetic TRH (protirelin) is administered by I.V. bolus in a dose of 200 to 500 mcg. As many as five samples (5 ml each) are then drawn at 5-, 10-, 15-, 20-, and 60-minute intervals to assess thyroid response. To facilitate blood collection and avoid multiple venipunctures, an indwelling (Foley) catheter can be used to obtain the required samples.

A sudden spike above the baseline TSH reading indicates a normally functioning pituitary but suggests hypothalamic dysfunction. If the TSH level fails to rise or remains undetectable, pituitary failure is likely. In thyrotoxicosis or thyroiditis, high concentrations of thyroid hormones inhibit TSH secretion. Consequently, TSH levels fail to rise when challenged by TRH.

• Hemolysis due to rough handling of the sample may affect test results.

Thyroxine
$[T_4]$

Purpose
• To evaluate thyroid function
• To aid in diagnosis of hyper- and hypothyroidism
• To monitor response to treatment with antithyroid medication in hyperthyroidism, and to monitor response to thyroid replacement therapy in hypothyroidism.

Normal results
Total T_4 levels range from 5 to 13.5 mcg/dl.

Abnormal results
Increased T_4 levels:
  Primary hyperthyroidism
  Secondary hyperthyroidism including excessive T_4 (L-thyroxine) replacement therapy.
Decreased T_4 levels:
  Primary hypothyroidism
  Secondary hypothyroidism
  T_4 suppression by normal, elevated, or replacement levels of triiodothyronine (T_3).

The basics
T_4 is secreted by the thyroid gland in response to thyroid-stimulating hormone (TSH) from the pituitary gland and, indirectly, to thyrotropin-releasing hormone (TRH) from the hypothalamus. The rate of secretion is normally regulated by a complex system of negative and positive feedback involving the thyroid, anterior pituitary, and hypothalamus. The suspected precursor, or prohormone, of T_3, T_4 is believed to convert to T_3 by a process known as monodeiodination, during which T_4 loses one of its four iodine atoms. The liver and kidneys—and to a lesser extent certain peripheral tissues—are the sites of this cru-

cial transformation. Only a fraction of T_4 (about 0.3%) circulates freely in the blood; the rest binds strongly to plasma proteins, primarily thyroxine-binding globulin (TBG). It is this minute fraction that is responsible for the clinical effects of thyroid hormone on body cells and tissues. This radioimmunoassay, one of the most common diagnostic indicators of thyroid function, measures the total circulating T_4 level when TBG is normal. The Murphy-Pattee, or T_4(D), a similar test based on competitive protein binding, also provides the same information and may be ordered as an alternate test. A normal T_4 level is no guarantee of euthyroidism; for example, normal readings occur in T_3 thyrotoxicosis. In the presence of overt signs of hyperthyroidism, therefore, further testing is necessary. Also, in doubtful cases of hypothyroidism, TSH level or TRH level tests may be indicated.

Procedure
Perform a venipuncture, and collect the sample in a 7-ml, red-top tube.

Patient care checklist
Before the test
☑ Explain or clarify test purpose, preparation, and procedure.
☑ Evaluate patient understanding.
☑ Withhold medications that may interfere with test results, as ordered. If they must be continued, note them on the laboratory slip. (If this test is being performed to monitor thyroid therapy, the patient continues to receive daily thyroid supplements.)

Interfering factors
• Hemolysis due to rough handling or stasis of the sample may interfere with accurate determination of test results.
• Hereditary factors and some hepatic diseases can decrease or increase TBG concentration; protein-wasting diseases (nephrotic syndrome) and androgens may also reduce TBG. Thus, TBG levels can affect determination of test results.

• Certain medications may interfere with test results: clofibrate, estrogens, levothyroxine, methadone, and progestins may increase T_4; clofibrate, ethionamide, free fatty acids, heparin, iodides, liothyronine sodium, lithium, methimazole, methylthiouracil, phenylbutazone, phenytoin, propylthiouracil, reserpine, salicylates (high dose), steroids, sulfonamides, and sulfonylureas may decrease T_4.

Thyroxine-binding globulin
(TBG)

Purpose
• To evaluate abnormal thyrometabolic states that do not correlate with thyroid hormone—triiodothyronine (T_3) or thyroxine (T_4)—values
• To identify TBG abnormalities.

Normal results
Values by electrophoresis range from 10 to 26 mcg T_4 (binding capacity)/100 ml to 16 to 24 mcg T_4 (binding capacity)/100 ml, depending on the laboratory; by radioimmunoassay, values range from 1.3 to 2 mg/100 ml. TBG levels normally rise during pregnancy and are high in neonates.

Abnormal results
Increased TBG levels:
  Hypothyroidism
  Some forms of hepatic disease
  Acute intermittent porphyria.
Decreased TBG levels:
  Hyperthyroidism
  Acromegaly
  Nephrotic syndrome
  Hypoproteinemia
  Acute illness
  Surgical stress.

The basics
This test measures the serum level of TBG, the predominant protein carrier for circulating T_4 and T_3. Any condition that affects TBG levels and subsequent binding capacity also affects the amount of free T_4 (FT_4) and free T_3 (FT_3) in circulation. This can be clinically significant, since only FT_4 and FT_3 are metabolically active. An underlying TBG abnormality renders tests for total T_3 and T_4 inaccurate, but does not alter tests for FT_3 and FT_4. Patients with TBG abnormalities require additional testing to evaluate thyroid function more precisely.

Procedure
Draw venous blood into a 10-ml, red-top tube.

Patient care checklist
Before the test
☑ Explain or clarify test purpose, preparation, and procedure.
☑ Evaluate patient understanding.
☑ Withhold medications that may interfere with test results, as ordered. If they must be continued, note them on the laboratory slip. (They may be continued to determine if prescribed drugs are affecting TBG levels.)

Interfering factors
• Estrogens (including oral contraceptives) and phenothiazines (perphenazine) elevate TBG levels.
• Androgens, prednisone, phenytoin, and high doses of salicylates depress TBG levels.
• Hemolysis due to rough handling of the sample may interfere with accurate determination of test results.

Tolbutamide tolerance test

Purpose
To diagnose insulinoma and rule out functional hyperinsulinism.

Normal results
After tolbutamide infusion, plasma glucose levels promptly drop to about half the fasting level, remain low for 30 minutes, and then gradually rise to pretest levels in 1½ to 3 hours.

Abnormal results

In insulinoma, glucose levels drop markedly and may take 3 hours or more to return to pretest levels.

The basics

I.V. infusion of tolbutamide stimulates the pancreatic beta cells and certain tumors to secrete insulin, and is used to evaluate patients with pancreatic disorders. (Oral tolbutamide is ineffective for this purpose.) Abnormal insulin secretion can be demonstrated indirectly by monitoring plasma glucose levels.

This test can help determine the cause of severe hypoglycemia shown in the fasting plasma glucose or 2-hour postprandial glucose test. The degree and duration of hypoglycemia help establish the diagnosis. In hyperinsulinism, plasma glucose levels mirror those found in normal persons. This does not occur with insulinoma.

Contraindications for this test include: patients with fasting glucose levels that fall below 50 mg/dl. Since tolbutamide depresses plasma glucose to about half the fasting level, it can cause such patients to develop severe hypoglycemia, leading to seizures and coma. The tolbutamide tolerance test is also contraindicated in patients with hypersensitivity to tolbutamide or other sulfonylureas, and should be used cautiously in patients with known hypersensitivity to sulfonamides.

Procedure

• Perform a venipuncture to obtain a fasting blood sample, and collect the sample in a 10-ml, gray-top tube.
• Prepare a mixture of 1 g tolbutamide and 20 ml sterile water; shake the solution to dissolve any crystals.
• Infuse this solution I.V. over 2 to 3 minutes.
• After the infusion, if insulinoma or hyperinsulinism is suspected, draw blood samples at 15, 30, 45, 60, 90, 120, 150, and 180 minutes.
• Specify the collection time of each sample on the laboratory slip, and send each sample to the laboratory immediately.

Special precautions

• The tolbutamide solution must be used within 1 hour of preparation.
• To avoid the multiple venipunctures required for this test, maintain the patency of the vein through a keep-vein-open (KVO) I.V. infusion with normal saline solution or by insertion of a heparin lock.

CLINICAL ALERT: **If the patient develops severe hypoglycemia, notify the physician. Record on the laboratory slip the time when symptoms developed, draw a blood sample, and discontinue the test. Give glucose I.V. to reverse this reaction.**

CLINICAL ALERT: **If the patient develops anaphylaxis, administer epinephrine S.C. or I.M., as ordered, to reverse the reaction, and notify the physician promptly.**

Patient care checklist

Before the test

☑ Explain or clarify test purpose, preparation, and procedure.
☑ Evaluate patient understanding.
☑ Instruct the patient to maintain a high-carbohydrate diet (150 to 300 mg/day) for 3 days before the test.
☑ Instruct the patient to fast overnight before the test and to avoid smoking during the fast.
☑ Withhold medications that may interfere with test results, as ordered. If they must be continued, note them on the laboratory slip.
☑ Alert the patient to the symptoms of hypoglycemia—weakness, restlessness, nervousness, hunger, and sweating—and tell him to report such symptoms immediately.
☑ Review the patient history for contraindications to this test, including very severe hypoglycemia and hypersensitivity to tolbutamide or other sulfonylureas and possibly to sulfonamides. Consult with the physician, as needed.

☑ Provide the patient with books, games, or puzzles for diversion, if necessary, since the procedure takes about 3 hours.

After the test

☑ Notify the physican if phlebitis has developed at the I.V. site; elevate the arm, and apply warm soaks.

☑ Provide the patient with a balanced meal or snack.

Interfering factors

• Hypoglycemic action of tolbutamide may be enhanced by salicylates, chloramphenicol, phenylbutazone, monoamine oxidase inhibitors, and sulfonamides.

• False-positive test results may result from hepatic dysfunction, the ingestion of excessive amounts of alcohol, malnutrition, azotemia, sarcoma, and some nonpancreatic tumors.

Transferrin
[Siderophilin]

Purpose

• To determine the iron-transporting capacity of the blood

• To evaluate iron metabolism in iron deficiency anemia.

Normal results

Serum transferrin values range from 250 to 390 mcg/dl, of which 65 to 170 mcg/dl are usually bound to iron.

Abnormal results

Decreased serum transferrin levels:
   Hepatic damage
   Renal disease (with excessive protein loss)
   Acute or chronic infection
   Cancer.
Increased serum transferrin levels:
   Severe iron deficiency.

The basics

A quantitative analysis of serum transferrin levels, this test evaluates iron metabolism. Transferrin, formed in the liver, transports circulating iron obtained from dietary sources and from the breakdown of red blood cells by reticuloendothelial cells. Most of this iron is transported to bone marrow for use in hemoglobin synthesis; some is converted to hemosiderin and ferritin, and is stored in these forms in the liver, the spleen, and bone marrow. Inadequate transferrin levels may therefore lead to impaired hemoglobin synthesis and, possibly, anemia. Transferrin, normally about 30% saturated with iron, is measured directly by immunoelectrophoresis; a serum iron level is usually obtained simultaneously.

Procedure

Perform a venipuncture, and collect the sample in a 10- to 15-ml, red-top tube.

Patient care checklist

Before the test

☑ Explain or clarify test purpose and procedure.

☑ Evaluate patient understanding.

Interfering factors

• Late pregnancy or the use of oral contraceptives may raise transferrin levels.

• Hemolysis due to rough handling of the sample may affect test results.

T_3 resin uptake $(T_3 \, RU)$
[Resin triiodothyronine uptake, T_3 uptake ratio $(T_3 \, UR)$]

Purpose

• To aid in diagnosis of hypo- and hyperthyroidism when thyroxine-binding globulin (TBG) levels are normal

• To aid in diagnosis of primary disorders of TBG levels.

Normal results

25% to 35% of radioactive T_3 (T_3*) binds to the resin.

Abnormal results

A high resin uptake percentage in the presence of elevated thyroxine (T_4) levels indicates:

Hyperthyroidism.

A low resin uptake percentage, together with low T_4 levels, indicates:

Hypothyroidism.

A high resin uptake percentage and a low or normal free T_4 (FT_4) suggest:

decreased TBG levels, as in:

Nephrotic syndrome

Androgen excess

Administration of certain drugs (salicylates, phenylbutazone, phenytoin).

A low resin uptake percentage and a high or normal FT_4 suggest:

increased TBG levels, as in:

Pregnancy.

The basics

This test indirectly measures FT_4 levels by demonstrating the availability of serum protein-binding sites for T_4. A known amount of T_3*, which exceeds the capacity of TBG to bind to it, and a resin are added to a serum sample. The radioactive hormone combines with unoccupied sites on the TBG; any leftover hormone remains free and available for binding to the resin particles. When the resin is separated from the serum, the amount of radioactivity left on the TBG or bound to resin—measured by radioimmunoassay—is expressed as a percentage of the total amount of the T_3* added initially. The results of T_3 resin uptake are frequently combined with a T_4 radioimmunoassay or T_4 (D) (competitive protein-binding test) to determine the FT_4 index, a mathematical calculation that is thought to reflect FT_4 by correcting for TBG abnormalities. The T_3 RU is considered a valuable ancillary test for thyroid gland dysfunction.

Procedure

Draw venous blood into a 7-ml, red-top tube.

Patient care checklist

Before the test

☑ Explain or clarify test purpose, preparation, and procedure.

☑ Evaluate patient understanding.

☑ Withhold medications that may interfere with test results, as ordered. If they must be continued, note them on the laboratory slip.

Interfering factors

• Therapy with phenylbutazone, phenytoin, high doses of aspirin, anabolic steroids, anticoagulants (heparin), or T_4 may produce a falsely elevated T_3* binding percentage.

• T_3 therapy, oral contraceptives, or estrogen replacement therapy produces a falsely decreased T_3* binding percentage. (In these cases, FT_4 and FT_3 tests are more valuable in assessing thyroid homeostasis.)

• Serious illness may influence test results; severe hepatic disease, nephrotic syndrome, or metastatic disease may cause abnormal elevations in T_3* binding percentage.

• Hemolysis caused by rough handling of the sample may interfere with accurate determination of test results.

Triglycerides

Purpose

• To screen for hyperlipemia
• To help identify nephrotic syndrome
• To determine the risk of coronary artery disease (CAD).

Normal results

Triglyceride values are age-related. Some controversy exists over the most appropriate normal ranges, but the following are fairly widely accepted:

Age	Triglycerides (mg/dl)
0 to 29	10 to 140
30 to 39	10 to 150
40 to 49	10 to 160
50 to 59	10 to 190

Abnormal results

Increased serum triglycerides and increased cholesterol:
Exaggerated risk of CAD.

Mildly to moderately increased serum triglycerides:
Biliary obstruction
Diabetes
Nephrotic syndrome
Endocrinopathies
Overconsumption of alcohol.

Markedly increased serum levels (without an identifiable cause):
Congenital hyperlipoproteinemia.

Decreased serum levels:
Malnutrition
Abetalipoproteinemia.

The basics

This test provides quantitative analysis of triglycerides—the main storage form of lipids—which constitute about 95% of fatty tissue. Increased or decreased serum triglyceride levels merely suggest a clinical abnormality, and additional tests are required for definitive diagnosis. However, serum triglyceride analysis permits early identification of hyperlipemia (characteristic in nephrotic syndrome and other conditions) and risk of CAD.

Procedure

Perform a venipuncture, and collect a serum sample in a 7-ml, red-top tube. A plasma sample is acceptable if a serum sample cannot be collected, but gives values that are usually slightly lower and that do not correlate reliably with the normal range in serum.

Patient care checklist

Before the test
☑ Explain or clarify test purpose, preparation, and procedure.
☑ Evaluate patient understanding.

☑ Restrict food (not water) for 12 to 14 hours before the test.
☑ Advise the patient to abstain from alcohol for 24 hours before the test.
☑ Withhold medications that may interfere with test results, as ordered. If they must be continued, note them on the laboratory slip.

Interfering factors

• A plasma sample may produce slightly lower values than a serum sample.
• Failure to comply with dietary restrictions may interfere with accurate determination of test results.
• Ingestion of alcohol within 24 hours of the test may cause elevated triglyceride levels.
• Certain drugs lower cholesterol levels but raise or have no effect on triglyceride levels. All antilipemics lower serum lipid concentration in the bloodstream, although their mechanisms of action may differ. Cholestyramine lowers cholesterol; it raises or may have no effect on triglycerides. Colestipol lowers cholesterol; it raises or may have no effect on triglycerides.
• Long-term use of corticosteroids raises triglyceride levels, as does use of oral contraceptives, estrogen, ethyl alcohol, furosemide, and miconazole.
• Clofibrate, dextrothyroxine, gemfibrozil, and niacin lower cholesterol and triglyceride levels.
• Certain drugs have a variable effect: probucol lowers cholesterol but has a variable effect on triglycerides.

Triiodothyronine
[T_3]

Purpose

• To aid in diagnosis of T_3 toxicosis
• To aid in diagnosis of hypo- and hyperthyroidism
• To monitor clinical response to thyroid replacement therapy in hypothyroidism.

Normal results

Serum T_3 levels range from 90 to 230 ng/dl. These values may vary with the laboratory performing this test. A rise in serum T_3 levels normally occurs during pregnancy.

Abnormal results

Increased serum T_3 levels:
Hyperthyroidism
T_3 toxicosis
Thyroid replacement therapy.
Decreased serum T_3 levels:
Hypothyroidism (T_3 levels may be normal in some patients)
Trauma or major surgery
Severe acute illness.

The basics

This highly specific radioimmunoassay measures total (bound and free) serum content of T_3 to investigate clinical indications of thyroid dysfunction. T_3, the more potent thyroid hormone, is derived primarily from thyroxine (T_4) through the process of monodeiodination. Like T_4 secretion, T_3 secretion occurs in response to thyroid-stimulating hormone released by the pituitary and, secondarily, to thyrotropin-releasing hormone from the hypothalamus through a complex negative feedback system. Although T_3 is present in the bloodstream in minute quantities and is metabolically active for only a short time, its impact on body metabolism dominates that of T_4. Another significant difference between the two major thyroid hormones is that T_3 binds less firmly to thyroxine-binding globulin (TBG). Consequently, T_3 persists in the bloodstream for a short time; half disappears in about 1 day, while half of T_4 disappears in 6 days. Generally, T_3 levels appear to be more accurate than T_4 levels in diagnosing hyperthyroidism.

Procedure

Draw venous blood into a 7-ml, red-top tube.

Patient care checklist

Before the test
☑ Explain or clarify test purpose, preparation, and procedure.
☑ Evaluate patient understanding.
☑ Withhold medications that may interfere with test results, as ordered. If they must be continued, note them on the laboratory slip.

Interfering factors

• Markedly increased or decreased TBG levels, regardless of cause, may alter test results.
• Hemolysis due to rough handling of the sample may alter test results.
• Clofibrate, estrogen, methadone, liothyronine sodium (T_3), and progestins increase T_3 levels.
• Clofibrate, ethionamide, free fatty acids, heparin, iodides, lithium, methimazole, methylthiouracil, phenylbutazone, phenytoin, propranolol, propylthiouracil, reserpine, salicylates (high doses), steroids, and sulfonamides decrease T_3 levels.

Two-hour postprandial plasma glucose
[2-hour postprandial blood sugar]

Purpose

• To aid in diagnosis of diabetes mellitus
• To monitor drug or diet therapy in patients with diabetes mellitus.

Normal results

In a person without diabetes, postprandial glucose values are less than 145 mg/dl by the glucose oxidase or hexokinase method; levels are slightly elevated in persons over age 50.

Abnormal results

Increased 2-hour postprandial blood glucose:
with values of 200 mg/dl or above on two tests:

Diabetes mellitus.
may also occur with:
Pancreatitis
Cushing's syndrome
Acromegaly
Pheochromocytoma
Hyperlipoproteinemia
Chronic hepatic disease
Nephrotic syndrome
Brain tumor
Sepsis
Gastrectomy with dumping syndrome
Eclampsia
Anoxia
Convulsive disorders.
Decreased glucose levels:
Hyperinsulinism
Insulinoma
Von Gierke's disease
Hypoglycemia
Myxedema
Adrenal insufficiency
Congenital adrenal hyperplasia
Hypopituitarism
Malabsorption syndrome
Hepatic insufficiency.

The basics

The 2-hour postprandial plasma glucose test is a valuable screening tool for detecting diabetes mellitus. This procedure is performed when the patient demonstrates symptoms of diabetes (polydipsia and polyuria) or when results of the fasting plasma glucose test suggest diabetes. In the oral glucose tolerance test (OGTT), plasma glucose measurements are obtained at regular intervals, but the 2-hour measurement reliably indicates the body's insulin response to carbohydrate ingestion. The postprandial test relies solely on the 2-hour glucose level. The greatest difference in normal and diabetic insulin responses, and thus in plasma glucose concentration, occurs about 2 hours after a glucose challenge. Values of this test, however, can fluctuate according to the patient's age. After age 50, for example, normal levels rise markedly and steadily, sometimes reaching 160 mg/dl or higher.

In younger patients, glucose concentration over 145 mg/dl suggests incipient diabetes and requires further evaluation. When postprandial test results are borderline, the OGTT may confirm diagnosis.

Procedure

• Perform a venipuncture, and collect the sample in a 5-ml, gray-top tube.
• Specify on the laboratory slip the time when the patient last ate, the sample collection time, and the time the last pretest insulin or hypoglycemic dose (if applicable) was given.
• If the sample is to be drawn by a technician, tell him the exact time the venipuncture must be performed.

Patient care checklist
Before the test
☑ Explain or clarify test purpose, preparation, and procedure.
☑ Evaluate patient understanding.
☑ Instruct the patient to eat a balanced meal or one containing 100 g of carbohydrate, then fast for 2 hours before the test.
☑ Advise the patient to avoid smoking and strenuous exercise after the meal.

Interfering factors
• False-positive results may be caused by acetaminophen when the glucose oxidase or hexokinase method is used. Other drugs known to cause plasma glucose elevations are chlorthalidone, thiazide diuretics, furosemide, triamterene, oral contraceptives (estrogen-progestogen combination), benzodiazepines, phenytoin, phenothiazines, lithium, epinephrine, arginine, phenolphthalein, dextrothyroxine, diazoxide, large doses of nicotinic acid, corticosteroids, and recent I.V. glucose infusions. Ethacrynic acid may also cause hyperglycemia, but large doses can cause hypoglycemia in patients with uremia.
• Depressed glucose levels may result from the use of beta-adrenergic blockers, amphetamines, ethanol, clofi-

brate, insulin, oral hypoglycemics, and monoamine oxidase inhibitors.

• Recent illness, infection, or pregnancy may raise glucose levels; strenuous exercise or stress may reduce them.

• Glycolysis caused by failure to refrigerate the sample or to send it to the laboratory immediately can depress glucose levels.

Uric acid

Purpose
• To confirm diagnosis of gout
• To help detect kidney dysfunction.

Normal results
Uric acid concentrations in men normally range from 4.3 to 8 mg/dl; in women, from 2.3 to 6 mg/dl.

Abnormal results
Increased serum uric acid levels:
  Gout
  Impaired renal function
  Congestive heart failure
  Von Gierke's disease
  Infections
  Hemolytic anemia
  Sickle cell anemia
  Polycythemia
  Neoplasms
  Psoriasis.
Decreased serum uric acid levels:
  Fanconi's syndrome
  Wilson's disease
  Acute hepatic atrophy.

The basics
Used primarily to detect gout, this test measures serum levels of uric acid, the major end metabolite of purine. Large amounts of purines are present in nucleic acids and derive from dietary and endogenous sources. Uric acid clears the body by glomerular filtration and tubular secretion. However, uric acid is not very soluble at a pH of 7.4 or

lower. Disorders of purine metabolism, rapid destruction of nucleic acids, and conditions marked by impaired renal excretion characteristically raise serum uric acid levels.

Procedure
Perform a venipuncture and collect the sample in a 10- to 15-ml, red-top tube.

Patient care checklist
Before the test
☑ Explain or clarify test purpose and procedure.
☑ Evaluate patient understanding.

Interfering factors
• Loop diuretics, ethambutol, vincristine, pyrazinamide, thiazides, and low doses of aspirin may raise uric acid levels. When uric acid is measured by the colorimetric method, false elevations may be caused by acetaminophen, ascorbic acid, levodopa, and phenacetin. Aspirin in high doses may decrease uric acid levels.

• Starvation, a high-purine diet, stress, and abuse of alcohol may raise uric acid levels.

Uroporphyrinogen I synthase
[Uroporphyrinogen I synthetase, porphobilinogen deaminase]

Purpose
To aid in diagnosis of latent or active acute intermittent porphyria (AIP).

Normal results
Values for uroporphyrinogen I synthase are 8.1 to 16.8 nm/second/liter for females and 7.9 to 14.7 nm/second/liter for males.

Abnormal results
Decreased uroporphyrinogen I synthase levels:
  Latent or active AIP.

The basics

This test measures blood levels of uro-porphyrinogen I synthase, an enzyme that converts porphobilinogen to uro-porphyrinogen during heme biosynthesis. However, a hereditary deficiency can reduce uroporphyrinogen I synthase levels by 50% or more, resulting in AIP. An autosomal-dominant disorder of heme biosynthesis, AIP can be latent indefinitely, until certain factors (some sex hormones and drugs, a low-carbohydrate diet, or an infection) precipitate active disease. An improvement over traditional urine tests that can detect AIP only during an acute episode, the uropor-phyrinogen I synthase test can detect AIP even during its latent phase. Thus, it can identify affected individuals before their first acute episode. Because it is specific for AIP, this test can also differentiate AIP from other types of porphyria. Levels below 6.0 nm/second/liter confirm AIP, but levels between 6.0 and 8.0 nm/second/liter are indeterminate. When levels are indeterminate, urine and stool tests for aminolevulinic acid and porphobilinogen may be ordered to support the diagnosis, since excretion of these porphyrin precursors increases substantially during an acute episode of AIP and may increase slightly during the latent phase.

Procedure

• Perform a venipuncture and collect the sample in a 10 ml, green-top tube.
• Place the sample on dry ice and send it frozen to the laboratory. (If frozen immediately, the sample will remain stable for up to 1 month.)

Patient care checklist

Before the test
☑ Explain or clarify test purpose, preparation, and procedure.
☑ Evaluate patient understanding.
☑ Restrict food and fluid for 12 to 14 hours before the test (the patient may drink water).
☑ If the patient's hematocrit is available, record it on the laboratory slip.
☑ Withhold medications that may interfere with test results, as ordered. If they must be continued, note them on the laboratory slip.

After the test
☑ If the patient has AIP, provide nutritional counseling. Teach him to avoid low-carbohydrate diets, alcohol, and such drugs as steroid hormones, estrogens, barbiturates, sulfonamides, phenytoin, griseofulvin, chlordiazepoxide, meprobamate, glutethimide, methyprylon, and ergot, which may precipitate an acute episode. Remind him to seek care for all infections promptly, since these may also precipitate an acute episode. Advise the patient about obtaining genetic counseling.

Interfering factors

• Hemolytic and hepatic diseases may elevate uroporphyrinogen I synthase levels.
• Hemolysis caused by rough handling of the sample may interfere with accurate interpretation of test results.
• Failure to freeze the sample will cause false-positive results.
• Failure to fast before the test may increase enzyme levels.
• A low-carbohydrate diet, alcohol, infections, and certain drugs, such as those listed above, may decrease enzyme levels.

Vitamin A *[retinol]* and carotene

Purpose

• To investigate suspected vitamin A deficiency or toxicity
• To aid in diagnosis of visual disturbances, especially night blindness and xerophthalmia
• To aid in diagnosis of skin diseases, such as keratosis follicularis or ichthyosis
• To screen for malabsorption.

Normal results
Using colorimetry, serum vitamin A values normally range from 125 to 150 IU/dl; carotene, from 48 to 200 mcg/dl.

Abnormal results
Decreased serum vitamin A levels:
 Celiac disease
 Infectious hepatitis
 Cystic fibrosis of the pancreas
 Obstructive jaundice
 Protein-calorie malnutrition
 Chronic nephritis.
Increased serum vitamin A levels:
 Excessive intake of vitamin A
 Uncontrolled diabetes mellitus.
Decreased serum carotene levels:
 Celiac disease
 Infectious hepatitis
 Cystic fibrosis of the pancreas
 Obstructive jaundice
 Insufficient intake of carotene (rare)
 Pregnancy.
Increased serum carotene levels:
 Grossly excessive dietary intake.

The basics
This test measures serum levels of vitamin A (retinol) and its precursor, carotene. A fat-soluble vitamin normally supplied by diet, vitamin A is important for reproduction, vision (especially night vision), and epithelial tissue and bone growth. It also maintains cellular and subcellular membranes and synthesis of mucopolysaccharides. The body absorbs vitamin A from the intestines as a fatty acid ester; chylomicrons in the lymphatic system then transport it to the liver, where nearly 90% is stored. Absorption of vitamin A requires the presence of adequate amounts of dietary fat and bile salts. Thus, impaired fat absorption or biliary obstruction inhibits vitamin A absorption, causing a deficiency of this vitamin. Serum levels of vitamin A can remain normal as long as the liver retains even a low reserve of vitamin A.

Procedure
Perform a venipuncture, and collect the sample in a 15-ml, red-top tube (this test requires 6 ml of serum).

Special precautions
Protect the sample from light, since vitamin A characteristically absorbs light.

Patient care checklist
Before the test
☑ Explain or clarify test purpose, preparation, and procedure.
☑ Evaluate patient understanding.
☑ Restrict food and fluid overnight before the test. (The patient may drink water.)

Interfering factors
• Patient failure to observe an overnight fast may influence test results.
• Hemolysis caused by rough handling of the sample may alter test results.

Vitamin B₂
[Riboflavin]

Purpose
To detect vitamin B_2 deficiency.

Normal results
Glutathione reductase has an activity index of 0.9 to 1.3.

Abnormal results
An index of 1.4 or greater indicates: vitamin B_2 deficiency due to:
 Insufficient dietary intake of vitamin B_2
 Malabsorption syndrome
 Increased metabolic demands, as in stress.

The basics
This test evaluates the nutritive status and metabolism of vitamin B_2, helping to detect vitamin B_2 deficiency. Absorbed from the intestinal tract and excreted in the urine, vitamin B_2 is essential for growth and tissue func-

tion. In the tissues, this vitamin combines with phosphate to produce the coenzymes flavin mononucleotide and flavin-adenine dinucleotide (FAD); these coenzymes subsequently participate in oxidation-reduction reactions with oxidative enzymes, such as glutathione reductase. In this test, glutathione reductase activity is measured before and after administration of exogenous FAD. Normally, glutathione reductase binds with FAD. If vitamin B_2 supply is inadequate, glutathione reductase activity and the degree of FAD unsaturation will markedly increase, inversely proportional to vitamin B_2 concentration. This serum test is considered more reliable than the urine vitamin B_2 test, which can produce artificially high values in patients after surgery or prolonged fasting.

Procedure
• Perform a venipuncture and collect the sample in a 7-ml, red-top tube.
• Mix the blood immediately with an equal amount of Alsever's solution, a preservative.
• Send the sample to the laboratory immediately; do not refrigerate or freeze the sample.

Patient care checklist
Before the test
☑ Explain or clarify test purpose, preparation, and procedure.
☑ Evaluate patient understanding.
☑ Advise the patient to maintain a normal diet before the test.
After the test
☑ Inform the patient with vitamin B_2 deficiency that good dietary sources of vitamin B_2 are milk products, organ meats (liver and kidneys), fish, green leafy vegetables, and legumes.

Interfering factors
• Hemolysis caused by rough handling of the sample may alter test results.
• Failure to add Alsever's solution to the sample may cause vitamin B_2 to deteriorate before testing.

Vitamin B_{12}
[Cyanocobalamin, antipernicious anemia factor, extrinsic factor]

Purpose
• To aid in differential diagnosis of megaloblastic anemia, which may be due to a deficiency of vitamin B_{12} or folic acid
• To aid in differential diagnosis of central nervous system (CNS) disorders that are affecting peripheral and spinal myelinated nerves.

Normal results
Serum vitamin B_{12} values range from 200 to 1,100 pg/ml.

Abnormal results
Decreased serum vitamin B_{12} levels: result from:
    Inadequate dietary intake of vitamin B_{12} (especially with strict vegetarians)
    Malabsorption syndrome
    Isolated malabsorption of vitamin B_{12}
    Hypermetabolic states, such as hyperthyroidism
    Pregnancy
    CNS damage.
result in:
    Megaloblastic anemia.
Increased serum vitamin B_{12} levels result from:
    Excessive dietary intake
    Hepatic disease
    Myeloproliferative disorders, such as myelocytic leukemia.

The basics
Serum vitamin B_{12} is usually performed concurrently with measurement of serum folic acid levels, since deficiencies of vitamin B_{12} and folic acid are the two most common causes of megaloblastic anemia. A water-soluble vitamin containing cobalt, vitamin B_{12} is essential to hematopoiesis,

DNA synthesis and growth, and myelin synthesis and CNS integrity. Ingested almost exclusively in animal products, vitamin B_{12} is absorbed from the ileum, after forming a complex with intrinsic factor, and is stored in the liver. A clinical vitamin B_{12} deficiency takes years to develop, since almost total conservation is provided by a cyclic pathway (enterohepatic circulation) that allows reabsorption of the vitamin B_{12} normally excreted in bile. Deficiency of intrinsic factor, however, causes malabsorption of vitamin B_{12} and may result in pernicious anemia.

Procedure
Perform a venipuncture, and collect the sample in a 7-ml, red-top tube.

Patient care checklist
Before the test
☑ Explain or clarify test purpose, preparation, and procedure.
☑ Evaluate patient understanding.

Cobalt: Critical Trace Element

A trace element found mainly in the liver, cobalt is an essential component of vitamin B_{12} and therefore is a critical factor in hematopoiesis. A balanced diet supplies sufficient cobalt to maintain hematopoiesis, primarily through foods containing vitamin B_{12}. However, excessive ingestion of cobalt may have toxic effects. Toxicity has occurred, for example, in persons who consumed large quantities of beer containing cobalt as a stabilizer, resulting in congestive heart failure from cardiomyopathy. Since quantitative analysis of cobalt alone is difficult because of the minute amount found in the body, cobalt is often measured by bioassay as part of vitamin B_{12}.

The normal cobalt concentration of human plasma is about 60 to 80 pg/ml.

☑ Restrict food and fluid overnight before the test.

Interfering factors
• Patient failure to observe the overnight fast can alter test results.
• Drugs such as para-aminosalicylic acid, phenytoin, neomycin, and colchicine may alter test results.
• Hemolysis caused by rough handling of the sample may alter test results.
(See *Cobalt: Critical Trace Element*.)

Vitamin C
[Ascorbic acid]

Purpose
To aid in diagnosis of scurvy, scurvy-like conditions, and metabolic disorders.

Normal results
Plasma vitamin C values range from 0.2 to 2 mg/dl.

Abnormal results
Decreased plasma vitamin C levels:
result from:
    Pregnancy and immediate postpartum period
    Infection
    Anemia.
result in:
    Scurvy.
Increased plasma vitamin C levels:
result from:
    Excessive ingestion of vitamin C.

The basics
This chemical assay measures plasma levels of vitamin C, a water-soluble vitamin required for collagen synthesis and cartilage and bone maintenance. Vitamin C also promotes iron absorption, influences folic acid metabolism, and may be necessary for withstanding the stresses of injury and infection. After vitamin C is absorbed from the small intestine, it is transported in the blood to the kidneys and

oxidized to dehydroascorbic acid. Then, it is stored in the adrenal and salivary glands, pancreas, spleen, testes, and brain. However, because the adrenal glands contain high concentrations of vitamin C, stimulation of these glands by adrenocorticotropic hormone may deplete stores of vitamin C. Severe vitamin C deficiency, or scurvy, causes capillary fragility, joint abnormalities, and multiple systemic symptoms. Excess vitamin C is converted to oxalate, which is excreted in the urine. Excessive concentration of oxalate can produce urinary calculi.

Procedure

• Perform a venipuncture, and collect the sample in a 15-ml, black-top tube containing oxalate.
• Send the sample to the laboratory immediately. If transport is delayed, place the sample on ice.

Patient care checklist

Before the test

☑ Explain or clarify test purpose, preparation, and procedure.
☑ Evaluate patient understanding.
☑ Restrict food and fluid intake overnight before the test.

Interfering factors

Failure to follow dietary restrictions or to transport the sample to the laboratory promptly, or hemolysis due to rough handling of the sample, may alter test results.

Vitamin D₃
[Cholecalciferol]

Purpose

• To evaluate skeletal disease, such as rickets and osteomalacia
• To aid in diagnosis of hypercalcemia
• To detect vitamin D toxicity.

Normal results

The range for serum 25-hydroxycholecalciferol is 10 to 55 ng/ml.

Abnormal results

Decreased or undetectable serum 25-hydroxycholecalciferol levels indicate:

vitamin D deficiency due to:
    Poor diet
    Decreased exposure to the sun
    Malabsorption of vitamin D.
vitamin D deficiency that can result in:
    Rickets or osteomalacia.
Increased levels indicate:
toxicity (over 100 ng/ml) due to:
    Excessive self-medication or prolonged therapy.
when associated with hypercalcemia:
    Hypersensitivity to vitamin D₃, as in sarcoidosis.

The basics

Vitamin D₃, the major form of vitamin D, is endogenously produced in the skin by the sun's ultraviolet rays and occurs naturally in fish liver oils, egg yolks, liver, and butter. Like all other fat-soluble vitamins, vitamin D₃ is absorbed from the intestine in the presence of bile salts and is stored in the liver. To become active, this vitamin must undergo conversion to 25-hydroxycholecalciferol, its circulating metabolite; and then to 1,25-dihydroxycholecalciferol, a potent compound—often called a hormone—that controls bone mineralization.

The hormonal function of vitamin D₃ closely parallels that of parathyroid hormone in maintaining calcium and phosphorus homeostasis. Low serum calcium and phosphorus levels stimulate production of parathyroid hormone, which then stimulates renal secretion of 1,25-dihydroxycholecalciferol to promote intestinal absorption of calcium and phosphate. Together, the two hormones stimulate renal absorption of calcium and mobilization of calcium from bone. This test determines serum levels of 25-hydroxycholecalciferol after chromatography has separated it from other vitamin D metabolites and contaminants. Clinically useful in evaluating nutritional status and biologic activity of vitamin D_3, this test is commonly combined with measurement of serum calcium and alkaline phosphatase levels.

Procedure
Perform a venipuncture, and collect the sample in a 7-ml, red-top tube.

Patient care checklist
Before the test
☑ Explain or clarify test purpose and procedure.
☑ Evaluate patient understanding.

Interfering factors
• Anticonvulsants and corticosteroids may lower serum levels.
• Hemolysis may alter test results.

Zinc

Purpose
To detect zinc deficiency or toxicity.

Normal results
Serum zinc values range from 0.75 to 1.4 mcg/ml.

Abnormal results
Decreased serum zinc levels:
   Hereditary deficiency
   Insufficient dietary intake
   Leukemia (markedly depressed)
   Alcoholic cirrhosis
   Myocardial infarction
   Ileitis
   Chronic renal failure
   Rheumatoid arthritis
   Anemia.
Increased (potentially toxic) serum zinc levels:
   Accidental ingestion
   Industrial exposure.
   (See *Industrial Exposure to Zinc Oxide*.)

The basics
This test measures serum levels of zinc, an important trace element. Zinc is found throughout the body but con-

---

Industrial Exposure to Zinc Oxide

Approximately 50,000 industrial workers risk toxic exposure to zinc oxide. Such overexposure can result from inhalation of dust or fumes in the following industries and occupations:

• Alloy manufacturing

• Brass foundry work

• Bronze foundry work

• Electric fuse manufacturing

• Gas welding

• Electroplating

• Galvanizing

• Junk metal refining

• Paint manufacturing

• Metal cutting

• Metal spraying

• Rubber manufacturing

• Roof making

• Zinc manufacturing

Information from *NIOSH Criteria for a Recommended Standard Occupational Exposure to Zinc Oxide* (Washington, D.C.: Department of Health, Education and Welfare, 1975), #76104.

centrates primarily in the blood cells, especially in leukocytes. This element is an integral compound of more than 80 enzymes and proteins, and plays a critical role in enzyme catalytic reactions. Zinc deficiency (hypozincemia) can seriously impair body metabolism, growth, and development. This defect is most apt to develop in patients with certain diseases, such as chronic alcoholism or renal disease, that tend to deplete zinc body stores. Zinc toxicity is rare but can occur after inhalation of zinc oxide during industrial exposure.

Procedure

Perform a venipuncture, and collect the sample in a metal-free collection tube. Laboratories provide special kits for this test on request.

Patient care checklist

Before the test

☑ Explain or clarify purpose and procedure.

☑ Evaluate patient understanding.

Interfering factors

• Zinc-chelating agents (such as penicillinase) and corticosteroids decrease serum zinc levels and may interfere with determination of results.

• Hemolysis caused by rough handling of the sample, or failure to use a metal-free collection tube or to send the sample to the laboratory immediately, can alter test results.

Selected References

American Diabetes Association. *The Physician's Guide to Type II Diabetes (NIDDM)—Diagnosis and Treatment,* 1984.

Beare, P.G., et al. *Nursing Implications of Diagnostic Tests,* 2nd ed. Philadelphia: J.B. Lippincott Co., 1985.

Bryer, J.B., et al. "The Dexamethasone Suppression Test in Depression: Some Correlates," *Biological Psychiatry* 20:814-18, 1985.

Burke, M.D. "Thyroid Function Studies," *Postgraduate Medicine,* December 1980.

Byrne, C.J., et al. *Laboratory Tests: Implications for Nursing Care,* 2nd ed. Menlo Park, Calif.: Addison-Wesley Publishing Co., 1986.

Carroll, B.J. "The Dexamethasone Suppression Test for Melancholia," *British Journal of Psychiatry* 140:292-304, 1982.

Cohen, Judith A., et al. "A Message from the Heart: What Isoenzymes Can Tell You about Your Cardiac Patient," *Nursing82* 12:46-49, April 1982.

Diagnostics, 2nd ed. Nurse's Reference Library. Springhouse, Pa.: Springhouse Corp., 1986.

Diseases, 2nd ed. Nurse's Reference Library. Springhouse, Pa.: Springhouse Corp., 1987.

Endocrine Disorders. Nurse's Clinical Library. Springhouse, Pa.: Springhouse Corp., 1984.

Given, Barbara A., and Simmons, Sandra J. *Gastroenterology in Clinical Nursing,* 4th ed. St. Louis: C.V. Mosby Co., 1983.

Goodhart, Robert, and Shils, Maurice E., eds. *Modern Nutrition in Health and Disease,* 6th ed. Philadelphia: Lea & Febiger, 1980.

Hansten, Philip D. *Drug Interactions,* 5th ed. Philadelphia: Lea & Febiger, 1984.

Hartung, G. Harley, et al. "Relation of Diet to High-Density Lipoprotein Cholesterol in Middle-Aged Marathon Runners, Joggers, and Inactive Men," *New England Journal of Medicine* 302:1357-61, February 14, 1980.

Henry, John Bernard, ed. *Todd-Sanford-Davidsohn Clinical Diagnosis and Management by Laboratory Methods,* vol. 1, 17th ed. Philadelphia: W.B. Saunders Co., 1984.

Hirschfeld, R.M.A., et al. "The Clinical Utility of the Dexamethasone Suppression Test in Psychiatry," *Journal of the American Medical Association* 250(16):2172-74, 1983.

Krishnan, K.R.R., et al. "What Does the Dexamethasone Suppression Test Identify?" *Biological Psychiatry* 20:957-64, 1985.

Leavelle, Dennis E., ed. *Mayo Medical Laboratories Test Catalog.* Rochester, Minn.: Mayo Medical Laboratories, 1984.

Maxwell, Morton H., and Kleeman, Charles R. *Clinical Disorders of Fluid and Electrolyte Metabolism,* 3rd ed. New York: McGraw-Hill Book Co., 1983.

McNeely, Michael D. "Drug Interference with Laboratory Tests of Endocrine Function," *Drug Therapy* 11(1):105-14, 1981.

Monitoring Fluid and Electrolytes Precisely, 2nd ed. New Nursing Skillbook Series. Springhouse, Pa.: Springhouse Corp., 1983.

Petersdorf, Robert G., and Adams, Raymond D., eds. *Harrison's Principles of Internal Medicine,* 10th ed. New York: McGraw-Hill Book Co., 1983.

Stanbury, John B., and Wyngaarden, James B. *The Metabolic Basis of Inherited Disease,* 5th ed. New York: McGraw-Hill Book Co., 1983.

Sumner, Sara M. "Refining Your Technique for Drawing Arterial Blood Gases," *Nursing80* 10:65-69, April 1980.

Tulchinsky, Dan, and Ryan, Kenneth J. *Maternal-Fetal Endocrinology.* Philadelphia: W.B. Saunders Co., 1980.

Watts, Nelson B., and Keffer, Joseph H. *Practical Endocrine Diagnosis,* 3rd ed. Philadelphia: Lea & Febiger, 1982.

Wegener, Lee T., ed. *Mayo Medical Laboratories Interpretive Handbook.* Rochester, Minn.: Mayo Medical Laboratories, 1984.

Williams, Robert H. *Textbook of Endocrinology,* 6th ed. Philadelphia: W.B. Saunders Co., 1981.

Williams, Sue Rodwell. *Mowry's Basic Nutrition and Diet Therapy,* 7th ed. St. Louis: C.V. Mosby Co., 1984.

Witzun, Joseph L., et al. "Normalization of Triglycerides in Type IV Hyperlipoproteinemia Fails to Correct Low Levels of High-Density Lipoprotein Cholesterol," *New England Journal of Medicine* 303:907-13, October 16, 1980.

3 IMMUNODIAGNOSTIC TESTING

Introduction

A normally functioning immune system provides continuous physiologic surveillance. When a foreign agent penetrates the body, a specific immune mechanism takes over, destroying the invading organism through the specialized activity of the lymphocytes and macrophages.

Immune response

The immune response is the mechanism by which the body recognizes an antigen as nonself, then proceeds to destroy it. Two distinct types of immune responses cooperate to protect the body. The humoral response involves antibodies that are products of the B cell (lymphocyte) line. These antibodies, or immunoglobulins, which attack the antigen, are classified as follows: IgM (provides the initial response); IgG (provides long-term immunity); IgA (provides antiviral antibodies, which are also known as secretory Ig); IgD (serves an unknown function); and IgE (operates primarily in allergic conditions). The cell-mediated response involves T cells (lymphocytes), which react with the antigen directly. T cells provide cellular immunity, inhibit tumor growth, cause the body to reject organ transplants, and produce autoimmune disorders. The antigen-antibody reactions of the immune system activate the complement system, which removes antigens from the body.

Immunologic disorders

Immunodeficiency disorders result from impaired development of the immune system's structural components (cells) or from defective expression of the immune response. Either can increase susceptibility to infection and cancer. Acquired immune deficiency syndrome (AIDS) has brought public attention to one of many types of immunodeficiencies. Hypersensitivity disorders (allergies) have been appropriately described as "immunity gone wrong" because they involve normal immune mechanisms with a hair-trigger sensitivity to substances that are not intrinsically harmful. Examples of such sensitivities include asthma and contact dermatitis. Autoimmunity results from an inability to distinguish self from nonself. The immune response is misdirected against the body's own tissues; autoantibodies usually attack intracellular "self-antigens." Examples of autoimmunity include rheumatoid arthritis and systemic lupus erythematosus. Immunoproliferative disorders may occur with overproduction of one immune response component. Examples of immunoproliferative disorders include leukemia and lymphoma.

Diagnostic uses

Serological diagnosis (one made through laboratory examination of antigen-antibody reactions in the serum) may be instrumental in uncovering infection, cancer, or other immune disorders such as allergy or autoimmune conditions. Successful blood transfusions also require tests that identify antigens and antibodies to make correct matching of donor and recipient blood possible.

Testing techniques
Most immunologic tests use combinations of techniques to evaluate humoral and cell-mediated immune responses or their individual components. The most commonly used laboratory methods include:

Precipitation
Forms interlocking aggregates caused by interactions between soluble antigens and antibodies.

Immunodiffusion
Relies on the tendency of antigen and antibody particles to diffuse in an agar matrix and to form a precipitin line where they meet. This test may be performed using single diffusion, double diffusion, or immunoelectrophoresis techniques. The latter uses an electrical current to speed diffusion of the reactants.

Agglutination
Occurs when large, insoluble parti-

Screening Blood For AIDS Antibodies

Tests that measure serum antibodies for human T-cell lymphotrophic virus type III (HTLV-III), the AIDS virus, have been licensed by the Food and Drug Administration and are now commercially available. The tests are used to screen donated blood for AIDS, preventing contamination of the nation's blood supply. However, these tests only confirm the presence of antibodies to the AIDS virus. They do not confirm that an individual has AIDS or is likely to develop it. The initial screening test is an enzyme-linked immunosorbent assay, commonly called by its acronym ELISA.

Drawbacks
The ELISA test is not 100% accurate, though, and sometimes gives false results. For instance, because test sensitivity varies among laboratories, a negative result does not necessarily mean that HTLV-III antibodies are absent. Also, in an asymptomatic patient, a positive result may result from immunity, subclinical infection, or cross-reactivity with other viral antigens. A false-positive result may also reflect a laboratory error. As a result, the U.S. Public Health Service recommends confirmation of any positive result before the patient is notified, using the Western blot test to detect antibodies for viral proteins. This test is more reliable than the ELISA test, but is technically more difficult and used primarily for research.

Clinical implications of a positive test for an asymptomatic patient are currently unknown.

Your role
Encourage the patient with positive screening tests to seek medical follow-up care, even if he is asymptomatic. Instruct him to report early signs of AIDS, such as fever, weight loss, axillary or inguinal lymphadenopathy, rash, and persistent cough or diarrhea.

Assume that he can transmit AIDS to others, until further or more conclusive evaluation proves otherwise. To prevent possible contagion, instruct him not to share razors, toothbrushes, or utensils (which may be contaminated with blood) and to cleanse such items with household bleach diluted 1:10 in water. Advise the patient to avoid donating blood, tissues, or an organ. If you suspect I.V. drug abuse, warn the patient not to share needles.

Encourage the patient to inform his doctor and dentist about his condition, so they can take proper precautions.

cles, such as bacteria or RBCs, are clumped together by antibodies to the particles, or to the antigens attached to the particles.

Immunofluorescence

Identifies an antigen by observing its antigen-antibody reaction with known antibodies flagged with fluorescent dye.

Radioimmunoassay

Relies on the competition between radiolabeled and unlabeled antigens for binding sites on antibodies to determine the amount of antigen in a serum sample.

Enzyme-linked immunosorbent assay (ELISA)

Identifies antibody or antigen, based on enzyme activation that occurs due to antigen-antibody reaction. (See *Screening Blood for AIDS Antibodies*.)

Complement fixation

Determines the presence and extent of antigen-antibody reaction, performed by adding a known antigen or antibody directed against an unknown antigen or antibody to a patient's serum and incubating the sample. RBCs coated with this same known antigen or antibody are added. If hemolysis does not occur, complement must have been depleted in the original reaction; in other words, the unknown antibody or antigen was present in the sample. The unknown antibody-antigen is assayed.

Monoclonal antibody assays

Monoclonal antibodies (homogeneous groups of a single type of antibody made against a specific antigen) have been used extensively for typing cells and cell subsets, detecting specific antigens, and differentiating malignant from nonmalignant cells. (See *Collection Techniques: Blood and Urine Samples*, pp. xii to xx, and *Understanding Titers*, p. 162.)

Patient-Learner guidelines

Patient-learner objectives:

• Define the test.

• State the specific purpose of the test.
• Explain the procedure.
• Discuss test preparation, procedure, and post-test care.

Teaching content:

• Define the test in terms the patient can understand.
• Explain the specific purpose of the test.
• Describe the procedure, if the patient is unfamiliar with it. If a venipuncture is necessary, explain that the patient's vein will be punctured, usually by a steel needle attached to a tube or syringe, so that blood can be collected for testing.
• Explain that collection of the blood sample causes some discomfort; however, the procedure is brief.
• Inform the patient that mild pressure will be applied to the puncture site following the procedure. Usually, a few minutes' pressure at most is sufficient. If the patient has a bleeding tendency, inform him that the pressure may be necessary for a longer period to control bleeding.
• Tell the patient that a clean, dry bandage will be applied to the puncture site, and to avoid infection, he should keep the site clean and dry for at least 24 hours. Patients with some immune diseases have a compromised immune system.
• Identify any dietary or medication restrictions necessary before the test. List items to be avoided, and give a definite time period. Explain that these steps are necessary to provide accurate test results. Verbal instructions should be accompanied by written instructions for outpatients.
• When appropriate, explain to the patient that test results may not be available immediately, but may take several days, especially if the sample is sent to another facility for testing.

Evaluation:

After the patient-teaching session is completed, evaluate whether the patient has satisfactorily met each

Understanding Titers

The titer is an index of the degree of immune responsiveness to a particular antigen. Titers are obtained for two purposes: 1) to determine if immunity exists to viruses (such as rubella, mumps, and smallpox) and bacteria or to bacterial by-products (such as streptolysin-O produced by A-betahemolytic streptococci); or 2) to determine whether a person has recently been exposed to a specific infectious agent.

There are two different laboratory tests employed to measure titers. One is agglutination, which is an antigen-antibody reaction that can be visibly observed as a clumping of particulate matter in the test system. The serum to be tested is diluted in increasing amounts (i.e., 1:8, 1:16, 1:32, 1:64, etc.) and mixed with the antigen (usually bacteria). If the serum contains antibodies to this antigen, agglutination will occur. The reciprocal of the lowest concentration in which an agglutination reaction still occurs is reported as the titer. For example, if the last dilution in which clumping occurred was 1:16, the titer is reported as 16. The higher the dilution, the stronger the immunity.

In most titer determinations for viral infections, another type of laboratory test—inhibition of agglutination or, more specifically, hemagglutination inhibition (HI)—is used. Ordinarily, viruses agglutinate goose red blood cells. Antibodies to these viruses in the patient's serum, however, will inhibit this re-action. Serial dilutions of the patient's serum are tested for the ability to inhibit the agglutination of the goose red blood cells. The titer is reported as the highest dilu-tion in which agglutination failed to occur. Again, the higher the dilution, the stronger the immunity.

When titers are performed to determine whether a person is immune to a particular infectious agent, the laboratory will inform you of the lowest titer necessary for immunity. This value may differ from laboratory to laboratory. When titers are used to determine whether or not a patient has been infected with or exposed to a particular antigen, obtaining read-ings during the acute and conva-lescent phases is helpful, as an increase in titer (usually fourfold) from acute to convalescent con-firms infection.

patient-learner objective by obtaining necessary patient feedback. Refocus teaching as needed.

ABO blood typing

Purpose
• To establish blood group according to the ABO system
• To check compatibility of donor and recipient blood before transfusion.

Normal results
Patient's blood group is identified as Group A, B, AB, or O.

The basics
This test classifies blood according to the presence of major antigens A and B on red cell surfaces and according to serum antibodies anti-A and anti-B. In forward typing, if agglutination occurs when the patient's red cells are mixed with anti-A serum, the A an-tigen is present and the blood is typed A. If agglutination occurs when the patient's red cells are mixed with anti-B serum, the B antigen is present and the blood is typed B. If agglutination occurs in both mixes, both A and B antigens are present and the blood is typed AB. If it does not occur in either

Identification of Blood Groups

Principal Blood Group	Antigens on Red Cell	Antibodies in Blood Serum
O	None	Anti-A and Anti-B
A	A	Anti-B
B	B	Anti-A
AB	AB	None

mix, no antigens are present and the blood is typed O. In reverse typing, if agglutination occurs when B cells are mixed with the patient's serum, anti-B is present and the blood is typed A. If agglutination occurs when A cells are mixed, anti-A is present and the blood is typed B. If agglutination occurs when both A and B cells are mixed, anti-A and anti-B are present and the blood is typed O. If agglutination does not occur when both A and B cells are mixed, neither anti-A nor anti-B are present and the blood is typed AB.

Because group O blood lacks both

Blood Group Compatibility Chart

Recipient's Blood Type	Compatible Donor Type
A	A, O
B	B, O
AB	A, B, AB, O
O	O

A and B antigens, it can be transfused in limited amounts to any recipient in an emergency, with little risk of agglutination. For this reason, a person with group O blood is called a universal donor. Such transfusion should be given as packed RBCs, from which the plasma has been removed. Because a person with AB blood has neither anti-A nor anti-B antibodies, he can receive A, B, or O blood (packed cells) and is called a universal recipient. (See *Blood Group Compatibility Chart*.)

Procedure
Perform a venipuncture, and collect the sample in a 10-ml lavender-top tube or red-top tube, as ordered (one tube per three units of blood).

Patient care checklist
Before the test
☑ Explain or clarify test purpose and procedure.
☑ Evaluate patient understanding.

Interfering factors
• Recent administration of dextran or I.V. contrast media causes cellular aggregation that resembles agglutination.
• Hemolysis due to rough handling of the sample may alter test results.
• If a patient has received blood in the past three months, antibodies to this donor blood may develop and linger, interfering with the patient's compatibility testing.

Acetylcholine receptor antibodies
(AChR) [Barre Test]

Purpose
• To confirm diagnosis of myasthenia gravis (MG)
• To monitor the effectiveness of immunosuppressive therapy for MG.

Normal results

AChR-binding antibodies: negative or less than or equal to 0.03 nmol/liter.
AChR-blocking antibodies: negative.

Abnormal results

Positive AChR antibodies:
  Confirm MG.

The basics

This is the most useful immunologic test to confirm a diagnosis of acquired (autoimmune) MG, a disorder of neuromuscular transmission. In normal muscle contraction, acetylcholine (ACh) is released from the terminal end of the nerve and binds to AChR sites on the muscle motor end plate. In MG, however, antibodies block and destroy AChR sites, causing muscle weakness that can be either generalized or localized to the ocular muscles. Patients who have only ocular symptoms of MG tend to have lower antibody titers than those who have generalized symptoms.

Procedure

• Perform a venipuncture, and collect the sample in a 7-ml red-top tube.
• Maintain the sample at room temperature.
• Immediately send the sample to the laboratory.

Patient care checklist

Before the test
☑ Explain or clarify test purpose and procedure.
☑ Evaluate patient understanding.
After the test
☑ Examine venipuncture site for infection. (If the patient has an autoimmune disease, he has a compromised immune system.)

Interfering factors

• Failure to maintain the sample at room temperature and to send it to the laboratory immediately may affect the accurate determination of test results.
• Patients undergoing thymectomy, thoracic duct drainage, immunosuppressive therapy, or plasmapheresis may show reduced AChR-antibody levels.
• Patients with amyotrophic lateral sclerosis may show false-positive test results.

Alpha-fetoprotein *(AFP)*

Purpose

To monitor the effectiveness of therapy in malignant conditions, such as hepatomas and germ cell tumors, and in certain nonmalignant conditions, such as ataxia-telangiectasia.

Normal results

Adults: less than 15 ng/ml.
Pregnant women: the normal level is computed based on gestational age, mother's age, mother's weight, the presence of a multiple pregnancy, and other factors.

Abnormal results

Increased alpha-fetoprotein levels in nonpregnant persons:
  Hepatocellular carcinoma
  Germ cell tumor of gonadal, retroperitoneal, or mediastinal origin
  Ataxia-telangiectasia
  Occasionally, cancer of the pancreas, stomach, or biliary system.
Slightly increased AFP levels in nonpregnant persons:
  Acute or chronic hepatitis
  Alcoholic cirrhosis.
Increased levels in pregnant women (found in maternal serum after 14 weeks' gestation):
  Fetal neural tube defects (such as spina bifida or anencephaly)
  Intrauterine death
  Other anomalies, such as duodenal atresia, omphalocele, tetralogy of Fallot, and Turner's syndrome.

The basics

AFP is a glycoprotein produced by fetal tissue and tumors that differentiate from midline embryonic structures.

During fetal development, AFP levels in serum and amniotic fluid rise; since this protein crosses the placenta, it also appears in maternal serum. After 14 weeks' gestation, AFP levels rise sharply in approximately 90% of fetuses with anencephaly and in 50% of those with spina bifida. Definitive diagnosis, however, necessitates ultrasonography and amniocentesis. In late stages of pregnancy, AFP concentrations in fetal and maternal serum and in amniotic fluid begin to diminish. During the first year of life, serum AFP levels continue to decline, and characteristically persist at a low level thereafter.

In hepatocellular carcinoma, a gradual decrease in elevated serum AFP levels indicates a favorable response to therapy. In germ cell tumors, serum AFP levels and serum human chorionic gonadotropin levels should be measured concurrently to assess therapy.

Procedure
Perform a venipuncture, and collect the sample in a 7-ml red-top tube.

Patient care checklist
Before the test
☑ Explain or clarify test purpose and procedure.
☑ Evaluate patient understanding.

Interfering factors
• Hemolysis caused by rough handling of the sample may alter serum AFP levels, thereby interfering with accurate determination of test results.
• Multiple pregnancy may cause false-positive test results.

Antibody screening test
[Indirect Coombs' test, indirect antiglobulin test]

Purpose
• To detect unexpected circulating antibodies to red cell antigens in the recipient's or donor's serum before transfusion
• To determine the presence of anti-Rho(D) (Rh-positive) antibody in maternal blood
• To evaluate the need for Rho(D) immune globulin administration
• To aid diagnosis of acquired hemolytic anemia.

Normal results
Agglutination does not occur, indicating that the patient's serum contains no circulating antibodies (other than anti-A and/or anti-B).

Abnormal results
Positive for agglutination:
Indicates the presence of unexpected circulating antibodies to red cell antigens. Such a reaction demonstrates donor and recipient incompatibility.
May indicate acquired hemolytic anemia.
Positive result in pregnant patient with Rh-negative blood:
Indicates the presence of antibodies to the Rh factor from previous transfusion with incompatible blood or from a previous pregnancy with an Rh-positive fetus.
Above a titer of 1:8:
Indicates that the fetus may develop hemolytic disease of the newborn. (Repeated testing throughout the patient's pregnancy is then necessary for evaluating progressive development of circulating antibody levels.)

The basics
The antibody screening test detects 95% to 99% of unexpected circulating antibodies in a patient's serum. After incubating the serum with group O red cells, which are unaffected by anti-A or anti-B antibodies, an antiglobulin (Coombs') serum is added. Agglutination occurs if the patient's serum contains an antibody to one or more antigens on the red cells. After this

Antibody Identification Test

This test identifies unexpected circulating antibodies detected by the antibody screening test (indirect Coombs' test). Group O red cells—at least three with and three without a specific antigen—are combined with serum containing unknown antibodies and are observed for agglutination. If the serum contains the corresponding antibody to the red cell antigen, a positive reaction occurs with RBCs that have the antigen but not with those that lack the antigen. Serum that reacts with Rh-positive cells, for example, but not with Rh-negative cells, probably contains the anti-$Rh_o(D)$ antibody. At least three red cells containing the antigen and three without it are used in each test to reduce error. Serum that contains rare or multiple antibodies requires more complicated procedures.

of the sample may interfere with accurate determination of test results.

• If a patient has received blood transfusions within the past 3 months, antibodies to this donor blood may develop and linger, thus interfering with the patient's compatibility testing.

• Failure to send the sample to the laboratory immediately will interfere with test results because the antibody screening must be done within 48 hours after the sample is drawn.

---

screening procedure detects the antibodies, the antibody identification test can determine the specific identity of the antibodies present. (See *Antibody Identification Test*.)

Procedure
Perform a venipuncture, and collect the sample in two 10-ml red-top tubes. (Some laboratories require 20 ml of clotted blood to perform this test.)

Patient care checklist
Before the test
☑ Explain or clarify test purpose and procedure.
☑ Evaluate patient understanding.

Interfering factors
• Previous administration of blood, dextran, or I.V. contrast media causes aggregation that resembles agglutination.
• Hemolysis caused by rough handling

Anti-deoxyribonucleic acid antibodies
(Anti-DNA antibodies)

Purpose
• To confirm systemic lupus erythematosus (SLE) after a positive antinuclear antibody test
• To monitor response to immunosuppressive therapy.

Normal results
Less than 1 mcg of native DNA bound/ml of serum.

Abnormal results
Increased anti-DNA levels:
A value of 1 to 2.5 mcg/ml:
  Remission phase of SLE; presence of other autoimmune disorders.
A value of 10 to 15 mcg/ml:
  Active SLE.
A decrease in elevated levels following immunosuppressive therapy:
  Demonstrates effective treatment of SLE.

The basics
This test measures antinative DNA antibody levels in a serum sample, using radioimmunoassay or a less sensitive technique, such as agglutination, complement fixation, or immunoelectrophoresis.

Procedure
Perform a venipuncture, and collect

the sample in a 7-ml red-top tube. (Some laboratories may specify a lavender- or gray-top tube.)

Patient care checklist
Before the test
☑ Explain or clarify test purpose and procedure.
☑ Evaluate patient understanding.

Interfering factors
A radioactive scan performed within 1 week of collecting the sample may alter the test results.

Antimitochondrial antibodies

Purpose
• To aid diagnosis of primary biliary cirrhosis
• To distinguish between extrahepatic jaundice and biliary cirrhosis.

Normal results
Negative for antimitochondrial antibodies at a 1:5 dilution.

Abnormal results
Positive for antimitochondrial antibodies:
  Primary biliary cirrhosis
  Chronic active hepatitis
  Drug-induced jaundice
  Cryptogenic cirrhosis
  Autoimmune diseases, such as systemic lupus erythematosus (SLE), rheumatoid arthritis, pernicious anemia, and idiopathic Addison's disease.

The basics
This test for antimitochondrial antibodies, which is usually performed with the test for anti-smooth-muscle antibodies, detects antibodies in serum by indirect immunofluorescence. Antimitochondrial antibodies react with mitochondria in the renal tabules, gastric mucosa, and other organs in which cells expend large amounts of energy.

These autoantibodies are present in several hepatic diseases, although their etiologic role is unknown, and there is no evidence that they cause hepatic damage.

Antimitochondrial antibodies appear in 79% to 94% of patients with primary biliary cirrhosis, but this test alone does not confirm diagnosis. Further tests, such as serum alkaline phosphatase, serum bilirubin, SGOT, SGPT, or cholangiography, may also be necessary. Since antimitochondrial antibodies rarely appear in patients with extrahepatic biliary obstruction, a positive test helps rule out this condition.

Procedure
Perform a venipuncture, and collect the sample in a 7-ml red-top tube.

Patient care checklist
Before the test
☑ Explain or clarify test purpose and procedure.
☑ Evaluate patient understanding.
After the test
CLINICAL ALERT: Apply pressure to venipuncture site until all bleeding has stopped. (Patients with hepatic disease may bleed excessively.)

Interfering factors
• Confusion of antimitochondrial antibodies with heterophil antibodies, cardiolipin antibodies to syphilis, ribosomal antibodies, or microsomal hepatic or renal antibodies, can cause inaccurate determination of test results.
• Oxyphenisatin can produce antimitochondrial antibodies in patients taking this drug.

Antinuclear antibodies
(ANA)

Purpose
• To screen for systemic lupus erythematosus (SLE)

• To monitor the effectiveness of immunosuppressive therapy for SLE.

Normal results

Negative for antinuclear antibodies at a titer of 1:32 or below.

Abnormal results

High antinuclear antibody titers:
  SLE.
Lower but still elevated titers may occur in patients with:
  Viral diseases
  Chronic hepatic diseases
  Collagen vascular diseases
  Autoimmune diseases
  Some healthy adults (incidence increases with age).

The basics

In conditions such as SLE, scleroderma, and certain infections, the body's immune system may perceive portions of its own cell nuclei as foreign, and may produce ANA. Specific ANA include antibodies to DNA, nucleoprotein, histones, nuclear ribonucleoprotein, and other nuclear constituents. Although ANA are harmless in themselves, since they do not penetrate living cells, they sometimes form antigen-antibody complexes that cause tissue damage (as in SLE). Because of multiorgan involvement, test results are not diagnostic, and can only partially confirm clinical evidence. Although it cannot confirm SLE, the higher the titer, the more specific the test is for SLE. This test measures the relative concentration of ANA in a serum sample, through indirect immunofluorescence. The pattern of nuclear immunofluorescence helps identify the type of immune disease present.

Procedure

Perform a venipuncture, and collect the sample in a 7-ml red-top tube.

Patient care checklist

Before the test
☑ Explain or clarify test purpose and procedure.
☑ Evaluate patient understanding.
After the test
☑ Observe venipuncture site for signs of infection. Report any changes to the physician. (Patients with an autoimmune disease have a compromised immune system.)
☑ Apply a clean, dry bandage to the site for at least 24 hours.

Interfering factors

Certain drugs—most commonly isoniazid, hydralazine, and procainamide—can produce a syndrome resembling SLE; other such drugs include para-aminosalicylic acid, chlorpromazine, clofibrate, phenytoin, griseofulvin, ethosuximide, gold salts, methyldopa, oral contraceptives, penicillin, propylthiouracil, phenylbutazone, methysergide, streptomycin, sulfonamides, tetracyclines, mephenytoin, quinidine, primidone, reserpine, and trimethadione.

Anti-smooth-muscle antibodies

Purpose

To aid diagnosis of chronic active hepatitis and primary biliary cirrhosis.

Normal results

Anti-smooth-muscle antibodies titer less than 1:20.

Abnormal results

High anti-smooth-muscle antibody titers:
  Chronic active hepatitis
  Primary biliary cirrhosis
  Infectious mononucleosis
  Acute viral hepatitis
  Malignant tumor of liver
  Intrinsic asthma.

The basics

This test measures the relative concentration of anti-smooth-muscle antibodies in serum using direct immunofluorescence and is usually performed with the test for antimitochondrial antibodies. Although the anti-smooth-muscle antibodies are most commonly associated with hepatic diseases, their etiologic role is unknown, and there is no evidence that they cause hepatic damage. This test is not very specific; these antibodies appear in about 66% of patients with chronic active hepatitis and 30% to 40% of patients with primary biliary cirrhosis.

Procedure

Perform a venipuncture, and collect the sample in a 7-ml red-top tube.

Patient care checklist

Before the test

☑ Explain or clarify test purpose and procedure.

☑ Evaluate patient understanding.

After the test

CLINICAL ALERT: **Apply pressure to the venipuncture site until bleeding stops, since patients with hepatic disease may bleed excessively.**

Antistreptolysin-O test

(ASO test) [Streptococcal antibody test]

Purpose

• To confirm recent or ongoing infection with beta-hemolytic streptococci
• To help diagnose rheumatic fever and post-streptococcal glomerulonephritis in the presence of clinical symptoms
• To distinguish between rheumatic fever and rheumatoid arthritis when joint pains are present.

Normal results

Adults and preschool-age children:
   ASO titer less than 85 Todd units/ml.

School-age children:
   ASO titer less than 170 Todd units/ml.

Abnormal results

High ASO titers:
Low-elevation titers:
   Uncomplicated streptococcal disease.
Titers to 250 Todd units/ml:
   Inactive rheumatic fever.
Titers of 500 to 5,000 Todd units/ml:
   Acute rheumatic fever
   Acute post-streptococcal glomerulonephritis.

The basics

Because streptococcal infections are often overlooked, serologic testing is valuable in patients with glomerulonephritis and acute rheumatic fever to confirm antecedent infection by showing serologic response to streptococcal antigen. The ASO test measures the relative serum concentrations of the antibody to streptolysin O, an oxygen-

---

Detecting Pathogens Quickly

Commercially available antigen/antibody test kits use direct antigen-testing techniques to detect certain pathogens in serum, urine, or cerebrospinal fluid (CSF) specimens quickly.

For example, products that use either monoclonal or polyclonal antibody technology to detect pathogens causing meningitis are currently available. Results on CSF may be available within 15 minutes. The following pathogens causing meningitis may be detected by using either a separate kit or a combination kit:

• *Hemophilus influenzae* type B
• *Streptococcus pneumoniae*
• *Neisseria meningitidis* group B
• Group B streptococcus
• *Neisseria meningitidis* groups A, C, and Y
• W 135

labile enzyme produced by group A beta-hemolytic streptococci. High ASO titers usually occur only after prolonged or recurrent infections. Serial titers, determined at 10- to 14-day intervals, provide more reliable information than a single titer. A rise in titer 2 to 5 weeks after the acute infection, which peaks 4 to 6 weeks after the initial rise, confirms poststreptococcal disease. Even healthy persons have some detectable ASO titer from previous minor streptococcal infections.

Procedure
Perform a venipuncture, and collect the sample in a 7-ml red-top tube.

Test For Anti-DNase B

The antideoxyribonuclease B (anti-DNase B) test, a process similar to the antistreptolysin-O (ASO) test, detects antibodies to DNase B, a potent antigen produced by all group A streptococci.

For adults, normal anti-DNase B titer is less than 85 Todd units/ml; for school-age children, less than 170 Todd units/ml; and for preschoolers, less than 60 Todd units/ml. Elevated anti-DNase B titers appear in 80% of patients with acute rheumatic fever, in 75% of those with poststreptococcal glomerulonephritis (following streptcoccal pharyngitis), and 60% of those with glomerulonephritis (following group A streptococcal pyoderma). This is a much higher percentage than those with ASO titer elevations (25%), making the test for anti-DNase B especially valuable in detecting a reaction to group A streptococcal pyoderma. Other streptococcal antigens are of limited diagnostic value, or their use is controversial.

Patient care checklist
Before the test
☑ Explain or clarify test purpose and procedure.
☑ Evaluate patient understanding.

Interfering factors
• Since patients with streptococcal skin infections rarely have abnormal ASO titers, even with poststreptococcal disease, false-negative results are likely in such patients.
• Antibiotic or corticosteroid therapy may suppress the streptococcal antibody response, and may interfere with accurate determination of test results.
• Hemolysis due to rough handling of the sample may interfere with accurate determination of test results.
(See *Detecting Pathogens Quickly*, p. 169, and *Test for Anti-DNase B*.)

Antithyroid antibodies

Purpose
To detect circulating antithyroglobulin antibodies when clinical evidence indicates Hashimoto's thyroiditis, Graves' disease, or other thyroid diseases.

Normal results
Titer less than 1:100 for both antithyroglobulin and antimirosomal antibodies.

Abnormal results
High antithyroid antibody titers:
    Subclinical autoimmune thyroid disease
    Graves' disease
    Idiopathic myxedema
    Adenomatous goiter
    Thyroid carcinoma
    Pernicious anemia
    Other autoimmune disorders, such as systemic lupus erythematosus, rheumatoid arthritis, and autoimmune hemolytic anemia.

Incidence of Thyroid Autoantibodies in Various Diseases

Disorder	Presence of Antithyroglobulin	Presence of Antimicrosomal Antibodies
Hashimoto's disease	60% to 95%	70% to 90%
Idiopathic myxedema	75%	65%
Graves' disease	30% to 40%	50% to 85%
Adenomatous goiter	20% to 30%	20%
Thyroid carcinoma	40%	15%
Pernicious anemia	25%	10%

Very high titers (may be in millions):
Strongly suggest Hashimoto's thyroiditis.
(See *Incidence of Thyroid Autoantibodies in Various Diseases.*)

The basics
In autoimmune disorders, such as Hashimoto's thyroiditis, thyroglobulin, the major colloidal storage compound, is released into the blood. Because thyroxine usually separates from thyroglobulin before its release into the blood, thyroglobulin does not normally enter the circulation. When it does, antithyroglobulin antibodies come into existence to attack this foreign substance; the ensuing autoimmune response damages the thyroid gland. The serum of a patient whose autoimmune system produces antithyroglobulin antibodies usually contains antimicrosomal antibodies, which react with the microsomes of the thyroid epithelial cells.

The tanned red cell hemagglutination test detects antithyroglobulin and antimicrosomal antibodies. Another laboratory technique, immunofluorescence, can detect antimicrosomal antibodies.

Procedure
Perform a venipuncture, and collect the sample in a 7-ml red-top tube.

Patient care checklist
Before the test
☑ Explain or clarify test purpose and procedure.
☑ Evaluate patient understanding.

C-reactive protein (CRP)

Purpose
• To detect the acute phase of inflammatory disease, such as exacerbations of rheumatoid arthritis and rheumatic fever
• To monitor response to therapy, especially in acute rheumatic fever and rheumatoid arthritis.

Normal results
Negative CRP.

Abnormal results
Positive CRP:
Bacterial infections, such as tuberculosis and pneumococcal pneumonia

Noninfectious inflammatory conditions, such as acute rheumatic fever, acute rheumatoid arthritis, systemic lupus erythematosus, malignancy, and myocardial infarction

During last half of pregnancy

With use of oral contraceptives.

The basics

Absent in the sera of healthy persons, C-reactive protein (CRP) is an abnormal specific glycoprotein produced by the liver and excreted into the bloodstream during the acute phase of inflammation from any cause. Thus, the test for CRP is nonspecific. CRP was initially discovered in the sera of patients with pneumococcal pneumonia, where it was shown to react with the C-mucopolysaccharide of the bacterial capsule—hence the name C-reactive protein. The major function of CRP is its interaction with the complement system. Antiserum is used to detect CRP in several immunoassays—radioimmunoassay, capillary precipitation, gel diffusion, and latex agglutination.

Procedure

Perform a venipuncture, and collect the sample in a 7-ml red-top tube.

Patient care checklist

Before the test

☑ Explain or clarify test purpose, preparation, and procedure.

☑ Evaluate patient understanding.

☑ Restrict food and fluids (except water) for at least four hours prior to the test.

Interfering factors

Pregnancy, ingestion of oral contraceptives, or the use of an intrauterine device may cause positive test results, due to production of CRP because of tissue stress.

Carcinoembryonic antigen
(CEA)

Purpose

• To monitor the effectiveness of cancer therapy

• To assist in preoperative staging of colorectal cancers

• To test for recurrence of colorectal cancers.

Normal results

Serum CEA values less than 5 ng/ml in healthy nonsmokers.

Abnormal results

Increased CEA levels:

Malignant conditions:

  Endodermally derived neoplasms of the gastrointestinal organs and the lungs

  Nonendodermal carcinoma, such as breast cancer and ovarian cancer.

Nonmalignant conditions:

  Benign hepatic disease

  Hepatic cirrhosis

  Alcoholic pancreatitis

  Inflammatory bowel disease

  Chronic heavy smoking.

The basics

CEA, a glycoprotein secreted onto the glycocalyx surface of cells lining the gastrointestinal tract, appears during the first or second trimester of fetal life. Normally, production of CEA is halted before birth, but may begin again later if a neoplasm develops. Since CEA levels are raised by conditions other than malignant neoplasms, this test cannot be used as a general indicator of cancer. However, this test is useful for staging, assessing the adequacy of surgical resection, and monitoring colorectal cancer therapy, since serum CEA levels, measured by enzyme immunoassay, usually return to normal within 6 weeks if cancer treatment is successful. Persistent elevation of CEA levels, however, suggests residual or recurrent tumor.

Procedure
Perform a venipuncture, and collect the sample in a 7-ml red-top tube.

Patient care checklist
Before the test
☑ Explain or clarify test purpose and procedure.
☑ Evaluate patient understanding.

Interfering factors
• Chronic cigarette smoking may elevate serum CEA levels, causing inaccurate interpretation of test results.
• Hemolysis caused by rough handling of the sample may elevate serum CEA levels, thereby altering test results.

Cold agglutinins

Purpose
• To help confirm primary atypical pneumonia
• To provide additional diagnostic evidence for cold agglutinin disease associated with many viral infections or lymphoreticular malignancy.

Normal results
Titer for cold agglutinins less than 1:16 (in elderly, titer may be higher).

Abnormal results
High titers for cold agglutinins:
  Infectious mononucleosis
  Cytomegalovirus infection
  Hemolytic anemia
  Multiple myeloma
  Scleroderma
  Malaria
  Cirrhosis
  Congenital syphilis
  Peripheral vascular disease
  Pulmonary embolism
  Tympanosomiasis
  Tonsillitis
  Staphylococcemia
  Occasionally in pregnancy.
Chronically high titers:
  Pneumonia
  Lymphoreticular malignancy.

Acute transiently high titers:
  Certain infectious diseases, notably primary atypical pneumonia.
Extremely high titers (1: 1,000 to 1: 1,000,000):
  Can occur with idiopathic cold agglutinin disease that precedes the development of lymphoma.

The basics
Cold agglutinins are antibodies (usually of the IgM type) that cause RBCs to aggregate at low temperatures and may occur in small amounts in healthy persons. In primary atypical pneumonia, cold agglutinins appear in serum of one-half to two-thirds of all patients during the first week of acute infection, even before antimycoplasmal antibodies can be detected by complement fixation or metabolic inhibition tests. Thus, titers usually become positive at 7 days, peak above 1:32 in 4 weeks, and commonly disappear quite rapidly after 6 weeks. When sequential titers verify this pattern and clinical evidence of pneumonia exists, diagnosis is confirmed. Patients with high cold agglutinin titers, such as those with primary atypical pneumonia, may develop acute transient hemolytic anemia after repeated exposure to cold; patients with persistently high titers may develop chronic hemolytic anemia. Patients with extremely high titers are susceptible to intravascular agglutination, which causes significant clinical problems, possibly leading to frostbite, anemia, Raynaud's phenomenon, or, rarely, focal gangrene.

Procedure
Perform a venipuncture, and collect the sample in a 7-ml red-top tube that has been prewarmed to 98.6° F. (37° C.).

Patient care checklist
Before the test
☑ Explain or clarify test purpose and procedure.

☑ Evaluate patient understanding.

After the test

<u>CLINICAL ALERT</u>: **Keep the patient warm if cold agglutinin disease is suspected. (If the patient is exposed to low temperatures, agglutination may occur within peripheral vessels, possibly leading to frostbite, anemia, Raynaud's phenomenon, or, rarely, focal gangrene.)**

☑ Observe the patient for signs of vascular abnormalities, such as mottled skin, purpura, jaundice, or pallor; pain or swelling of the extremities; and cramping of fingers and toes. (Hemoglobinuria may result from severe intravascular hemolysis on exposure to severe cold.)

Interfering factors

• Hemolysis caused by rough handling of the sample can falsely depress titers, as can refrigeration of the sample before serum is separated from RBCs.

• Antibiotics can interfere with the development of cold agglutinins.

Complement assays

Purpose

• To help detect immunomediated disease and genetic complement deficiency

• To monitor the effectiveness of therapy.

Normal results

Total complement: 41 to 90 hemolytic units

C1 esterase inhibitor: 16 to 33 mg/dl

C3: in males, 88 to 252 mg/dl; in females, 88 to 206 mg/dl.

C4: in males, 12 to 72 mg/dl; in females, 13 to 75 mg/dl.

Abnormal results

Increased total complement levels:
  Obstructive jaundice
  Thyroiditis
  Acute rheumatic fever

  Rheumatoid arthritis
  Acute myocardial infarction
  Ulcerative colitis
  Diabetes.

Decreased total complement levels:

Characteristic in:
  Systemic lupus erythematosus (SLE)
  Acute post-streptococcal glomerulonephritis
  Acute serum sickness.

May occur in:
  Advanced cirrhosis of the liver
  Multiple myeloma
  Hypogammaglobulinemia
  Rapidly rejecting allografts.

Decreased C1 esterase inhibitor:
  Hereditary angioedema.

Decreased C3:
  Recurrent pyrogenic infection.

Decreased C4:
  SLE.

The basics

Complement is a collective term for a system of at least 20 serum proteins designed to destroy foreign cells and to help remove foreign materials. The system may be triggered by contact with antigen-antibody complexes or by clotting factor XIIa. A cascade of events follows, which results in the formation of a complex that ruptures cell membranes. Complement components are numerically designated as C1 through C9, with C1 having three subcomponents: C1q, C1r, and C1s. Complement comprises 3% to 4% of total serum globulins, and plays a key role in antibody-mediated immune reactions. Complement can function as a defense by promoting the removal of infectious agents, or as a threat by triggering destructive reactions in host tissues. Therefore, complement deficiency can increase susceptibility to infection, and can predispose to other diseases. Complement assays are indicated in patients with known or suspected immunomediated disease or repeatedly abnormal response to infection.

Complement Cascade: Two Pathways

Classical Pathway

Initiated by antigen-antibody complexes
▼
$\overline{C1qrs}$ generates an enzyme that cleaves C4 and C2
▼
$\overline{C142}$ is formed, which cleaves C3
▼
C3a (anaphylatoxin) and C3b are formed; C3a is released and functions in inflammation; C3b is an opsonin and is active in the enzyme $\overline{C1423b}$
▼
$\overline{C1423b}$ induces cleavage of C5

Alternative Pathway

Initiated by IgA, some IgG, and certain polysaccharides, lipopolysaccharides, and trypsin-like enzymes
▼
Factor B combines with C3b in the presence of Factor D
▼
C3bBb (stabilized by properdin) is formed, which acts on C3
▼
C3bBbC3b (stabilized by properdin) is formed, which induces cleavage of C5

Forms C5a (anaphylatoxin) and C5b; C5a is released and functions in inflammation; C5b binds to C6,7
▼
C5b,6,7 binds to C8
▼
C5b,6,7,8 binds to C9
▼
C5b,6,7,8,9 causes cell lysis

The complement system plays an indispensable role in the humoral immune response. Activation of the complement cascade follows one of two pathways: the *classical pathway*, initiated by antigen-antibody complexes, or the *alternative pathway*, triggered by IgA; some IgG molecules; and certain polysaccharides, lipopolysaccharides, and trypsin-like enzymes.

Classical: Upon activation of the classical pathway by antigen-antibody complexes, C1qrs generates an enzyme that cleaves C4 and C2, producing C142 (the classical pathway C3 convertase). C142 then cleaves C3 into C3a (anaphylatoxin) and C3b. This forms C1423b, the classical pathway C5 convertase.

Alternative: C3b, spontaneously cleaved from C3 continuously in the blood, is inactivated by Factors I

and H. However, in the presence of certain activators (such as polysaccharides), Factors I and H are less able to inactivate C3b. This initiates the alternative pathway. Factor B combines with C3b in the presence of Factor D to form the alternative pathway C3 convertase, C3bBb. C3bBb, in turn, acts on C3 to form C3bBbC3b, the alternative pathway C5 convertase. Properdin stabilizes both C3bBb and C3bBbC3b, causing cleavage of C3 into C3a and C3b. C3bBbC3b induces cleavage of C5, producing C5a and C5b.

The binding of C5b to C6,7 initiates the membrane attack phase. C5b,6,7 causes leakage of intracellular fluid. Leakage increases dramatically when C5b,6,7 binds with C8. Rapid cytolysis occurs when the final complement component, C9, binds to C5b,6,7,8.

Normally, complement is present in serum in an inactive state until "fixed" or activated in the classic pathway by binding to an antibody-coated surface. In the classic pathway, a specific antibody identifies and coats an antigen that enters the body. C1 recognizes and binds with this specific antibody, activating the complement cascade (a series of enzymatic reactions involving all complement components), producing a coordinated inflammatory response, and usually resulting in cell lysis.

In the alternate pathway, substances such as polysaccharides, bacterial endotoxins, and aggregated immunoglobulins react with properdin and Factors B, D, H, and I, producing an enzyme that activates C3. In turn, C3 activates the remainder of the complement cascade.

In both pathways, specific inhibitors regulate the sequential activation of complement components. The C1 esterase inhibitor, the most commonly studied inhibitor, regulates the classic pathway; the C3b inhibitor can regulate either pathway, since C3 is a pivotal component of both.

Complement abnormalities may be genetic or acquired; acquired abnormalities are more common. Depressed total complement levels are clinically more significant than elevations. Although various laboratory methods are used to evaluate and measure total complement and its components, hemolytic assay, laser nephelometry, and radial immunodiffusion are the most common. Complement assays provide valuable information about the patient's immune system, but the results must be considered in light of serum immunoglobulin and autoantibody tests for definitive diagnosis of immunomediated disease or abnormal response to infection. (See *Complement Cascade: Two Pathways*, p. 175.)

Procedure
Perform a venipuncture, and collect the sample in a 7-ml red-top tube.

Patient care checklist
Before the test
☑ Explain or clarify test purpose and procedure.
☑ Evaluate patient understanding.
After the test
☑ Keep the venipuncture site clean and dry. (Patient may have a compromised immune system.)

Interfering factors
• Hemolysis caused by rough handling of the sample, or, since complement is heat-labile and deteriorates rapidly, failure to send the sample to the laboratory immediately may interfere with accurate determination of test results.

• A history of recent heparin therapy can affect test results.

Crossmatching

Purpose
To serve as the final check for compatibility between the donor's blood and the recipient's blood.

Normal results
Negative crossmatch (the absence of agglutination):
Indicates probable compatibility between the donor's blood and the recipient's blood, so transfusion of donor blood can proceed.
Positive crossmatch (agglutination occurs):
Indicates incompatibility between the donor's blood and the recipient's blood, so the donor's blood cannot be transfused to the recipient.

The basics
Crossmatching establishes compatibility or incompatibility of the donor's and the recipient's blood. It is the best antibody detection test available for avoiding lethal transfusion reactions.

After the donor's and the recipient's ABO blood type and Rh factor type are determined, major crossmatching tests are needed for compatibility between the donor's RBCs and the recipient's serum. The donor's RBCs and the recipient's serum are compatible if the recipient's serum has no antibodies that would destroy transfused cells and possibly cause an acute hemolytic reaction. Agglutination, the sign of a positive crossmatch, indicates an undesirable antigen-antibody reaction. The donor's blood must be withheld, and the crossmatch continued to determine the cause of the incompatibility and to identify the antibody.

Minor crossmatching tests determine compatibility between the donor's serum and the recipient's RBCs. This crossmatch is less important, however, because the donor's antibodies are greatly diluted in the recipient's plasma. Since the antibody-screening test is routinely performed on all blood donors, minor crossmatching is often omitted.

Procedure
• Perform a venipuncture, and collect the sample in a 10-ml red-top tube (one tube for three units of blood ordered).
• Label the sample with the patient's name, room number, and hospital or blood bank number. Also include the amount and type of blood component desired.

Patient care checklist
Before the test
☑ Explain or clarify test purpose and procedure.
☑ Evaluate patient understanding.
☑ Note date and time of any previous transfusions. If more than 48 hours have elapsed since the previous transfusion, previously crossmatched donor blood must be re-crossmatched with a new recipient serum sample to detect newly acquired incompatibilities before transfusion.

Interfering factors
• Previous administration of dextran

or I.V. contrast media causes aggregation resembling agglutination.
• Previous blood administration may produce antibodies to the donor blood that may interfere with compatibility testing.
• Hemolysis due to rough handling of the sample may interfere with accurate determination of test results.
• Failure to send the sample to the laboratory immediately may cause false results, because crossmatching must be performed on the sample within 48 hours.

Cryoglobulins

Purpose
To detect cryoglobulinemia in patients with Raynaud-like vascular symptoms.

Normal results
Negative for cryoglobulins.

Abnormal results
Positive for cryoglobulins:
  Cryoglobulinemia.
  (See *Cryoglobulin Levels in Associated Diseases*, p. 178.)

The basics
Cryoglobulins are abnormal serum proteins that precipitate at low laboratory temperatures ($32.9°$ F. [$4°$ C.]) and redissolve after being warmed. The presence of cryoglobulins in the blood (cryoglobulinemia) is usually associated with immunologic disease, but can also occur in the absence of known immunopathology. Cryoglobulinemia occurs in three forms: Type I, in which the reaction of a single monoclonal immunoglobulin is involved; Type II, in which a monoclonal immunoglobulin shows antibody activity against a polyclonal immunoglobulin; and Type III, in which both components are polyclonal immunoglobulins. If patients with cryoglobulinemia are subjected to cold, they

Cryoglobulin Levels In Associated Diseases

Type of Cryoglobulin	Serum Level	Associated Diseases
Type I Monoclonal cryoglobulin	> 5 mg/ml	• Myeloma • Waldenström's macroglobulinemia • Chronic lymphocytic leukemia
Type II Mixed cryoglobulin	> 1 mg/ml	• Rheumatoid arthritis • Sjögren's syndrome • Mixed essential cryoglobulinemia
Type III Mixed polyclonal cryoglobulin	< 1 mg/ml (50% below 80 mcg/ml)	• Systemic lupus erythematosus • Rheumatoid arthritis, Sjögren's syndrome • Infectious mononucleosis • Cytomegalovirus infections • Acute viral hepatitis • Chronic active hepatitis • Primary biliary cirrhosis • Poststreptococcal glomerulonephritis • Infective endocarditis • Leprosy • Kala-azar • Tropical splenomegaly syndrome

may experience Raynaud-like symptoms (pain, cyanosis, and coldness of fingers and toes), which generally result from precipitation of cryoglobulins in cooler parts of the body. The cryoglobulin test involves refrigerating a serum sample at 39.2° F. (4° C.) for at least 72 hours and observing for formation of a heat-reversible precipitate. Such a precipitate requires further study by immunoelectrophoresis or double diffusion, to identify cryoglobulin components. Although the presence of cryoglobulins in the blood confirms cryoglobulinemia, this finding does not always mean the presence of clinical disease.

Procedure
• Warm the syringe and collection tube to 98.6° F. (37° C.) before venipuncture, and keep them at that temperature.
• Perform a venipuncture, and collect the sample in the warm 10-ml red-top tube.

Patient care checklist
Before the test
☑ Explain or clarify test purpose, preparation, and procedure.
☑ Evaluate patient understanding.
☑ Restrict food and fluids for 4 to 6 hours before the test.

After the test
☑ If the test is positive for cryoglobulins, tell the patient to avoid cold temperatures or contact with cold objects.
☑ Observe the patient for intravascular coagulation (decreased color and temperature in distal extremities; increased pain).

Interfering factors
• Failure to adhere to dietary restrictions may interfere with the accurate determination of test results.
• Failure to maintain the sample at 98.6° F. (37° C.) before centrifugation may cause loss of cryoglobulins.
• Reading the sample before the end of the 72-hour precipitation period may cause test results to be reported incorrectly, since some cryoglobulins take several days to precipitate.

Direct antiglobulin test
[Direct Coombs' test]

Purpose
• To diagnose hemolytic disease of the newborn (HDN)
• To investigate hemolytic transfusion reactions
• To aid differential diagnosis of hemolytic anemias, which may result from an autoimmune reaction, drugs, underlying disease (such as lymphoma), or anemias (which may be congenital).

Normal results
Negative; neither antibodies nor complement appear on RBCs.

Abnormal results
Positive for immunoglobulins:
When performed on umbilical cord blood:
  HDN.
When performed using venipuncture:
  Hemolytic anemia
  Sepsis.

Weakly positive test:
  Transfusion reaction in which the patient's antibodies react with the transfused RBCs containing the corresponding antigen.

The basics
The direct antiglobulin test detects immunoglobulins (antibodies) on the surfaces of RBCs. These immunoglobulins coat RBCs when they become sensitized to an antigen, such as the Rh factor. In this test, antiglobulin (Coombs') serum added to saline-washed RBCs results in agglutination if immunoglobulins or complement are present. This test is "direct" because it requires only one step—the addition of Coombs' serum to washed cells. If an infant has HDN, transfusion of compatible Rh-negative blood may be necessary to prevent anemia. In addition to indicating the presence of hemolytic anemia, a positive test result can help differentiate between autoimmune and secondary hemolytic anemia, which can be drug-induced or associated with underlying disease, such as lymphoma.

Procedure
• For an adult, perform a venipuncture and collect the sample in two 5-ml red-top tubes.
• For a neonate, after the cord is clamped and cut, draw 5 ml of cord blood into a red-top or lavender-top tube, as ordered.

Patient care checklist
Before the test
☑ Explain or clarify test purpose and procedure to the patient or to the parents of the newborn.
☑ Evaluate patient/parent understanding.
☑ Withhold medications that can induce autoimmune hemolytic anemia, as ordered.
After the test
☑ Inform the patient or the parents of an infant with HDN that further test-

ing will be necessary to monitor anemia.

Interfering factors

• Hemolysis caused by rough handling of the sample may interfere with accurate determination of test results.

• False-positive results may follow use of quinidine, methyldopa, cephalosporin, sulfonamide, chlorpromazine, diphenylhydantoin, dipyrone, ethosuximide, hydralazine, levodopa, mefenamic acid, melphalan, penicillin, procainamide, rifampin, streptomycin, tetracyclines, and isoniazid.

• Failure to send the sample to the laboratory immediately may cause false results, because the test must be performed within 24 hours after the sample is drawn.

Extractable nuclear antigen (ENA) antibodies
[Ribonucleoprotein (RNP) antibodies; anti-Smith (Sm) antibodies; Sjögren's (SS-B) antibodies]

Purpose

• To aid differential diagnosis of autoimmune disease

• To distinguish between anti-RNP and anti-Sm antibodies

• To screen for anti-RNP antibodies (common in mixed connective tissue disease [MCTD])

• To screen for anti-Sm antibodies (common in systemic lupus erythematosus [SLE])

• To support diagnosis of collagen vascular autoimmune diseases

• To monitor response to therapy.

Normal results

Serum is negative for anti-RNP, anti-Sm, and SS-B antibodies.

Abnormal results

Positive for anti-Sm antibodies:
  SLE (highly diagnostic).

Positive for anti-RNP antibodies:
  SLE
  Progressive systemic sclerosis
  Other rheumatic disorders.
High levels of anti-RNP antibodies, with a low titer of anti-Sm antibodies:
  MCTD.
Positive for SS-B antibodies:
  Sjögren's syndrome.

The basics

ENA is a complex of at least two, and possibly three, antigens. Antibodies to these antigens are associated with certain autoimmune disorders. Tests to detect ENA antibodies help differentiate autoimmune disorders with similar signs and symptoms. The RNP antibody test detects RNP antibodies. This test aids in the differential diagnosis of systemic rheumatic disease, and is a useful follow-up test for collagen vascular autoimmune disease. The anti-Sm antibody test detects Sm antibodies, a specific marker for SLE. This test, too, helps monitor collagen vascular autoimmune disease. The Sjögren's antibody test detects the SS-B autoantibodies produced in Sjögren's syndrome, an immunologic abnormality sometimes associated with rheumatoid arthritis and SLE. However, this test is not diagnostic for Sjögren's syndrome. Anti-ENA tests are most useful in tandem with anti-DNA, serum complement, and antinuclear antibody tests.

Procedure

Perform a venipuncture, and collect the sample in a 7-ml red-top tube.

Patient care checklist

Before the test
☑ Explain or clarify test purpose and procedure.
☑ Evaluate patient understanding.
After the test
☑ Check venipuncture site for infection, since the patient with an autoimmune disease has a compromised immune system.

☑ Keep a clean, dry bandage over the site for at least 24 hours.

Interfering factors
Failure to send the sample to the laboratory immediately may interfere with accurate determination of test results.

Febrile agglutination tests

Purpose
• To support clinical findings in diagnosis of disorders caused by *Salmonella,* rickettsiae, *F. tularensis,* or *Brucella* organisms in which isolation from the blood or excreta is difficult
• To identify the cause of fever of unknown origin (FUO).

Normal results
Normal dilutions are as follows:
Salmonella antibody: less than 1:80
Brucellosis antibody: less than 1:80
Tularemia antibody: less than 1:40
Rickettsial antibody: less than 1:40.

Abnormal results
In **Salmonella** *infection:*
  H and O agglutinins usually appear in serum after one week, and titers continue to rise for 3 to 6 weeks. O agglutinins usually fall to insignificant levels in 6 to 12 months. H agglutinin titers may remain elevated for several years.
In brucellosis:
  Titers usually rise after 2 or 3 weeks, and reach their highest levels between 4 and 8 weeks. (Nevertheless, absence of *Brucella* agglutinins does not rule out brucellosis.)
In tularemia:
  Titers usually become positive in the second week of infection, exceed 1:320 by the third week, peak in 4 to 7 weeks, and usually decline gradually 1 year after recovery.

In rickettsial infections, including Rocky Mountain spotted fever and typhus:
  The Weil-Felix reaction is positive with antibodies to *Proteus* (not the causal agent) 6 to 12 days after infection; titers peak in 1 month and usually drop to negative in 5 or 6 months. (However, this test cannot be used for diagnosing rickettsialpox or Q fever, since the antibodies of these diseases do not cross-react with *Proteus* antigens.)

The basics
The Weil-Felix reaction for rickettsial disease, Widal's test for *Salmonella,* and tests for brucellosis and tularemia are essentially the same. With these tests, the observed rise and fall of titers is crucial for detecting active infection. If this is not possible, certain titer levels can suggest the disorder. For all febrile agglutinins, a fourfold increase in titers is strong evidence of infection.

Special precautions
<u>CLINICAL ALERT:</u> **Use standard hospital isolation procedures when collecting and handling samples.**

Patient care checklist
Before the test
☑ Explain or clarify test purpose and procedure.
☑ Evaluate patient understanding.
After the test
☑ In FUO and suspected infection, contact the hospital infection control department. Isolation may be necessary.

Interfering factors
• Failure to send the sample to the laboratory immediately may affect the accurate determination of test results.
• Vaccination or continuous exposure to bacterial or rickettsial infection (resulting in immunity) causes high titers.
• Many antibodies cross-react with bacteria that cause other infectious diseases. For example, tularemia an-

tibodies cross-react with Brucella antigens.

• Immunodeficient patients may show infectious symptoms but be unable to produce antibodies. In such cases, titers remain negative, even during infection.

• Patients receiving antibiotic therapy show depressed titers early in the course of the disorder.

• Patients with elevated immunoglobulin levels due to hepatic disease, or those who use drugs excessively, often have high *Salmonella* titers.

• Patients who have had skin tests with *Brucella* antigen may show elevated *Brucella* titers.

• Patients with *Proteus* infections may show positive Weil-Felix titers for rickettsial disease.

Fluorescent treponemal antibody absorption test
(FTA-ABS; FTA)

Purpose
• To confirm primary or secondary syphilis
• To screen for suspected false-positive results of Venereal Disease Research Laboratory (VDRL) tests.

Normal results
Negative (no fluorescence) or nonreactive FTA-ABS test.

Abnormal results
Reactive test (indicating presence of treponemal antibodies):
    Primary syphilis (positive in 80% to 90% of affected patients)
    Secondary syphilis (positive in 100% of affected patients).
Minimally reactive test:
    Systemic lupus erythematosus
    Genital herpes
    Increased or abnormal globulins
    Pregnancy.

The basics
This test uses indirect immunofluorescence to detect antibodies to the cause of syphilis—the spirochete *Treponema pallidum*—in serum. The presence of treponemal antibodies in the serum does not indicate the stage or the severity of infection. (However, the presence of these antibodies in CSF is strong evidence of tertiary neurosyphilis.) Higher antibody levels persist for several years, with or without treatment. Because antibody levels remain constant for long periods, the FTA-ABS test is not recommended for monitoring response to therapy. The absence of treponemal antibodies—a nonreactive test—does not necessarily rule out syphilis. *T. pallidum* causes no detectable immunologic changes in the blood for 14 to 21 days after initial infection. Organisms may be detected earlier by examining suspicious lesions with a dark-field microscope. Low antibody levels or other nonspecific factors produce borderline findings. In such cases, repeated testing and a thorough review of patient history may be productive. In addition, the FTA-ABS test does not always distinguish between *T. pallidum* and certain other treponemas, such as those that cause pinta, yaws, and bejel. (See *Two New Tests for* Treponema Pallidum.)

Procedure
Perform a venipuncture, and collect the sample in a 7-ml red-top tube.

Patient care checklist
Before the test
☑ Explain or clarify test purpose and procedure.
☑ Evaluate patient understanding.
After the test
☑ If the test is reactive, implement health teaching concerning syphilis.
☑ If the test is nonreactive or borderline, but syphilis has not been ruled out, instruct the patient concerning the importance of follow-up testing.

Two New Tests For *Treponema Pallidum*

The recently developed microhemagglutination assay for *Treponema pallidum* antibody increases the specificity of syphilis testing by eliminating methodologic interference. In this assay, tanned sheep RBCs are coated with *T. pallidum* antigen and are combined with absorbed test serum. Hemagglutination occurs in the presence of specific anti–*T. pallidum* antibodies in the serum.

In the enzyme-linked immunosorbent assay (ELISA), tubes coated with *T. pallidum* are washed and then treated with enzyme-labeled antihuman globulin. After the substrate for the enzymes is added to the tubes, the enzymatic activity is measured by quantitating the reaction product formed.

Interfering factors
Hemolysis caused by rough handling of the sample may alter test results.

Fungal serology
[Blastomycosis, coccidioidomycosis, histoplasmosis, aspergillosis, and sporotrichosis antibodies; cryptococcosis antigen]

Purpose
• To rapidly detect the presence of antifungal antibodies, aiding in the diagnosis of mycosis
• To monitor the effectiveness of therapy for mycosis.

Normal results
Depending on the test method, a negative finding, or normal titer, usually indicates the absence of mycosis. (See *Serum Test Methods for Fungal Infections*, p. 184.)

Abnormal results
Serum Test Methods for Fungal Infections, p. 184, summarizes the clinical significance of abnormal serologic test values for complement fixation, immunodiffusion, precipitin, latex agglutination, and agglutination techniques.

The basics
Most healthy persons easily overcome initial mycotic infection, but the elderly and those with deficient immune systems are more susceptible to acute or chronic mycotic infection and to disorders secondary to such infection. Mycosis can be deep-seated or superficial: deep-seated mycosis occurs primarily in the lungs; superficial mycosis, in the skin or the mucosal linings. Although cultures are usually performed to diagnose mycosis by identifying the causative organism, occasionally serologic tests provide the sole evidence for mycosis. Such serologic tests employ immunodiffusion, complement fixation, precipitin, latex agglutination, or agglutination methods to demonstrate the presence of specific mycotic antibodies.

Procedure
Perform a venipuncture, and collect the sample in a 10-ml sterile red-top tube.

Patient care checklist
Before the test
☑ Explain or clarify test purpose, preparation, and procedure.
☑ Evaluate patient understanding.
☑ Restrict food and fluids for 12 to 24 hours before the test.

Interfering factors
• Some antigens, such as the blastomycosis and histoplasmosis antigens, may cross-react to produce false-positive readings or high titers.
• Recent skin testing with fungal antigens may elevate titers.

Serum Test Methods For Fungal Infections

Disease and Normal Values	Clinical Significance of Abnormal Results
Blastomycosis Complement fixation: titers < 1:8	Titers ranging from 1:8 to 1:16 suggest infection; titers > 1:32 denote active disease. A rising titer in serial samples taken every 3 to 4 weeks indicates disease progression; a falling titer indicates regression. This test has limited diagnostic value due to high percentage of false-negatives.
Immunodiffusion: negative	A more sensitive test for blastomycosis; detects 80% of infected persons
Coccidioidomycosis Complement fixation: titers < 1:2	Most sensitive test for this fungus. Titers ranging from 1:2 to 1:4 suggest active infection; titers > 1:16 usually denote active disease. Test may remain negative in mild infections.
Immunodiffusion: negative	Most useful for screening, followed by complement fixation test for confirmation
Precipitin: titers < 1:16	Good screening test; titers > 1:16 usually indicate infection. 80% of infected persons show positive titers by 2 weeks: most revert to negative by 6 months. Early primary disease is shown by positive precipitin and negative complement fixation test. A positive complement fixation and negative precipitin test indicate chronic disease.
Histoplasmosis Complement fixation (histoplasmin): titers < 1:8	Titers ranging from 1:8 to 1:16 suggest infection; titers > 1:32 indicate active disease. Antibodies generally appear 10 to 21 days after initial infection. Test is positive in 10% to 15% of cases.
Complement fixation (yeast): titers < 1:18	More sensitive than histoplasmin complement fixation test; gives positive results in 75% to 80% of cases. (Both histoplasmin and yeast antigens are positive in 10% of cases.) A rising titer in serial samples taken every 2 to 3 weeks indicates progressive infection; a decreasing titer indicates regression. Titers ranging from 1:8 to 1:16 suggest infection; titers > 1:32 indicate active disease.
Immunodiffusion (histoplasmin): negative	Appearance of both H and M bands indicates active infection. If the M band appears first and lasts longer than the H band, the infection may be regressing. The M band alone may indicate early infection, chronic disease, or a recent skin test.

(continued)

Serum Test Methods For Fungal Infections *(continued)*

Disease and Normal Values	Clinical Significance of Abnormal Results
Aspergillosis Complement fixation: titers < 1:8	Titers of > 1:8 suggest infection. Approximately 70% to 90% of patients with known pulmonary aspergillosis and/or aspergillus allergy present antibodies, and so do about 5% of the general population. This test cannot detect invasive aspergillosis, because patients with this disease do not present antibodies; biopsy is required.
Immunodiffusion: negative	One or more precipitin bands suggests infection; precipitins appear in 95% of patients with pulmonary fungus balls and in 50% of those with allergic bronchopulmonary disorders. The number of bands is related to complement fixation titers; the more precipitin bands, the higher the titer.
Sporotrichosis Agglutination: titers < 1:40	Titers > 1:80 usually indicate active disease. The test usually is negative in cutaneous infections, positive in extracutaneous infections.
Cryptococcosis Latex agglutination for cryptococcal antigen: negative	About 90% of patients with cryptococcal meningoencephalitis present capsular antigen in CSF serum. (Serum is less frequently positive than CSF.) Culturing is definitive since false-positives do occur. (Presence of rheumatoid factor may cause a positive reaction.) Serum antigen tests are positive in 33% of patients with pulmonary cryptococcosis; biopsy is usually required.

• Many mycoses depress the immune system, causing low titers or false-negative test results.

• Failure to send a sterile sample to the laboratory immediately, or to store the sample properly if transport is delayed, may interfere with accurate determination of test results.

• A nonfasting specimen may alter test results.

Ham test
[Acidified serum lysis test]

Purpose
• To determine the cause of undiagnosed hemolytic anemia, hemoglobinuria, and bone marrow aplasia.

• To establish a diagnosis of paroxysmal nocturnal hemoglobinuria (PNH), a rare hematologic disease.

Normal results
RBCs do not undergo hemolysis.

Abnormal results
Hemolysis of RBCs indicates:
   PNH.

The basics
The Ham test relies on the susceptibility of RBCs to lysis: RBCs from patients with PNH are unusually susceptible to lysis by complement.

Procedure

Laboratory personnel will perform the venipuncture and collect the sample because the blood sample must be defibrinated immediately.

Patient care checklist

Before the test

☑ Explain or clarify test purpose and procedure.

☑ Evaluate patient understanding.

Interfering factors

• Blood containing large numbers of spherocytes may produce false-positive results.

• Blood from patients with congenital dyserythropoietic anemia or HEM-PAS (a rare hematologic disorder) will show false-positive results.

Hepatitis B surface antigen *(HB$_s$Ag)* *[Hepatitis-associated antigen; Australia antigen]*

Purpose

• To screen blood donors for hepatitis B

• To screen persons at high risk for contracting hepatitis B (such as hemodialysis nurses)

• To aid differential diagnosis of viral hepatitis.

Viral Hepatitis Test Panel

The three types of viral hepatitis produce similar symptoms but differ in terms of transmission, course of treatment, prognosis, and carrier status. When clinical history is insufficient for differentiation, serologic tests can aid diagnosis. Hepatitis A and hepatitis B antigens induce type-specific antibodies detectable by radioimmunoassay. The third hepatitis virus--non-A, non-B--is identified only by distinguishing it from A and B types. All tests require only a small sample of blood.

Typical Sequence of Hepatitis A Markers After Exposure

Testing for Hepatitis A: Present in blood and feces only briefly before symptoms appear, hepatitis A virus may elude detection. However, anti-HAV, the antibody to hepatitis A virus, appears early in the acute phase of the disease, persists for many years after recovery, and ultimately gives the patient immunity. A single positive anti-HAV test may indicate previous exposure to the virus, but because this antibody persists so long in the bloodstream, only evidence of *rising* anti-HAV titers confirms hepatitis A as the cause of current or very recent infection. Determining recent infection relies on identifying the antibody as IgM (associated with recent infection). A negative anti-HAV test rules out hepatitis A.

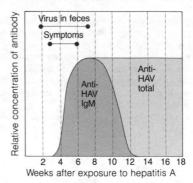

Courtesy of Abbott Laboratories, Abbott Park, Ill., *Serodiagnostic Assessment of Acute Viral Hepatitis.*

Normal results
Negative.

Abnormal results
Positive for HB$_s$Ag:
Hepatitis B (confirming)
Hemophilia, Hodgkin's disease, leukemia (more than 5% of patients with these disorders have positive HB$_s$Ag)

The basics
HB$_s$Ag appears in the sera of patients with hepatitis B virus (formerly called serum hepatitis or long-incubation hepatitis). It can be detected during the extended incubation period and usually during the first 3 weeks of acute infection or if the patient is a carrier. Since transmission of hepatitis is one of the gravest complications associated with blood transfusion, all donors must be screened for hepatitis B before their blood is stored. This screening, required by the Food and Drug Administration's Bureau of Biologics, has helped reduce the incidence of hepatitis. However, this test does not screen for hepatitis A virus (infectious hepatitis). If hepatitis B antigens are found in donor blood, this blood must be discarded, because it carries a 40% to 70% risk of transmitting hepatitis. Blood samples that test positive should be retested, since inaccurate results do occur. (For related tests to diagnose viral hepatitis, see *Viral Hepatitis Test Panel*.)

Typical Sequence of Hepatitis B Markers After Exposure

Testing for Hepatitis B: Hepatitis B viral cells are composed of a core protein and a surface protein. The surface antigen (HB$_s$Ag) appears in serum during the long incubation period (up to 26 weeks) or during the early acute phase of infection (2 to 3 weeks) and normally peaks after symptoms begin. High levels of HB$_s$Ag, continuing 3 or more months after onset of acute infection, suggest the development of chronic hepatitis or carrier status. Potential blood donors are screened for this antigen to prevent transmission of hepatitis B to recipients.

Another antibody to develop after exposure to hepatitis B is anti-HB$_c$, induced by the core component of the B antigen. An early indicator of acute infection, antibody (IgM) to core antigen (anti-HB$_c$ IgM) is rarely detected in chronic infection. Thus, it is also useful in distinguishing acute from chronic infection and hepatitis B from non-A, non-B.

Anti-HB$_s$, antibody to the surface component of the B virus, appears long after symptoms have subsided and after the antigen itself (HB$_s$Ag) has disappeared from blood. Detection of the antibody signals late convalescence or recovery from infection. Anti-HB$_s$ remains in the blood to provide immunity to reinfection.

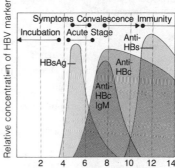

Courtesy of Abbott Laboratories, Abbott Park, Ill., *Serodiagnostic Assessment of Acute Viral Hepatitis.*

Procedure
Perform a venipuncture, and collect the sample in a 7-ml red-top tube.

Special precautions
CLINICAL ALERT: **Wash your hands carefully after the procedure, or wear gloves when drawing blood. Be sure you dispose of the needle properly.**

Patient care checklist
Before the test
☑ Explain or clarify test purpose and procedure.
☑ Evaluate patient understanding.
After the test
☑ Notify blood donor if test results are positive for the antigen. Report confirmed viral hepatitis to public health authorities (this is a reportable disease in most states).

Heterophil agglutination tests
[Paul-Bunnell test or "presumptive" test, and Davidsohn's differential absorption test]

Purpose
To aid differential diagnosis of infectious mononucleosis.

Normal results
Negative, no reaction; titer less than 1:56 (may be higher in the elderly).

Abnormal results
Positive, or titer greater than 1:56:
  Infectious mononucleosis
  Systemic lupus erythematosus
  Cryoglobulinemia
  Presence of antibodies to nonsyphilitic treponema (yaws, pinta, bejel).

The basics
Heterophil agglutination tests detect and identify two IgM antibodies in human serum that react against foreign RBCs. In the Paul-Bunnell test—also called the "presumptive" test—Epstein-Barr virus (EBV) antibodies, found in the sera of patients with infectious mononucleosis, agglutinate with sheep RBCs in a test tube. However, Forssman antibodies, present in some normal serum as well as in conditions such as serum sickness, also agglutinate with sheep RBCs, thus rendering test results inconclusive for infectious mononucleosis. If the Paul-Bunnell test establishes a presumptive titer, Davidsohn's differential absorption test can then distinguish between EBV antibodies and Forssman antibodies.

Although heterophil antibodies are present in the sera of approximately 80% of patients with infectious mononucleosis 1 month after onset, a positive finding—a titer higher than 1:56—does not confirm this disorder. (Confirmation of infectious mononucleosis depends on heterophil agglutination tests that show absolute lymphocytosis, with 10% to 30% or more atypical lymphocytes.)

In infectious mononucleosis, a gradual increase in titer to about 1:224 during week 3 or 4, followed by a gradual decrease during weeks 4 to 8, proves most conclusive. However, a negative titer does not always rule out this disorder; occasionally, the titer becomes reactive 2 weeks later. Therefore, if symptoms persist, the test should be repeated in 2 weeks. (See *Spot Test for Infectious Mononucleosis.*)

Procedure
Perform a venipuncture, and collect the sample in a 7-ml red-top tube.

Patient care checklist
Before the test
☑ Explain or clarify test purpose and procedure.
☑ Evaluate patient understanding.
After the test
☑ If the titer is positive and infectious

Spot Test For Infectious Mononucleosis

Several screening tests can detect the heterophil infectious mononucleosis (IM) antibody. One of these tests—the Monospot—converts the Paul-Bunnell and the Davidsohn's differential absorption tests into one rapid slide test without titration. Monospot relies on agglutination of horse RBCs by heterophil antibodies. Since horse RBCs contain both Forssman and IM antigens, differential absorption of the patient's serum is necessary to distinguish between them. This is done by mixing the serum sample with guinea pig kidney antigen (containing only Forssman antigen) on one end of a slide, and with beef RBC stroma (containing only IM antigen) on the other. Each absorbs only the heterophil antibody specific to it. After addition of horse RBCs to each spot, agglutination on the beef cell end of the slide indicates the presence of the IM heterophil antibody and confirms IM. Monospot rivals the classic heterophil agglutination test for sensitivity. False-positives may occur in the presence of lymphoma, hepatitis A and hepatitis B, leukemia, and pancreatic cancer.

mononucleosis is confirmed, instruct the patient in the treatment plan.
☑ If the titer is positive but infectious mononucleosis is not confirmed, or if the titer is negative but symptoms persist, explain that additional testing will be necessary in a few days or weeks to confirm diagnosis and to plan effective treatment.

Interfering factors
• If treatment for mononucleosis begins before development of heterophil antibodies, the titer is usually negative.
• Patients addicted to narcotics may have high titers.

Human leukocyte antigen test (HLA test)

Purpose
• To provide histocompatibility typing of tissue recipients and donors
• To aid genetic counseling
• To aid paternity testing.

Results
Incompatible HLA-A, HLA-B, HLA-C, or HLA-D groups:
 May cause unsuccessful tissue transplantation.
Some diseases associated with certain types of HLAs:
 HLA-DR5—Hashimoto's thyroiditis
 HLA-B27—Ankylosing spondylitis (detectable in 88% of affected patients)
 HLA-B8 and Dw3—Graves' disease
 HLA-B8—Chronic autoimmune hepatitis, celiac disease, and myasthenia gravis
 HLA-Dw3—Addison's disease, Sjögren's syndrome, dermatitis herpetiformis, and systemic lupus erythematosus
 HLA-B27, Dw2, A3, and B18—Multiple sclerosis.
Paternity testing:
 A putative father who presents a phenotype (two haplotypes: one from the father and one from the mother) with no haplotype or antigen pair identical to one of the child's is excluded as the father. A putative father with one haplotype identical to one of the child's *may* be the father; the probability varies with the incidence of the haplotype in the population.

The basics

The HLA test identifies a group of antigens present on the surfaces of all nucleated cells, but most easily detected on lymphocytes. These antigens are essential to immunity, and determine the degree of histocompatibility between transplant recipients and donors. Numerous antigenic determinants (over 60, for instance, at the HLA-B locus) are present for each site; one set of each antigen is inherited from each parent. Three types of HLA (HLA-A, HLA-B, and HLA-C) are measured with a lymphocyte microcytotoxicity assay. A fourth type of HLA, HLA-D, is measured by a mixed leukocyte reaction. High incidences of specific HLA types have been linked to specific diseases, but these findings have little diagnostic significance. Thus, HLA testing is best used as an adjunct to diagnosis.

Procedure

Perform a venipuncture and collect the sample in an ACD collection tube.

Patient care checklist

Before the test

☑ Explain or clarify test purpose and procedure.

☑ Evaluate patient understanding.

Interfering factors

• Hemolysis caused by rough handling of the sample may interfere with accurate determination of test results.

• HLA from blood transfused within 72 hours before collection of a blood sample may interfere with accurate determination of test results.

Immune complex assays

Purpose

• To demonstrate circulating immune complexes in serum

• To monitor response to therapy

• To estimate the severity of disease.

Normal results

Immune complexes are not detectable in serum.

Abnormal results

Immune complexes are present in:

Systemic lupus erythematosus (SLE)

Rheumatoid arthritis

Postinfectious syndromes

Serum sickness

Drug sensitivity.

The basics

When immune complexes are produced faster than they can be cleared by the lymphoreticular system, immune complex disease may occur. Immune complexes can develop when a certain ratio of antigen reacts with antibody of isotopes IgG 1, 2, 3, or IgM in tissues. These complexes can fix the first component of complement (C1) and activate the complement cascade. Subsequent complement-mediated activity leads to inflammation and local tissue necrosis. In the blood, soluble circulating immune complexes may also activate complement and eventually cause damage, usually in the renal glomeruli, the aorta, and other large blood vessels.

Histologic examination of tissue obtained by biopsy and the use of fluorescence or peroxidase staining with antibodies specific for immunologic types generally detect immune complexes. However, since tissue biopsies cannot provide information about titers or complexes still in circulation, serum assays, which detect circulating immune complexes indirectly, may be required. Because of the inherent variability of these complexes, several serum test methods may be appropriate, using C1, the rheumatoid factor (RF), or cellular substrates, such as Raji cells, as reagents. Since most immune complex assays have not been standardized, more than one test may be required to achieve accurate results.

For definitive diagnosis, the presence of these complexes must be considered with the results of other studies. For example, in SLE, immune complexes are associated with high titers of antinuclear antibodies and circulating antinative deoxyribonucleic acid antibodies. Because of their filtering function, renal glomeruli seem most vulnerable to immune complex deposition, although blood vessel walls and choroid plexuses (vascular folds in the ventricles of the brain) can be affected. Renal biopsy to detect immune complexes can provide conclusive evidence for immune complex (Type III) glomerulonephritis, differentiating it from other types of glomerulonephritis.

Procedure

Perform a venipuncture and collect the sample in a 7-ml red-top tube.

Patient care checklist

Before the test

☑ Explain or clarify test purpose and procedure.

☑ Evaluate patient understanding.

After the test

☑ Take special care to keep the venipuncture site clean and dry, since many patients with immune complexes have compromised immune systems.

Interfering factors

• Failure to send the serum sample to the laboratory immediately can result in the deterioration of immune complexes, and therefore can interfere with accurate determination of test results.

• Recent heparin therapy may affect test results if the patient is scheduled for C1q assays.

• The presence of cryoglobulins in the patient's serum can interfere with the accurate determination of test results.

• Inability to standardize RF inhibition tests and platelet aggregation assays can interfere with accurate determination of test results.

Immunoglobulins G, A, and M
[Quantitative AGM test for immunoglobulins IgG, IgA, and IgM]

Purpose

• To diagnose paraproteinemias, such as multiple myeloma and Waldenström's macroglobulinemia

• To detect hypo- and hypergammaglobulinemia, as well as nonimmunologic diseases, such as cirrhosis and hepatitis, that are associated with abnormally high immunoglobulin levels

• To assess the effectiveness of chemotherapy or radiation therapy.

Normal results

Using nephelometry, serum immunoglobulin levels for adults range as follows:

IgG: 6.4 to 14.3 mg/ml
IgA: 0.3 to 3 mg/ml
IgM: 0.2 to 1.4 mg/ml.

Abnormal results

See *Serum Immunoglobulin Levels in Various Disorders,* p. 192, which shows IgG, IgA, and IgM levels in various disorders.

Findings confirm diagnosis in:
    Congenital and acquired hypogammaglobulinemias
    Myelomas
    Macroglobulinemia.

Findings can support diagnoses based on other tests in:
    Hepatic and autoimmune diseases
    Leukemias
    Lymphomas.

The basics

Immunoglobulins, proteins that can function as specific antibodies in response to antigen stimulation, are responsible for the humoral aspects of immunity. They are classified into five groups—IgG, IgA, IgM, IgD, and IgE—that are normally present in serum in predictable percentages. IgG

Serum Immunoglobulin Levels In Various Disorders

Disorder	IgG	IgA	IgM
Immunoglobulin disorders			
Lymphoid aplasia	D	D	D
Agammaglobulinemia	D	D	D
Type I dysgammaglobulinemia (selective IgG and IgA deficiency)	D	D	N or I
Type II dysgammaglobulinemia (absent IgA and IgM)	N	D	D
IgA globulinemia	N	D	N
Ataxia-telangiectasia	N	D	N
Multiple myeloma, macroglobulinemia, lymphomas			
Heavy chain disease (Franklin's disease)	D	D	D
IgG myeloma	I	D	D
IgA myeloma	D	I	D
Macroglobulinemia	D	D	I
Acute lymphocytic leukemia	N	D	N
Chronic lymphocytic leukemia	D	D	D
Acute myelocytic leukemia	N	N	N
Chronic myelocytic leukemia	N	D	N
Hodgkin's disease	N	N	N
Hepatic disorders			
Hepatitis	I	I	I
Laennec's cirrhosis	I	I	N
Biliary cirrhosis	N	N	I
Hepatoma	N	N	D
Other disorders			
Rheumatoid arthritis	I	I	I
Systemic lupus erythematosus	I	I	I
Nephrotic syndrome	D	D	N
Trypanosomiasis	N	N	I
Pulmonary tuberculosis	I	N	N

KEY: N = Normal; I = Increased; D = Decreased

Adapted with permission from Jacques B. Wallach, *Interpretation of Diagnostic Tests: A Handbook Synopsis of Laboratory Medicine* (3rd ed.; Boston: Little, Brown & Co., 1978), p. 71.

comprises about 75% of serum immunoglobulins and includes the warm-temperature type; IgA, about 15% of the total; IgM, 5% to 7% and includes cold agglutinins, rheumatoid factor, and ABO blood group isoagglutinins; IgD and allergen-specific IgE comprise less than 2%. Deviations from these normal immunoglobulin percentages are characteristic in many immune disorders—cancer, hepatic disorders, rheumatoid arthritis, and systemic lupus erythematosus, to name a few. Immunoelectrophoresis identifies IgG, IgA, and IgM in a serum sample; the level of each is measured by radial immunodiffusion or nephelometry. Some laboratories detect immunoglobulin by indirect immunofluorescence and radioimmunoassay. (See *Insulin Antibodies Test*.)

Procedure

Perform a venipuncture, and collect the sample in a 7-ml red-top tube.

Patient care checklist

Before the test

☑ Explain or clarify test purpose, preparation, and procedure.

☑ Restrict food and fluids, except for water, for 12 to 14 hours before the test.

☑ Evaluate patient understanding.

After the test

☑ Tell the patient how to protect himself from bacterial infection if findings show abnormally low immunoglobulin levels (especially IgG or IgM).

☑ Observe patients with abnormally low immunoglobulin levels for signs of infection (fever, chills, rash, or skin ulcers).

☑ Instruct patients with abnormally high immunoglobulin levels and symptoms of monoclonal gammopathies to report any bone pain or tenderness. (Such a patient has numerous antibody-producing malignant plasma cells in bone marrow, which hamper production of other blood components.)

☑ Observe patients with abnormally high immunoglobulin levels and symptoms of monoclonal gammopathies for signs of hypercalcemia, renal failure, and spontaneous pathologic fractures.

Interfering factors

• Radiation therapy or chemotherapy—with methotrexate, for example—may reduce immunoglobulin levels, due to the suppressive effects of these treatments on bone marrow.

• Aminophenazone, anticonvulsants, asparaginase, hydralazine, hydantoin derivatives, oral contraceptives, and phenylbutazone may raise all immunoglobulin levels. Methotrexate and severe hypersensitivity to BCG (bacille Calmette-Guerin) vaccine may lower all levels. Dextrans, phenytoin, and high doses of methylprednisolone lower IgG and IgA levels; dextrans and methylprednisolone lower IgM levels. Methadone raises IgG levels; alcoholism raises IgA levels; narcotic addiction may raise IgM levels.

• Failure to send the sample to the laboratory immediately may cause deterioration of immunoglobulins.

Insulin Antibodies Test

Using radioimmunoassay, this test detects insulin antibodies in the blood of patients who receive insulin for treatment of diabetes mellitus. Most insulin preparations are derived from beef and pork pancreases and contain insulin-related peptides, impurities that are the major immunogenic components in insulin. IgG antibodies that form in response to these peptides complex with subsequent insulin injections and neutralize the insulin so it cannot regulate glucose metabolism. Detection of insulin antibodies confirms this process as the cause of insulin resistance and suggests the need for alternate therapy to control hyperglycemia.

Detection of insulin antibodies may also confirm "factitious hypoglycemia," an unusual condition that results from insulin injection rather than from a disorder, such as insulinoma.

Leukoagglutinin test
[White cell antibodies]

Purpose

• To detect leukoagglutinins in blood recipients who develop transfusion reactions, thus differentiating between hemolytic and febrile nonhemolytic transfusion reactions

• To detect leukoagglutinins in blood donors after transfusion of donor blood causes a reaction in the recipient.

Normal results

Negative for white cell antibodies (agglutination does not occur because serum contains no antibodies).

Abnormal results

Positive—in a recipient's blood:

Indicates the presence of leukoagglutinins, identifying recipient's transfusion reaction as a febrile nonhemolytic reaction to these antibodies.

Positive—in a donor's blood:

Indicates the presence of leukoagglutinins, identifying the cause of a recipient's reaction as an acute, noncardiogenic pulmonary edema.

The basics

Leukoagglutinins are antibodies that react with white blood cells and may cause a transfusion reaction. These antibodies usually develop after exposure to foreign white cells through transfusions, pregnancies, or allografts. If a blood recipient has these antibodies, a febrile nonhemolytic reaction may occur 1 to 4 hours after the start of whole blood, red blood cell, platelet, or granulocyte transfusion. (All of these blood products contain some granulocytes, which react with the antibodies.) This nonhemolytic reaction (marked by fever and severe chills, sometimes with nausea, headache, and transient hypertension) must be distinguished from a true hemolytic reaction before further transfusion can proceed.

If a blood donor has these antibodies, the recipient may develop acute, noncardiogenic pulmonary edema after transfusion of the donor's blood. In this case, the donor's blood must be tested for leukoagglutinins to determine if these have caused the recipient's reaction. A pretransfusion blood sample taken from the blood bank's crossmatch sample is preferred for this test.

Procedure

If a pretransfusion sample is not available from the blood bank, perform a venipuncture and collect a blood sample in a 10-ml red-top tube. (The laboratory will require 3 to 4 ml of serum for testing.)

Patient care checklist

Before the test

☑ Explain or clarify test purpose and procedure.

☑ Evaluate patient understanding.

☑ Review patient history for pregnancy and past transfusions. (Pregnant patients who have had several transfusions experience febrile reactions more often than other patients.)

After the test

CLINICAL ALERT: **If a transfusion recipient has a positive leukoagglutinin test, continued transfusions require premedication with acetaminophen 1 to 2 hours before the transfusion; specially prepared leukocyte-poor blood; or both, to prevent further reactions.**

☑ If a donor has a positive leukoagglutinin test, explain the meaning of this result to him to help prevent further transfusion reactions.

Interfering factors

Previous administration of dextran or I.V. contrast media causes aggregation resembling agglutination.

Lupus erythematosus *(LE)* cell preparation

Purpose

• To aid diagnosis of systemic lupus erythematosus (SLE)

• To monitor treatment of SLE (about 60% of successfully treated patients fail to show LE cells after 4 to 6 weeks of therapy).

Normal results

Negative. (No LE cells are present.)

Abnormal results
Positive for LE cells:
LE—two or more LE cells are found in 75% to 80% of patients with LE.
Chronic active hepatitis
Rheumatoid arthritis
Scleroderma
Drug reactions.

The basics
LE cell preparation is an in vitro procedure used in the diagnosis of SLE. This test is less sensitive and reliable than either the antinuclear antibody (ANA) or the anti-deoxyribonucleic acid (anti-DNA) antibody test, and it is seldom used today. Occasionally, it is used because it requires minimal equipment and reagents. However, up to 25% of patients with SLE demonstrate no LE cells. Apart from supportive clinical signs, definitive diagnosis of SLE may necessitate a confirming ANA or anti-DNA test.

Procedure
Perform a venipuncture, and collect the sample in a 7-ml red-top tube.

Patient care checklist
Before the test
☑ Explain or clarify test purpose and procedure.
☑ Evaluate patient understanding.
After the test
☑ Observe venipuncture site for infection and keep a clean, dry bandage over the site for at least 24 hours because many patients with SLE have compromised immune systems.

Interfering factors
• Hemolysis caused by rough handling of the sample may interfere with accurate determination of test results.
• Certain drugs—most commonly isoniazid, hydralazine, and procainamide—can produce a syndrome resembling SLE. Other such drugs include para-aminosalicylic acid, chlorpromazine, clofibrate, phenytoin, griseofulvin, ethosuximide, gold salts, methyldopa, oral contraceptives, penicillin, propylthiouracil, phenylbutazone, methysergide, streptomycin, sulfonamides, tetracyclines, mephenytoin, quinidine, primidone, reserpine, and trimethadione.

Lymphocyte transformation tests
[Mitogen assay, antigen assay, mixed lymphocyte culture (MLC) assay]

Purpose
• To assess and monitor genetic and acquired immunodeficiency states
• To provide histocompatibility typing of both tissue transplant recipients and donors
• To detect exposure to various pathogens, such as those causing malaria, hepatitis, and mycoplasmal pneumonia. (See *Lymphocyte Marker Assays*, p. 196.)

Normal results
Mitogen assay:
Normal stimulation index greater than 10.
Antigen assay:
Normal stimulation index greater than 3.
MLC assay:
Unresponsiveness indicates histocompatibility for the D locus antigens.

Abnormal results
Mitogen assay:
Low stimulation assay or unresponsiveness:
Depressed or defective immune system.
Antigen assay:
A high stimulation index (with intact immune system):
Exposure to relevant pathogen
Disorders such as malaria, hepatitis, mycoplasmal pneumonia, peri-

Lymphocyte Marker Assays

A normal immune response requires a balance between several interacting cell types—most notably, T-helper and T-suppressor cells. By using highly specific monoclonal antibodies, levels of lymphocyte differentiation can be defined, and both normal and malignant cell populations can be analyzed. The chart below lists some lymphocyte marker assays and their indications.

Lymphocyte Marker Assay	Purpose
Pan T-cell marker	• To measure mature T-cells in immune dysfunction
T-helper/inducer subset marker	• To identify and characterize the proportion of T-helper cells in autoimmune or immunoregulatory disorders • To detect immunodeficiency disorders, such as AIDS • To differentiate T-cell acute lymphoblastic leukemia from T-cell lymphomas and other lymphoproliferative disorders
T-suppressor/cytotoxic subset marker	• To identify and characterize the proportion of T-suppressor cells in autoimmune and immunoregulatory disorders • To characterize lymphoproliferative disorders
T-cell/E-Rosette receptor	• To differentiate lymphoproliferative disorders of T-cell origin, such as T-cell lymphocytic leukemia and lymphoblastic lymphoma, from those of non-T-cell origin
Pan-B (B-1) marker	• To differentiate lymphoproliferative disorders of B-cell origin, such as B-cell chronic lymphocytic leukemia, from those of T-cell origin
Pan-B (BA-1) marker	• To identify B-cell lymphoproliferative disorders, such as B-cell chronic lymphocytic leukemia
CALLA (common acute lymphocytic leukemia antigen) marker	• To identify bone marrow regeneration • To identify non-T-cell acute lymphocytic leukemia
Lymphocyte subset panel (B, pan-T, T-helper/inducer, T-suppressor/cytotoxic, and T-helper/T-suppressor ratio)	• To evaluate immunodeficiencies • To identify immunoregulation associated with autoimmune disorders • To characterize lymphoid malignancies
Lymphocytic leukemia marker panel (T-cell markers [E-Rosette receptor and Leu-9], B-cell markers [B-1 and BA-1], and CALLA)	• To characterize lymphocytic leukemias as T, B, non-T, or non-B, regardless of the stage of differentiation of the malignant cells

odontal disease, and certain viral infections in patients who no longer have detectable antibodies.

A low stimulation index:
Defective immune system
Lack of exposure to disorders listed above.

MLC assay:
High stimulation index:
Poor compatibility (between recipients and donors).

The basics

Transformation tests evaluate lymphocyte competency without injection of antigens into the patient's skin. These in vitro tests eliminate the risk of adverse effects, but can still accurately assess the ability of lymphocytes to proliferate and to recognize and respond to antigens. (Serial testing can be performed to monitor the effectiveness of therapy in a patient with an immunodeficiency disease.) The

mitogen assay evaluates the mitotic response of T and B lymphocytes to a foreign antigen. Lymphocyte responsiveness, or the extent of mitosis, is reported as a stimulation index. The antigen assay uses specific antigens, such as PPD, Candida, mumps, tetanus toxoid, and streptokinase, to stimulate lymphocyte transformation. This too is reported as a stimulation index. The MLC assay tests the response of lymphocytes to histocompatibility antigens. The MLC assay is useful in matching transplant recipients and donors, and in testing immunocompetence. In this test, the stimulation index is a measure of compatibility. (See *Neutrophil Function Tests.*)

Procedure

Perform a venipuncture. If the patient is an adult, collect the sample in a 7-ml green-top (heparinized) tube; for a child, use a 5-ml green-top tube.

Neutrophil Function Tests

Normal neutrophils—the body's primary defense against bacterial invasion—engulf and destroy bacteria and foreign particles by a process known as phagocytosis. In patients who suffer from repeated bacterial infections, neutrophil function tests may reveal the inability of neutrophils to kill a target bacteria or to migrate to the bacterial site (chemotaxis).

Neutrophil killing ability can be evaluated by the *nitroblue tetrazolium (NBT) test,* which relies on neutrophil generation of bactericidal enzymes and toxins during killing. This action results in increased oxygen consumption and glucose metabolism, which reduces colorless NBT to blue formazan. The reduced dye is then extracted with pyridine and measured photometri-

cally; the level of reduction indicates phagocytic activity.

Neutrophil killing activity can also be evaluated by noting the *chemiluminescence*—or ability to emit light—of neutrophils. After a neutrophil phagocytizes a microorganism, oxygen-containing substances form within phagocytic vacuoles. As the cell is stimulated, it emits light in proportion to the amount of oxygen-containing substances that are formed, providing an indirect measurement of phagocytosis.

Chemotaxis can be assessed in vitro by placing bacteria in the lower half of a two-part chamber and phagocytic neutrophils in the upper half. After incubation, migrating cells are counted microscopically and compared to standard values.

Patient care checklist
Before the test
☑ Explain or clarify test purpose and procedure.
☑ Evaluate patient understanding.
After the test
☑ Keep venipuncture site clean and dry. (Many of these patients have a compromised immune system.)

Interfering factors
• Pregnancy or the use of oral contraceptives depresses lymphocyte response to PHA, and thus causes a low stimulation index.
• Chemotherapy may hinder accurate determination of test results, unless pretherapy baseline values are available for comparison.
• A radioisotope scan performed within 1 week before the test may alter test results.
• Failure to send the sample to the laboratory immediately may alter test results.

Radioallergosorbent test
(RAST)

Purpose
• To identify allergens to which the patient has an immediate (IgE-mediated) hypersensitivity
• To monitor response to therapy.

Normal results
RAST results are interpreted in relation to a control or reference serum that differs among laboratories.

Abnormal results
Elevated serum IgE levels suggest hypersensitivity to the specific allergen or allergens used.

The basics
The RAST measures IgE antibodies in serum by radioimmunoassay and iden-tifies specific allergens that cause rashes, asthma, hay fever, drug reactions, or other atopic complaints. Before RAST was developed, skin testing was the only reliable method for identifying allergens. RAST is easier to perform and is an accurate substitute for skin testing; it is also less painful for and less dangerous to the patient. However, careful selection of specific allergens, based on the patient's clinical history, is crucial for effective testing. Although skin testing is still the preferred means of diagnosing IgE-mediated hypersensitivities, RAST may be more useful when a skin disorder makes accurate reading of skin tests difficult, when a patient requires continual antihistamine therapy, or when skin tests are negative but the patient's clinical history supports IgE-mediated hypersensitivity.

Procedure
Perform a venipuncture, and collect the sample in a 7-ml red-top tube. Generally, 1 ml of serum is sufficient for five allergen assays. Note on the laboratory slip the specific allergen(s) to be tested.

Patient care checklist
Before the test
☑ Explain or clarify test purpose and procedure.
☑ Evaluate patient understanding.

Interfering factors
A radioactive scan within 1 week before sample collection may affect the accuracy of test results.

Rh typing

Purpose
• To establish blood type according to the Rh system

- To help determine the compatibility of a donor before transfusion
- To determine if the patient needs a RhoGAM (Rh immunoglobulin) injection.

Normal results

Patient blood is classified as Rh-positive, Rh-negative, or Rh-positive D^u. (See *Implications of $Rh_o(D)$ Typing Test Results.*)

The basics

The Rh system classifies blood by the presence or absence of the $Rh_o(D)$ antigen on the surface of RBCs. In this test, a patient's RBCs are mixed with serum containing anti-$Rh_o(D)$ antibodies and are observed for agglutination. If agglutination occurs, the $Rh_o(D)$ antigen is present, and the patient's blood is typed Rh-positive; if agglutination does not occur, the antigen is absent, and the patient's blood is typed Rh-negative. Rh typing is performed routinely on prospective blood donors and on recipients before transfusion. Only prospective blood donors are fully tested to exclude the D^u variant of the $Rh_o(D)$ antigen before being classified as having Rh-negative blood. Persons who have this antigen are considered Rh-positive donors, but are generally transfused as Rh-negative recipients. If an Rh-negative woman delivers an Rh-positive baby, or aborts a fetus whose Rh-type is unknown, she should receive a RhoGAM (Rh immunoglobulin) injection within 72 hours, to prevent hemolytic disease of the newborn in future births.

Procedure

- Perform a venipuncture, and collect the sample in a 10- to 15-ml lavender-top tube or red-top tube, as ordered (one tube for each three units of blood ordered).
- If a transfusion is ordered, a transfusion request form must accompany the sample to the laboratory.

Patient care checklist

Before the test

☑ Explain or clarify test purpose and procedure.

Implications of $RH_o(D)$ Typing Test Results

Classified as $Rh_o(D)$-positive, $Rh_o(D)$-negative, or $Rh(D^u)$-positive, donor blood may be transfused only if it is compatible with the recipient's blood, as follows:

$Rh_o(D)$ Recipient Types	Compatible $Rh_o(D)$ Donor Types	Incompatible $Rh_o(D)$ Donor Types
$Rh_o(D)$-positive	$Rh_o(D)$-positive or $Rh_o(D)$-negative	None
$Rh_o(D)$-negative	$Rh_o(D)$-negative	$Rh_o(D)$-positive
RhD^u-positive	RhD^u-positive, $Rh_o(D)$-negative, or $Rh_o(D)$-positive (the least desirable choice, as it may cause a mild hemolytic reaction)	None

☑ Encourage patient to carry a blood group identification card in his wallet to protect him in an emergency. (Most laboratories will provide such a card on request.)
☑ Evaluate patient understanding.

Interfering factors
• Recent administration of dextran or I.V. contrast media results in cellular aggregation resembling agglutination.
• If the patient has received blood in the past 3 months, antibodies to this donor blood may develop and linger, interfering with compatibility testing.
• Methyldopa, cephalosporins, or levodopa may cause false-positive results of the direct antiglobulin (Coombs') test for the D^u antigen.
• Failure to send the sample to the laboratory immediately, since the test must be performed within 48 hours, may affect the results.

Rheumatoid factor (RF)

Purpose
To confirm rheumatoid arthritis (RA), especially when clinical diagnosis is doubtful. It is the most useful test for confirming this disorder.

Normal results
Normal RF titer is less than 1:20; normal rheumatoid screening test is nonreactive or negative.

Abnormal results
Positive for rheumatoid factor:
Titers above 1:80:
  RA (usually considered confirming if patient also meets criteria for clinical diagnosis).
Titers between 1:20 and 1:80:
  Systemic lupus erythematosus
  Scleroderma
  Polymyositis
  Tuberculosis
  Infectious mononucleosis
  Leprosy
  Syphilis
  Sarcoidosis
  Chronic hepatic disease
  Subacute bacterial endocarditis
  Chronic interstitial fibrosis
  (See *Presence of Rheumatoid Factor [RF] in Various Diseases When Both SCAT and Latex Test Used.*)

The basics
In RA, "renegade" IgG antibodies, produced by lymphocytes in the synovial joints, react with other IgG or IgM to produce immune complexes, complement activation, and tissue destruction. How IgG molecules become antigenic is still unknown, but they may be altered by aggregating with viruses or other antigens. These immune complexes can migrate from the synovial fluid to other areas of the body, causing vasculitis, subcutaneous nodules, or lymphadenopathy. The IgG or IgM molecules that react with altered IgG are called rheumatoid factors.

Agglutination and flocculation tests—the sheep cell agglutination test (SCAT) and the latex fixation test—can detect RF. The SCAT is the better diagnostic method for confirming RA; the latex fixation test is the better screening method. It is important to recognize that a negative RF titer does not rule out RA; 20% to 25% of patients with RA lack reactive RF titers, and RF itself is not reactive until 6 months after onset of active disease. Repeating the test is sometimes useful. In addition, 5% of the general population, including as many as 25% of the elderly, have positive RF titers. Correlation between RF and RA is inconclusive, and positive diagnosis always requires correlation with clinical status.

Procedure
Perform a venipuncture, and collect the sample in a 7-ml red-top tube.

Presence of Rheumatoid Factor (RF) in Various Diseases When Both SCAT and Latex Test Used

Disease	RF
Classic rheumatoid arthritis (RA)	80%
Early or atypical RA	50%
Juvenile RA	20%
Infectious diseases	10%
Healthy adults	5%
Elderly persons	25%

Adapted with permission from Henry J. Smith and Robert G. Blaker, *Laboratory Aids for the Diagnosis of Autoimmune Disorders* (Van Nuys, Calif.: Bio-Science Laboratories, 1975), p. 13. Used by permission of the publisher.

Patient care checklist
Before the test
☑ Explain or clarify test purpose and procedure.
☑ Evaluate patient understanding.
After the test
☑ Cover venipuncture site with a clean dry bandage for 24 hours. Check regularly for infection, since a patient with RA may be immunologically compromised from the disease or from corticosteroid therapy.

Interfering factors
• Inadequately activated complement may cause false-positive results.
• Serum with high lipid or cryoglobulin levels may cause false-positive test results, and requires repetition of the test after restriction of fat intake.
• Serum with high IgG levels may cause false-negative results, through competition with IgG on the surface of latex particles or sheep RBCs used as substrate.

Rubella antibodies

Purpose
• To diagnose rubella (German measles) infection, especially congenital infection
• To determine susceptibility to rubella in children and in women of childbearing age.

Results
For immunity:
Titer of less than 1:8 or 1:10 (depending on the test) indicates:
    Susceptibility to rubella.
Titer of greater than 1:10 indicates:
    Adequate protection against rubella.
For rubella infection:
    Acute serum titers range from 1:8 to 1:16.
    Convalescent serum titers range from 1:64 to 1:1,024 + .
An antibody titer greater than 1:8 in an infant aged 6 months or older, who has not been exposed to rubella postnatally, confirms congenital rubella.

The basics
Although rubella is generally a mild viral infection in children and young adults, it can produce severe infection in the fetus, resulting in spontaneous abortion, stillbirth, or birth defects. Generally, the earlier the infection occurs during pregnancy, the greater the damage to the fetus. When rubella infection occurs during the first trimester, cataracts, deafness, and cardiac defects—congenital rubella syndrome—can result. Low birth weight, microcephaly, and mental retardation are other common manifestations. Since rubella infection normally in-

duces IgG and IgM antibody production, measuring rubella antibodies can determine present infection and immunity resulting from past infection. The rubella antibodies normally appear 2 to 4 days after the onset of the rash, peak in 2 to 3 weeks, then slowly decline but remain detectable for life. Since maternal antibodies cross the placenta and persist in the infant's serum for up to 6 months, congenital rubella can be detected only after this period. The test for rubella requires two serum samples: one 3 days after onset of rash (acute titer); another, 2 to 3 weeks later (convalescent titer). A fourfold or greater rise from the acute to the convalescent titer indicates a recent rubella infection. The test for immunity requires one sample.

Procedure
Perform a venipuncture and collect the sample in a 7-ml red-top tube.

Patient care checklist
Before the test
☑ Explain or clarify test purpose and procedure. Provide emotional support, as needed, to parents when congenital rubella is suspected.
☑ Evaluate patient/parent understanding.
After the test
☑ Instruct patient to return for an additional blood test when appropriate.
☑ If a woman of childbearing age (or a child) is found susceptible to rubella (titer of 1:8 or less), explain to the patient (or to the patient's parents) that vaccination can prevent rubella, and that she must wait at least 3 months after vaccination before becoming pregnant, or risk permanent damage or death to the fetus.
☑ If a pregnant patient is found susceptible to rubella, instruct the patient to return for follow-up rubella antibody tests, as ordered, to detect possible subsequent infection.

☑ If the test confirms rubella in a pregnant patient, provide emotional support. As needed, refer her for appropriate counseling.

Interfering factors
Hemolysis caused by rough handling of the specimen may interfere with accurate determination of test results.

T- and B-lymphocyte assays

Purpose
• To aid diagnosis of primary and secondary immunodeficiency diseases
• To distinguish benign from malignant lymphocytic proliferative diseases
• To monitor response to therapy.

Normal results
Currently, T and B cell assays are being standardized, and values may differ from one laboratory to another, depending on the test technique.
Generally, of the total number of lymphocytes:
T cells comprise 68% to 75%
B cells comprise 10% to 20%
Null cells comprise 5% to 20%.
Total lymphocyte count—1,500 to 3,000/mm^3
T cell count—1,400 to 2,700/mm^3
B cell count—270 to 640/mm^3
NOTE: These counts are higher in children.

Abnormal results
Elevated B-cell count:
    Chronic lymphocytic leukemia
    Multiple myeloma
    Waldenström's macroglobulinemia
    DiGeorge's syndrome (a congenital T-cell deficiency).
Decreased B-cell count:
    Acute lymphocytic leukemia
    Certain congenital or acquired immunoglobulin deficiency diseases

(in other immunoglobulin deficiency diseases, especially if only one immunoglobulin class is deficient, the B-cell count remains normal).

Elevated T-cell count:
  Multiple myeloma
  Acute lymphocytic leukemia
  Occasionally, infectious mononucleosis.

Decreased T-cell count:
  Acquired T-cell deficiency diseases, such as AIDS (Acquired Immune Deficiency Syndrome)
  Congenital T-cell deficiency diseases, such as DiGeorge's, Nezelof's, and Wiskott-Aldrich syndromes
  Certain B-cell proliferative disorders, such as chronic lymphocytic leukemia and Waldenström's macroglobulinemia.

The basics

Lymphocytes—key cells in the immune system—have the capacity to recognize antigens through special receptors found on their surfaces. The two main kinds of lymphocytes, T and B cells, originate in the bone marrow. The T cells mature under the influence of the thymus gland; B cells evolve without thymic influence. Cell separation is used to isolate lymphocytes from other cellular blood elements. The percent of T and B cells is determined by attaching a label or a marker, and by using different identification techniques. The E rosette test identifies T cells. Direct immunofluorescence detects B cells. Unlike T cells, B cells present receptors for complement as well as for Fc portions of immunoglobulin. Null cells, which make up the remainder of the lymphocytes, possess Fc receptors but no other detachable surface markers, and have no known diagnostic significance. Null cells are usually determined by subtracting the T and B cells from the total lymphocytes. Normal T-cell and B-cell counts do not necessarily ensure a competent immune system. In autoimmune diseases, such as systemic lupus erythematosus and rheumatoid arthritis, T and B cells, though present in normal numbers, may not be functionally competent. An abnormal T-cell or B-cell count suggests, but does not confirm, specific diseases.

Procedure

Perform a venipuncture, and collect the sample in a 7-ml green-top (heparinized) tube.

Patient care checklist
Before the test
☑ Explain or clarify test purpose and procedure.
☑ Evaluate patient understanding.
After the test
☑ Keep the venipuncture site clean and dry, since many patients with T- and B-cell changes have a compromised immune system.

Interfering factors
• Failure to use the proper collection tube, to mix the sample and anticoagulant adequately, or to send the sample to the laboratory immediately can interfere with accurate testing.
• T- and B-cell counts can change rapidly with changes in health status, from the effects of stress, or after surgery, chemotherapy, steroid or immunosuppressive therapy, and X-rays.
• The presence of immunoglobulins, such as autologous antilymphocyte antibodies that sometimes occur in autoimmune disease, can alter test results.

Terminal deoxynucleotidyl transferase (TdT) test

Purpose
• To help differentiate acute lympho-

cytic leukemia (ALL) from acute non-lymphocytic leukemia
• To help differentiate lymphoblastic lymphomas from non-Hodgkin's lymphomas
• To monitor response to therapy.

Normal results
Serum TdT levels:
   0 to 10 IU/10^{13} cells.
Bone marrow:
   Not established, but similar to serum TdT levels.

Abnormal results
Elevated TdT levels:
   ALL
   Blastic phase of chronic myelogenous leukemia
   Lymphoblastic lymphoma
   Acute lymphoblastic leukemia
   Acute nonlymphocytic leukemias (small percentage).

The basics
Using indirect immunofluorescence, this test measures levels of TdT, an intranuclear enzyme found in certain primitive lymphocytes in the normal thymus and bone marrow. Since TdT acts as a biochemical marker for these lymphocytes, it can help to classify the origin of a particular tissue. Thus, the TdT test is useful in differentiating certain types of leukemias and lymphomas marked by primitive cells that cannot be identified by histology alone. Measurement of TdT may also help determine prognosis for these diseases, and may provide early diagnosis of a relapse. For example, although TdT levels are elevated in ALL, TdT positive cells are absent in patients who are in remission.

Procedure
• Contact the laboratory before performing the test, to ensure that they are able to process the sample and to find out how much blood to draw if a blood test will be performed.
• Cleanse the site thoroughly, since patients with leukemia are more susceptible to infection.
• In a blood test: Perform the venipuncture, and collect the sample in two 7-ml green-top (heparinized) tubes. In bone marrow aspiration: Inject 1 ml of bone marrow into a 7-ml green-top (heparinized) tube and dilute it with 5 ml of sterile saline. (Also see "Bone marrow aspiration and biopsy," pp. 444 to 448.)
• Wrap the tubes in a paper towel.
• Refrigerate the tubes on cold packs or wet ice, and send them to the laboratory immediately.

Patient care checklist
Before the test
☑ Explain or clarify test purpose, preparation, and procedure.
☑ Evaluate patient understanding.
☑ Restrict food and fluids for 12 to 14 hours prior to venipuncture.
(For patient care prior to bone marrow aspiration, see Chapter 9.)
After the test
CLINICAL ALERT: **Apply pressure to the venipuncture site until bleeding stops, since patients with leukemia may bleed excessively.**

Interfering factors
• Failure to obtain a representative sample may interfere with accurate determination of bone marrow aspiration results.
• Performing a bone marrow aspiration on a child may produce false-positive results, since TdT is normally present in bone marrow during the proliferation of prelymphocytes.
• Bone marrow regeneration, idiopathic thrombocytopenic purpura, and neuroblastoma may produce false-positive bone marrow aspiration results, since these conditions cause TdT-positive bone marrow.

TORCH test *(Tests for toxoplasmosis, rubella, cytomegalovirus [CMV], and herpes simplex)*

Purpose

To detect toxoplasmosis, rubella, CMV, or herpes simplex congenital infection.

Results

Normal maternal serum shows absent or low and stable IgG antibody titers to a TORCH agent; absence of specific IgM class antibodies.

Normal infant serum shows absent or declining (over 8 to 12 weeks) IgG antibody titers to a TORCH agent; absence of specific IgM class antibodies.

Initial IgG antibody titers are usually obtained from both maternal and infant serum and then compared, as follows:

If maternal titers and infant titers are both negative:

Rules out congenital TORCH infection.

If maternal titers are higher than infant titers:

Congenital TORCH infection highly unlikely.

If infant titers are higher than maternal titers:

Congenital TORCH infection suspected (follow-up titers warranted).

If maternal and infant titers are equal:

Congenital TORCH infection unlikely (follow-up titers possible).

Follow-up IgG antibody titers are obtained from infant serum, usually 8 to 12 weeks later, and interpreted as follows:

Declining titers:

No congenital TORCH infection.

Persistently high or increased titers:

Congenital TORCH infection.

Specific IgM class antibody levels to TORCH agents may also be obtained from infant serum:

If specific IgM absent:

No congenital TORCH infection.

If specific IgM present:

Congenital TORCH infection.

The basics

TORCH is an abbreviation for toxoplasmosis, rubella, CMV, and herpes simplex virus. A complete TORCH screen refers to serological assays for these agents in maternal and infant serum.

When TORCH infections occur during pregnancy, they can cross the placenta and result in abortion, stillbirth, or mild to severe congenital malformation and disease. The severity of the effects depends on the period of fetal development in which infection occurs, and on individual fetal response as well as maternal response. Immature cells are believed to be more easily infected and to support the growth of virus better than older cells. In general, chances of maternal transmission of these agents to the fetus decrease sharply after the 8th week of gestation. Once the fetus is infected, however, the organisms persist throughout gestation and for months postnatally.

The routine use of complete TORCH screening prenatally is no longer indicated as much as in the past. However, individual testing for a suspected TORCH agent, such as rubella screening, is very much warranted prenatally. (See "Rubella antibodies," p. 201.)

More commonly today, the complete TORCH screen is performed when congenital infection in the infant is suspected. Serum is obtained from mother and infant, and compared. If infant IgG antibody levels are acquired passively from the mother, they should decline considerably within 8 to 12 weeks. Therefore, if these titers remain unchanged (high) or are even increased in serial sera from the infant, congenital infection is indicated. Also, if the IgG titer is exceptionally high, congenital infection is suspected, but should be confirmed by other measures, such as cultures and follow-up serology, if warranted.

Detection of IgM-specific antibody may also be helpful in diagnosing congenital infections. Unlike IgG antibodies, which may be transferred to the fetus across the placenta, IgM antibodies do not cross the placenta. Instead, these antibodies are actively produced by the fetus in response to the infectious agent.

The advantage of IgM testing is that it can be performed from one serum specimen and does not require the time essential for either viral cultures or for serial titers. Both false-positive and false-negative IgM titers may occur, however, so laboratory results are not always conclusive and must be correlated with the patient history and clinical presentation.

If any serological TORCH testing in the infant is positive, it is often confirmed by other measures. For example, if CMV congenital infection is suspected, isolating CMV from infant urine is the preferred confirming diagnostic method.

Procedure
Perform a venipuncture, or collect cord blood. Collect the specimen in a 7-ml red-top tube.

Patient care checklist
Before the test
☑ Explain or clarify test purpose and procedure to the parents of the infant.
☑ Explain that serial blood samples may be needed to detect changing antibody titers.
☑ Evaluate parents' understanding.
After the test
☑ If tests indicate congenital TORCH infection, provide support and help with referrals.

Interfering factors
• Hemolysis of blood samples caused by rough handling of the specimen may alter test results.

• Testing infant serum without testing maternal serum may interfere with accurate interpretation of test results.

VDRL *(Venereal Disease Research Laboratory)* test

Purpose
• To screen for primary and secondary syphilis
• To confirm primary or secondary syphilis in the presence of syphilitic lesions
• To monitor response to treatment.

Normal results
Nonreactive test.

Abnormal results
Reactive test:
Primary syphilis (reactive in 50% of affected patients)
Secondary syphilis (reactive in nearly all affected patients)
Tertiary syphilis (reactive in only

Rapid Plasma Reagin (RPR) Card Test

This rapid, macroscopic serologic test is an acceptable substitute for the VDRL test in diagnosis of syphilis. The RPR test, available as a kit, employs a cardiolipin antigen to detect reagin, the antibody relatively specific to the causative agent of syphilis. In the RPR test, the patient's serum is mixed with cardiolipin on a plastic-coated card, rotated mechanically, and examined with the unaided eye. If flocculation occurs, the test sample is diluted until no visible reaction occurs. The last dilution to show visible flocculation is the titer of the reagin antibody.

In the RPR test, like the VDRL test, normal serum shows no flocculation.

some affected patients, using CSF specimen)

Biologic false positives can occur in conditions such as infectious mononucleosis, malaria, leprosy, hepatitis, systemic lupus erythematosus, rheumatoid arthritis, and nonsyphilitic treponemal diseases, such as pinta or yaws.

The basics

This flocculation test demonstrates the presence of reagin—an antibody relatively specific for *Treponema pallidum*, the spirochete that causes syphilis—in a serum sample. Definitive flocculation is reported as a reactive test; slight flocculation is reported as a weakly reactive test. If syphilitic lesions exist, a reactive VDRL test is diagnostic. If no lesions are evident, a reactive VDRL test necessitates repeated testing. However, transient or permanent biologic false-positive reactions can make accurate interpretation difficult. A nonreactive test does not rule out syphilis, because *T. pallidum* causes no detectable immunologic changes in the serum for 14 to 21 days after infection. However, dark-field microscopic examination of exudate from suspicious lesions can provide early diagnosis by identifying the causative spirochetes. A serum sample is used in the VDRL test, but this test may also be performed on a specimen of CSF, obtained by lumbar puncture, to test for tertiary syphilis. However, the VDRL test of CSF is less sensitive than the fluorescent treponemal antibody absorption test. (See *Rapid Plasma Reagin (RPR) Card Test* and *Tests for Syphilis*.)

Procedure

Perform a venipuncture, and collect the sample in a 7-ml red-top tube.

Patient care checklist

Before the test

☑ Explain or clarify test purpose, preparation, and procedure.

☑ Evaluate patient understanding.

Tests For Syphilis

The fluorescent treponemal antibody absorption (FTA-ABS) test—which uses a strain of the *Treponema pallidum* antigen itself as a reagent—is more sensitive than the VDRL (Venereal Disease Research Laboratory) test or the rapid plasma reagin (RPR) test in detecting all stages of untreated syphilis, but its complex testing method and incidence of false-positive results make it an impractical screening tool. The VDRL and RPR tests are preferred for wide-scale screening and also when primary- and secondary-stage disease are suspected. In advanced syphilis, when the VDRL test may be negative for more than one third of infected persons, the FTA-ABS test is preferred for sensitivity and is also the most reliable confirmation of a positive VDRL.

The VDRL test can be used to monitor response to treatment. Untreated syphilis produces titers that are low in the primary stage (<1:32), elevated in the secondary stage (>1:32), and variable in the tertiary stage. Successful therapy markedly reduces titers, with two thirds of patients reverting to a negative VDRL, especially during the first two stages of disease. Third-stage therapy seldom produces a nonreactive VDRL, but maintenance of low-reactive values during the 6- to 12-month post-therapy period indicates success. A subsequent rise signals reinfection. By comparison, FTA-ABS test results usually remain positive following treatment.

Many patients with infectious diseases show temporary false-positive VDRL test results. Chronic false-positive VDRL and FTA-ABS test readings are associated with the immune complex diseases.

Adapted with permission from Allen L. Pusch, "Serodiagnostic Tests," in *Todd-Sanford-Davidsohn Clinical Diagnosis and Management by Laboratory Methods*, Vol. 2, edited by John Bernard Henry (16th ed.; Philadelphia: W.B. Saunders Co., 1979), p. 1890.

☑ Restrict patient's alcoholic intake for 24 hours before the test.

After the test

☑ If the test is nonreactive or borderline, but syphilis has not been ruled out, instruct patient to return for follow-up testing. Explain that borderline results do not necessarily mean he is free of the disease.

☑ If the test is reactive, explain the importance of proper treatment. Provide patient with further information about venereal disease and how it is spread, and stress the need for antibiotic therapy. Also, prepare patient for mandatory inquiries from public health authorities.

☑ If the test is reactive, but the patient shows no clinical signs of syphilis, inform the patient that many uninfected persons show false-positive reactions. However, stress the need for further specific tests to rule out syphilis.

Interfering factors

• Ingestion of alcohol within 24 hours of the test can produce transient, nonreactive results.

• A faulty immune system can cause non-reactive results.

• Hemolysis of the sample can interfere with test results.

Selected References

Bryant, Neville J. *An Introduction to Immunohematology*, 2nd ed. Philadelphia: W.B. Saunders Co., 1982.

Circular of Information for the Use of Human Blood and Blood Components by Physicians. Washington, D.C.: American Association of Blood Banks, September 1978.

Diagnostics, 2nd ed. Nurse's Reference Library. Springhouse, Pa.: Springhouse Corp., 1986.

Fischbach, Frances. *A Manual of Laboratory Diagnostic Tests*, 2nd ed. Philadelphia: J.B. Lippincott Co., 1984.

Guyton, Arthur C. *Textbook of Medical Physiology*, 6th ed. Philadelphia: W.B. Saunders Co., 1981.

Hansten, Philip D. *Drug Interactions*, 5th ed. Philadelphia: Lea & Febiger, 1984.

Harvey, A. McGehee, ed. *The Principles and Practice of Medicine*, 21st ed. East Norwalk, Conn.: Appleton-Century-Crofts, 1984.

Henry, John Bernard, ed. *Todd-Sanford-Davidsohn Clinical Diagnosis and Management by Laboratory Methods*, vol. 1, 17th ed. Philadelphia: W.B. Saunders Co., 1984.

Immune Disorders. Nurse's Clinical Library. Springhouse, Pa.: Springhouse Corp., 1985.

Lamb, Jane O. *Laboratory Tests for Clinical Nursing.* Bowie, Md.: Robert J. Brady Co., 1984.

Leavelle, Dennis E., ed. *Mayo Medical Laboratories Test Catalog.* Rochester, Minn.: Mayo Medical Laboratories, 1984.

McNeeley, M.D. "Drug Interference with Laboratory Tests of Immunologic Status," *Drug Therapy* 73-76, March 1981.

Milgrom, Felix, et al., eds. *Principles of Immunological Diagnosis in Medicine.* Philadelphia: Lea & Febiger, 1981.

Miller, William V., ed. *Technical Manual of the American Association of Blood Banks*, 7th ed. Philadelphia: J.B. Lippincott Co., 1977.

Miller, William V., et al. *Technical Methods and Procedures of the American Association of Blood Banks.* Washington, D.C.: American Association of Blood Banks, 1974.

Rose, Noel R., and Friedman, Herman, eds. *Manual of Clinical Immunology*, 2nd ed. Washington, D.C.: American Society for Microbiology, 1980.

Stites, Daniel P., et al., eds. *Basic and Clinical Immunology*, 4th ed. Los Altos, Calif.: Lange Medical Pubs., 1982.

Wegener, Lee T., ed. *Mayo Medical Laboratories Interpretive Handbook.* Rochester, Minn.: Mayo Medical Laboratories, 1984.

Wyngaarden, James, and Smith, Lloyd. *Cecil Textbook of Medicine*, 16th ed. Philadelphia: W.B. Saunders Co., 1982.

4 URINE TESTING

Introduction

The renal system's main function is to maintain the body's internal homeostasis. It does this through glomerular filtration and tubular reabsorption and secretion. The major outcome is filtration of wastes and conservation of essential solutes. In implementing these functions, the kidneys also exert an important influence on regulation of electrolytes and water, blood pressure, acid-base balance, calcium and phosphate balance, and erythropoiesis.

Urine volume reflects overall fluid homeostasis. Actual volume depends on fluid intake, the concentration of solutes in the filtrate, cardiac output, hormonal influences, and fluid loss through the lungs, the large bowel, and the skin. In adults, urine volume normally ranges from 800 to 2,000 ml/day, and averages 1,200 to 1,500 ml/day. In children, volume ranges from 300 to 1,300 ml/day; however, a child's urine output is three to four times greater per kilogram of body weight than that of an adult.

Actual composition of normal urine changes—depending on diet, physical activity, and emotional stress; however, it always includes water, urea, uric acid, and sodium chloride. Urine also usually contains other nonprotein nitrogen compounds, citric acid, other organic acids, catecholamines, sulfur-containing compounds, phosphate, potassium, calcium, magnesium, reducing substances, mucoproteins, vitamins, and hormones. In the presence of disease, urine may contain protein, glucose, ketone bodies, hemoglobin, lipids, bacteria, pus, urobilinogen, or calculi.

Routine urinalysis and special studies of renal function provide valuable information about the integrity of renal and urinary functions, and also serve as sensitive indicators of overall health. These tests often begin the diagnostic workup and may reveal abnormal findings before clinical symptoms appear. Abnormal findings suggest the presence of disease and usually mandate further tests to identify a specific disorder.

Special tests for filtration, reabsorption, and secretion permit precise evaluation of renal function. Clearance, the volume of plasma that can be cleared of a substance per unit of time, is the principle used to assess these urine-forming mechanisms; it is also a measure of renal plasma flow, which, if diminished, impairs renal function. Clearance depends on how efficiently the renal tubular cells handle the substance that has been filtered by the glomerulus. If the tubules do not reabsorb or secrete the substance, clearance equals the glomerular filtration rate (GFR). If the tubules reabsorb it, clearance is less than the GFR. If the tubules secrete it, clearance is greater than the GFR. If the tubules reabsorb and secrete the substance, clearance is less than, equal to, or greater than the GFR.

Accurate urine testing depends on careful collection techniques. (See pp. xii to xx.)

Patient-teaching guidelines

Patient-learner objectives:
- Define the test.
- State the specific purpose of the test.
- Explain the procedure.
- Discuss test preparation, procedure, and post-test care.

Teaching content:
- Define the test in terms the patient can understand.
- Explain the specific purpose of the test.
- Describe the procedure.
  —To collect a random urine specimen, instruct the ambulatory patient to urinate directly into a clean, dry specimen container. Tell the nonambulatory patient to void into a clean bedpan or urinal and to notify appropriate personnel, who will transfer the urine to a specimen container.
  —To collect a second-voided specimen, instruct the patient to void and discard the urine. Then, after he drinks at least one glass of fluid to stimulate urine production, tell him to void 30 minutes later into a clean, dry specimen container or clean bedpan or urinal.
  —To collect a timed urine specimen, such as a 24-hour sample, instruct the patient to void and discard the urine; then begin timed collection with the next voiding. Stress that he must collect *all* urine during the test period. Tell the patient not to void directly into the container, since it may contain a preservative that can cause irritation or injury. When appropriate, inform the patient to keep the container refrigerated or on ice during the collection period. Just before the end of the collection period, instruct the patient to void and to add the last specimen to the container.
  —To collect a pediatric urine specimen, explain to the parents that it will be necessary to place the child on his back with knees flexed. The perineal area should then be cleaned and dried. For a boy, the collection device will be applied over his penis and scrotum, with the flaps of the collection bag pressed against his perineum to ensure a tight fit. For a girl, the collection bag will be applied to her perineum. Explain that the child should wear a diaper over the collection bag to discourage tampering with it.
- When indicated, tell the patient to save the first urine specimen of the morning. Explain that, since this is the most concentrated specimen, it is the specimen of choice for analyzing urinary sediment.
- Instruct the patient not to include toilet tissue or stool in any urine specimen, since this can interfere with accurate test results.
- Identify any dietary or medication restrictions necessary before the test. List items to be avoided, and give a definite time period. When these restrictions are applicable, explain that they will help provide more accurate test results.
- For home patients, provide written instructions as well; stress that the specimen should be brought to the designated laboratory immediately upon completion of collection, or it should be kept refrigerated.

Evaluation:
After the patient-teaching session is completed, evaluate whether or not the patient has satisfactorily met each patient-learner objective by obtaining necessary patient feedback. Refocus teaching as needed.

Acid mucopolysaccharides
(AMPs)

Purpose
To diagnose mucopolysaccharidosis, a deficiency in carbohydrate metabolism.

Normal results
Normal AMP values vary with age.

	AMPs	
Age	(mg glucuronic acid) / g creatinine	/24 hours
2	8 to 30	
4	7 to 27	
6	6 to 24	
8	4 to 22	
10	2 to 18	
12	0 to 15	
14	0 to 12	

Abnormal results
Increased AMP levels reliably indicate:
   Mucopolysaccharidosis.

The basics
This quantitative test for mucopolysaccharidosis measures the urine level of AMPs, a group of polysaccharides or carbohydrates, in infants with family histories of the disease. When an inborn error of metabolism causes enzymatic deficiencies, AMPs—especially dermatan sulfate and heparitin sulfate—accumulate in the tissues, producing a rare disorder called mucopolysaccharidosis. Its severest form, Hurler's syndrome (gargoylism), results from deposition of these macromolecular complexes in several organs, particularly the heart and kidneys, and excretion of large amounts of mucopolysaccharides in the urine. Supplementary quantitative analysis and detailed blood studies can identify the defective enzyme.

Procedure
• Obtain a 24-hour urine specimen. Add 20 ml toluene as a preservative at the start of the collection. (See "Timed collection," pp. xviii and xix.)
• Indicate the patient's age on the laboratory slip.

Special precautions
During the collection period, refrigerate the specimen or place it on ice.

Patient care checklist
Before the test
☑ Explain or clarify test purpose, preparation, and procedure.
☑ Evaluate parents' understanding.
☑ Instruct parents of the patient on proper way to collect specimen at home.
After the test
☑ Wash the child's perineum with soap and water to remove the adhesive remaining from the urine collector.

Interfering factors
• Failure to collect all urine during the test period can alter test results.
• Improper specimen storage can alter test results.
• Heparin elevates urine levels of AMPs.

Aldosterone

Purpose
To aid in diagnosis of primary and secondary aldosteronism.

Normal results
Urine aldosterone levels range from 2 to 16 mcg/24 hours.

Abnormal results
Increased urine aldosterone levels (30 to 60 mcg/24 hours):
   Primary hyperaldosteronism resulting from an aldosterone-secreting adenoma or adrenocortical hyperplasia.
Increased urine aldosterone levels (50 to 150 mcg/24 hours):
   Secondary hyperaldosteronism resulting from malignant hypertension, congestive heart failure, cirrhosis, nephrotic syndrome, or idiopathic cyclic edema.
Decreased urine aldosterone levels:
   Addison's disease
   Salt-losing syndrome
   Toxemia of pregnancy.

The basics

This test measures urine levels of aldosterone, the principal mineralocorticoid secreted by the zona glomerulosa of the adrenal cortex. Aldosterone promotes retention of sodium and excretion of potassium by the renal tubules, thereby helping to regulate blood pressure and fluid and electrolyte balance. In turn, aldosterone secretion is controlled by the renin-angiotensin system. Renin, an enzyme released in the kidneys in response to low plasma volume, stimulates production of angiotensin I, which is converted to angiotensin II, a powerful vasopressor that directly stimulates the adrenal cortex to secrete aldosterone. Potassium levels also influence aldosterone secretion: increased potassium concentration stimulates the adrenal cortex, triggering a substantial increase in aldosterone secretion to promote potassium excretion. This feedback mechanism is vital to maintaining fluid and electrolyte balance. Urine aldosterone levels, measured through radioimmunoassay, are usually evaluated after measurement of serum electrolyte and renin levels.

Procedure

Collect a 24-hour urine specimen in a bottle containing a preservative to keep the specimen at a pH of 4.0 to 4.5. (See "Timed collection," pp. xviii and xix.)

Special precautions

Refrigerate the specimen or place it on ice during the collection period.

Patient care checklist

Before the test

☑ Explain or clarify test purpose, preparation, and procedure.

☑ Evaluate patient understanding.

☑ Instruct the patient to maintain a normal sodium diet (3 g/day) and to avoid sodium-rich foods.

☑ Instruct the patient to avoid strenuous exercise and stressful situations during the collection period.

Interfering factors

● Antihypertensive drugs promote sodium and water retention and may suppress urine aldosterone levels.

● Diuretics and most steroids promote sodium excretion and may raise aldosterone levels.

● Some corticosteroids, such as fludrocortisone, mimic mineralocorticoid activity and consequently may lower aldosterone levels.

● Patient failure to maintain a normal dietary intake of sodium can alter test results.

● Failure to collect *all* urine during the 24-hour specimen collection period may interfere with accurate determination of test results.

● Failure to store the urine specimen properly may affect test results.

● Excessive physical exercise or emotional stress stimulates adrenocortical secretion and thus increases aldosterone levels.

● A radioactive scan performed within 1 week before the test may interfere with accurate determination of aldosterone levels using this radioimmunoassay method.

Amino acid screening

Purpose

● To screen for renal aminoaciduria, an amino acid disorder

● To follow up plasma test findings when results of these tests suggest certain overflow aminoacidurias.

Normal results

Patterns on thin-layer chromatography are reported as normal.

Abnormal results

Thin-layer chromatography shows gross changes or abnormal patterns:
   Aminoaciduria.

The basics

This test screens for aminoaciduria—elevated urine amino acids—a condition that may result from inborn errors of metabolism due to the absence of specific enzymatic activities. Normally, up to 200 mg of amino acids may be excreted in the urine in 24 hours. Abnormal metabolism causes an excess of one or more amino acids to appear in plasma and, as the renal threshold is exceeded, in urine. Aminoacidurias may be classified as either primary (overflow) aminoacidopathies or secondary (renal) aminoacidopathies. The latter type is associated with conditions marked by defective tubular reabsorption from congenital disorders. A more specific defect, such as cystinuria, may cause one or more amino acids to appear in urine.

To screen newborns, children, and adults for congenital aminoacidurias, plasma or urine specimens may be used. The plasma test is the better indicator of overflow aminoacidurias; urine testing is used to confirm or monitor certain amino acid disorders and to screen for renal aminoacidurias.

Various laboratory techniques are available to screen for aminoacidurias, but chromatography is the preferred method. Positive findings on chromatography can be elaborated by fractionation to show specific amino acid levels. Testing for specific amino acid levels is also necessary for infants or young children with acidosis, severe vomiting and diarrhea, and abnormal urine odor. Such testing is especially important in newborns, because early diagnosis of certain aminoacidurias may prevent mental retardation by allowing prompt treatment. (See also *Chromatographic Identification of Amino Acid Disorders*, pp. 214 and 215.)

Procedure
• If the patient is an infant, clean and dry the genital area, attach the collection device, and observe for voiding. Transfer urine—at least 20 ml—to a specimen container.
• If the patient is an adult or a child, collect a fresh random specimen.

Patient care checklist
Before the test
☑ Explain or clarify test purpose and procedure.
☑ Evaluate patient/parent understanding.

Interfering factors
• Failure to send the urine specimen to the laboratory immediately may alter test results.
• Results are invalid in a newborn who has not ingested dietary protein in the 48 hours preceding the test.

Amylase

Purpose
• To diagnose acute pancreatitis when serum amylase levels are normal or borderline
• To aid diagnosis of chronic pancreatitis and salivary gland disorders.

Normal results
Urine amylase is reported in various units of measure, so values differ from laboratory to laboratory. The Mayo Clinic reports urinary excretion of 10 to 80 amylase units/hour as normal.

Abnormal results
Increased urine amylase levels:
  Acute pancreatitis
  Destruction of pancreatic duct
  Intestinal obstruction
  Obstruction of salivary duct
  Carcinoma of head of pancreas
  Mumps
  Acute spleen injury
  Renal disease with impaired absorption
  Perforated peptic or duodenal ulcers
  Gallbladder disease.
Decreased urine amylase levels:
  Chronic pancreatitis
  Cachexia
  Alcoholism
  Cancer of the liver

Chromatographic Identification of Amino Acid Disorders

Chromato-graphic band no.	Amino acids	PKU		Maple syrup urine disease		Cystinuria	
		Plasma	Urine	Plasma	Urine	Plasma	Urine
1	Leucine, isoleucine			+	+		
2	Phenylalanine	+	+				
3	Valine, methionine			+	+		
4	Tryptophan, beta-aminoisobutyric acid						
5	Tyrosine						
6	Proline			+			
7	Alanine, ethanolamine						
8	Threonine, glutamic acid						
9	Homocitrulline, glycine, serine, hydroxy-proline, aspartic acid, glutamine, citrulline			+			
10	Homocystine, asparagine						
11	Argininosuccinic acid, histidine, arginine, lysine, ornithine, cystathionine, cystine, cysteine, hydroxylysine						+

KEY: + = Increased amino acids in the plasma and/or urine

In chromatography—the preferred method for screening aminoacidurias—amino acids migrate into multicolored bands. (The sequence of amino acids and their corresponding band numbers, as listed above, reflects these standard migratory

Cirrhosis
Hepatitis
Hepatic abscess.

The basics

Amylase is a starch-splitting enzyme primarily produced in the pancreas and salivary glands, usually secreted into the alimentary tract, and absorbed into the blood; small amounts of amylase are also absorbed into the blood directly from these organs. Following glomerular filtration, amylase is excreted in the urine. In the presence of adequate renal function, serum and urine levels usually rise in tandem. However, within 2 or 3 days of onset of acute pancreatitis, serum amylase levels fall to normal, but elevated urine amylase persists for 7 to 10 days. One method for determining urine amylase levels is the dye-coupled starch method. The laboratory requires 2 days to complete the analysis. If the

		Metabolic amino acid disorders									
Homocystinuria		Hartnup disease		Arginino-succinicacidemia		Histidinemia		Hyperprolin-emia Type A		Citrullinuria	
Plasma	Urine	Plasma	Urine	Plasma	Urine	Plasma	Urine	Plasma	Urine	Plasma	Urine
			+								
			+								
+		+								+	
			+								
								+			
							+				
			+					+		+	+
+											
			+	+		+	+				+

patterns.) When congenital enzyme deficiencies and subsequent metabolic disorders increase plasma and urine amino acid levels, these bands intensify.

female patient is menstruating, the test may have to be rescheduled.

Procedure
Collect a 2-, 6-, 8-, or 24-hour urine specimen. (See "Timed collection," pp. xviii and xix.)

Special precautions
Cover and refrigerate the specimen during the collection period. If the pa-tient is catheterized, keep the collection bag on ice.

Patient care checklist
Before the test
☑ Explain or clarify test purpose and procedure.
☑ Evaluate patient understanding.
☑ Withhold medications that may interfere with test results for 24 hours prior to the test. If they must be continued, note on laboratory slip.

Interfering factors

• Heavy bacterial contamination of the specimen or blood in the urine may alter test results.

• Ingestion of morphine, meperidine, codeine, pentazocine, bethanechol, thiazide diuretics, indomethacin, or alcohol within 24 hours of the test may raise urine amylase levels.

• Fluorides may lower urine amylase levels.

• Salivary amylase in the urine, caused by coughing or talking over the sample, may raise urine amylase levels.

• Failure to collect all urine during the test period may alter test results.

• Improper storage of the specimen may affect test results.

Arylsulfatase A (ARS A)

Purpose

To aid in diagnosis of cancer of the bladder, the colon, or the rectum; of myeloid (granulocytic) leukemia; and of metachromatic leukodystrophy (an inherited lipid storage disease).

Normal results

ARS A values in men range from 1.4 to 19.3 units/liter; in women, from 1.4 to 11 units/liter; and in children, over 1 unit/liter.

Abnormal results

Increased ARS A levels:
  Cancer of the bladder
  Cancer of the colon
  Cancer of the rectum
  Myeloid leukemia.
Decreased ARS A levels:
  Metachromatic leukodystrophy.

The basics

ARS A, a lysosomal enzyme found in every cell except the mature erythrocyte, is principally active in the liver, the pancreas, and the kidneys, where exogenous substances are detoxified into ester sulfates. When ARS A is present in large amounts, it reverses this process by catalyzing the release of free phenylsulfates, such as benzidine and naphthyline, from the ester sulfates. Research has not resolved whether elevated ARS A levels provoke malignant growths or are simply an enzymatic response to their presence.

This test measures urine ARS A levels by colorimetric or kinetic techniques. Test results are generally available in 2 to 3 days. If the female patient is menstruating, the test may have to be rescheduled, since increased numbers of epithelial cells in the urine raise ARS A levels.

Procedure

Collect a 24-hour urine specimen. (See "Timed collection," pp. xviii and xix.)

Special precautions

Keep the collection container refrigerated or on ice during the collection period. If the patient is catheterized, keep the collection bag on ice for the duration of the test; it is advisable to change the continuous urinary drainage apparatus before beginning the test.

Patient care checklist
Before the test
☑ Explain or clarify test purpose and procedure.
☑ Evaluate patient understanding.

Interfering factors

• Failure to collect all urine during the test period may alter test results.

• Contamination of the urine specimen by stool, menses, or improper storage may interfere with accurate determination of test results.

• Surgery performed within 1 week before the test may raise ARS A levels.

Bence Jones protein

Purpose

To aid in the diagnosis of multiple myeloma in patients with characteristic clinical signs, such as bone pain (especially in the back and thorax) and persistent anemia and fatigue.

Normal results

Urine should contain no Bence Jones proteins.

Abnormal results

The presence of Bence Jones proteins in urine suggests multiple myeloma or Waldenström's macroglobulinemia. Very low levels, in the absence of other symptoms, may result from benign monoclonal gammopathy. However, clinical evidence figures prominently in diagnosis of multiple myeloma.

The basics

Bence Jones proteins are abnormal light-chain immunoglobulins of low molecular weight that are derived from the clone of a single plasma cell (monoclonal). This globulin appears in the urine of 50% to 80% of patients with multiple myeloma and in most patients with Waldenström's macroglobulinemia.

In most cases, these proteins—thought to be synthesized by malignant plasma cells in the bone marrow—are rapidly cleared from the plasma and do not usually appear in serum. When these proteins exceed renal tubular capacity to break down and reabsorb them, they overflow and are excreted in the urine (overflow proteinuria). Eventually, the renal tubular cells degenerate from the effort to reabsorb excess amounts of protein. Consequently, protein precipitates and inclusions occur in the renal tubular cells. If renal failure results from such precipitation or from hypercalcemia, increased uric acid, or infiltration by abnormal plasma cells, more Bence Jones proteins and other proteins then appear in the urine, since the dysfunctional nephrons no longer control protein excretion.

Urine screening tests, such as thermal coagulation and Bradshaw's test, can detect Bence Jones proteins, but urine immunoelectrophoresis is usually the method of choice for quantitative studies. Serum immunoelectrophoresis, which is sometimes used, is less sensitive than the urine tests. Nevertheless, both urine and serum studies are frequently used for patients suspected of having multiple myeloma.

Procedure

Collect an early-morning urine specimen of at least 50 ml.

Special precautions

Refrigerate the specimen if there is a delay in transporting it to the laboratory.

Patient care checklist

Before the test

☑ Explain or clarify test purpose and procedure.

☑ Evaluate patient understanding.

Interfering factors

- False-positive results may occur in connective tissue disease, renal insufficiency, or certain malignancies.
- Contamination of the specimen with menstrual blood, prostatic secretions, or semen may cause false-positive results.
- Failure to send the specimen to the laboratory immediately or to keep the specimen refrigerated may cause false-positive results, because heat-coagulable protein denatures or decomposes at room temperature.

Bilirubin

Purpose

To help identify the cause of jaundice.

Normal results

Bilirubin is not found in urine in a routine screening test.

Abnormal results

High concentrations of direct bilirubin in urine may be evident from the specimen's appearance (dark, with a yellow foam). To diagnose jaundice, however, the presence or absence of direct bilirubin in urine must be correlated with serum test results, and with urine and fecal urobilinogen levels (see *Comparative Values of Bilirubin and Urobilinogen*).

The basics

This screening test, based on a color reaction with a specific reagent, detects abnormally high urine concentrations of direct (conjugated) bilirubin. The reticuloendothelial system produces bilirubin from hemoglobin breakdown. The pigment bilirubin then combines with albumin, a plasma protein, and is transported to the liver as indirect (unconjugated) bilirubin. In the liver, most indirect bilirubin joins with glucuronic acid to form bilirubin glucuronide and bilirubin diglucuronide—water-soluble compounds almost totally excreted into the bile. In the intestine, bacterial action converts direct bilirubin to urobilinogen. Normally, only a small amount of direct bilirubin—unbound or bound to albumin—returns to plasma. The kidneys filter the unbound portion, which may appear in trace amounts in the urine. Fat-soluble indirect bilirubin cannot be filtered by the glomeruli and is never present in urine. Bilirubin in the urine may indicate liver disease caused by infections, biliary disease, or hepatotoxicity.

When combined with urobilinogen measurements, this test helps identify disorders that can cause jaundice. The analysis can be performed at bedside, using a bilirubin reagent strip, or in the laboratory. Highly sensitive spectrophotometric assays may be needed to detect trace amounts of urine bilirubin. This screening test does not detect such minute amounts. Laboratory analysis is completed in 1 day.

Procedure

Collect a random urine specimen in the container provided. For bedside analysis, use one of the following procedures:

Dipstrip:

Dip the reagent strip into the specimen and remove it immediately. After 20 seconds, and with adequate lighting, compare the strip color with the color standards. Record the test results on the patient's chart.

Ictotest:

This test is easier to read and more sensitive than the dipstrip method. Place five drops of urine on the asbestos-cellulose test mat. If bilirubin is present, it will be absorbed into the mat. Next, put a reagent tablet on the wet area of the mat, and place two drops of water on the tablet. If bilirubin is present, a blue-to-purple coloration will develop on the mat. Pink or red indicates absence of bilirubin— a negative test.

Special precautions

• Use only a freshly voided specimen. Bilirubin disintegrates after 30 minutes' exposure to room temperature or light.

• If the specimen is to be analyzed in the laboratory, send it to the laboratory immediately. Record the time of collection on the patient's chart.

• If hepatitis is suspected, affix the correct biohazard label to the specimen.

Patient care checklist

Before the test

☑ Explain or clarify test purpose and procedure.

☑ Evaluate patient understanding.

Interfering factors

• Dipstrip testing, such as with Chemstrip or N-Multistix, is affected by large amounts of ascorbic acid and nitrite, which may lower bilirubin levels and cause false-negative test results.

• Phenazopyridine and phenothiazine derivatives, such as chlorpromazine

Comparative Values of Bilirubin and Urobilinogen

Causes of jaundice	Serum		Urine		Feces
	Indirect bilirubin	Direct bilirubin	Bilirubin	Urobilinogen	Urobilinogen
Unconjugated hyperbilirubinemia					
• *Hemolytic disorders* (hemolytic anemia, erythroblastosis fetalis)	↑	N	O	N↑	↑
• *Gilbert's disease* (constitutional hepatic dysfunction)	↑ ↑	N	O	N↓	N↓
• *Crigler-Najjar syndrome* (congenital hyperbilirubinemia)	↑ ↑ ↑	N	O	N↓	N↓
Conjugated hyperbilirubinemia					
• Extrahepatic obstruction (calculi, tumor, scar tissue in common bile duct or hepatic excretory duct)	N	↑	+	↓O	↓O
• *Hepatocellular disorders* (viral, toxic, or alcoholic hepatitis; cirrhosis; parenchymal injury)	↑	↑	+	↓N↑	N↓
• *Hepatocanalicular disorders or intrahepatic obstruction* (drug-induced cholestasis; some familial defects, such as Dubin-Johnson and Rotor's syndromes; viral hepatitis; primary biliary cirrhosis)	↑	↑	+	↓N↑	N↓

Key

↑	Increased
N↑	May be increased
↑ ↑	Moderately increased
↑ ↑ ↑	Markedly increased
N	Normal
O	Absent
+	Present
N↓	Normal or reduced
↓O	Decreased or absent
↓N↑	Variable

and acetophenazine maleate, can cause false-positive results.

• Exposure of the specimen to room temperature or light can lower bilirubin levels, due to bilirubin degradation.

Calcium and phosphates

Purpose
• To evaluate calcium and phosphate metabolism and excretion
• To monitor treatment of calcium or phosphate deficiency.

Normal results
Values depend on dietary intake. Males excrete < 275 mg of calcium/24 hours; females, < 250 mg/24 hours. Normal excretion of phosphate is < 1,000 mg/24 hours.

Abnormal results
See *Disorders that Affect Urine Calcium and Urine Phosphorus Levels.*

The basics
This test measures the urine levels of calcium and phosphates, elements essential for the formation and resorp-

Disorders that Affect Urine Calcium and Urine Phosphorus Levels

Disorder	Urine calcium level	Urine phosphate level
Hyperparathyroidism	Elevated	Elevated
Vitamin D intoxication	Elevated	Suppressed
Metastatic carcinoma	Elevated	Normal
Sarcoidosis	Elevated	Suppressed
Renal tubular acidosis	Elevated	Elevated
Multiple myeloma	Elevated or normal	Elevated or normal
Paget's disease	Normal	Normal
Milk-alkali syndrome	Suppressed or normal	Suppressed or normal
Hypoparathyroidism	Suppressed	Suppressed
Acute nephrosis	Suppressed	Suppressed or normal
Chronic nephrosis	Suppressed	Suppressed
Acute nephritis	Suppressed	Suppressed
Renal insufficiency	Suppressed	Suppressed
Osteomalacia	Suppressed	Suppressed
Steatorrhea	Suppressed	Suppressed

tion of bone. Urine calcium and phosphate levels generally parallel serum levels.

Normally absorbed in the upper intestine and excreted in feces and urine, calcium and phosphates help maintain tissue and fluid pH, electrolyte balance in cells and extracellular fluids, and permeability of cell membranes. Calcium promotes enzymatic processes, aids blood coagulation, and lowers neuromuscular irritability; phosphates aid carbohydrate metabolism. Factors that affect the calcium level and, indirectly, the phosphate level include parathyroid hormone level, calcitonin, and plasma proteins.

Procedure
Collect a 24-hour urine specimen. (See "Timed collection," pp. xviii and xix.)

Special precautions
Observe a patient with low urine calcium levels for tetany.

Patient care checklist
Before the test
☑ Explain or clarify test purpose, preparation, and procedure.
☑ Evaluate patient understanding.
☑ Instruct the patient to adhere to Albright-Reifenstein diet (which contains about 130 mg of calcium/24 hours) for 3 days before the test.
☑ Encourage the patient to be as active as possible before the test.

Interfering factors
• Failure to collect all urine during the test period may alter test results.
• Thiazide diuretics decrease excretion of calcium.
• Prolonged inactivity and ingestion of corticosteroids, sodium phosphate, and calcitonin increase excretion.
• Vitamin D increases phosphate absorption and excretion.
• Parathyroid hormone increases urinary excretion of phosphates and decreases urinary excretion of calcium.

Catecholamines

Purpose
• To aid in diagnosis of pheochromocytoma in a patient with unexplained hypertension
• To aid in diagnosis of neuroblastoma, ganglioneuroma, and dysautonomia.

Normal results
Urine catecholamine values range from undetectable to 135 mcg/24 hours, or from undetectable to 18 mcg/dl in a random specimen.

Abnormal results
Increased urine catecholamine levels:
  Pheochromocytoma
  Neuroblastoma
  Ganglioneuroma
  Myasthenia gravis
  Muscular dystrophy.
Decreased urine catecholamine levels:
  Dysautonomia.

The basics
This test uses spectrophotofluorometry to measure urine levels of the major catecholamines—epinephrine, norepinephrine, and dopamine. Epinephrine is secreted by the adrenal medulla; dopamine, by the central nervous system; and norepinephrine, by both. Catecholamines help regulate metabolism and prepare the body for the fight-or-flight response to stress. Certain tumors can also secrete catecholamines. One of the most common of these tumors is a pheochromocytoma, which usually causes intermittent or persistent hypertension.

The specimen of choice for this test is a 24-hour urine specimen, since catecholamine secretion fluctuates diurnally and in response to pain, heat, cold, emotional stress, physical exercise, hypoglycemia, injury, hemorrhage, asphyxia, and drugs. However, a random specimen may be useful for evaluating catecholamine levels after a hypertensive episode.

For a complete diagnostic workup of catecholamine secretion, urine levels of catecholamine are measured concurrently. These metabolites—metanephrine, normetanephrine, homovanillic acid, and vanillylmandelic acid—normally appear in the urine in greater quantities than the catecholamines.

Procedure

Collect a 24-hour urine specimen in a bottle containing a preservative to keep the specimen acidified to a pH of 3.0 or less. (See "Timed collection," pp. xviii and xix.) If a random specimen is ordered, collect it immediately after a hypertensive episode.

Special precautions

Refrigerate a 24-hour specimen or place it on ice during the collection period.

Patient care checklist

Before the test

☑ Explain or clarify test purpose, preparation, and procedure.

☑ Evaluate patient understanding.

☑ Instruct the patient to avoid stressful situations and excessive physical activity during the collection period.

Interfering factors

• Caffeine, insulin, nitroglycerin, aminophylline, ethanol, sympathomimetics, methyldopa, tricyclic antidepressants, chloral hydrate, quinidine, quinine, tetracycline, B-complex vitamins, isoproterenol, levodopa, and monoamine oxidase inhibitors may raise urine catecholamine levels.

• Clonidine, guanethidine, reserpine, and iodine-containing contrast media may suppress the levels of urine catecholamines.

• Phenothiazines, erythromycin, and methenamine compounds may raise or suppress levels.

• Failure to comply with drug restrictions, to collect all urine during the test period, or to store the specimen properly may alter test results.

• Excessive physical exercise or emotional stress raises catecholamine levels.

Copper

Purpose

• To help detect Wilson's disease

• To screen infants with family histories of Wilson's disease.

Normal results

Urinary excretion of copper is 15 to 60 mcg/24 hours.

Abnormal results

Increased urine copper levels:

 Usually indicate:

  Wilson's disease.

 May also occur in:

  Nephrotic syndromes

  Chronic active hepatitis

  Biliary cirrhosis

  Rheumatoid arthritis.

The basics

This test measures the urine level of copper, an essential trace element and a component of several metalloenzymes and proteins necessary for hemoglobin synthesis and oxidation reaction. Urine normally contains only a small amount of free copper; only trace amounts of free copper exist in plasma. Most copper in plasma is bound to and transported by an alpha$_2$-globulin (plasma protein) called ceruloplasmin. When copper is unbound, the ions can inhibit many enzyme reactions, resulting in copper toxicity.

Determination of urine copper levels is frequently used to detect Wilson's disease, a rare, inborn metabolic error, most common among persons of eastern European Jewish, southern Italian, or Sicilian ancestry. Wilson's disease is marked by decreased ceruloplasmin, increased urinary excretion of copper, and accumulation of copper in the interstitial tissues of the liver and brain. The cause of this disorder is unclear. Early detection and treatment (low-copper diet and D-penicillamine) are vital to prevent irreversible changes, such as nerve tissue degeneration and cirrhosis of the liver.

Procedure
Collect a 24-hour urine specimen. (See "Timed collection," pp. xviii and xix.)

Patient care checklist
Before the test
☑ Explain or clarify test purpose and procedure.
☑ Evaluate patient understanding.

Interfering factors
• Failure to collect all urine during the test period may alter test results.
• Administration of D-penicillamine—rarely given before diagnosis—causes elevated urine levels of copper.

Copper reduction test
[Clinitest tablet test]

Purpose
• To detect mellituria
• To monitor urine glucose levels during insulin therapy, after determination that the sugar in the urine is glucose.

Normal results
No glucose in urine.

Abnormal results
Presence of glucose in urine:
  Usually indicates:
    Diabetes mellitus.
  Also occurs in:
    Adrenal disorders
    Thyroid disorders
    Hepatic disease
    Central nervous system disease
    Fanconi's syndrome

Conditions involving low renal threshold
Toxic renal tubular disease
Heavy metal poisoning
Glomerulonephritis
Nephrosis
Pregnancy.
  Occurs with administration of:
    Hyperalimentation
    Large amounts of glucose
    Asparaginase
    Corticosteroids
    Carbamazepine
    Ammonium chloride
    Thiazide diuretics
    Dextrothyroxine
    Large amounts of nicotinic acid
    Lithium carbonate
    Long-term phenothiazines.

The basics
The copper reduction test measures the concentration of reducing substances in the urine through the reaction of those substances with a commercially prepared tablet—Clinitest. Clinitest, which reacts to glucose and to other reducing substances (mostly sugars), has almost replaced Benedict's test. This test is most valuable for providing the diabetic patient with a simple, at-home method of monitoring urine glucose level. (See *Home Tests,* pp. 685 to 687.) However, it is sometimes used as a rapid laboratory screening tool.

Procedure
Collect a second-voided urine specimen. First, ask the patient to void; then give him a drink of water. About 30 minutes later, ask him to give another specimen. Test this second-voided specimen, according to the five-drop Clinitest tablet test.
Five-drop Clinitest tablet test:
• Pour one Clinitest tablet from the bottle into the lid. Do not touch the tablet.
• Hold the medicine dropper vertically, and instill five drops of urine from the specimen container into the test tube. Be sure all five drops reach

the bottom of the test tube to be tested.

• Flush the dropper with water to rinse it, then add 10 drops of water to the test tube.

• Hold the test tube at the top and add one Clinitest tablet.

• Observe the color change, especially during effervescence—the "pass-through" phase. (See *"Pass-Through" Phenomenon*.)

• Wait 15 seconds after effervescence subsides, and gently agitate the test tube. If color develops at the 15-second interval, read the color against the Clinitest color chart, and record the results. Ignore any changes that develop after 15 seconds. If rapid color changes occur in the pass-through phase of the five-drop test, record the results as over 2% without comparison to the color chart. Or, perform a two-drop Clinitest tablet test.

Two-drop Clinitest tablet test:
This test is performed when rapid color changes occur in the pass-through phase of the five-drop test. Follow the procedure for the five-drop test, but use only two drops of urine.

Special precautions
CLINICAL ALERT: **Do not handle the Clinitest tablets, since sodium hydroxide and moisture produce caustic burns. Wash your hands immediately if contact is made, and avoid touching your eyes.**

• Store tablets in a well-marked, child-proof bottle to avoid accidental ingestion.

• Do not use discolored (dark blue) tablets. The normal color of fresh tablets is light blue, with darker blue flecks.

CLINICAL ALERT: **During effervescence, hold the test tube near the top to avoid burning your hands; it becomes boiling hot.**

Patient care checklist
Before the test
☑ Explain or clarify test purpose and procedure.
☑ Instruct patient on how to obtain a second-voided urine specimen.
☑ Evaluate patient understanding.
After the test
☑ Teach the newly diagnosed diabetic how to perform this test.
☑ Evaluate return demonstration.

Interfering factors
• Presence of reducing substances other than glucose may alter test results. (See *Reducing Substances that Give False-Positive Results*.) Use a glucose-oxidase test instead.

• Failure to use freshly voided urine or to flush urine residue from the medicine dropper may alter test results.

"Pass-Through" Phenomenon

Color changes during the boiling or effervescent stage are important. If the color of the specimen in the five-drop test goes from blue-green to green to olive to orange to brick red to green-brown, do not compare the color of the specimen with the reference chart: the glucose concentration is 4+ (2 g/dl or more). Proceed with the two-drop test. Similar results with the two-drop test mean glycosuria greater than 10 g/dl.

**Negative
(Blue-green)**
↓
**¼%
(Green)**
↓
**½%
(Olive)**
↓
**¾%
(Brown-green)**
↓
**1%
(Tan)**
↓
**2%
(Green-brown)**

Acute or chronic glomerulonephritis
Polycystic kidney disease.

Reducing Substances that Give False-Positive Results

Aminosalicylic acid	Levodopa
Ascorbic acid	Maltose
Cephalosporins	Metolazone
Chloral hydrate	Nalidixic acid
Chloramphenicol	Nitrofurantoin
Creatinine	Penicillin G
Cysteine	Pentoses
Fructose	Probenecid
Galactose	Salicylates
Isoniazid	Streptomycin
Ketone bodies	Tetracycline
Lactose	Uric acid

• Failure to detect the pass-through phenomenon or to use the correct reference chart for color comparison of the specimen may alter test results.
• Failure to use whole or fresh Clinitest tablets or to keep the tablet container tightly closed to prevent absorption of light or moisture may alter test results.

Creatinine

Purpose
• To help assess glomerular filtration
• To check the accuracy of 24-hour urine collection, based on the relatively constant levels of creatinine excretion.

Normal results
Urine creatinine levels range from 1 to 1.9 g/24 hours for men, and from 0.8 to 1.7 g/24 hours for women.

Abnormal results
Decreased urine creatinine levels:
Conditions causing impaired renal perfusion, such as shock
Renal disease due to urinary tract obstruction
Chronic bilateral pyelonephritis

The basics
This test measures urine levels of creatinine, the chief metabolite of creatine. Produced in amounts proportional to total body muscle mass, creatinine is removed from the plasma primarily by glomerular filtration and is excreted in the urine. Since the body does not recycle it, creatinine has a relatively high, constant clearance rate, making it an efficient indicator of renal function. However, the creatinine clearance test, which measures both urine and plasma creatinine clearance, is a more precise index than this test. A standard method for determining urine creatinine levels is based on the Jaffé reaction, in which creatinine treated with an alkaline picrate solution yields a bright orange-red complex.

Procedure
Collect a 24-hour urine specimen in a specimen bottle that contains a preservative to prevent the degradation of creatinine. (See "Timed collection," pp. xviii and xix.)

Special precautions
Refrigerate the specimen or keep it on ice during the collection period. When the collection is completed, send the specimen to the laboratory immediately.

Patient care checklist
Before the test
☑ Explain or clarify test purpose, preparation, and procedure.
☑ Evaluate patient understanding.
☑ Instruct the patient not to eat an excessive amount of meat before the test.
☑ Instruct the patient to avoid strenuous physical exercise during the collection period.

Interfering factors
• Drugs that may affect urine creatinine levels include corticosteroids, gentamicin, tetracyclines, diuretics, and amphotericin B.
• Failure to observe pretest restrictions may interfere with accurate determination of test results.
• Failure to collect all urine during the test period may alter test results.
• Failure to store the specimen properly may alter test results.

Creatinine clearance

Purpose
• To assess renal function (primarily glomerular filtration)
• To monitor progression of renal insufficiency.

Normal results
For men (age 20), creatinine clearance is 90 ml/minute/1.73 m^2 of body surface; for women (age 20), 84 ml/minute/1.73 m^2. For older patients, concentrations normally decrease by 6 ml/minute/decade.

Abnormal results
Decreased creatinine clearance levels:
Conditions causing reduced renal blood flow, such as shock, congestive heart failure, severe dehydration, renal artery obstruction
Acute tubular necrosis
Acute or chronic glomerulonephritis
Advanced bilateral chronic pyelonephritis
Advanced bilateral renal lesions, as in polycystic kidney disease, renal tuberculosis, and malignancy
Nephrosclerosis.

The basics
Creatinine, an anhydride of creatine, is formed and excreted in constant amounts by an irreversible reaction, and functions solely as the main end product of creatine. Creatinine production is proportional to total muscle mass and is relatively unaffected by normal physical activity, diet, or urine volume.

An excellent diagnostic indicator of renal function, the creatinine clearance test determines how efficiently the kidneys are clearing creatinine from the blood. The rate of clearance is expressed in terms of the volume of blood (in ml) that can be cleared of creatinine in 1 minute. Creatinine levels become abnormal when more than 50% of the total nephron units have been damaged. High creatinine clearance rates generally have little diagnostic significance.

Procedure
• Collect a timed urine specimen over 2, 6, 12, or 24 hours in a bottle containing a preservative to prevent degradation of the creatinine. (See "Timed collection," pp. xviii and xix.)
• Perform a venipuncture any time during the collection period, and collect the sample in a 7-ml, red-top tube.

Special precautions
Refrigerate the urine specimen or keep it on ice during the collection period.

Patient care checklist
Before the test
☑ Explain or clarify test purpose, preparation, and procedure.
☑ Evaluate patient understanding.
☑ Instruct the patient not to eat an excessive amount of red meat before the test.
☑ Instruct the patient to avoid strenuous physical exercise during the collection period.

Interfering factors
• Drugs that may affect creatinine clearance include amphotericin B, thiazide diuretics, furosemide, and aminoglycosides.
• A high-protein diet before the test and strenuous physical exercise during

the collection period may increase creatinine excretion.
• Failure to observe pretest restrictions may alter test results.
• Failure to collect all urine during the test period may interfere with accurate determination of test results.
• Failure to store the specimen properly may alter test results.

Cyclic adenosine monophosphate (cAMP)

Purpose
To aid in differential diagnosis of pseudohypoparathyroidism and hypoparathyroidism.

Results
A ten- to twentyfold increase (3.6 to 4 micromoles) in cAMP demonstrates a normal response or hypoparathyroidism. Failure to respond to parathyroid hormone, indicated by normal urinary excretion of cAMP, suggests Type I pseudohypoparathyroidism.

The basics
Formed from adenosine triphosphate by the action of the enzyme adenylate cyclase, the nucleotide cAMP influences the protein synthesis rate within cells. As the messenger for parathyroid hormone, cAMP helps distinguish pseudohypoparathyroidism and hypoparathyroidism. In the patient with the latter and in a healthy person, urine cAMP rises minutes after a parathyroid hormone dose. But it fails to rise in pseudohypoparathyroidism, in which the glands produce sufficient or excessive hormone, but normal end organ response to it is blocked. Pseudohypoparathyroidism is a rare inherited disorder resulting from tissue resistance to parathyroid hormone, and produces hypocalcemia, hyperphosphatemia, and skeletal and constitutional abnormalities.
This test is contraindicated in patients with high calcium levels (since para-

thyroid hormone further raises calcium levels). It should be performed cautiously in patients receiving digitalis and in those with sarcoidosis or renal or cardiac disease.

Procedure
• Instruct the patient to empty his bladder. If the patient has an indwelling (Foley) catheter in place, change the collection bag. If ordered, send this specimen to the laboratory; otherwise, discard it.
• Prepare the parathyroid hormone for infusion, as directed, using sterile water for dilution.
• Start the I.V. with 5% dextrose in water, and infuse the parathyroid hormone over 15 minutes. Record the start of the I.V. as time zero.
• Collect a urine specimen 3 to 4 hours after infusion, in a container to which hydrochloric acid has been added as a preservative. (See "Timed collection," pp. xviii and xix.)

Special precautions
• If transport of the specimen to the laboratory is delayed, refrigerate the specimen. If the patient has a catheter in place, keep the collection bag on ice.
CLINICAL ALERT: **Before the infusion begins, perform a skin test to detect a possible allergy to parathyroid hormone; keep epinephrine readily available in case of an adverse reaction.**

Patient care checklist
Before the test
☑ Explain or clarify test purpose and procedure.
☑ Evaluate patient understanding.
After the test
CLINICAL ALERT: **Observe the patient for symptoms of hypercalcemia: lethargy, anorexia, nausea, vomiting, vertigo, and abdominal cramps.**

Interfering factors

• Contamination of the specimen may interfere with accurate determination of test results.

• Improper storage of the specimen may alter test results.

• Failure to acidify the urine with hydrochloric acid may alter test results.

Delta-aminolevulinic acid
(ALA)

Purpose

• To screen for lead poisoning

• To aid in diagnosis of porphyrias and certain hepatic disorders, such as hepatitis and hepatic carcinoma.

Normal results

Urine ALA values range from 1.5 to 7.5 mg/dl/24 hours.

Abnormal results

Increased urine ALA levels:
  Lead poisoning
  Acute porphyria
  Hepatic carcinoma
  Hepatitis.

The basics

Using the colorimetric technique, this quantitative analysis of urine ALA levels helps diagnose porphyrias, hepatic disease, and lead poisoning. (In an emergency, a simple qualitative screening test can be performed.) ALA, the basic precursor of the porphyrins, normally converts to porphobilinogen through the action of the enzyme ALA-dehydrase during heme synthesis. Impaired conversion, as in porphyrias and lead poisoning, causes urine ALA levels to rise before other chemical or hematologic changes occur.

Procedure

Collect a 24-hour urine specimen in a light-resistant bottle containing a preservative (usually glacial acetic acid) to prevent degradation of ALA. (See "Timed collection," pp. xviii and xix.)

Special precautions

• Refrigerate the specimen or keep it on ice during the collection period. When the collection is completed, send the specimen to the laboratory immediately.

• Protect the specimen from direct sunlight. If the patient has an indwelling (Foley) catheter in place, insert the drainage bag into a dark plastic bag.

Patient care checklist

Before the test

☑ Explain or clarify test purpose and procedure.

☑ Evaluate patient understanding.

Interfering factors

• Barbiturates and griseofulvin cause porphyrins to accumulate in the liver and thus raise urine ALA levels. Vitamin E in pharmacologic doses may lower urine ALA levels.

• Failure to observe medication restrictions, if ordered, may interfere with accurate determination of test results.

• Failure to collect all urine during the test period may alter test results.

• Failure to store the specimen properly may alter test results.

D-xylose absorption test

Purpose

• To aid in differential diagnosis of malabsorption

• To determine the cause of malabsorption syndrome.

Normal results

For children: blood concentration, greater than 30 mg/dl in 1 hour; urine, 16% to 33% of ingested D-xylose excreted in 5 hours.

For adults under age 65: blood concentration, 25 to 40 mg/dl in 2 hours; urine, more than 4 g in 5 hours.

For adults aged 65 and older: blood concentration, 25 to 40 mg/dl in 2 hours; urine, more than 3.5 g excreted in 5 hours and more than 5 g excreted in 24 hours.

Abnormal results
Decreased blood and urine D-xylose levels:
  Sprue
  Celiac disease
  Enteritis involving jejunum
  Whipple's disease
  Multiple jejunal diverticula
  Myxedema
  Diabetic neuropathic diarrhea
  Rheumatoid arthritis
  Alcoholism
  Severe congestive heart failure
  Ascites.

The basics
One of the most important tests for malabsorption, D-xylose absorption evaluates patients with symptoms of malabsorption, such as weight loss and generalized malnutrition, weakness, and diarrhea. In this test, the patient ingests a standard dose of D-xylose—a pentose sugar that is absorbed in the small intestine without the aid of pancreatic enzymes, passed through the liver without being metabolized, and excreted in the urine. Because of its absorption in the small intestine without digestion, measurement of D-xylose in the urine and blood indicates the absorptive capacity of the small intestine. Patients may experience abdominal discomfort or diarrhea after D-xylose ingestion. Normally, blood levels of D-xylose peak 2 hours after ingestion, and 80% to 95% of the dose is excreted in 5 hours; the remaining dose, in 24 hours. Patients aged 65 and older, or those with borderline or elevated creatinine levels, tend to have low 5-hour urine levels but normal 24-hour levels.

Procedure
• Perform a venipuncture to obtain a fasting blood sample, and collect the sample in a 10-ml, red-top tube.
• Collect a first-voided morning urine specimen. Label this specimen, and send it to the laboratory immediately to serve as a baseline.
• Give the patient 25 g of D-xylose dissolved in 8 oz (240 ml) of water, followed by an additional 8 oz (240 ml) of water. If the patient is a child, administer 0.5 g D-xylose/lb of body weight, up to 25 g. Record the time of D-xylose ingestion.
• In an adult, draw a blood sample 2 hours after D-xylose ingestion; in a child, 1 hour after. Collect the sample in a 10-ml red-top tube (or a 10-ml gray-top tube if the sample will not be tested immediately). Occasionally, a 5-hour sample may be drawn to support the findings of the 1- or 2-hour sample.
• Collect and pool all urine during the 5 or 24 hours following D-xylose ingestion, as ordered. (See "Timed collection," pp. xviii and xix.)
• Maintain bed rest and withhold food and fluids (other than administration of D-xylose) throughout the test period.

Special precautions
Be sure to collect all urine and to refrigerate the specimen during the collection period.

Patient care checklist
Before the test
☑ Explain or clarify test purpose and procedure.
☑ Evaluate patient understanding.

Interfering factors
• Failure to adhere to restrictions of diet and activity affects absorption of D-xylose.
• Aspirin decreases D-xylose excretion by the kidneys.
• Indomethacin depresses intestinal absorption.
• Failure to obtain a complete urine specimen may alter test results.

• Failure to collect blood samples at designated times may alter test results.
• Intestinal overgrowth of bacteria or renal retention or insufficiency may cause depressed urine levels.

Free cortisol

Purpose
To aid in diagnosis of Cushing's syndrome.

Normal results
Free cortisol values range from 24 to 108 mcg/24 hours.

Abnormal results
Increased urine free cortisol levels:
  Cushing's syndrome due to adrenal hyperplasia, or adrenal or pituitary tumor
  Ectopic adrenocorticotropic hormone (ACTH) production.

The basics
Used as a screen for adrenocortical hyperfunction, this test measures urine levels of the portion of cortisol not bound to the corticosteroid-binding globulin transcortin. It is one of the best diagnostic tools for detecting Cushing's syndrome. The major glucocorticoid secreted by the adrenal cortex in response to ACTH stimulation, cortisol helps regulate fat, carbohydrate, and protein metabolism; it also helps promote glyconeogenesis, anti-inflammatory response, and cellular permeability. Only about 10% of this hormone is unbound and physiologically active; this small portion is known as free cortisol. Urine cortisol concentrations increase significantly when the amount secreted exceeds the binding capacity of transcortin, which is normally almost saturated.

Radioimmunoassay determinations of free cortisol levels in a 24-hour urine specimen—unlike a single measurement of plasma cortisol—reflect overall secretion levels instead of diurnal variations. Concurrent measurements of plasma cortisol and ACTH, with urine 17-hydroxycorticosteroids and the dexamethasone suppression test, may be used to confirm diagnosis.

Hepatic disease and obesity, which can raise plasma cortisol levels, generally do not appreciably raise urine levels of free cortisol. Low levels have little diagnostic significance and do not necessarily indicate adrenocortical hypofunction.

Procedure
Collect a 24-hour urine specimen in a bottle containing a preservative to keep the specimen at a pH of 4.0 to 4.5. (See "Timed collection," pp. xviii and xix.)

Special precautions
Refrigerate the specimen or place it on ice during the collection period.

Patient care checklist
Before the test
☑ Explain or clarify test purpose and procedure.
☑ Evaluate patient understanding.
☑ Instruct the patient to avoid stressful situations and excessive physical activity during the collection period.

Interfering factors
• Prolonged steroid therapy and drugs such as reserpine, phenothiazines, morphine, and amphetamines may elevate free cortisol levels.
• Failure to collect all urine during the test period may interfere with accurate determination of test results.
• Failure to store the specimen properly may alter test results.

Glucose oxidase test

Purpose
• To detect glycosuria
• To monitor urine glucose levels during insulin therapy.

Normal results
No glucose is present in urine.

Abnormal results
Presence of glucose in urine:
  Usually indicates:
    Diabetes mellitus.
  Also occurs in:
    Adrenal disorders
    Thyroid disorders
    Hepatic disease
    Central nervous system disease
    Fanconi's syndrome
    Conditions involving low renal
      threshold
    Toxic renal tubular disease
    Heavy metal poisoning
    Glomerulonephritis
    Nephrosis
    Pregnancy.
  Occurs with administration of:
    Hyperalimentation
    Large amounts of glucose
    Asparaginase
    Corticosteroids
    Carbamazepine
    Ammonium chloride
    Thiazide diuretics
    Dextrothyroxine
    Large amounts of nicotinic acid
    Lithium carbonate
    Phenothiazines (long-term).

The basics
The glucose oxidase test—which involves the use of commercial, plastic-coated reagent strips (Clinistix, Diastix) or Tes-Tape—is a specific, qualitative test for glycosuria. Although indicated in routine urinalysis, the test is used primarily to monitor urine glucose in patients with diabetes. Because of this test's simplicity and convenience, patients can perform it at home. There is no standardization in how results are recorded, so it is necessary to note the type of test used along with the results. (Also see *Home Tests,* pp. 685 to 687.)

Procedure
Collect a second-voided urine specimen: First ask the patient to void; then give him a drink of water. About 30 minutes later, ask him to give another specimen. Test this second-voided specimen according to one of the following procedures:
Clinistix test:
• Dip the test area of the reagent strip in the specimen for 2 seconds. Remove excess urine by tapping the strip against a clean surface or the side of the container, and begin timing.
• Hold the strip in the air, and "read" the color *exactly 10 seconds* after taking the strip out of the urine by comparing it with the reference color blocks on the label of the container.
• Record the results and the type of test used. Ignore color changes that develop after 10 seconds.
Diastix test:
• Dip the reagent strip in the specimen for 2 seconds. Remove excess urine by tapping the strip against the container, and begin timing.
• Hold the strip in the air, and compare the color to the color chart *exactly 30 seconds* after taking the strip out of the urine. Ignore color changes that develop after 30 seconds.
• Record the results and the type of test used.
Tes-Tape:
• Withdraw about 1½″ (3.8 cm) of the reagent tape from the dispenser.
• Dip ¼″ (0.6 cm) in the specimen for 2 seconds. Remove excess urine by tapping the strip against the side of the container, and begin timing.
• Hold the tape in the air, and compare the color of the darkest part of the tape to the color chart *exactly 60 seconds* after taking the strip out of the urine. If the tape indicates 0.5% or higher, wait an additional 60 seconds to make the final color comparison.
• Record the results and the type of test used.

Special precautions
• Keep the test strip container tightly closed to prevent deterioration of strips by exposure to light or moisture. Store

it in a cool place (under 86° F. [30° C.]) to avoid heat degradation.

• Do not use discolored or darkened Clinistix or Diastix, or dark yellow or yellow-brown Tes-Tape.

Patient care checklist

Before the test

☑ Explain or clarify test purpose and procedure.

☑ Instruct the patient on how to obtain a second-voided urine specimen.

☑ Evaluate patient understanding.

CLINICAL ALERT: Check to see if the patient is receiving levodopa, ascorbic acid, phenazopyridine, salicylates, or hypochlorites. If so, use Clinitest tablets instead.

After the test

☑ Teach the newly diagnosed diabetic how to perform this test.

☑ Evaluate return demonstration.

Interfering factors

• Dilute, stale urine may interfere with accurate determination of test results.

• Bacterial contamination of the specimen may alter test results.

• Reducing substances such as levodopa, ascorbic acid, phenazopyridine, methyldopa, tetracyclines, or salicylates may cause false-negative results.

• Using reagent strips after the expiration date may alter test results.

• Failure to keep the reagent strip container tightly closed may alter test results.

• Failure to record the reagent strip method used may adversely affect test results.

Hemoglobin

Purpose

To aid in diagnosis of hemolytic anemias or severe intravascular hemolysis from a transfusion reaction.

Normal results

Hemoglobin is not present in the urine.

Abnormal results

Hemoglobinuria may result from:

Severe intravascular hemolysis caused by a blood transfusion reaction, burns, or a crushing injury

Acquired hemolytic anemia caused by chemical or drug intoxication or malaria

Hemolytic anemia known as paroxysmal nocturnal hemoglobinuria

Congenital hemolytic anemias

Renal epithelial damage caused by acute glomerulonephritis or pyelonephritis

Renal tumor

Tuberculosis.

Hemoglobinuria is less commonly associated with:

Cystitis

Ureteral calculi

Urethritis.

The basics

Contained within red blood cells (RBCs), hemoglobin consists of heme—an iron-protoporphyrin complex—and globin—a polypeptide. Hemoglobin combines with oxygen and carbon dioxide to allow RBCs to transmit these gases between the lungs and the tissues. Aging RBCs are constantly being destroyed by normal mechanisms within the reticuloendothelial system. However, when RBC destruction occurs within the circulation, as in intravascular hemolysis, free hemoglobin enters the plasma and binds with haptoglobin, a plasma $alpha_2$-globulin. If the plasma level of hemoglobin exceeds that of haptoglobin, the excess of unbound hemoglobin is excreted in the urine (hemoglobinuria).

This test is based on the fact that heme proteins act like enzymes that catalyze oxidation of organic substances, such as guaiac or orthotoluidine. This reaction produces a blue coloration; the intensity of color varies with the amount of hemoglobin present. Microscopic examination is required to identify intact RBCs in urine (hematuria), which can occur in the presence of unbound hemoglobin. If the female patient is menstruating, reschedule the test.

Procedure
Collect a random urine specimen.

Patient care checklist
Before the test
☑ Explain or clarify test purpose and procedure.
☑ Evaluate patient understanding.

Interfering factors
• Lysis of RBCs in stale or alkaline urine may adversely affect test results.
• Contamination of the specimen with menstrual blood may alter test results.
• Bacterial peroxidases in highly infected specimens can produce false-positive test results.
• Large doses of vitamin C or of drugs that contain vitamin C as a preservative (such as certain antibiotics) can inhibit reagent activity, producing false-negative results.
• Nephrotoxic drugs (such as amphotericin B) or anticoagulants (such as warfarin) may cause a positive result for hemoglobinuria or hematuria.

Hemosiderin

Purpose
To aid in diagnosis of hemochromatosis.

Normal results
Hemosiderin is not found in urine.

Abnormal results
The presence of hemosiderin:
  Usually indicates:
    Hemochromatosis.
  May also suggest:
    Pernicious anemia
    Chronic hemolytic anemia
    Multiple blood transfusions
    Paroxysmal nocturnal hemoglobinuria.

The basics
This test measures the urine level of hemosiderin, a colloidal iron oxide and one of the two forms of storage iron deposited in body tissue. When iron storage mechanisms fail to manage iron overload, excess iron may escape to cells unaccustomed to high iron concentrations and may produce toxic effects. Particularly vulnerable to such toxicity are the liver, myocardium, bone marrow, pancreas, kidneys, and skin, which tend to develop tissue damage known as hemochromatosis. This disorder may occur in a rare hereditary form known as primary hemochromatosis, and in exogenous forms. Liver or bone marrow biopsy is necessary for confirmation of primary hemochromatosis. Elevated tissue storage of iron without associated tissue damage is called hemosiderosis and is often confused with hemochromatosis.

Procedure
Collect a random urine specimen of approximately 30 ml.

Patient care checklist
Before the test
☑ Explain or clarify test purpose and procedure.
☑ Evaluate patient understanding.

Interfering factors
Failure to send the specimen to the laboratory immediately may alter test results.

Homovanillic acid
(HVA)

Purpose
• To aid in diagnosis of neuroblastoma and ganglioneuroma
• To rule out pheochromocytoma.

Normal results
Urine HVA value for adults is less than 8 mg/24 hours. In children, the range

of normal urine HVA values (mcg/mg creatinine) varies with age:

Age (years)	HVA
15 to 17	0.5 to 2
10 to 15	0.25 to 12
5 to 10	0.5 to 9
2 to 5	0.5 to 13.5
1 to 2	4 to 23
0 to 1	1.2 to 35

Abnormal results
Increased urine HVA levels suggest:
  Neuroblastoma
  Ganglioneuroma.

The basics
This test is a quantitative analysis of urine levels of HVA, which is a metabolite of dopamine, one of the three major catecholamines. Synthesized primarily in the brain, dopamine is a precursor to epinephrine and norepinephrine, the other principal catecholamines. The liver breaks down most dopamine into HVA, for eventual excretion; a minimal amount of dopamine appears in the urine.

Using two-dimensional chromatography, urine HVA levels are usually measured simultaneously with the major catecholamines and other catecholamine metabolites—metanephrine, normetanephrine, and vanillylmandelic acid. The principal indication for this test is suspected neuroblastoma or ganglioneuroma, which usually affects children and adolescents. HVA levels do not usually rise in patients with pheochromocytoma because this tumor secretes mainly epinephrine, which metabolizes primarily into vanillylmandelic acid. Thus, an abnormally high urine HVA level generally rules out pheochromocytoma.

Procedure
Collect a 24-hour urine specimen in a bottle containing a preservative, to keep the specimen at a pH of 2.0 to 4.0. (See "Timed collection," pp. xviii and xix.)

Special precautions
Refrigerate the specimen or keep it on ice during the collection period.

Patient care checklist
Before the test
☑ Explain or clarify test purpose and procedure.
☑ Evaluate patient understanding.
☑ Instruct the patient to avoid stressful situations and excessive physical exercise during the collection period.

Interfering factors
• Monoamine oxidase inhibitors decrease urine HVA levels by inhibiting dopamine metabolism.
• Aspirin, methocarbamol, and levodopa may raise or lower HVA levels.
• Failure to observe drug restrictions, if ordered, may alter test results.
• Failure to collect all urine during the test period may alter test results.
• Failure to store the specimen properly may adversely affect test results.
• Excessive physical exercise or emotional stress during the collection period may raise HVA levels.

Human chorionic gonadotropin (hCG) [Pregnancy test]

Purpose
• To detect and confirm pregnancy
• To aid in diagnosis of hydatidiform mole or hCG-secreting tumors.

Normal results
In qualitative analysis, if agglutination fails to occur, test results are positive, indicating pregnancy. In quantitative analysis, urine hCG levels in the first trimester of a normal pregnancy may be as high as 500,000 IU/24 hours; in the second trimester, they range from 10,000 to 25,000 IU/24 hours; and in the third trimester, from 5,000 to 15,000 IU/24 hours. After delivery, hCG levels decline rapidly and within a few days are undetectable. Measur-

able hCG should not be found in the urine of males or nonpregnant females.

Abnormal results
Increased urine hCG levels during pregnancy may indicate:
  Multiple pregnancy
  Erythroblastosis fetalis.
Decreased hCG levels during pregnancy may indicate:
  Threatened abortion
  Ectopic pregnancy.
Measurable levels of hCG in males and nonpregnant females may indicate:
  Choriocarcinoma
  Ovarian or testicular tumors
  Melanoma
  Multiple myeloma
  Gastric, hepatic, pancreatic, or breast cancer.

The basics
As a qualitative analysis of urine levels of hCG, this test can detect pregnancy as early as 10 days after a missed menstrual period. Quantitative measurements can evaluate suspected hydatidiform mole or hCG-secreting tumors. After conception, placental trophoblastic cells start to produce hCG, a glycoprotein, which prevents degeneration of the corpus luteum at the end of the normal menstrual cycle. The corpus luteum then secretes large quantities of progesterone and estrogen, promoting early development of the endometrium, placenta, and fetus. During the first trimester, hCG levels rise steadily and rapidly, peaking around the 10th week of gestation, and subsequently tapering off to less than 10% of peak levels.

The most common method of evaluating hCG in urine is hemagglutination inhibition. This laboratory procedure, based on an antigen-antibody reaction, can provide both qualitative and quantitative information. The qualitative urine test is easier and less expensive than the serum hCG test (beta-subunit assay), so it is used

more frequently to detect pregnancy. (Also see *"Home Tests,"* p. 686.)

Procedure
• For verification of pregnancy (qualitative analysis), collect a first-voided morning urine specimen. If this is not possible, collect a random specimen.
• For quantitative analysis of hCG, collect a 24-hour urine specimen. (See "Timed collection," pp. xviii and xix.)
• Specify the date of the patient's last menstrual period on the laboratory slip.

Special precautions
Refrigerate the 24-hour specimen or keep it on ice during the collection period.

Patient care checklist
Before the test
☑ Explain or clarify test purpose and procedure.
☑ Evaluate patient understanding.

Interfering factors
• Gross proteinuria (in excess of 1 g/24 hours), hematuria, or an elevated erythrocyte sedimentation rate may produce false-positive results, depending on the laboratory method used.
• Early pregnancy, ectopic pregnancy, or threatened abortion may produce false-negative test results.
• Phenothiazines may cause false-negative or false-positive results.
• Tap water or soap in the specimen may produce false-positive results.

17-hydroxycorticosteroids
(17-OHCS)

Purpose
To assess adrenocortical function.

Normal results
Urine 17-OHCS values range from 4.5 to 12 mg/24 hours in males, and from 2.5 to 10 mg/24 hours in females.

Children aged 8 to 12 years normally excrete less than 4.5 mg/24 hours; younger children excrete less than 1.5 mg/24 hours. Levels normally increase slightly during the first trimester of pregnancy. Patients who are obese or very muscular may excrete slightly higher amounts of 17-OHCS because of increased cortisol catabolism.

Abnormal results
Increased urine 17-OHCS levels:
  May indicate:
    Cushing's syndrome
    Adrenal carcinoma or adenoma
    Pituitary tumor.
  May also occur in:
    Hyperthyroidism
    Severe hypertension
    Virilism
    Acute pancreatitis
    Eclampsia.
Decreased urine 17-OHCS levels may indicate:
    Addison's disease
    Hypopituitarism
    Myxedema.

The basics
This test measures urine levels of 17-OHCS, metabolites of the hormones that regulate glyconeogenesis. More than 80% of all urinary 17-OHCS are metabolites of cortisol, the primary adrenocortical steroid. Test findings thus reflect cortisol secretion and, indirectly, adrenocortical function. Since cortisol secretion varies diurnally and in response to stress and many other factors, urine 17-OHCS levels are most accurately determined from a 24-hour specimen. Column chromatography and spectrophotofluorometry with the Porter-Silber reagent are used to measure 17-OHCS levels. Levels of plasma cortisol, urine free cortisol, and urine 17-ketosteroids may be measured, and adrenocorticotropic hormone stimulation and suppression testing performed, to confirm results of this test.

Procedure
Collect a 24-hour urine specimen in a bottle containing a preservative to prevent deterioration of the specimen. (See "Timed collection," pp. xviii and xix.)

Special precautions
Refrigerate the specimen or place it on ice during the collection period.

Patient care checklist
Before the test
☑ Explain or clarify test purpose and procedure.
☑ Evaluate patient understanding.
☑ Instruct the patient to avoid stressful situations and excessive physical activity during the collection period.

Interfering factors
• Drugs such as the following may elevate urine 17-OHCS levels: meprobamate, phenothiazines, spironolactone, ascorbic acid, chloral hydrate, glutethimide, chlordiazepoxide, penicillin G, hydroxyzine, quinidine, quinine, iodides, and methenamine.
• Drugs such as the following may suppress levels: hydralazine, phenytoin, thiazide diuretics, ethinamate, nalidixic acid, and reserpine.
• Failure to follow drug restrictions, if ordered, may interfere with accurate determination of test results.
• Failure to collect all urine during the test period may alter test results.
• Failure to store the specimen properly may alter test results.

5-hydroxyindoleacetic acid
(5-HIAA)

Purpose
To aid in diagnosis of carcinoid tumors (argentaffinomas).

Normal results
Urine 5-HIAA values are less than 6 mg/24 hours.

Abnormal results

Marked increase in urine 5-HIAA levels, possibly as high as 200 to 600 mg/24 hours, indicates a carcinoid tumor. However, since these tumors vary in their capacity to store and secrete serotonin, some patients with carcinoid syndrome (metastatic carcinoid tumors) may not show elevated levels. Repeated testing is often necessary.

The basics

This quantitative analysis of urine levels of 5-HIAA is used mainly to screen for carcinoid tumors (argentaffinomas). Urine 5-HIAA levels reflect plasma concentrations of serotonin (5-hydroxytryptamine). This powerful vasopressor is produced by argentaffin cells, primarily in the intestinal mucosa, and is metabolized through oxidative deamination into 5-HIAA. Carcinoid tumors, found generally in the intestine or appendix, secrete an excessive amount of serotonin, which is reflected by high 5-HIAA levels. This test measures 5-HIAA levels by the colorimetric technique and is most accurately performed with a 24-hour urine specimen, which can detect small or intermittently secreting carcinoid tumors.

Procedure

Collect a 24-hour urine specimen in a bottle containing a preservative to keep the specimen at a pH of 2.0 to 4.0. (See "Timed collection," p. xviii.)

Special precautions

Refrigerate the specimen or keep it on ice during the collection period.

Patient care checklist
Before the test
☑ Explain or clarify test purpose and procedure.
☑ Evaluate patient understanding.
☑ Instruct the patient to avoid foods containing serotonin, such as bananas, plums, pineapples, avocados, eggplants, tomatoes, or walnuts, for 4 days before the test.

Interfering factors

● Melphalan, reserpine, and fluorouracil raise urine 5-HIAA levels.
● Ethanol, tricyclic antidepressants, monoamine oxidase inhibitors, methyldopa, and isoniazid characteristically suppress 5-HIAA levels.
● Methenamine compounds, phenothiazines, salicylates, guaifenesin, mephenesin, methocarbamol, and acetaminophen may raise or lower 5-HIAA levels.
● Failure to observe drug and dietary restrictions may interfere with accurate determination of test results.
● Failure to collect all urine during the test period may alter test results.
● Failure to store the specimen properly may alter test results.
● Severe gastrointestinal disturbance or diarrhea may adversely affect test results.

Hydroxyproline

Purpose
● To monitor treatment for disorders characterized by bone resorption, primarily Paget's disease
● To aid in diagnosis of disorders characterized by bone resorption.

Normal results

Values for adults are 14 to 45 mg/24 hours; or 0.4 to 5 mg/2-hour specimen (males) and 0.4 to 2.9 mg/2-hour specimen (females). Normal values for children are much higher and peak between ages 11 and 18. Values also rise during the third trimester of pregnancy, reflecting fetal skeletal growth.

Abnormal results
Increased urine hydroxyproline levels may indicate:
  Bone disease such as Paget's disease
  Metastatic bone tumors
  Endocrine disorders that stimulate hormonal secretion.

Decreased urine hydroxyproline levels are seen:

During therapy for bone resorption disorders.

The basics

This test measures total urine levels of hydroxyproline, an amino acid found mainly in collagen (a component of skin and bone). Urine hydroxyproline levels are a good index of bone matrix turnover, because levels increase when collagen breaks down during bone resorption. Bone matrix turnover and hydroxyproline levels normally rise in children during periods of rapid skeletal growth; however, they also rise in disorders that increase bone resorption. This test helps diagnose these disorders, but it is more commonly used to monitor response to drug therapy in conditions marked by rapid bone resorption.

Hydroxyproline levels are most often determined colorimetrically on a timed urine sample; they may also be determined by ion-exchange or gas-liquid chromatography. A collagen-restricted diet is essential for this test, because hydroxyproline levels reflect collagen intake. Free hydroxyproline, a small component of total hydroxyproline and a sensitive indicator of dietary collagen intake, may be measured to validate results.

Procedure

Collect a 2-hour or 24-hour urine specimen, as ordered, in a container that has a preservative to prevent degradation of hydroxyproline. (See "Timed collection," pp. xviii and xix.)

Special precautions

Refrigerate the specimen or keep it on ice during the collection period.

Patient care checklist

Before the test

☑ Explain or clarify test purpose and procedure.

☑ Evaluate patient understanding.

☑ Instruct the patient to adhere to a collagen-restricted diet for 24 hours before the test and during the test period by avoiding meat, fish, poultry, jelly, or any foods containing gelatin.

☑ Note the patient's age and sex on the laboratory slip.

Interfering factors

• Ascorbic acid, vitamin D, aspirin, and glucocorticoids, as well as calcitonin and mithramycin (used to treat Paget's disease), can decrease levels.

• Failure to observe dietary restrictions may alter test results.

• Failure to collect all urine during the test period may alter test results.

• Failure to store the specimen properly may adversely affect test results.

• Psoriasis and burns can promote collagen turnover, elevating urine hydroxyproline levels.

Inulin clearance

Purpose

• To measure glomerular filtration rate (GFR)

• To evaluate renal function.

Normal results

Clearance is normally 90 to 130 ml/minute for age 21 and older; 86 to 126 ml/minute for ages 11 to 20; and 82 to 122 ml/minute from birth to age 10. Clearance may decrease as much as 45% after age 70.

Abnormal results

Decreased inulin clearance is characteristic in:

Congestive heart failure

Decreased renal blood flow

Acute tubular necrosis

Acute and chronic glomerulonephritis

Advanced chronic bilateral pyelonephritis

Nephrosclerosis

Advanced bilateral renal lesions

Bilateral ureteral obstruction
Dehydration.

The basics

Inulin, a polysaccharide of fructose obtained from dahlias and artichokes, is metabolically inert within the body. When injected I.V., inulin is almost entirely filtered by the glomeruli but is reabsorbed by the tubules. Inulin clearance is, therefore, practically an exact measure of the GFR.

Despite its sensitivity and low incidence of adverse effects, the inulin clearance test is time-consuming, complex, and uncomfortable for the patient, and thus is infrequently performed. Less accurate tests, such as urea and creatinine clearance, are used instead. Iothalamate (^{125}I) can be substituted for inulin and usually follows the same procedure as inulin clearance. Because the iodine content is negligible, ^{125}I can be given to patients with iodine hypersensitivity but is contraindicated during pregnancy, lactation, and periods of growth.

Procedure

• Perform a venipuncture, and collect 10 ml of blood in a green-top (heparinized) tube, to be used as a control sample.
• Catheterize the patient. Make sure the bladder is empty, and save the urine for a baseline specimen.
• Start an I.V. using 250 ml of 5% dextrose in water.
• Infuse the recommended priming dose of 25 ml of 10% inulin by I.V. bolus over 4 minutes. Allow 30 minutes for distribution.
• Using an I.V. pump, infuse the maintenance solution of 500 ml of 1.5% inulin at a constant rate of 4 ml/minute.
• Collect a urine specimen 30 minutes after starting the I.V., and collect three additional specimens at 20-minute intervals thereafter. Clamp the catheter between collections.
• Draw a blood sample in a 10-ml, green-top (heparinized) tube at the midpoint of each 20-minute period and at the end of the test.
• Record the inulin dosage on the laboratory slip. Properly label each specimen, and include the collection time.

Special precautions

• Inulin clearance should be used cautiously in patients with cardiac disease, since increased fluid intake may cause congestive heart failure.
• Use the solution for I.V. bolus within 1 hour of preparation. Before administration, shake the ampul and heat it in boiling water to dissolve all crystals. Then, cool to body temperature.
• If the patient already has a catheter in place, do not use the urine in the drainage bag. Empty the bag, and clamp the catheter for 1 hour before obtaining a baseline specimen.
• Handle blood samples gently to prevent hemolysis, and send specimens to the laboratory immediately after each collection. If more than 10 minutes will elapse before transport, refrigerate the urine specimen.

Patient care checklist
Before the test
☑ Explain or clarify test purpose and procedure.
☑ Evaluate patient understanding.
☑ Instruct the patient to abstain from food for 4 hours before the test.
☑ Instruct the patient to abstain from exercise the morning of the test.
☑ Instruct the patient to drink 1 liter of water 1 hour before the test, and encourage him to drink during the test to maintain adequate urine flow.

Interfering factors

• Failure to infuse inulin at a constant rate.
• Failure to collect blood and urine specimens at the proper intervals.
• Failure to adhere to dietary and exercise restrictions.
• Hemolysis caused by rough handling of blood samples.

17-ketogenic steroids
(17-KGS)

Purpose
- To evaluate adrenocortical function
- To aid in diagnosis of Cushing's syndrome and Addison's disease.

Normal results
Urine 17-KGS levels range from 4 to 14 mg/24 hours in men, and from 2 to 12 mg/24 hours in women. Children aged 11 to 14 excrete 2 to 9 mg/24 hours; younger children and infants excrete 0.1 to 4 mg/24 hours.

Abnormal results
Increased urine 17-KGS levels:
   Cushing's syndrome
   Congenital adrenal hyperplasia
   Adrenal carcinoma or adenoma.
Decreased urine 17-KGS levels:
   Addison's disease.
   May reflect:
      Panhypopituitarism
      Cretinism
      General wasting.

The basics
Using spectrophotofluorometry, this test determines urine levels of 17-KGS, which consist of the 17-hydroxycorticosteroids—cortisol and its metabolites, for example—and other adrenocortical steroids, such as pregnanetriol, that can be oxidized in the laboratory to 17-ketosteroids. Because 17-KGS represent such a large group of steroids, this test provides an excellent overall assessment of adrenocortical function. For accurate diagnosis of specific disease, 17-KGS must be compared with results of other tests, including plasma adrenocorticotropic hormone (ACTH), plasma cortisol, ACTH stimulation, single-dose metyrapone, and dexamethasone suppression. Levels rise with severe physical or emotional stress.

Procedure
Collect a 24-hour urine specimen in a bottle containing a preservative to keep the specimen at a pH of 4.0 to 4.5. (See "Timed collection," p. xviii.)

Special precautions
Refrigerate the specimen or keep it on ice during the collection period.

Patient care checklist
Before the test
☑ Explain or clarify test purpose and procedure.
☑ Instruct the patient to avoid excessive physical exercise and stressful situations during the collection period.
☑ Evaluate patient understanding.

Interfering factors
- Urine 17-KGS levels may be elevated by ACTH therapy and by drugs such as meprobamate, phenothiazines, spironolactone, penicillin, oleandomycin, and hydralazine.
- Levels may be suppressed by estrogens, quinine, reserpine, and thiazides, as well as by long-term corticosteroid therapy.
- Nalidixic acid and dexamethasone may elevate or suppress urine 17-KGS levels.
- Failure to observe drug restrictions, if ordered, may adversely affect test results.
- Failure to collect all urine during the collection period may alter test results.
- Failure to store the specimen properly may alter test results.

Ketone test

Purpose
- To screen for ketonuria
- To identify diabetic ketoacidosis and carbohydrate deprivation
- To distinguish between a diabetic and a nondiabetic coma
- To monitor control of diabetes mellitus, ketogenic weight reduction, and treatment of diabetic ketoacidosis.

Normal results
No ketones are present in urine.

Abnormal results
Ketonuria is present in uncontrolled diabetes mellitus, starvation, and as a metabolic complication of hyperalimentation.

The basics
In this routine, semiquantitative screening test, which has largely replaced Rothera's and Gerhardt's tests, the action of urine on a commercially prepared product (Acetest tablet, Chemstrip K, Ketostix, or Keto-Diastix) measures the urine level of ketone bodies. Each product measures a specific ketone body; for example, Acetest measures acetone, while Ketostix measures acetoacetic acid. Urine determinations reflect serum concentration.

Excess amounts of ketone bodies (acetoacetic acid, acetone, and beta-hydroxybutyric acid)—the by-products of fat metabolism—follow carbohydrate deprivation, such as with starvation or diabetic ketoacidosis. (Also see *Home Tests,* pp. 685 to 687.)

Procedure
Collect a second-voided urine specimen: First ask the patient to void; then give him a drink of water. About 30 minutes later, ask him to give another specimen. Test this second-voided specimen according to one of the following procedures:
Acetest:
• Pour one tablet into the lid of the bottle, and then place the tablet on a piece of white paper.
• Place one drop of urine on the tablet.
• After 30 seconds, compare the tablet color (white, lavender, or purple) with the color chart, and record the results.
Ketostix:
• Dip the reagent stick into the specimen and remove it immediately.

• After 15 seconds, compare the stick color (buff or purple) with the color chart.
• Record the results as negative or as small, moderate, or large amounts of ketones.
Keto-Diastix:
(Urine glucose concentration is usually measured at the same time using this dipstick.)
• Dip the reagent stick into the specimen, and remove it immediately. Tap the edge of the stick against the container or a clean, dry surface to remove excess urine.
• Hold the stick horizontally to prevent mixing the chemicals from the two areas. Interpret each area of the stick separately.
• After exactly 15 seconds, compare the color of the ketone section (buff or purple) with the appropriate color chart.
• After 30 seconds, compare the color of the glucose section. Ignore color changes that occur after the specified waiting periods.
• Record the results as negative or as small, moderate, or large amounts of ketones.

Special precautions
• The specimen must be tested within 60 minutes after it is obtained, or it must be refrigerated. Allow refrigerated specimens to return to room temperature before testing.
• Do not use tablets or strips that have become discolored or darkened.

Patient care checklist
Before the test
☑ Explain or clarify test purpose and procedure.
☑ Instruct the patient on how to obtain a second-voided urine specimen.
☑ Evaluate patient understanding.
After the test
☑ Teach the newly diagnosed diabetic how to perform this test.
☑ Evaluate return demonstration.

Interfering factors
• Failure to keep the reagent container tightly closed to prevent absorption of light or moisture, or bacterial contamination of the specimen, causes false-negative results.
• Levodopa, phenazopyridine, and sulfobromophthalein produce false-positive test results when Ketostix or Keto-Diastix is used.

17-ketosteroids
(17-KS)

Purpose
• To aid in diagnosis of adrenal and gonadal dysfunction
• To aid in diagnosis of adrenogenital syndrome (congenital adrenal hyperplasia)
• To monitor cortisol therapy in the treatment of adrenogenital syndrome.

Normal results
Urine 17-KS values range from 6 to 21 mg/24 hours in men, and from 4 to 17 mg/24 hours in women. Children between the ages of 11 and 14 excrete 2 to 7 mg/24 hours; younger children and infants excrete 0.1 to 3 mg/24 hours. (See *17-Ketosteroid Fractionation Normal Test Values*, p. 243, for specific steroid values.)

Abnormal results
Increased urine 17-KS:
  May result from:
    Adrenal hyperplasia, carcinoma, or adenoma
    Adrenogenital syndrome.
  May indicate:
    Stein-Leventhal syndrome
    Lutein cell tumor of the ovary
    Androgenic arrhenoblastoma
    Interstitial cell tumor of the testes
Decreased urine 17-KS levels:
  May result from:
    Addison's disease
    Panhypopituitarism
    Eunuchoidism
    Castration.

May occur in:
  Cretinism
  Myxedema
  Nephrosis.

The basics
This test uses the spectrophotofluorometric technique to measure urine levels of 17-KS. Steroids and steroid metabolites characterized by a ketone group on carbon 17 in the steroid nucleus, 17-KS originate primarily in the adrenal glands but also in the testes, which produce one-third of 17-KS in males, and in the ovaries, which produce a minimal amount of 17-KS in females. Although not all 17-KS are androgens, they cause androgenic effects. For example, excessive secretion of 17-KS may result in hirsutism and may increase clitoral or phallic size; in utero, elevated 17-KS levels may cause a female fetus to develop a male urogenital tract. Because 17-KS do not include all of the androgens (testosterone, for example, the most potent androgen, is not a 17-KS), these levels provide only a rough estimate of androgenic activity. To provide additional information about androgen secretion, plasma testosterone levels may be measured concurrently; 17-KS fractionation may also be appropriate.

Characteristically, 17-KS levels rise during pregnancy, severe stress, chronic illness, or debilitating disease. When this test is used to monitor cortisol therapy for adrenogenital syndrome, 17-KS levels typically return to normal with adequate cortisol administration. If the female patient is menstruating, the urine collection may have to be postponed, since the presence of blood in the specimen interferes with test findings.

Procedure
Collect a 24-hour urine specimen in a bottle containing a preservative to keep the specimen at a pH of 4.0 to 4.5. (See "Timed collection," pp. xviii and xix.)

17-Ketosteroid Fractionation Normal Test Values

Steroid	Adult male	Adult female	Male (age 10 to 15)	Female (age 10 to 15)	Both sexes (age 0 to 9)
Androsterone	2.2 to 5	0.5 to 2.4	0.2 to 2	0.2 to 2.5	≤ 1
Dehydroepiandrosterone	0 to 2.3	0 to 1.2	< 0.4	< 0.4	< 0.2
Etiocholanolone	1.9 to 4.7	1.1 to 3	0.1 to 1.6	0.7 to 3	≤ 1
11-hydroxyandrosterone	0.5 to 1.3	0.2 to 0.6	0.1 to 1.1	0.2 to 1	≤ 1
11-hydroxyetiocholanolone	0.3 to 0.7	0.2 to 0.6	< 0.3	0.1 to 0.5	≤ 0.5
11-ketoandrosterone	0 to 0.1	0 to 0.2	< 0.1	< 0.1	< 0.1
11-ketoetiocholanolone	0.2 to 0.7	0.2 to 0.6	0.2 to 0.6	0.1 to 0.6	≤ 0.7
Pregnanediol	0.6 to 1.6	0.2 to 2.4	0.1 to 0.7	0.1 to 1.2	< 0.5
Pregnanetriol	0.6 to 1.3	0.1 to 1	0.2 to 0.6	0.1 to 0.6	< 0.3
5-pregnanetriol	0 to 0.3	0 to 0.3	< 0.3	< 0.3	< 0.2
11-ketopregnanetriol	0 to 0.2	0 to 0.4	< 0.3	< 0.2	< 0.2

Through gas-liquid chromatography, this fractionation test shows which specific steroids in the 17-ketosteroid (KS) group are elevated or suppressed, and thus aids differential diagnosis of conditions suggested by abnormal 17-KS levels.

Special precautions
Refrigerate the specimen or place it on ice during the collection period.

Patient care checklist
Before the test
☑ Explain or clarify test purpose and procedure.
☑ Instruct the patient to avoid excessive physical exercise and stressful situations during the collection period.
☑ Evaluate patient understanding.

Interfering factors
• Meprobamate, phenothiazines, spironolactone, and oleandomycin may elevate urine 17-KS levels.
• Estrogens, penicillin, ethacrynic acid, and phenytoin may suppress 17-KS levels.
• Nalidixic acid and quinine may elevate or suppress 17-KS levels.
• Failure to observe drug restrictions, if ordered, may adversely affect test results.
• Failure to collect all urine during the collection period may alter test results.

• Failure to store the specimen properly may alter test results.
• Contamination of the urine specimen by menses may interfere with test findings.

Lysozyme
[Muramidase]

Purpose
• To aid in diagnosis of acute monocytic or granulocytic leukemia, and to monitor the progression of these diseases
• To evaluate proximal tubular function and to diagnose renal impairment
• To detect rejection or infarction of kidney transplantation.

Normal results
Urine lysozyme values are less than 3 mg/24 hours.

Abnormal results
Increased urine lysozyme levels:
  Impaired renal proximal tubular reabsorption
  Acute pyelonephritis
  Nephrotic syndrome
  Tuberculosis of the kidney
  Severe extrarenal infection
  Rejection or infarction of kidney transplantation
  Polycythemia vera
  Acute onset or relapse of monocytic or myelomonocytic leukemia
  Acute onset or relapse of granulocytic leukemia.
Decreased urine lysozyme levels:
  Lymphocytic leukemia.

The basics
Lysozyme, a low-molecular-weight enzyme, is present in mucus, saliva, tears, skin secretions, and various internal body cells and fluids. This enzyme splits, or lyses, the cell walls of gram-positive bacteria and, with complement and other blood factors, acts to destroy them. Lysozyme seems to be synthesized in granulocytes and monocytes, and it first appears in serum after destruction of such cells. When serum lysozyme levels exceed three times normal, the enzyme appears in urine. However, since renal tissue also contains lysozyme, renal injury alone can cause measurable excretion of this enzyme.

This test measures urine lysozyme levels turbidimetrically. Serum lysozyme determinations, using the same method, confirm the results of urine testing. Test results should be available in 1 day. If the female patient is menstruating, the test may have to be rescheduled for a later date.

Procedure
Collect a 24-hour urine specimen. (See "Timed collection," pp. xviii and xix.)

Special precautions
Cover and refrigerate the specimen throughout the collection period. If the patient has an indwelling (Foley) catheter in place, keep the collection bag on ice.

Patient care checklist
Before the test
☑ Explain or clarify test purpose and procedure.
☑ Evaluate patient understanding.

Interfering factors
• The presence of bacteria in the specimen decreases urine lysozyme levels.
• The presence of blood or saliva in the specimen increases lysozyme levels.
• Failure to collect all urine during the test period may alter test results.

Magnesium

Purpose
• To rule out magnesium deficiency in patients with symptoms of central nervous system irritation
• To detect excessive urinary excretion of magnesium

• To help evaluate glomerular function in renal disease.

Normal results
Urinary excretion of magnesium is less than 150 mg/24 hours (atomic absorption).

Abnormal results
Increased urine magnesium levels may result from:
   Early chronic renal disease
   Adrenocortical insufficiency
   Chronic alcoholism
   Chronic ingestion of magnesium-containing antacids.
Decreased urine magnesium levels may result from:
   Malabsorption
   Acute or chronic diarrhea
   Diabetic acidosis
   Dehydration
   Advanced renal failure
   Primary aldosteronism
   Decreased dietary intake of magnesium.

The basics
This test measures the urine level of magnesium, an important cation absorbed in the intestinal tract and excreted in the urine. It is especially useful because magnesium deficiency is detectable in urine before it changes serum magnesium levels. Measurement of urine magnesium was rarely used in the past but is becoming more important, especially in large clinics, to rule out magnesium deficiency as the cause of neurologic symptoms and to help evaluate glomerular function in suspected renal disease.

Procedure
Collect a 24-hour urine specimen. (See "Timed collection," pp. xviii and xix.)

Patient care checklist
Before the test
☑ Explain or clarify test purpose and procedure.
☑ Evaluate patient understanding.

☑ If the patient is receiving magnesium-containing antacids, diuretics (for example, ethacrynic acid and spironolactone), or aldosterone, note this on the laboratory slip.

Interfering factors
• Failure to collect all urine during the test period may alter test results.
• Ethacrynic acid, thiazide diuretics, aldosterone, or excessive amounts of magnesium-containing antacids elevate urine magnesium levels.
• Spironolactone lowers urine magnesium levels.
• Increased calcium intake reduces urinary excretion of magnesium.

Melanin

Purpose
To aid in diagnosis of malignant melanomas.

Normal results
Urine does not contain melanogens or melanin.

Abnormal results
In the presence of a visible skin tumor, large quantities of melanin or melanogens in urine indicate advanced internal metastasis. Since malignant melanomas may also develop in internal organs, large quantities of melanin or melanogens in a urine specimen, in the absence of a visible skin tumor, indicate an internal melanoma.

The basics
This relatively rare test measures urine levels of melanin, the brown black pigment that colors the skin, hair, and eyes. An end product of tyrosine metabolism, melanin is normally elaborated by specialized cells called melanocytes. Cutaneous melanomas—malignant tumors that produce excessive amounts of melanin—develop most often around the head and neck, but may also originate in mu-

cous membranes (as in the rectum), the retinas, or the central nervous system, where melanocytes appear. Patients with these tumors may excrete melanin precursors—melanogens—in their urine. If the urine is left standing, exposure to air converts the melanogens to melanin in about 24 hours.

Thormählen's test uses sodium nitroprusside (nitroferricyanide) to detect melanogens or melanin in urine, based on characteristic color changes. More specific tests for melanin, such as chromatography, isolate and measure the pigment. Test results are generally available on the same day.

Procedure
Collect a random urine specimen.

Patient care checklist
Before the test
☑ Explain or clarify test purpose and procedure.
☑ Evaluate patient understanding.

Interfering factors
Failure to send the urine specimen to the laboratory immediately may alter test results.

Myoglobin

Purpose
• To aid in diagnosis of muscular disease
• To detect extensive infarction of muscle tissue
• To assess the extent of muscular damage from crushing trauma.

Normal results
Myoglobin does not appear in the urine.

Abnormal results
Myoglobinuria occurs in:
Acute or chronic muscular disease
Alcoholic polymyopathy
Familial myoglobinuria
Extensive myocardial infarction (MI).
Myoglobinuria results from:
Severe trauma to the skeletal muscles.
Transient myoglobinuria may follow:
Strenuous or prolonged exercise.

The basics
This test detects the presence of myoglobin—a red pigment found in the cytoplasm of cardiac and skeletal muscle cells—in the urine. Myoglobin probably serves as a reservoir of oxygen, facilitating its movement within muscle. When muscle cells are extensively damaged, as by disease or severe crushing trauma, myoglobin is released into the blood, quickly cleared by renal glomerular filtration, and eliminated in the urine (myoglobinuria). For example, myoglobin appears in the urine within 24 hours after MI. Because of the marked structural similarities of urine myoglobin and urine hemoglobin, they are not satisfactorily differentiated by qualitative assays.

The test method most commonly used to detect myoglobinuria is the differential precipitation test. Hemoglobin, bound to haptoglobin, precipitates when urine is mixed with ammonium sulfate. Myoglobin, however, remains soluble and can be measured. Test results are generally available in 1 day if the specimen is sent to the laboratory. (See *Bedside Testing for Urine Blood Pigments*, p. 247, if the specimen is not to be sent to the laboratory.)

Procedure
Collect a random urine specimen.

Patient care checklist
Before the test
☑ Explain or clarify test purpose and procedure.
☑ Evaluate patient understanding.

Interfering factors
• If this test is performed with reagent strips—Hemastix, for example—the

Bedside Testing for Urine Blood Pigments

To test a patient's urine for blood pigments at bedside, use one of the following methods:

Dipstick (Hemastix):
• Collect a urine specimen.
• Dip the stick into the specimen, and withdraw it.
• After 30 seconds, compare the stick with the color chart. Blue indicates a positive reaction; the intensity of color indicates pigment concentration.

Occult tablet:
• Collect a urine specimen.
• Put one drop of urine on the filter paper. Place the tablet on the urine, and then put two drops of water on the tablet.
• After 2 minutes, inspect the filter paper around the tablet. Blue indicates a positive reaction; the intensity of color indicates pigment concentration.

Occult solution:
• Collect a urine specimen.
• After placing one drop of urine on the filter paper, close the package and turn it over. Open the opposite side, and place two drops of solution on the filter paper.
• After 30 seconds, inspect the filter paper. Blue indicates a positive reaction; the intensity of color indicates pigment concentration.
   Because these methods detect only blood pigments, immunochemical studies are necessary to differentiate hemoglobin from other blood pigments, such as myoglobin.

Osmolality

Purpose
• To evaluate the diluting and concentrating ability of the kidneys
• To aid in differential diagnosis of the syndrome of inappropriate antidiuretic hormone (SIADH)
• To aid in differential diagnosis of polyuria
• To aid in differential diagnosis of oliguria.

Normal results
Range: 50 to 1,400 mOsm/kg.
Average: 300 to 800 mOsm/kg.

Abnormal results
Increased osmolality (concentrated urine):
   Intracellular dehydration
   Hypovolemia
   SIADH
   Emotional stress
   Surgical or accidental trauma
   Increased plasma colloid osmotic
      pressure
   Administration of hypertonic saline
   Increased dietary intake of salt
   Hyperglycemia
   Addison's disease.
Fixed osmolality (approximately 300 mOsm/kg regardless of hydration status):
   Advanced renal medullary disease
   Obstructive uropathy with hydro-
      nephrosis
   Chronic renal failure (advanced).
Decreased osmolality (dilute urine):
   Water diuresis
   Inhibition of antidiuretic hormone
      (ADH) release
   Diabetes insipidus
   Elevated blood pressure in patients
      with high renin-aldosterone levels
   Decreased sympathetic stimulation
   Thyroid hormone release
   Hyponatremia

recent ingestion of large amounts of vitamin C can inhibit the test reaction.
• Extremely dilute urine can reduce test sensitivity.

Acute alcohol ingestion
Chronic renal failure (early).

The basics

Osmolality refers to the measurement of the exact number of osmotically active particles per kilogram of water. The total osmolality of extracellular fluid is primarily determined by the number of sodium and chloride ions. The total osmolality of intracellular fluid is determined primarily by the presence of potassium ions. Both extracellular and intracellular fluid compartments are approximately 300 mOsm. The kidney can normally concentrate urine to an osmolality four times that of plasma if there is a need to conserve fluid, and can dilute urine to an osmolality one-fourth that of plasma when large volumes of water must be eliminated.

Plasma osmolality regulates the release of ADH from the pituitary gland. The effect of ADH on the permeability of the epithelium of the loop of Henle and the collecting tubules of the kidneys regulates urine osmolality. Thus, simultaneous determinations of serum and urine osmolality can help evaluate the distal tubular response to circulating ADH.

Urine volume, as well as specific gravity, bears considerable relationship to osmolality, but the relationship is not absolute. Generally, a patient who increases fluid intake will excrete more urine with a low specific gravity and low urine osmolality; a patient who decreases fluid intake will excrete less urine with a higher specific gravity and increased urine osmolality. However, if urine contains large amounts of high-molecular-weight solutes such as protein or intravenous dyes, the specific gravity would be high, and the osmolality could be low.

Any factor that stimulates ADH release, such as dehydration, emotional stress, or surgical trauma, will ordinarily produce concentrated urine with increased osmolality. Factors that inhibit ADH release, such as alcohol consumption, increased water intake, and increased blood volume, produce dilute urine with a decreased osmolality. SIADH is characterized by a continuous release of ADH in spite of low plasma osmolality and the production of urine with increased osmolality.

Urine osmolality varies greatly with diet and hydration status and should always be evaluted in relation to serum osmolality. The ratio of urine osmolality to serum osmolality should exceed 1.0, and following an overnight fast should be 3.0 or more.

Since the ability to concentrate urine is one of the first kidney functions to be lost in early renal failure, a urine concentration test may be ordered. In this test, urine osmolality is determined following an overnight 8- to 10-hour period of fluid restriction.

In a urine dilution test, urine osmolality is determined following a period of increased fluid intake.

Procedure

Collect a random sample of urine free of preservatives. If possible, obtain a first-voided morning specimen.

Patient care checklist

Before the test

☑ Explain or clarify test purpose, preparation, and procedure.
☑ Evaluate patient understanding.
☑ Restrict fluids overnight before the test.

Interfering factors

• Failure to account for the hydration status of the patient will make accurate interpretation of the results impossible.

• Diuretics decrease urine osmolality.
• Radiocontrast dye decreases osmolality.
• Barbiturates, morphine, and anesthetics increase urine osmolality.

Oxalate

Purpose
• To detect primary hyperoxaluria in infants
• To rule out hyperoxaluria in renal insufficiency.

Normal results
Urine oxalate levels up to 40 mg/24 hours are considered normal.

Abnormal results
Increased urine oxalate levels:
    Primary hyperoxaluria
    Pancreatic insufficiency
    Diabetes mellitus
    Cirrhosis
    Pyridoxine deficiency
    Crohn's disease
    Ileal resection
    Ingestion of antifreeze or stain remover
    Reaction to a methoxyflurane anesthetic.

The basics
This test measures urine levels of oxalate, a salt of oxalic acid. Oxalate is an end product of metabolism and is excreted almost exclusively in the urine. Most important, the test detects hyperoxaluria, a disorder in which oxalate accumulates in the soft and connective tissue, especially in the kidneys and bladder, causing chronic inflammation and fibrosis. Calcium oxalate deposits are the most common cause of renal calculi, which may produce kidney damage. The laboratory requires at least 2 days to complete the analysis.

Procedure
Collect a 24-hour urine specimen in a light-protected container with hydrochloric acid. (See "Timed collection," pp. xviii and xix.)

Special precautions
Refrigerate the urine specimen or keep it on ice during the collection period.

Patient care checklist
Before the test
☑ Explain or clarify test purpose and procedure.
☑ Instruct the patient or the parents of the patient to restrict intake of tomatoes, strawberries, rhubarb, and spinach for about 1 week before the test.
☑ Evaluate patient/parent understanding.

Interfering factors
• Failure to collect all urine during the test period may alter test results.
• Improper storage of the specimen during the collection period may alter test results.
• Ingestion of strawberries, tomatoes, rhubarb, or spinach increases urine oxalate levels.

Para-aminohippuric acid excretion *(PAH)*

Purpose
To evaluate renal function by determining the effective renal plasma flow (ERPF).

Normal results
PAH excretion is normally 400 to 700 ml/minute at age 20; excretion decreases 17 ml/minute each decade thereafter.

Abnormal results
Decreased PAH levels:
    Decreased cardiac output or arterial blood pressure
    Organic disease of renal vascular system
    Increased resistance to blood flow resulting from early essential hypertension or systemic arterial hypotension
    Diminished functional renal tissue.

The basics

When plasma PAH levels are maintained at 10 to 20 mcg/ml by I.V. infusion, almost all PAH is cleared in one passage through the kidneys by glomerular filtration and by tubular secretion. However, since a small fraction of this flow normally fails to perfuse the proximal tubules and a corresponding fraction of PAH fails to be excreted, PAH clearance merely approximates the actual renal plasma flow. Consequently, PAH excretion measures the *effective* renal plasma flow (ERPF) and is indicated for patients in whom impaired renal function is suspected.

This test takes approximately 2 hours to perform and requires frequent collection of blood and urine specimens and an I.V. infusion. Because this test is technically complex and is uncomfortable for the patient, it is infrequently used.

Procedure

• Perform a venipuncture, and collect 10 ml of blood in a green-top (heparinized) tube, to be used as a baseline sample.
• Catheterize the patient. Make sure the bladder is empty, and save the urine for a baseline specimen.
• Start an I.V. and infuse the recommended priming dose of 25 ml of 10% PAH by I.V. bolus over 4 minutes, allowing 30 minutes for distribution.
• Then, using an I.V. pump, infuse the maintenance solution of 500 ml of 1.5% PAH at a constant rate of 4 ml/minute.
• Collect a urine specimen after the I.V. is started and three additional specimens at 20-minute intervals thereafter. Clamp the catheter between collections.
• Draw a blood sample at the midpoint of each 20-minute period and at the end of the test.
• Record the PAH dosage on the laboratory slip. Properly label each specimen, and include the collection times.

Special precautions

• This test is used cautiously in patients with cardiac dysfunction, since the increased blood volume accompanying enforced hydration and PAH infusion may precipitate congestive heart failure.
• If the patient already has a catheter in place, do not use the urine in the drainage bag. Empty the bag, and clamp the catheter for 1 hour before obtaining a baseline specimen.
• Administer the priming dose of PAH slowly and cautiously, observing the patient closely for adverse reactions.
• Wrap the I.V. bottle of maintenance solution in foil to protect it from light.
• If more than 10 minutes will elapse before transport, refrigerate the urine specimen.

Patient care checklist

Before the test

☑ Explain or clarify test purpose, preparation, and procedure.

☑ Instruct the patient to refrain from eating solid foods for at least 4 hours before the test, if ordered, and to abstain from exercise the morning of the test.

☑ Encourage fluid intake before and during the test to maintain adequate urine flow.

☑ Tell the patient to watch for and report possible adverse effects of PAH administration: nausea, vomiting, cramping, vasomotor disturbances, and flushing.

☑ Evaluate patient understanding.

After the test

☑ Continue to observe the patient for adverse reactions to PAH.

Interfering factors

• Pyrogenic agents or a high-protein diet can increase PAH excretion.
• Diuretics, penicillin, phenolsulfonphthalein, probenecid, and salicylates can depress excretion.
• Procaine and sulfonamides interfere with the laboratory methodology.

- Failure to infuse PAH at a constant rate may adversely affect test results.
- Failure to collect blood and urine specimens at the proper intervals may invalidate test results.
- Failure to adhere to dietary and exercise restrictions may alter test results.
- Hemolysis caused by rough handling of the blood samples may alter test results.

Phenolsulfonphthalein excretion (PSP)

Purpose
- To determine renal plasma flow
- To evaluate tubular function.

Normal results
Twenty-five percent of the PSP dose is excreted in 15 minutes; 50% to 60% in 30 minutes; 60% to 70% in 1 hour; and 70% to 80% in 2 hours. Normal excretion for children (excluding infants) is 5% to 10% higher than for adults.

Abnormal results
Increased PSP excretion is characteristic in:
  Hypoalbuminemia
  Hepatic disease
  Multiple myeloma.
Decreased PSP excretion is characteristic in:
  Renal vascular disease
  Urinary tract obstruction
  Congestive heart failure
  Gout.

The basics
Although the PSP excretion test is less accurate than the para-aminohippuric acid excretion test or the inulin clearance test, it is a simpler method for evaluating kidney function. This test is indicated in a patient with abnormal results in the urine concentration test,

one of the earliest signs of renal dysfunction. When PSP is administered I.V., the kidneys normally clear 70% of the dose in one passage, primarily by proximal tubular excretion. Glomerular filtration removes 5%, and the liver removes an additional 10% to 20%. The PSP excretion rate, which equals 70% of renal plasma flow, is determined by alkalinizing the urine, diluting the samples to equal volumes, and comparing the results with a normal colorimetric graph.

Procedure
- Instruct the patient to void, and then discard the urine. The physician will administer exactly 1 ml of PSP (6 mg of dye) I.V.
- Collect a urine specimen at 15 minutes, 30 minutes, 1 hour, and if ordered, 2 hours after the injection. If the patient is catheterized, be sure to clamp the catheter between collections.
- Encourage fluid intake, since 40 ml is required for each specimen.
- Record the PSP dosage on the laboratory slip. Properly label each specimen, and include the collection times.

Special precautions
- This test should be used cautiously in a patient with cardiac dysfunction or renal insufficiency, since the increased fluid intake necessary for proper hydration may precipitate congestive heart failure.
- Keep epinephrine available, since allergic reactions to PSP develop occasionally.
- If the patient already has a catheter in place, do not use the urine in the drainage bag. Empty the bag, and clamp the catheter for 1 hour before the test.
- Send specimens to the laboratory immediately after each collection. If more than 10 minutes will elapse before transport, refrigerate the specimen.

Patient care checklist
Before the test
☑ Explain or clarify test purpose and procedure.
☑ Tell the patient to increase fluid intake before and during the test to maintain adequate urine flow.
☑ Inform the patient that his urine will temporarily turn red.
☑ Evaluate patient understanding.

Interfering factors
• Inexact measurement of PSP dosage may interfere with accurate determination of test results.
• Failure to collect urine specimens at the designated times may invalidate test results.
• The patient's inability to void at specified intervals may adversely affect test results.
• Collection of insufficient specimens (less than 40 ml) may alter test results.
• Decreased PSP excretion may result from administration of I.V. pyelography radiopaque fluid, or from chlorothiazide, aspirin, phenylbutazone, penicillin, sulfonamides, and probenecid.
• Azo dyes and sulfobromophthalein interfere with colorimetric measurement of PSP.
• Abnormal drainage sites, such as fistulas, or hematuria may alter test results.

Placental estriol

Purpose
To assess fetoplacental status, especially in high-risk pregnancy.

Normal results
Values vary considerably, but serial measurements of urine estriol levels, when plotted on a graph, should describe a steadily rising curve (see *Urine Estriol Levels in a Typical Pregnancy*).

Abnormal results
A 40% drop from baseline values that occurs on 2 consecutive days strongly suggests placental insufficiency and impending fetal distress. A 20% drop over 2 weeks, or failure of consecutive estriol levels to rise in a normal curve, similarly indicates inadequate placental function and undesirable fetal status.

A chronically low urine estriol curve may result from fetal adrenal insufficiency, congenital anomalies (such as anencephaly), Rh isoimmunization, or placental sulfatase deficiency. A high-risk pregnancy in which maternal glomerular filtration rate (GFR) decreases, as in hypertension or diabetes mellitus, may cause a low-normal estriol curve. In such a case, the pregnancy may continue, as long as no complications develop and estriol levels continue to rise. However, falling estriol levels or a sudden drop from baseline values indicates severe fetal distress. High urine estriol levels are possible in multiple pregnancy.

The basics
This test monitors fetal viability by measuring urine levels of placental estriol, the predominant estrogen excreted in urine during pregnancy. Toward the end of the first trimester, placental constituents combine with estriol precursors from the fetal adrenal cortex and liver to steadily increase estriol production. This steady rise in estriol reflects a properly functioning placenta and, in most cases, a healthy, growing fetus. Normally, estriol is secreted in much smaller amounts by the ovaries in nonpregnant females, by the testes in males, and by the adrenal cortex in both sexes.

The usual clinical indication for this test is high-risk pregnancy, such as one complicated by maternal hypertension, diabetes mellitus, preeclampsia, toxemia, or a history of stillbirth. Serial testing is necessary to plot the expected rise in estriol levels or to show the absence of such a rise. The spec-

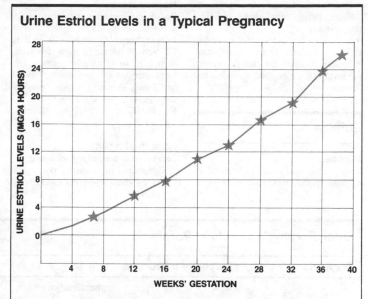

Urine Estriol Levels in a Typical Pregnancy

URINE ESTRIOL LEVELS (MG/24 HOURS)

WEEKS' GESTATION

Since urine estriol rises as normal gestation proceeds, any significant changes in serial urine determinations suggest abnormal conditions that may require prompt medical intervention.

imen of choice for this test is a 24-hour urine specimen, since estriol levels fluctuate diurnally. Radioimmunoassay is the usual test method. Generally, serum estriol levels are considered more reliable than urine levels. Serum levels are not influenced by maternal GFR, nor are they as readily affected by drugs, some of which actually destroy urinary estriol.

Procedure
• Collect a 24-hour urine specimen in a bottle containing a preservative to keep the specimen at a pH of 3.0 to 5.0. (See "Timed collection," pp. xviii and xix.)
• Note the week of gestation on the laboratory slip, and send the specimen to the laboratory.

Special precautions
Refrigerate the specimen or keep it on ice during the collection period.

Patient care checklist
Before the test
☑ Explain or clarify test purpose and procedure.
☑ Evaluate patient understanding.

Interfering factors
• Administration of the following drugs may influence urine estriol levels: steroid hormones (including estrogens, progesterone, and corticosteroids), methenamine mandelate, phenothiazines, ampicillin, phenazopyridine hydrochloride, tetracyclines, cascara sagrada, senna, phenolphthalein, hydrochlorothiazide, and meprobamate.
• Maternal hemoglobinopathy, anemia, malnutrition, and hepatic or intestinal disease characteristically decrease estriol levels.

- Failure to collect all urine during the 24-hour period may adversely affect test results.
- Failure to refrigerate the specimen or keep it on ice may alter test results.
- Failure to maintain the prescribed pH level in the specimen may alter test results.

Porphyrins

Purpose

To aid in diagnosis of congenital or acquired porphyrias.

Normal results

Porphyrin and precursor values for urine fall in these ranges:

Uroporphyrins: in women, from 1 to 22 mcg/24 hours; in men, from undetectable to 42 mcg/24 hours.

Coproporphyrins: in women, from 1 to 57 mcg/24 hours; in men, from undetectable to 96 mcg/24 hours.

Porphobilinogen (PBG): in both sexes, up to 1.5 mg/24 hours.

Abnormal results

Increased urine porphyrin levels:
  Congenital or acquired porphyrias (see *Urine Porphyrin Levels in Porphyria*)

Urine Porphyrin Levels in Porphyria

Porphyria	Porphyrin precursors	
	ALA	Porphobilinogen
Erythropoietic porphyria	Normal	Normal
Erythropoietic protoporphyria	Normal	Normal
Acute intermittent porphyria	Highly increased	Highly increased
Variegate porphyria	Highly increased during acute attack	Normal or slightly increased; highly increased during acute attack
Coproporphyria	Increased during acute attack	Increased during acute attack
Porphyria cutanea tarda (assumed to be acquired in association with other hepatic diseases; genetic causes possible)	Variable	Variable

Defective heme biosynthesis increases urinary porphyrins and their corresponding precursors.

Infectious hepatitis
Hodgkin's disease
Central nervous system disorders
Cirrhosis
Heavy metal, benzene, or carbon
tetrachloride toxicity.

The basics

This test is a quantitative analysis of urine porphyrins (most notably, uroporphyrins and coproporphyrins) and their precursors (porphyrinogens, such as PBG). Porphyrins are red-orange fluorescent compounds, consisting of four pyrrole rings, that are produced during heme biosynthesis. They are present in all protoplasm, figure in energy storage and utilization, and are normally excreted in urine in small amounts. Elevated urine levels of porphyrins or porphyrinogens, therefore, reflect impaired heme biosynthesis. Such impairment may result from inherited enzyme deficiencies (congenital porphyrias) or from defects caused by disorders such as hemolytic anemias and hepatic disease (acquired porphyrias). Because heme synthesis occurs primarily in bone marrow and the liver, porphyrias are classified as erythropoietic or hepatic.

Determination of the specific porphyrins and porphyrinogens found in a urine specimen can help identify the impaired metabolic step in heme biosynthesis. Occasionally, a preliminary qualitative screening is performed on a random specimen; a positive finding on the screening test must be confirmed by the quantitative analysis of a 24-hour specimen. For correct diagnosis of a specific porphyria, urine porphyrin levels should be correlated with plasma and fecal porphyrin levels.

Procedure

Collect a 24-hour urine specimen in a light-resistant specimen bottle containing a preservative to prevent degradation of the light-sensitive porphyrins and their precursors. (See "Timed collection," pp. xviii and xix.)

Special precautions

- Refrigerate the specimen or keep it on ice during the collection period. Then send it to the laboratory immediately.
- If a light-resistant container is not available, protect the specimen from light exposure. If an indwelling (Foley) catheter is in place, put the collection bag in a dark plastic bag.

Patient care checklist

Before the test

☑ Explain or clarify test purpose and procedure.

☑ Evaluate patient understanding.

Porphyrins

Uroporphyrins	Coproporphyrins
Highly increased	Increased
Normal	Normal
Variable	Variable
Normal or slightly increased; may be highly increased during acute attack	Normal or slightly increased; may be highly increased during acute attack
Not applicable	May be highly increased during acute attack
Highly increased	Increased

☑ Withhold medications that interfere with test results for at least 10 to 12 days before the test. If they must be continued, note the medications on the laboratory slip.

Interfering factors
• Elevated urine urobilinogen levels can affect the reagent used in the PBG screening test.
• Oral contraceptives and griseofulvin can elevate levels.
• Rifampin turns urine red-orange, interfering with results.
• Pregnancy and menstruation may increase porphyrin levels.
• Barbiturates, chloral hydrate, chlorpropamide, sulfonamides, meprobamate, and chlordiazepoxide generally induce porphyria or porphyrinuria.
• If the urine specimen is left standing for a few hours, PBG levels decline.

Potassium

Purpose
To determine whether hypokalemia is caused by renal or extrarenal disorders.

Normal results
Potassium excretion is 25 to 125 mEq/24 hours, with an average potassium concentration of 25 to 100 mEq/liter.

Abnormal results
Increased urine potassium levels:
  Dehydration
  Starvation
  Cushing's disease
  Salicylate intoxication.
Decreased urine potassium levels:
  Gastrointestinal disorders
  Aldosteronism
  Renal tubular acidosis
  Chronic renal failure.

The basics
This quantitative test measures urine levels of potassium, a major intracellular cation that helps regulate acid-base balance and neuromuscular function. Potassium imbalance may cause such signs and symptoms as muscle weakness, nausea, diarrhea, confusion, hypotension, and EKG changes; severe imbalance may lead to cardiac arrest.

Most commonly, a serum potassium test is performed to detect hyperkalemia (abnormally high levels) or hypokalemia (abnormally low levels). A urine potassium test may be performed to evaluate hypokalemia when a history and physical examination fail to uncover the cause. Since the kidneys regulate potassium balance through potassium excretion in the urine, measuring urine levels can determine whether hypokalemia results from a renal disorder, such as renal tubular acidosis, or an extrarenal disorder, such as malabsorption syndrome. If results suggest a renal disorder, additional renal function tests may be ordered.

Procedure
Collect a 24-hour urine specimen. (See "Timed collection," pp. xviii and xix.)

Special precautions
Refrigerate the specimen or place it on ice during the collection period.

Patient care checklist
Before the test
☑ Explain or clarify test purpose and procedure.
☑ Evaluate patient understanding.
After the test
CLINICAL ALERT: **Monitor the hypokalemic patient for diminished reflexes; rapid, weak, irregular pulse; mental confusion; hypotension; anorexia; muscle weakness; and paresthesias. Watch for EKG changes, especially a flattened T wave, ST depression, and U-wave elevation. Severe potassium imbalance may lead to ventricular fibrillation, respiratory paralysis, and cardiac arrest.**

Interfering factors

• Excess dietary potassium raises urine potassium levels.

• Excessive vomiting or stomach suctioning produces urine potassium levels that do not reflect actual potassium depletion.

• Potassium-wasting medications, such as ammonium chloride, thiazide diuretics, and acetazolamide, raise urine potassium levels.

• Failure to collect all urine during the test period may alter test results.

• Incorrect storage of the specimen may adversely affect test results.

Pregnanediol

Purpose

• To evaluate placental function in pregnant females

• To evaluate ovarian function in nonpregnant females.

Normal results

In nonpregnant females, urine pregnanediol values normally range from 0.5 to 1.5 mg/24 hours during the proliferative phase of the menstrual cycle. Within 24 hours after ovulation, pregnanediol levels begin to rise and continue to rise for 3 to 10 days, as the corpus luteum develops. During this luteal phase, normal urine pregnanediol values range from 2 to 7 mg/24 hours. In the absence of fertilization, levels drop sharply, as the corpus luteum degenerates and menstruation begins.

During pregnancy, urine pregnanediol levels rise markedly (see *Urine Pregnanediol in Normal Pregnancy*, p. 258), peaking around the 36th week of gestation and returning to prepregnancy levels by day 5 to 10 postpartum.

Normal postmenopausal values range from 0.2 to 1 mg/24 hours. In males, urine pregnanediol levels rarely rise above 1.5 mg/24 hours.

Abnormal results

During pregnancy, a marked decrease in urine pregnanediol levels based on a single 24-hour urine specimen, or a steady decrease in pregnanediol levels in serial measurements, may indicate placental insufficiency and necessitates immediate investigation. A precipitous drop in pregnanediol values may suggest fetal distress, as in threatened abortion or preeclampsia, or fetal death.

In nonpregnant females, abnormally low urine pregnanediol levels may occur with anovulation, amenorrhea, or other menstrual abnormalities. Low-to-normal pregnanediol levels may be associated with hydatidiform mole. Elevations may indicate luteinized granulosa or theca cell tumors, diffuse thecal luteinization, or metastatic ovarian cancer.

Adrenal hyperplasia or biliary tract obstruction may elevate urine pregnanediol values in males or females. Some forms of primary hepatic disease produce abnormally low levels in both sexes.

The basics

Using gas chromatography or radioimmunoassay, this test measures urine levels of pregnanediol, the chief metabolite of progesterone. Although biologically inert, pregnanediol has diagnostic significance because it reflects about 10% of the endogenous production of its parent hormone. Progesterone is produced in nonpregnant females by the corpus luteum during the latter half of each menstrual cycle, preparing the uterus for implantation of a fertilized ovum. If implantation does not occur, progesterone secretion drops sharply; if implantation does occur, the corpus luteum secretes more progesterone to further prepare the uterus for pregnancy and to begin development of the placenta. Toward the end of the first trimester, the placenta becomes the primary source of progesterone secretion, producing the

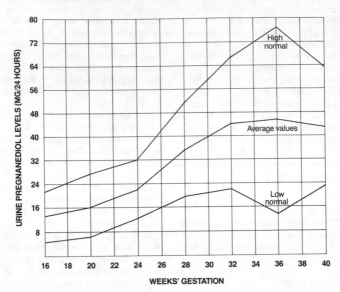

Urine Pregnanediol in Normal Pregnancy

Serial determinations of the *average* levels (middle line on chart) of pregnanediol rise steadily until about 32 weeks' gestation, then level off. Excretion decreases 24 hours postpartum and drops to prepregnancy levels within 5 to 10 days. A wide range of normal values is possible—high normal, low normal, and average levels.

Adapted with permission from R. P. Sherman, *Journal of Obstetrics and Gynecology.* 66:1, 1959.

progressively larger amounts needed to maintain pregnancy.

Normally, urine levels of pregnanediol reflect variations in progesterone secretion during the menstrual cycle and during pregnancy. However, pregnanediol measurements are not reliable indicators of fetal viability, since levels can remain normal even after fetal death, as long as maternal circulation to the placenta remains adequate. Direct measurement of plasma progesterone levels by radioimmunoassay may also be done. Pregnanediol

is present in the urine as a metabolite of progesterone and is produced in small amounts by the adrenal cortex, the principal site of secretion in males, postmenopausal women, and menstruating females before ovulation.

Procedure
● Collect a 24-hour urine specimen. (See "Timed collection," pp. xviii and xix.)
● If the patient is pregnant, note the approximate week of gestation on the laboratory slip. For other premenopausal females, note the stage of the menstrual cycle on the laboratory slip.

Special precautions
Refrigerate the specimen or keep it on ice during the collection period.

Patient care checklist
Before the test
☑ Explain or clarify test purpose and procedure.
☑ Evaluate patient understanding.
After the test
☑ Advise the pregnant patient that this test may be repeated several times to obtain serial measurements.

Interfering factors
• Methenamine mandelate, methenamine hippurate, and drugs containing adrenocorticotropic hormone elevate urine pregnanediol levels.
• Progestogens and combination oral contraceptives characteristically lower pregnanediol levels.
• Failure to collect all urine during the collection period may alter test results.
• Failure to refrigerate the specimen or keep it on ice may alter test results.

Pregnanetriol

Purpose
• To aid in diagnosis of adrenogenital syndrome
• To monitor cortisol replacement.

Normal results
The rate of pregnanetriol excretion for adults is less than 3.5 mg/24 hours; for children aged 7 to 16, the rate ranges from 0.3 to 1.1 mg/24 hours; and for children younger than age 6 (including infants), the excretion rate is up to 0.2 mg/24 hours.

Abnormal results
Increased urine pregnanetriol levels suggest:
   Adrenogenital syndrome.

The basics
Using spectrophotometry, this test determines urine levels of pregnanetriol, the metabolite of the cortisol precursor 17-hydroxyprogesterone. Pregnanetriol is normally excreted in the urine in minute amounts. However, when cortisol biosynthesis is impaired at the point of 17-hydroxyprogesterone conversion, urinary excretion of pregnanetriol rises significantly. Such impairment results from the absence or deficiency of particular biosynthetic enzymes that convert 17-hydroxyprogesterone to cortisol; in turn, low plasma cortisol levels interfere with the negative feedback mechanism that inhibits secretion of adrenocorticotropic hormone (ACTH). Consequently, excessive 17-hydroxyprogesterone accumulates in the plasma, leading to increased formation and excretion of pregnanetriol in urine.

Urine pregnanetriol levels may be measured concomitantly with urine 17-ketosteroids and urine 17-ketogenic steroids to assess androgen levels, which also rise with impairment of cortisol biosynthesis. Elevated androgen levels, which occur in adrenogenital syndrome (congenital adrenal hyperplasia), result from conversion of excessive 17-hydroxyprogesterone to androgens and from hypersecretion of adrenal androgens in response to excessive ACTH stimulation. When cortisol replacement adequately inhibits hypersecretion of ACTH and subsequent overproduction of 17-hydroxyprogesterone, pregnanetriol levels fall within the normal range.

Procedure
Collect a 24-hour urine specimen in a bottle containing a preservative to keep the specimen at a pH of 4.0 to 4.5. (See "Timed collection," p. xviii.)

Special precautions
Refrigerate the specimen or keep it on ice during the collection period.

Patient care checklist
Before the test
☑ Explain or clarify test purpose and procedure.

☑ Evaluate patient/parent understanding.

Interfering factors
• Failure to collect all urine during the test period may adversely affect test results.
• Failure to store the specimen properly may alter test results.

Protein

Purpose
To aid in diagnosis of pathologic states characterized by proteinuria, primarily renal disease.

Normal results
Up to 150 mg of protein is excreted in 24 hours.

Abnormal results
Persistent proteinuria indicates renal disease resulting from increased glomerular permeability. *Minimal* proteinuria (less than 0.5 g/24 hours), however, is most often associated with renal diseases in which glomerular involvement is not a major factor, such as chronic pyelonephritis. *Moderate* proteinuria (0.5 to 4 g/24 hours) occurs in several types of renal disease—acute or chronic glomerulonephritis, amyloidosis, toxic nephropathies—or in diseases in which renal failure often develops as a late complication (diabetes or heart failure, for example). *Heavy* proteinuria (more than 4 g/24 hours) is commonly associated with nephrotic syndrome.

When accompanied by an elevated white blood cell (WBC) count, proteinuria indicates urinary tract infection; with hematuria, proteinuria indicates local or diffuse urinary tract disorders. Other pathologic states (infections and lesions of the central nervous system, for example) can also result in detectable amounts of proteins in the urine.

The basics
This is a quantitative test for proteinuria. Normally, the glomerular membrane allows only proteins of low molecular weight to enter the filtrate. The renal tubules then reabsorb most of these proteins, normally excreting a small amount that is undetectable by a screening test. Proteinuria can result from glomerular leakage of plasma proteins (a major cause of protein excretion), from overflow of filtered proteins of low molecular weight (when these are present in excessive concentrations), from impaired tubular reabsorption of filtered proteins, and from the presence of renal proteins derived from the breakdown of kidney tissue. However, not all forms of proteinuria have pathologic significance. *Benign* proteinuria can result from changes in body position. *Functional* proteinuria is associated with emotional or physiologic stress, and is usually transient.

Many drugs (such as amphotericin B, gold preparations, aminoglycosides, polymyxins, and trimethadione) inflict renal damage, causing true proteinuria. This makes the routine evaluation of urine proteins essential during such treatment.

A qualitative screening often precedes this test. (See *Random Specimen Screening for Protein*.) A positive result requires quantitative analysis of a 24-hour urine specimen by acid precipitation tests. In all forms of proteinuria, fractionation results obtained by electrophoresis provide more precise information than the screening test. For example, excessive hemoglobin in the urine indicates intravascular hemolysis; elevated myoglobin suggests muscle damage; albumin suggests increased glomerular permeability; and Bence Jones protein suggests multiple myeloma.

Procedure
Collect a 24-hour urine specimen. A special specimen container can be ob-

tained from the laboratory. (See "Timed collection," pp. xviii and xix.)

Special precautions
Refrigerate the specimen or place it on ice during the collection period.

Random Specimen Screening for Protein

Qualitative screening tests for proteinuria include reagent strips (dipsticks) and acids that precipitate proteins (sulfosalicylic acid, or acetic acid with heat).

To perform such a test, collect a clean-catch urine specimen, preferably in the morning, when the urine is most concentrated and yields the most reliable information. Commonly, a reagent strip (such as Combistix) is used. Dip the strip into the urine; remove excess urine by tapping the strip against a clean surface or the edge of the container; hold the strip in a horizontal position to prevent mixing of chemicals from adjacent areas. Immediately place the strip close to the color block on the bottle and carefully compare colors. The results correspond to mg/dl of protein (usually albumin, since strips are most sensitive to albumin).

Negative = 0 to 5 mg/dl
Trace = 5 to 20 mg/dl
1+ = 30 mg/dl
2+ = 100 mg/dl
3+ = 300 mg/dl
4+ = 1,000 mg/dl

Normally, no detectable protein is present in a random specimen, although normal kidneys do excrete a minute amount. A positive result requires quantitative analysis of a 24-hour urine specimen.

Phenazopyridine can alter the color reaction of certain brands of reagent strips; so can high salt or alkaline content of the urine specimen. Acetazolamide and sodium bicarbonate can cause false-positive results with some reagent strips.

Patient care checklist
Before the test
☑ Explain or clarify test purpose and procedure.
☑ Evaluate patient understanding.

Interfering factors
• Administration of tolbutamide, para-aminosalicylic acid, acetazolamide, sodium bicarbonate, penicillin, sulfonamides, iodine contrast media, and cephalosporins may cause false-positive results in acid preparation tests.
• Contamination of the urine specimen with heavy mucus, vaginal or prostatic secretions, or the presence of numerous WBCs can alter test results, regardless of laboratory method.
• Very dilute urine (which may result from forcing fluids) may depress protein values and cause false-negative results.

Sodium and chloride

Purpose
• To help evaluate fluid and electrolyte imbalance
• To monitor the effects of a low-salt diet
• To help evaluate renal and adrenal disorders.

Normal results
Urine sodium excretion is 30 to 280 mEq/24 hours; normal urine chloride excretion, 110 to 250 mEq/24 hours; and normal urine sodium-chloride excretion, 5 to 20 g/24 hours.

Abnormal results
Increased urine sodium levels may reflect:
    Increased salt intake
    Adrenal failure
    Salicylate toxicity
    Diabetic acidosis
    Salt-losing nephritis
    Water-deficient dehydration.

Decreased urine sodium levels suggest:
   Decreased salt intake
   Primary aldosteronism
   Acute renal failure
   Congestive heart failure.
Increased urine chloride levels may result from:
   Water-deficient dehydration
   Salicylate toxicity
   Diabetic acidosis
   Addison's disease
   Salt-losing renal disease.
Decreased urine chloride levels may result from:
   Excessive diaphoresis
   Congestive heart failure
   Hypochloremic metabolic alkalosis.

The basics

This test determines urine levels of sodium, the major extracellular cation, and of chloride, the major extracellular anion. Less significant than serum levels (and, consequently, performed less frequently), measurement of urine sodium and urine chloride concentrations is used to evaluate renal conservation of these two electrolytes and to confirm serum sodium and chloride values.

Sodium and chloride help maintain osmotic pressure and water and acid-base balance. After these ions are absorbed by the intestinal tract, they are regulated by the kidneys and rise and fall in tandem. The kidneys conserve constant serum levels of sodium and of chloride—even at the risk of dehydration or edema—or excrete excessive amounts. Normal ranges of sodium and chloride in the urine vary greatly with dietary salt intake and perspiration.

Procedure

Collect a 24-hour urine specimen. (See "Timed collection," pp. xviii and xix.)

Special precautions

Refrigerate the specimen or keep it on ice during the collection period.

Patient care checklist

Before the test
☑ Explain or clarify test purpose and procedure.
☑ Evaluate patient understanding.

Interfering factors

• Failure to collect all urine during the test period may alter test results.
• Ammonium chloride and potassium chloride elevate urine chloride levels.
• Sodium bicarbonate and thiazide diuretics raise urine sodium levels.
• Steroids suppress urine sodium levels.

Total urine estrogens

Purpose

• To evaluate ovarian activity and help determine the cause of amenorrhea and female hyperestrogenism
• To aid in diagnosis of testicular tumors
• To assess fetoplacental status.

Normal results

Values for nonpregnant females are as follows:
Preovulatory phase: 5 to 25 mcg/24 hours
Ovulatory phase: 24 to 100 mcg/24 hours
Luteal phase: 12 to 80 mcg/24 hours.

In postmenopausal females, values are less than 10 mcg/24 hours; in males, from 4 to 25 mcg/24 hours.

Abnormal results

Increased total urine estrogen levels in nonpregnant females may indicate tumors of ovarian or adrenocortical origin, adrenocortical hyperplasia, or a metabolic or hepatic disorder. In males, elevated total estrogen levels are associated with testicular tumors.

Increased total urine estrogen levels are normal during pregnancy; serial determinations should show a rising titer (see "Placental estriol," p. 252).

Decreased total urine estrogen levels may reflect ovarian agenesis, primary ovarian insufficiency (caused by Stein-Leventhal syndrome, for example), or secondary ovarian insufficiency (caused by pituitary or adrenal hypofunction, or by metabolic disturbances).

The basics

This test is a quantitative analysis of total urine levels of estradiol, estrone, and estriol—the major estrogens present in significant amounts in urine. In females who are past puberty, these estrogens are secreted by the theca interna cells of the ovarian follicle and by the corpus luteum; in pregnancy, by the placenta; and after menopause, primarily by the adrenal gland. In males, two-thirds of estradiol and of estrone is derived from testosterone; the remaining third of estradiol and smaller quantities of estrone are secreted by the testes. In both sexes, the liver, which oxidizes or converts hormones to glucuronide and sulfate conjugates, is the major organ of estrogen metabolism. A common method for measuring total urine estrogen levels involves purification by gel filtration, followed by spectrophotofluorometry.

Procedure

• Collect a 24-hour urine specimen in a bottle containing a preservative to keep the specimen at a pH of 3.0 to 5.0. (See "Timed collection," p. xviii.)
• If the patient is pregnant, note the approximate week of gestation on the laboratory slip. If the patient is a nonpregnant female, note the stage of her menstrual cycle.

Special precautions

Refrigerate the specimen or keep it on ice during the collection period.

Patient care checklist

Before the test

☑ Explain or clarify test purpose and procedure.
☑ Evaluate patient understanding.

Interfering factors

• Drugs that may influence total urine estrogen levels include steroids (such as estrogens, progesterone, and high-dose corticosteroids), methenamine mandelate, phenazopyridine hydrochloride, phenothiazines, tetracyclines, phenolphthalein, ampicillin, meprobamate, senna, cascara sagrada, and hydrochlorothiazide.
• Failure to collect all urine during the 24-hour period may alter test results.
• Failure to refrigerate the specimen or keep it on ice may alter test results.
• Improper pH control of the specimen may lead to inaccurate test results.

Tryptophan challenge test

Purpose

To detect vitamin B_6 deficiency.

Normal results

Excretion of xanthurenic acid after a tryptophan challenge dose is less than 50 mg/24 hours.

Abnormal results

Urine levels of xanthurenic acid exceeding 100 mg/24 hours indicate vitamin B_6 deficiency.

The basics

Since direct assay of vitamin B_6 is not currently available, measurement of urine xanthurenic acid after a challenge dose of tryptophan can confirm deficiency long before symptoms appear.

Although vitamin B_6 is not directly involved in energy metabolism, it is essential for reactions that occur in protein metabolism and for amino acid synthesis. Vitamin B_6 comprises three compounds—pyridoxine, pyridoxal, and pyridoxamine—that function as coenzymes in many biochemical reactions, including the conversion of tryptophan to niacin. Normally, this conversion prevents formation of xanthurenic acid; however, when vitamin

B_6 is deficient, xanthurenic acid levels rise.

Procedure
• Administer L-tryptophan P.O. (usually, 50 mg/kg for children, and up to 2 g/kg for adults).
• Ask the patient to void; discard the urine, and immediately begin collection of a 24-hour urine specimen in a specimen bottle containing a crystal of thymol, a preservative. (See "Timed collection," pp. xviii and xix.)

Special precautions
Refrigerate the specimen or place it on ice during the collection period.

Patient care checklist
Before the test
☑ Explain or clarify test purpose and procedure.
☑ Evaluate patient understanding.

Interfering factors
• Failure to collect all urine during the test period.
• Improper specimen storage.

Tubular reabsorption of phosphate

Purpose
• To evaluate parathyroid function
• To aid in diagnosis of primary hyperparathyroidism
• To aid in differential diagnosis of hypercalcemia.

Normal results
Renal tubules normally reabsorb 80% or more of phosphate.

Abnormal results
Increased reabsorption of phosphate may result from:
    Uremia
    Renal tubular disease
    Osteomalacia
    Sarcoidosis
    Myeloma.

Decreased reabsorption of phosphate suggests:
    Primary hyperparathyroidism.

The basics
Since tubular reabsorption of phosphate is closely regulated by parathyroid hormone (PTH), measuring urine and plasma phosphate, with creatinine clearance, provides an indirect method of evaluating parathyroid function. (See *Equation for Tubular Reabsorption of Phosphate*.) PTH helps maintain optimum blood levels of ionized calcium and controls renal excretion of calcium and phosphate. Specifically, PTH stimulates reabsorption of calcium and inhibits reabsorption of phosphate from the glomerular filtrate. A regulatory feedback mechanism causes PTH secretion to diminish as ionized calcium levels return to normal. In primary hyperparathyroidism,

---

Equation for Tubular Reabsorption of Phosphate (TRP)

Using the equation in Figure 1, phosphate reabsorption is calculated by comparing creatinine clearance with phosphate clearance. Figure 2 is an example of a normal value for TRP; Figure 3 is an example of an abnormal value.

$$TRP\ (\%) = 100 \times \frac{1 - \dfrac{\text{urine phosphate} \times \text{serum creatinine}}{\text{urine creatinine} \times \text{serum phosphate}}}{}$$

$$TRP\ (\%) = 100 \times \frac{1 - 1.0 \times 1.0}{1.5 \times 4} = 83\%$$

$$TRP\ (\%) = 100 \times \frac{1 - 1.8 \times 8}{1.6 \times 3} = 70\%$$

excessive secretion of PTH disrupts this calcium-phosphate balance.

This test is indicated to detect hyperparathyroidism in persons with clinical signs of this disorder and with borderline or normal values for serum calcium, phosphate, and alkaline phosphatase. Reabsorption of less than 74% of phosphate strongly suggests primary hyperparathyroidism. Depressed reabsorption occurs in a small number of patients with renal calculi but without parathyroid tumor. However, normal reabsorption occurs in roughly one-fifth of patients with parathyroid tumor.

Procedure
• Perform a venipuncture, and collect the sample in a 10-ml, red-top tube.
• Instruct the patient to empty his bladder, and discard the urine; record this as time zero. Collect a 24-hour urine specimen. (See "Timed Collection," pp. xviii and xix.)
• After the venipuncture, allow the patient to eat, and encourage fluid intake to maintain adequate urine flow.

Special precautions
Keep the urine specimen container refrigerated or on ice during the collection period.

Patient care checklist
Before the test
☑ Explain or clarify test purpose, preparation, and procedure.
☑ Instruct the patient to maintain a normal phosphate diet for 3 days before the test. This diet includes a moderate amount of legumes, nuts, milk, egg yolks, meat, poultry, fish, cereals, and cheese.
☑ Evaluate patient understanding.
☑ Restrict food and fluids from midnight the night before the test.
☑ Withhold medications that interfere with test results during the test itself. If they must be continued, note this on the laboratory slip.

Interfering factors
• Hemolysis caused by rough handling of the sample may alter test results.
• Failure to collect and refrigerate all urine during the test period may alter test results.
• The patient's failure to follow guidelines for diet restrictions and phosphate intake may alter test results, since low phosphate intake (less than 500 mg/day) may elevate tubular reabsorption values and a high-phosphate diet (3,000 mg/day) may lower them.
• Amphotericin B and chlorothiazide diuretics may diminish reabsorption.
• Furosemide and gentamicin may enhance reabsorption.

Urea clearance

Purpose
To assess total renal function.

Normal results
The urea clearance rate ranges from 64 to 99 ml/minute with maximal clearance. If the flow rate is less than 2 ml/minute, normal clearance is 41 to 68 ml/minute. (If the urine flow rate is less than 1 ml/minute, this test should not be performed.)

Abnormal results
Decreased urea clearance:
  May indicate:
    Decreased renal blood flow
    Acute or chronic glomerulonephritis
    Acute tubular necrosis
    Nephrosclerosis.
  May result from:
    Polycystic kidney disease
    Renal tuberculosis
    Malignancy involving the kidneys
    Bilateral ureteral obstruction
    Congestive heart failure
    Dehydration.

The basics

The urea clearance test is a quantitative analysis of urine levels of urea, the main nitrogenous component in urine and the end product of protein metabolism. After filtration by the glomeruli, roughly 40% of the urea is reabsorbed by the renal tubules. Because of this reabsorption, urea clearance was once considered a precise fraction (60%) of the glomerular filtration rate (GFR). However, since the reabsorption rate of urea varies with the amount of water reabsorbed, this test actually assesses overall renal function; the creatinine clearance test provides a more accurate evaluation of the GFR. In urea clearance, blood urea content and the total amount of urea excreted in the urine are proportional only when the rate of urine flow is 2 ml/minute or higher (maximal clearance). At lower flow rates, the accuracy of the test decreases. The equation for determining urea clearance is $C = (U \times V)$ divided by P; C represents the clearance rate; U equals the urine concentration of urea; V, the volume of urine collected during the test period (converted to ml/minute); and P, the plasma concentration of urea. High urea clearance usually is not diagnostically significant.

Procedure

• Instruct the patient to empty his bladder. Discard the urine. If the patient is catheterized, empty the drainage bag before beginning the specimen collection.
• Give the patient water to drink to ensure adequate urine output.
• Collect two specimens 1 hour apart, and mark the collection time on the laboratory slip.
• Perform a venipuncture anytime during the collection period, and collect the sample in a 7-ml, red-top tube.

Special precautions

Since this is a clearance test, make sure that the patient empties his bladder and that the total amount of urine is collected from each hour's specimen.

Patient care checklist

Before the test

☑ Explain or clarify test purpose, preparation, and procedure.
☑ Instruct the patient to refrain from physical exercise before and during the test.
☑ Evaluate patient understanding.
☑ Restrict food and fluids from midnight the night before the test.

Interfering factors

• The patient's failure to empty his bladder completely—the most common error in this test—and to observe pretest restrictions may lead to inaccurate test results.
• Caffeine, milk, or small doses of epinephrine increase urea clearance.
• Antidiuretic hormone or large doses of epinephrine decrease urea clearance.
• Corticosteroids, amphotericin B, thiazide diuretics, and streptomycin may also affect test results.
• Hemolysis caused by rough handling of the blood sample may alter test results.

Uric acid

Purpose

• To detect enzyme deficiencies and metabolic disturbances that affect uric acid production
• To help measure the efficiency of renal clearance.

Normal results

Urine uric acid values vary with diet, but generally range from 250 to 750 mg/24 hours.

Abnormal results

Increased urine uric acid levels:
   May result from:
      Chronic myeloid leukemia
      Polycythemia vera

Multiple myeloma
Early remission in pernicious anemia
Fanconi's syndrome
Wilson's disease.
May occur in:
Lymphosarcoma and lymphatic leukemia during radiotherapy.
Decreased urine uric acid levels occur in:
Gout
Conditions causing severe renal damage.

The basics

A quantitative analysis of urine uric acid levels, this test supplements serum uric acid testing for identifying disorders that alter production or excretion of uric acid (such as leukemia, gout, and renal dysfunction). Derived from dietary purines in organ meats (liver, kidney, and sweetbread) and from endogenous nucleoproteins, uric acid (as urate) is found normally in the blood and in other tissues in amounts totaling about 1 g. Its primary site of formation is the liver, although the intestinal mucosa is also involved in urate production. As the chief end product of purine catabolism, urate passes from the liver through the bloodstream to the kidneys, where roughly 50% is excreted daily in the urine. Renal urate metabolism is complex, involving glomerular filtration, tubular secretion, and a second reabsorption by the renal tubules.

The most specific laboratory method for detecting uric acid is spectrophotometric absorption, after treatment of the specimen with the enzyme uricase.

Procedure

Collect a 24-hour urine specimen. (See "Timed collection," pp. xviii and xix.)

Special precautions

Refrigerate the specimen or keep it on ice during the collection period.

Patient care checklist
Before the test
☑ Explain or clarify test purpose and procedure.
☑ Evaluate patient understanding.

Interfering factors

• Drugs that decrease urine uric acid excretion include diuretics, such as benzthiazide, furosemide, and ethacrynic acid, as well as pyrazinamide.
• Low doses of salicylates, phenylbutazone, and probenecid also lower uric acid levels; high doses of these drugs cause levels to rise above normal.
• Allopurinol, a drug used to treat gout, increases uric acid excretion.
• Urine uric acid concentrations rise with a high-purine diet and fall with a low-purine diet.
• Failure to observe drug restrictions, if ordered, may alter test results.
• Failure to collect all urine during the test period may alter test results.

Urinalysis

Purpose

• To screen for renal or urinary tract disease
• To help detect metabolic or systemic disease unrelated to renal disorders.

Normal results

See *Normal Findings in Routine Urinalysis,* p. 268.

Abnormal results
Color:
Changes in color can result from diet, drugs, and many metabolic, inflammatory, or infectious diseases.
Odor:
In diabetes mellitus, starvation, and dehydration, a fruity odor accompanies formation of ketone bodies. In urinary tract infection, a fetid odor is common, especially if *Escherichia coli* is present. Maple

Normal Findings in Routine Urinalysis

Element	Findings
Macroscopic	
Color	Straw
Odor	Slightly aromatic
Appearance	Clear
Specific gravity	1.005 to 1.020
pH	4.5 to 8.0
Protein	None
Glucose	None
Ketones	None
Other sugars	None
Microscopic	
Red blood cells	0 to 3/high-power field
White blood cells	0 to 4/high-power field
Epithelial cells	Few
Casts	None, except occasional hyaline casts
Crystals	Present
Yeast cells	None
Parasites	None
Bacteria	None

syrup urine disease and phenyl-ketonuria also cause distinctive odors.

Turbidity:

Turbid urine may contain red or white cells, bacteria, fat, or chyle and may reflect renal infection.

Specific gravity:

Low specific gravity ($<$ 1.005) is characteristic of diabetes insipidus, nephrogenic diabetes insipidus, acute tubular necrosis, and pyelonephritis. Fixed specific gravity, in which values remain 1.010 regardless of fluid intake, occurs in chronic glomerulonephritis with severe renal damage. High specific gravity ($>$ 1.020) occurs in nephrotic syndrome, dehydration, acute glomerulonephritis, congestive heart failure, liver failure, and shock.

pH:

Alkaline urine pH may result from Fanconi's syndrome, urinary tract infection, and metabolic or respiratory alkalosis. Acid urine pH is associated with renal tuberculosis, pyrexia, phenylketonuria and alkaptonuria, and all forms of acidosis.

Protein:

Proteinuria suggests renal diseases, such as nephrosis, glomerulosclerosis, glomerulonephritis, nephrolithiasis, polycystic kidney disease, and renal failure. Proteinuria can also result from multiple myeloma.

Sugars:

Glycosuria usually indicates diabetes mellitus but may also result from pheochromocytoma, Cushing's syndrome, and increased intracranial pressure. Fructosuria, galactosuria, and pentosuria generally suggest rare hereditary metabolic disorders. However, an alimentary form of pentosuria and fructosuria may follow excessive ingestion of pentose or fructose, resulting in hepatic failure to metabolize the sugar. Since the renal tubules fail to reabsorb pentose or fructose, these sugars spill over into the urine.

Ketones:

Ketonuria occurs in diabetes mellitus when cellular energy needs exceed available cellular glucose. Ketonuria may also occur in starvation states and in conditions of acutely increased metabolic demand associated with decreased food intake, such as diarrhea or vomiting.

Cells:

Hematuria indicates bleeding within the genitourinary tract and may result from infection, obstruction, inflammation, trauma, tumors, glomerulonephritis, renal hypertension, lupus nephritis, renal tuberculosis, renal vein thrombosis, hydronephrosis, pyelonephritis, scurvy, malaria, parasitic infection of the bladder, subacute bacterial endocarditis, polyarteritis nodosa, and hemorrhagic disorders. Numerous white cells in urine usually imply urinary tract inflammation, especially cystitis or pyelonephritis. White cells and white cell casts in urine suggest renal infection. An excessive number of epithelial cells suggests renal tubular degradation.

Casts:

Casts, plugs of gelled proteinaceous material (high-molecular-weight mucoprotein), form in the renal tubules and collecting ducts by agglutination of protein cells or cellular debris and are flushed loose by urine flow. Excessive numbers of casts indicate renal disease. Hyaline casts are associated with renal parenchymal disease, inflammation, and trauma to the glomerular capillary membrane; epithelial casts, with renal tubular damage, nephrosis, eclampsia, amyloidosis, and heavy metal poisoning; coarse and fine granular casts, with acute or chronic renal failure, pyelonephritis, and chronic lead intoxication; fatty and waxy casts, with nephrotic syndrome, chronic renal disease, and diabetes mellitus; red blood cell casts, with renal parenchymal disease (especially glomerulonephritis), renal infarction, subacute bacterial endocarditis, vascular disorders, sickle cell anemia, scurvy, blood dyscrasias, malignant hypertension, collagen disease, and acute inflammation; and white blood cell casts, with acute pyelonephritis and glomerulonephritis, nephrotic syndrome, pyogenic infection, and lupus nephritis.

Crystals:

Some crystals normally appear in urine, but numerous calcium oxalate crystals suggest hypercalcemia. Cystine crystals (cystinuria) reflect an inborn error of metabolism.

Other components:

Bacteria yeast cells and parasites in urinary sediment reflect genitourinary tract infection, as well as contamination of external genitalia. Yeast cells, which may be mistaken for red cells, can be identified by their ovoid shape, lack of color, variable size, and frequently, signs of budding. The most common parasite in sediment is *Trichomonas vaginalis,* a flagellated protozoan that commonly causes vaginitis, urethritis, and prostatovesiculitis.

The basics

Routine urinalysis is an important, commonly used screening test for urinary and systemic pathologies. Normal urine findings suggest the absence of major disease, while abnormal findings suggest its presence and mandate further urine or blood tests to identify a specific disorder. The elements of routine urinalysis include the evaluation of physical characteristics (color, odor, and opacity); the determination of specific gravity and pH; the detection and rough measurement of protein, glucose, and ketone bodies; and the examination of sediment for red and white blood cells, casts, and crystals.

Nonpathologic variations in normal values may result from diet, nonpathologic conditions, specimen collection time, and other factors. For example, specific gravity influences urine color and odor: as specific gravity increases, urine becomes darker and its odor becomes stronger; as specific gravity decreases, urine lightens. Specific gravity is highest in the first-voided morning specimen.

Urine pH, which is greatly affected by diet and medications, influences the appearance of urine and the composition of crystals. An alkaline pH (above 7.0)—characteristic of a diet high in vegetables, citrus fruits, and dairy products but low in meat—causes turbidity, and formation of phosphate, carbonate, and amorphous crystals. An acid pH (below 7.0)—typical of a high-protein diet—produces turbidity, and formation of oxalate, cystine, amorphous urate, and uric acid crystals.

Although protein is usually absent from the urine, it can appear in urine in a benign condition known as orthostatic (postural) proteinuria. This condition is most common during the second decade of life, is intermittent, appears after prolonged standing, and disappears after recumbency.

Transient benign proteinuria can also occur with fever, exposure to cold, emotional stress, or strenuous exercise. Sugars, also usually absent from the urine, may appear under normal conditions. The most common sugar in urine is glucose. Transient, nonpathologic glycosuria may result from emotional stress or pregnancy and may follow ingestion of a high-carbohydrate meal. Other sugars—fructose, lactose, and pentose—rarely appear in urine under nonpathologic conditions. (Lactosuria, however, can occur during pregnancy and lactation.)

The three important elements present in centrifuged urine sediment are cells, casts, and crystals. Red cells do not commonly appear in urine without pathologic significance, but hematuria may occasionally follow strenuous exercise.

Laboratory methods for detecting or measuring these elements include visual examination for appearance; reagent strip screening for pH, protein, glucose, and ketone bodies; refractometry for specific gravity; and microscopic inspection of centrifuged sediment for cells, casts, and crystals.

Procedure

Collect a random urine specimen of at least 15 ml. If possible, obtain a first-voided morning specimen, since this contains the greatest concentration of solutes.

Drugs that Influence Routine Urinalysis Results

Drugs that Change Urine Color:

Alcohol (light, due to diuresis)
Chlorpromazine hydrochloride (black)
Chlorzoxazone (orange to purple-red)
Deferoxamine mesylate (red)
Fluorescein sodium I.V. (yellow-orange)
Furazolidone (brown)
Iron salts (black)
Levodopa (dark)
Metronidazole (dark)
Methylene blue (blue-green)
Nitrofurantoin (brown)
Oral anticoagulants, indanedione derivatives (orange)
Phenazopyridine (orange-red, orange-brown, or red)
Phenolphthalein (red to purple-red)
Phenolsulfonphthalein (pink or red)
Quinacrine (deep yellow)
Riboflavin (yellow)
Rifampin (red-orange)
Sulfasalazine (orange-yellow)
Sulfobromophthalein (red)

Drugs that Cause Urine Odor:

Antibiotics
Paraldehyde
Vitamins

Drugs that Increase Specific Gravity:

Albumin
Dextran
Glucose

Specific Gravity (continued)

Radiopaque contrast media

Drugs that Decrease pH:

Ammonium chloride
Ascorbic acid
Diazoxide
Methenamine
Metolazone

Drugs that Increase pH:

Acetazolamide
Amphotericin B
Mafenide
Sodium bicarbonate
Potassium citrate

Drugs that Show a False-Positive Result for Proteinuria:

Acetazolamide (Combistix or Labstix)
Aminosalicylic acid (sulfosalicylic acid or Extons method)
Cephalothin in large doses (sulfosalicylic acid method)
Nafcillin (sulfosalicylic acid method)
Sodium bicarbonate (all methods)
Tolbutamide (sulfosalicylic acid method)
Tolmetin (sulfosalicylic acid method)

Drugs that Cause True Proteinuria:

Amikacin
Amphotericin B
Bacitracin
Gentamicin
Gold preparations
Kanamycin
Neomycin

Proteinuria (continued)

Netilmicin
Phenylbutazone
Polymyxin B
Streptomycin
Tobramycin
Trimethadione

Drugs that Can Cause Either True Proteinuria or False-Positive Results:

Penicillin in large doses (except with Ames reagent strips); however, some penicillins cause true proteinuria.
Sulfonamides (sulfosalicylic acid method)

Drugs that Cause False-Positive Glycosuria:

Aminosalicylic acid (Benedict's test)
Ascorbic acid (Clinistix, Diastix, or Tes-Tape)
Ascorbic acid in large doses (Clinitest tablets)
Cephalosporins (Clinitest tablets)
Chloral hydrate (Benedict's test)
Chloramphenicol (Benedict's test or Clinitest tablets)
Isoniazid (Benedict's test)
Levodopa (Clinistix, Diastix, or Tes-Tape)
Levodopa in large doses (Clinitest tablets)
Methyldopa (Tes-Tape)
Nalidixic acid (Benedict's test or Clinitest tablets)
Nitrofurantoin (Benedict's test)

(continued)

Drugs that Influence Routine Urinalysis Results *(continued)*

False-Positive Glycosuria *(continued)*

Penicillin G in large doses (Benedict's test)

Phenazopyridine (Clinistix, Diastix, or Tes-Tape)

Probenecid (Benedict's test or Clinitest tablets)

Salicylates in large doses (Clinitest tablets, Clinistix, Diastix, or Tes-Tape)

Streptomycin (Benedict's test)

Tetracycline (Clinistix, Diastix, Tes-Tape)

Tetracyclines, due to ascorbic acid buffer (Benedict's test or Clinitest tablets)

Drugs that Cause True Glycosuria:

Ammonium chloride
Asparaginase
Carbamazepine
Corticosteroids
Dextrothyroxine
Lithium carbonate
Nicotinic acid (large doses)
Phenothiazines (long-term)
Thiazide diuretics

Drugs that Cause False-Positive Results for Ketonuria:

Levodopa (Ketostix or Labstix)

Phenazopyridine (Ketostix or Gerhardt's reagent strip shows atypical color)

Phenolsulfonphthalein (Rothera's test)

Phenothiazines (Gerhardt's reagent strip shows atypical color)

Salicylates (testing with Gerhardt's reagent strip shows reddish color)

Sulfobromophthalein (Bili-Labstix)

Drugs that Cause True Ketonuria:

Ether (anesthesia)
Isoniazid (intoxication)
Isopropyl alcohol (intoxication)
Insulin (excessive doses)

Drugs that Increase White Blood Cells:

Allopurinol
Ampicillin
Aspirin toxicity
Kanamycin
Methicillin

Drugs that Cause Hematuria:

Amphotericin B
Coumarin derivatives
Methenamine in large doses
Methicillin
Para-aminosalicylic acid
Phenylbutazone
Sulfonamides

Drugs that Cause Casts:

Amphotericin B
Aspirin toxicity
Bacitracin
Ethacrynic acid
Furosemide
Gentamicin
Griseofulvin
Isoniazid
Kanamycin
Neomycin
Penicillin
Radiographic agents
Streptomycin
Sulfonamides

Drugs that Cause Crystals (if urine is acidic):

Acetazolamide
Aminosalicylic acid
Ascorbic acid
Nitrofurantoin
Theophylline
Thiazide diuretics

Special precautions

• If the patient is being evaluated for renal colic, strain the specimen to catch stones or stone fragments. Place an unfolded 4″ x 4″ gauze pad or a fine-mesh sieve over the specimen container, and carefully pour the urine through the gauze or sieve.

• Send the specimen to the laboratory immediately, or refrigerate it if analysis will be delayed longer than 1 hour.

Patient care checklist

Before the test

☑ Explain or clarify test purpose and procedure.

☑ Evaluate patient understanding.

Interfering factors
• Failure to follow proper collection procedure may invalidate test results.
• Failure to send the specimen to the laboratory immediately may alter test results.
• Failure to refrigerate the specimen may alter test results.
• Strenuous exercise before routine urinalysis may cause transient myoglobinuria, producing misleading results.
• Many drugs can influence the results of this test. See *Drugs that Influence Routine Urinalysis Results,* p. 271.

Urobilinogen

Purpose
• To aid in diagnosis of extrahepatic obstruction, such as blockage of the common bile duct
• To aid in differential diagnosis of hepatic and hematologic disorders.

Normal results
Urine urobilinogen values in women range from 0.1 to 1.1 Ehrlich units/2 hours; in men, from 0.3 to 2.1 Ehrlich units/2 hours.

Abnormal results
See *Comparative Values of Bilirubin and Urobilinogen,* p. 219.

The basics
This test detects impaired liver function by measuring urine levels of urobilinogen, the colorless, water-soluble products that result from the reduction of bilirubin by intestinal bacteria. Up to 50% of intestinal urobilinogen returns to the liver, where some of it is resecreted into bile and, eventually, into the intestine through enterohepatic circulation. Small amounts of this reabsorbed urobilinogen also enter general circulation, for ultimate excretion in the urine (urobilinogenuria).

Eliminated in large amounts in the feces (50 to 250 mg/day) and in small amounts in the urine (1 to 4 mg/day), urobilinogen reflects bile pigment metabolism. Consequently, absent or altered urobilinogen levels can indicate hepatic damage or dysfunction. Urine urobilinogen can also indicate hemolysis of red blood cells, which increases bilirubin production and causes increased production and excretion of urobilinogen. Quantitative analysis of urine urobilinogen in the laboratory involves addition of Ehrlich's reagent to a 2-hour urine specimen. The resulting color reaction is read promptly by spectrophotometry. A quantitative test may also be performed using reagent strips (see *Random Specimen for Urobilinogen,* p. 274).

Procedure
Collect a random or 2-hour urine specimen, as ordered. A 2-hour specimen is ideally collected between 1 p.m. and 3 p.m., when urobilinogen levels peak.

Special precautions
Send the specimen to the laboratory *immediately*. This test must be performed within 30 minutes of collection, since urobilinogen quickly oxidizes to an orange compound called urobilin.

Patient care checklist
Before the test
☑ Explain or clarify test purpose, preparation, and procedure.
☑ Tell the patient to avoid eating bananas for 48 hours before the test.
☑ Evaluate patient understanding.

Interfering factors
• The following drugs affect the test reagent and may interfere with accurate determination of urobilinogen levels: para-aminosalicylic acid, phenazopyridine, procaine, mandelate, phenothiazines, and sulfonamides.
• Highly alkaline urine, which may be caused by acetazolamide or sodium bicarbonate, may elevate urobilinogen levels.

Random Specimen for Urobilinogen

Quantitative tests for urinary urobilinogen excretion can also be done with reagent strips, such as Bili-Labstix or N-Multistix (dip-and-read test).

To perform such tests, collect a clean-catch urine specimen in a clean, dry container—preferably during the afternoon when urine urobilinogen levels peak—and test the specimen immediately. A fresh urine specimen is essential for reliable results, because urobilinogen is very unstable when exposed to room temperature and light. Dip the strip into the urine, and as you remove it, start timing the reaction. Carefully remove excess urine by tapping the edge of the strip against the container or a clean, dry surface, to prevent color changes along the edge of the test area. When using N-Multistix (or a similar product for multiple testing), hold the strip in a horizontal position to prevent mixing of chemicals from adjacent reagent areas. Place the strip near the color block on the bottle, and carefully compare the colors. Read the results at 45 seconds. The results correspond to Ehrlich units/dl of urine.

(Normal)
yellow-green
to yellow = 0.1 to 1 Ehrlich unit/dl of urine

(Positive)
yellow-orange = 2 Ehrlich units/dl of urine

(Positive)
medium
yellow-orange = 4 Ehrlich units/dl of urine

(Positive)
light
brown-orange = 8 Ehrlich units/dl of urine

(Positive)
brown-orange = 12 Ehrlich units/dl of urine

Normally, a random specimen contains small amounts of urobilinogen. This test cannot determine the *absence* of urobilinogen in the specimen being tested.

Para-aminosalicylic acid may cause unreliable results with this reagent strip test. Drugs containing azo dyes (phenazopyridine), such as Azo Gantrisin, mask test results by causing a golden color.

• Bananas eaten up to 48 hours before the test may increase urobilinogen levels.

Vanillylmandelic acid
(VMA)

Purpose
• To help detect pheochromocytoma, neuroblastoma, and ganglioneuroma
• To evaluate the function of the adrenal medulla

Normal results
Urine VMA levels range from 0.7 to 6.8 mg/24 hours.

Abnormal results
Increased urine VMA levels may result from a catecholamine-secreting tumor. (See *Urine Determinations in Diagnosis of Catecholamine-Secreting Tumors,* and *Urinary Values in Pheochromocytoma,* p. 276.)

The basics
Using spectrophotofluorometry, this test determines urine levels of VMA, a phenolic acid. VMA is the catecholamine metabolite that is normally

most prevalent in the urine, and is the product of hepatic conversion of epinephrine and norepinephrine; urine VMA levels reflect endogenous production of these major catecholamines. Like the test for urine total catecholamines, this test helps detect catecholamine-secreting tumors—most prominently pheochromocytoma—and helps evaluate the function of the adrenal medulla, the primary site of catecholamine production. This test is preferably performed on a 24-hour urine specimen (not a random specimen) to overcome the effects of diurnal variations in catecholamine secretion. Other catecholamine metabolites—metanephrine, normetanephrine, and homovanillic acid—may be measured at the same time.

Procedure
Collect a 24-hour urine specimen in a bottle containing a preservative to keep the specimen at a pH of 3.0. (See "Timed collection," pp. xviii and xix.)

Special precautions
Refrigerate the specimen or keep it on ice during the collection period.

Patient care checklist
Before the test
☑ Explain or clarify test purpose, preparation, and procedure.
☑ Instruct the patient to restrict foods and beverages containing phenolic acid, such as coffee, tea, bananas, citrus fruits, chocolate, and vanilla, for 3 days before the test, and to avoid stressful situations and excessive physical activity during the urine collection period.
☑ Evaluate patient understanding.

Interfering factors
• Epinephrine, norepinephrine, lithium carbonate, and methocarbamol may raise urine VMA levels.
• Chlorpromazine, guinethidine, reserpine, monoamine oxidase inhibitors, and clonidine may lower VMA levels.

• Levodopa and salicylates may raise or lower VMA levels.
• Failure to observe drug restrictions,

Urine Determinations in Diagnosis of Catecholamine-Secreting Tumors

Although a pheochromocytoma is a catecholamine-producing tumor, causing hypersecretion of epinephrine and norepinephrine by the adrenal medulla, not every patient shows elevations of catecholamines in the urine. Moreover, hypertension, a prime clue in this condition, is sometimes absent. Thus, an analysis of one or more catecholamine metabolites offers diagnostic support to an analysis of total catecholamines.

When catecholamines remain normal in the presence of hypertension, elevated vanillylmandelic acid (VMA) may signal a tumor. Or metanephrine may be high, when VMA and catecholamines are essentially unchanged. VMA assay is also an alternate method, when catecholamine analysis has been compromised by interfering food or drugs. Elevated excretion of homovanillic acid (HVA) typically indicates malignant pheochromocytoma, although the incidence of malignancy is very low.

Measurement of urine VMA is diagnostically useful in two neurogenic tumors — neuroblastoma, a common soft-tissue tumor that is a leading cause of death in infants and young children, and ganglioneuroma, a well-defined tumor of the sympathetic nervous system that occurs in older children and young adults. Both tumors primarily produce dopamine and give the expected high readings of dopamine's metabolite HVA, especially in their malignant forms. But both disorders also show abnormal increases in urine VMA.

Urinary Values in Pheochromocytoma

Metabolite	Normal excretion rate (mg/24 hours)	Usual range in pheochromocytoma (mg/24 hours)
Free catecholamines	< 0.1	0.2 to 4
Metanephrines (normetanephrine plus metanephrine)	< 1.3	2.5 to 40
Vanillylmandelic acid	< 6.8	10 to 250

Adapted with permission from Karl Engelman, *Textbook of Medicine*, Vol. 2, edited by Paul B. Beeson and Walsh McDermott (15th ed.; Philadelphia: W.B. Saunders Co., 1979), p. 2204.

if ordered, may adversely affect test results.
• Failure to follow special dietary restrictions may alter test results.
• Failure to collect all urine during the test period may alter test results.
• Failure to store the specimen properly may alter test results.
• Excessive physical exercise or emotional stress may raise VMA levels.

Vitamin B₁
[Thiamine]

Purpose
To help confirm vitamin B₁ deficiency (beriberi) and to distinguish it from other causes of polyneuritis.

Normal results
Urinary excretion ranges from 100 to 200 mcg/24 hours.

Abnormal results
Decreased urine vitamin B₁ levels can result from:
    Inadequate dietary intake
    Hyperthyroidism
    Alcoholism
    Severe hepatic disease
    Chronic diarrhea
    Prolonged diuretic therapy.

The basics
This test is used to detect a deficiency of vitamin B₁ (beriberi). This water-soluble vitamin, which requires folic acid (folate) for effective uptake, is absorbed in the duodenum and excreted in the urine. Urine levels of vitamin B₁ reflect dietary intake and metabolic storage of thiamine. A coenzyme in decarboxylase reactions with citric acids, vitamin B₁ helps metabolize carbohydrates, fats, and proteins.

Rare in the United States, vitamin B₁ deficiency is most common in Orientals, in whom it results from subsistence on polished rice. Vitamin B₁ deficiency may result from inadequate dietary intake (usually associated with alcoholism), impaired absorption (malabsorption syndrome), impaired utilization (hepatic disease), or conditions that increase the metabolic demand (pregnancy, lactation, fever, exercise, hyperthyroidism, surgery, and high carbohydrate intake). High dietary intake of fats and protein spares the vitamin B₁ necessary for tissue respiration.

Procedure
Collect a 24-hour urine specimen. (See "Timed collection," pp. xviii and xix.)

Special precautions
Refrigerate the specimen or place it on ice during the collection period.

Patient care checklist
Before the test
☑ Explain or clarify test purpose and procedure.
☑ Evaluate patient understanding.
After the test
☑ Advise patients who are deficient in vitamin B_1 of good dietary sources of this vitamin: beef, pork, organ meats, fresh vegetables (especially peas and beans), and wheat and other whole grains.

Interfering factors
• Failure to collect all urine during the test period may alter test results.
• Improper specimen storage may alter test results.

Vitamin C
[Ascorbic acid]

Purpose
To aid diagnosis of scurvy, scurvylike conditions, and metabolic disorders, such as malnutrition, that interfere with oxidative processes.

Normal results
Urine vitamin C excretion is 30 mg/ 24 hours.

Abnormal results
Decreased urine vitamin C levels:
  Are associated with:
    Infection
    Cancer
    Burns
    Stress-producing conditions
    Prolonged I.V. therapy without vitamin C replacement.
  May indicate:
    Malnutrition
    Malabsorption
    Renal deficiencies
    Scurvy.

The basics
Through colorimetric measurement of urinary levels, this test determines body stores of vitamin C. This water-soluble vitamin, which is easily absorbed by the intestine, acts as a reversible reducing agent in metabolic processes, aids collagen formation, and helps maintain connective and osteoid tissues. This analysis is particularly useful in diagnosing scurvy, an extreme deficiency of vitamin C characterized by the degeneration of connective and osteoid tissues, dentin, and endothelial membranes. Scurvy is considered uncommon in the United States today. However, it may appear in alcoholics, persons who are on low-residue or low-citrus diets, and infants who have been weaned to cow's milk that does not contain a vitamin C supplement. A random urine sample is analyzed before a 24-hour urine sample is collected and tested.

Procedure
Collect a 24-hour urine specimen. (See "Timed collection," pp. xviii and xix.)

Special precautions
Refrigerate the specimen or place it on ice during the collection period.

Patient care checklist
Before the test
☑ Explain or clarify test purpose and procedure.
☑ Instruct the patient to maintain a normal diet during the collection period.
☑ Evaluate patient understanding.
After the test
☑ Advise the patient with vitamin C deficiency that citrus fruits, tomatoes, potatoes, cabbage, and strawberries are good dietary sources of vitamin C.

Interfering factors
Improper specimen collection and storage may alter test results.

Selected References

Bauer, John D. *Clinical Laboratory Methods.* St. Louis: C.V. Mosby Co., 1982.

Diagnostics, 2nd ed. Nurse's Reference Library. Springhouse, Pa.: Springhouse Corp., 1986.

Duarte, Cristobal G. *Renal Function Tests.* Boston: Little, Brown & Co., 1980.

Endocrine Disorders. Nurse's Clinical Library. Springhouse, Pa.: Springhouse Corp., 1984.

Engram, Barbara White. "Do's and Don'ts of Urologic Nursing: Ten Ways to Improve Your Urologic Nursing Care," *Nursing83* 13:49, October 1983.

Fischbach, Frances. *A Manual of Laboratory Diagnostic Tests,* 2nd ed. Philadelphia: J.B. Lippincott Co., 1984.

Flamenbaum, Walter, and Hamburger, Robert J. *Nephrology: An Approach to the Patient with Renal Disease.* Philadelphia: J.B. Lippincott Co., 1982.

Guyton, Arthur C. *Textbook of Medical Physiology,* 6th ed. Philadelphia: W.B. Saunders Co., 1981.

Hansten, Philip D. *Drug Interactions,* 5th ed. Philadelphia: Lea & Febiger, 1984.

Henry, John Bernard, ed. *Todd-Sanford-Davidsohn Clinical Diagnosis and Management by Laboratory Methods,* vol. 1, 17th ed. Philadelphia: W.B. Saunders Co., 1984.

Kunin, Calvin M. *Detection, Prevention, and Management of Urinary Tract Infections,* 3rd ed. Philadelphia: Lea & Febiger, 1979.

Lamb, Jane O. *Laboratory Tests for Clinical Nursing.* Bowie, Md.: Robert J. Brady Co., 1984.

Lancaster, Larry E. *The Patient with End Stage Renal Disease,* 2nd ed. New York: John Wiley & Sons, 1984.

Leavelle, Dennis E., ed. *Mayo Medical Laboratories Test Catalog.* Rochester, Minn.: Mayo Medical Laboratories, 1984.

Massry, Shaul G., and Glassock, Richard J. *Textbook of Nephrology,* vol. 2. Baltimore: Williams & Wilkins Co., 1983.

McConnell, Edwina A. "Urinalysis: A Common Test, But Never Routine," *Nursing82* 12:108-11, February 1982.

Price, Sylvia, and Wilson, Lorraine. *Pathophysiology: Clinical Concepts of Disease Processes,* 2nd ed. New York: McGraw-Hill Book Co., 1982.

Raphael, Stanley S. *Lynch's Medical Laboratory Technology,* 4th ed. Philadelphia: W.B. Saunders Co., 1983.

Ravel, Richard. *Clinical Laboratory Medicine,* 4th ed. Chicago: Year Book Medical Pubs., 1984.

Renal and Urologic Disorders. Nurse's Clinical Library. Springhouse, Pa.: Springhouse Corp., 1984.

Smith, Donald R. *General Urology,* 10th ed. Los Altos, Calif.: Lange Medical Pubs., 1981.

Stark, June L. "BUN/Creatinine: Your Keys to Kidney Function," *Nursing80* 10:33-38, May 1980.

Tilkian, Sarko M., et al. *Clinical Implications of Laboratory Tests,* 3rd ed. St. Louis: C.V. Mosby Co., 1983.

Widmann, Frances K. *Clinical Interpretation of Laboratory Tests,* 9th ed. Philadelphia: F.A. Davis Co., 1983.

Williams, Robert H. *Textbook of Endocrinology,* 6th ed. Philadelphia: W.B. Saunders Co., 1981.

5 ADDITIONAL BODY FLUID TESTING

Introduction

Body fluids are analyzed for a variety of reasons. Some analyses confirm a diagnosis; others identify the cause and nature of an effusion, and still others have more diverse purposes. In fact, hematologic, chemistry, cytologic, microbiologic, or serologic techniques may be needed. At times, analysis is secondary to therapeutic removal of fluid.

Some procedures to remove body fluids pose serious risks to the patient. An informed consent is needed. Careful assessment for complications during and following procedures is a major nursing function.

Patient-teaching guidelines
Patient-learner objectives:
• Define the test.
• State the specific purpose of the test.
• Explain the procedure.
• Discuss test preparation and procedure and post-test care.
• Identify possible risks or adverse effects.
Teaching content:
• Define the test in terms the patient can understand.
• Explain the specific purpose of the test.
• Describe the procedure. Be sure to describe any positions the patient may have to assume during or after the test. Describe the equipment, which may be unfamiliar and anxiety-producing.
• Inform the patient where the test will be performed. Many of these tests are performed at the bedside; others are performed in a special laboratory or the unit treatment room.
• If applicable, explain that the patient may experience some pain, discomfort, or other sensation, such as tingling, during or after the test. If a local anesthetic will be administered, explain that it will alleviate much discomfort.
• Caution the patient to follow directions carefully. For example, he may be instructed not to move suddenly during a test. Failure to follow the directions may result in a complication and may necessitate a repeat test.
• Inform the patient of any special preparation for the test. For some tests, food, fluids, and certain drugs are restricted for a period of time immediately prior to the test because they may interfere with test results.
• Describe any special care or restrictions following the test. Be sure to explain why they are necessary. If assessment measures will be implemented frequently, alleviate undue patient anxiety by explaining them as a routine precaution.
• Answer any questions the patient may still have after the physician explains the risks and adverse effects associated with the test.
Evaluation:
After the patient-teaching session has been completed, evaluate whether or not the patient has satisfactorily met each patient-learner objective by obtaining necessary patient feedback. Refocus teaching as needed.

Amniotic fluid analysis

Purpose

• To detect fetal abnormalities, particularly chromosomal and neural tube defects, especially Down's syndrome and spina bifida
• To detect hemolytic disease of the newborn
• To diagnose metabolic disorders, amino acid disorders, and mucopolysaccharidoses
• To determine fetal age and maturity, especially pulmonary maturity
• To assess fetal health by detecting the presence of meconium or blood, or measuring amniotic levels of estriol and fetal thyroid hormone
• To identify fetal gender when one or both parents are carriers of a sex-linked disorder.

Normal and abnormal results

For detailed analysis of the appearance and components of amniotic fluid, see *Analysis of Amniotic Fluid,* pp. 281-282.

The basics

Amniocentesis is the transabdominal needle aspiration of 10 to 20 ml of amniotic fluid for laboratory analysis. This test can be performed only when the amniotic fluid level reaches 150 ml, usually after the 16th week of pregnancy.

Amniotic fluid reflects important metabolic changes in the fetus, the placenta, or the mother. It protects the fetus from external trauma, allows fetal movement, and provides an even body temperature and limited source of protein (10% to 15%) for the fetus. Although the origin of amniotic fluid is uncertain, it may arise as a water-permeable transudate from fetal skin, or as a dialysate from the maternal serum through the fetal membranes into the amniotic cavity. Its original composition is essentially the same as that of interstitial fluid. As the fetus matures, however, the amniotic fluid becomes progressively more diluted with hypotonic fetal urine.

One of the chief differences between amniotic fluid and maternal plasma during intrauterine development is the amniotic fluid's relatively high levels of uric acid, urea, and creatinine. The volume of amniotic fluid steadily rises from 50 ml at the end of the first trimester to an average of 1,000 ml near term; at 40 weeks' gestation, the volume decreases to 700 to 800 ml.

Blood in amniotic fluid is usually of maternal origin and does not indicate abnormality. However, it does inhibit cell growth and changes the level of other amniotic fluid constituents.

Testing for *bilirubin* usually is not performed until the 26th week, since that is the earliest time successful therapy for Rh sensitization can begin. Bilirubin level is determined by spectrophotometric measurement of the optic density of the amniotic fluid.

Meconium, a semisolid, viscous material found in the fetal gastrointestinal tract, consists of mucopolysaccharides, desquamated cells, vernix, hair, and cholesterol. Meconium passes into the amniotic fluid when hypoxia causes fetal distress and relaxation of the anal sphincter. Meconium is a normal finding in breech presentation. Meconium in the amniotic fluid produces a peak of 410 mμ on the spectrophotometric analysis. However, serial amniocentesis may show a clearing of meconium over a 2- to 3-week period. If meconium is present during labor, the newborn's nose and throat require thorough cleaning to prevent meconium aspiration.

Alpha-fetoprotein is a fetal alpha globulin produced first in the yolk sac and, later, in the parenchymal cells of the liver and gastrointestinal tract. Although high amniotic fluid levels indicate neural tube defects, the alpha-fetoprotein level may remain normal if the defect is small and closed.

Analysis of Amniotic Fluid

Test	Normal Findings	Fetal Implications of Abnormal Results
Color	Clear, with white flecks of vernix caseosa in a mature fetus	Blood of maternal origin is usually harmless. "Port wine" fluid may indicate abruptio placentae. Fetal blood may indicate damage to the fetal, placental, or umbilical cord vessels by the amniocentesis needle.
Bilirubin	Increases from the 14th to the 24th week of pregnancy, then decreases, gradually reaching zero at term	High levels indicate hemolytic disease of the newborn in isoimmunized pregnancy.
Meconium	Absent (except in breech presentation)	Presence indicates fetal hypotension or distress.
Creatinine	More than 2 mg/100 ml in a mature fetus (increases gradually as fetal kidneys mature)	Decrease may indicate immature fetus (less than 37 weeks old).
Lecithin-sphingo-myelin (L/S) ratio	More than 2 generally indicates fetal pulmonary maturity	Less than 2 indicates pulmonary immaturity and subsequent respiratory distress syndrome.
Phosphatidylglycerol	Present	Absence indicates pulmonary immaturity.
Glucose	Less than 45 mg/100 ml	Excessive increases at term or near term indicate hypertrophied fetal pancreas and subsequent neonatal hypoglycemia.
Insulin	Normally increases from the 27th to the 40th week	Sharp increases (up to 27 times normal) indicate a poorly controlled diabetic patient.
Alpha-fetoprotein	Variable, depending on gestational age and laboratory technique. Highest concentration (about 18.5 mcg/ml) occurs at 13 to 14 weeks.	Inappropriate increases indicate multiple pregnancies, neural tube defects such as spina bifida or anencephaly, omphalocele, esophageal or duodenal atresia, cystic fibrosis, Turner's syndrome, fetal bladder neck obstruction with hydronephrosis, impending fetal death, congenital nephrosis, or contamination by fetal blood.

(continued)

Analysis of Amniotic Fluid (continued)

Test	Normal Findings	Fetal Implications of Abnormal Results
Bacteria	Absent	Presence indicates chorioamnionitis.
Chromosome	Normal karyotype	Abnormal karyotype may indicate fetal sex and chromosome disorders.
Acetylcholinesterase	Absent	Presence may indicate neural tube defects, exomphalos, or other serious malformations.
Uric acid	Increases as the fetus matures but wide fluctuations prevent its being an accurate predictor of fetal maturity	Levels are increased by severe erythroblastosis fetalis, familial hyperuricemia, and Lesch-Nyhan syndrome.
Estrone, estradiol, estriol, estriol conjugates	Occur in varying amounts. Estriol (most prevalent) increases from 25.7 ng/ml during 16th to 20th weeks to almost 1,000 ng/ml at term.	Estriol level is decreased if severe erythroblastosis fetalis occurs.
Enzymes	A total of 25 different enzymes can be identified (usually in low concentrations)	Increased acetylcholinesterase levels may occur with neural tube defects, exomphalos, or other serious malformations.

The Type II cells lining the fetal lung alveoli produce *lecithin* slowly in early pregnancy, and then markedly increase production around the 35th week.

The *sphingomyelin* level parallels that of lecithin until the 35th week, when it gradually decreases. Measuring the ratio of lecithin to sphingomyelin (L/S ratio) confirms fetal pulmonary maturity (L/S ratio > 2) or suggests a risk of respiratory distress (L/S ratio < 2). However, fetal respiratory distress may develop in the fetus of a patient with diabetes, even though the L/S ratio is greater than 2.

Measuring *glucose* levels in the fluid can aid in assessing glucose control in the patient with diabetes, but this is not done routinely.

When the mother carries an *X-linked disorder,* determination of fetal sex is important. If chromosome karyotyping identifies a male fetus, there is a 50% chance he will be affected; a female fetus will not be affected, but has a 50% chance of being a carrier.

Amniocentesis is indicated during pregnancy associated with advanced maternal age (over 35); family history of genetic, chromosomal, or neural tube defects; or previous miscarriage. Adverse effects from this test are rare; potential risks include spontaneous abortion, trauma to the fetus or placenta, bleeding, premature labor, infection, and Rh sensitization from fetal bleeding into the maternal circulation. However, because such complications are possible, amniocentesis is contraindicated as a general screening test.

Abnormal test results or failure of the tissue cultures to grow may necessitate repetition of the test.

Procedure
• Instruct the patient to fold her hands behind her head to prevent her from accidentally touching the sterile field and causing contamination.
• Fetal and placental position are determined, usually through palpation and ultrasonic visualization, and then the physician locates a pool of amniotic fluid.
• The patient's skin is prepared with an antiseptic and alcohol.
• 1 ml of 1% lidocaine is injected with a 25G needle, first intradermally and then subcutaneously.
• A 20G spinal needle with a stylet is inserted into the amniotic cavity and the stylet is withdrawn.
• A 10-ml syringe is attached to the needle; the fluid is aspirated and placed in an amber or foil-covered test tube; then the needle is withdrawn.
• An adhesive bandage is placed over the needle insertion site.

The APT Test

Blood in the amniotic fluid can be of maternal or fetal origin. The APT test, based on the premise that fetal hemoglobin is alkali-resistant and adult hemoglobin changes to alkaline hematin after the addition of alkali, can differentiate the two. This test may be performed on all bloody amniotic fluid samples.

Dilute 1 ml of amniotic fluid with water until it turns pink. Centrifuge for 10 minutes, and decant the supernatant. Add five parts supernatant to one part 0.25 N (1%) sodium hydroxide, and observe for 1 or 2 minutes. Fetal blood appears red; maternal blood, yellow-brown. To confirm results, repeat the test with known maternal blood.

Shake Test or Foam Stability Test

Amniotic fluid from mature fetal lungs contains surface-active material (surfactants). In this test, bubbles should appear on the surface of a test tube of amniotic fluid that is shaken vigorously if adequate amounts of surfactants are present.

Numerically label five clean, dry test tubes and add 1 ml, 0.75 ml, 0.50 ml, 0.25 ml, and 0.20 ml of amniotic fluid to test tubes 1, 2, 3, 4, and 5 respectively. Add normal saline: 0.25 ml, 0.50 ml, 0.75 ml, and 0.80 ml to tubes 2, 3, 4, and 5. Then add 1 ml of 95% ethanol to each test tube. Cap each test tube with a clean rubber stopper (do not use your finger since it contains surface-active material). Shake each test tube for 15 seconds and place upright in rack (undisturbed) for 15 minutes.

A complete ring of bubbles is a positive result. Negative results in tube 1 (the 1:1 dilution) indicate a high risk of respiratory distress syndrome (RDS). A positive result in tube 3 (1:2 dilution) indicates pulmonary maturity. Negative results in the other tubes indicate varying degrees of RDS risk (62% develop mild-to-severe respiratory problems). Blood or meconium in the fluid invalidates the test.

Patient care checklist
Before the test
☑ Explain or clarify test purpose and procedure.
☑ Evaluate patient understanding.
☑ Make sure the patient has signed a consent form.
☑ Instruct the patient to void immediately before the test. (This will minimize the risk of puncturing the bladder and aspirating urine instead of amniotic fluid.)
After the test
☑ Monitor fetal heart rate and ma-

Chorionic Villi Sampling

Chorionic villi sampling, or biopsy, is an experimental prenatal test that may someday replace amniocentesis for quick, safe detection of fetal chromosomal and biochemical disorders. Developed in Europe and now being tested in the United States, the procedure is performed during the first trimester of pregnancy. Preliminary results may be available within hours; complete results, within a few days. In contrast, amniocentesis cannot be performed before the 16th week of pregnancy, and the results are not available for at least 2 weeks. Thus, chorionic villi sampling offers the advantage of earlier detection of fetal abnormalities.

The chorionic villi are fingerlike projections that surround the embryonic membrane and eventually give rise to the placenta. Cells obtained from an appropriate sample are of fetal, rather than maternal, origin and thus can be analyzed for fetal abnormalities. Samples are best obtained between the 8th and 10th weeks of pregnancy. Before 7 weeks, the villi cover the embryo and make

selective sampling difficult. After 10 weeks, maternal cells begin to grow over the villi and the amniotic sac begins to fill the uterine cavity, making the procedure difficult and potentially dangerous.

To collect a chorionic villi sample, place the patient in the lithotomy position. The physician will check the placement of the patient's uterus bimanually and then insert a Graves speculum and swab the cervix with an antiseptic solution. If necessary, he may use a tenaculum to straighten an acutely flexed uterus, to permit cannula insertion. Guided by ultrasound and, possibly, endoscopy, he will direct the catheter through the cannula to the villi. Suction will be applied to the catheter to remove about 30 mg of tissue from the villi. The sample will be withdrawn, placed in a Petri dish, and examined with a dissecting microscope. Part of the specimen will then be cultured for further testing.

Results of a chorionic villi testing can be used to detect about 200 diseases prenatally. For example, direct analysis of rapidly dividing

---

ternal vital signs every 15 minutes for at least 30 minutes.

☑ If the patient feels faint or nauseated, or sweats profusely, position her on her left side to counteract uterine pressure on her vena cava.

CLINICAL ALERT: **Before the patient is discharged, instruct her to notify the physician immediately if she experiences abdominal pain or cramping, chills, fever, vaginal bleeding or leakage of serous vaginal fluid, or fetal hyperactivity or unusual fetal lethargy.**

☑ Evaluate patient understanding.

Interfering factors

• Failure to place the fluid specimen in an appropriate amber or foil-covered

tube may result in abnormally low bilirubin levels.

• Blood or meconium in the fluid adversely affects the L/S ratio.

• Maternal blood in the fluid may lower creatinine levels.

• Fetal blood in the fluid specimen invalidates the alpha-fetoprotein results, since even small amounts of fetal blood (50 μl/10 ml) can double alpha-fetoprotein concentrations.

• Several disorders that are not associated with pregnancy (including infectious mononucleosis, cirrhosis, hepatic cancer, teratoma, endodermal sinus tumor, gastric carcinoma, pancreatic carcinoma, and subacute hereditary tyrosinemia) can cause increased alpha-fetoprotein levels.

•

fetal cells can detect chromosome disorders; DNA analysis can detect hemoglobinopathies; and lysosomal enzyme assays can screen for lysosomal storage disorders, such as Tay-Sachs disease.

The test appears to provide reliable results except when the sample contains too few cells or the cells fail to grow in culture. Patient risks for this procedure are considered similar to those for amniocentesis—there is a slight chance of spontaneous abortion, cramps, infection, and bleeding.

Unlike amniocentesis, chorionic villi sampling cannot detect complications in cases of Rh sensitization, uncover neural tube defects, or determine pulmonary maturity. However, it may prove to be the best way to detect other serious fetal abnormalities early in pregnancy.

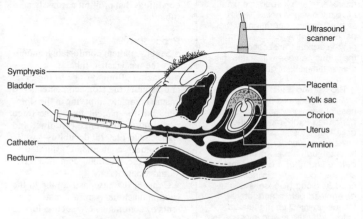

• Disposable plastic syringes can be toxic to amniotic fluid cells.
(See also *The APT Test*, p. 283; *Shake Test or Foam Stability Test*, p. 283; and *Chorionic Villi Sampling*.)

Basal gastric secretion test

Purpose
To determine gastric output in the fasting state.

Normal results
Basal secretion ranges:
Females: 0.2 to 3.8 mEq/hour
Males: 1 to 5 mEq/hour.

Abnormal results
Increased basal secretion:
   Duodenal or jejunal ulcer (after partial gastrectomy).
Markedly increased:
   Zollinger-Ellison syndrome.
Decreased secretion:
   Gastric carcinoma
   Benign gastric ulcer.
Absence of secretion:
   Pernicious anemia.

The basics
Although gastric secretion peaks after ingestion of food, small amounts of gastric juice are also secreted between meals. This secretion, known as basal secretion, results from psychoneurogenic influences mediated by the va-

gus nerves and by hormones, such as gastrin.

This test measures basal secretion under fasting conditions by aspirating stomach contents through a nasogastric tube, and is indicated in patients with obscure epigastric pain, anorexia, and weight loss. Since external factors—such as the sight or odor of food—and psychological stress stimulate gastric secretion, accurate testing requires that the patient be isolated from all sources of sensory stimulation. Although abnormal basal secretion can suggest various gastric and duodenal disorders, these findings are nonspecific, and complete evaluation of secretion requires the gastric acid stimulation test.

Contraindications to this test include: conditions that prohibit nasogastric intubation.

Procedure

• Seat the patient comfortably, and insert the nasogastric tube.
• Attach a 20-ml syringe to the tube, and aspirate the stomach contents. To ensure complete emptying of the stomach, ask the patient to assume three positions in sequence—supine, and right and left lateral decubitus—while the stomach contents are aspirated.
• Label the specimen container "Residual Contents."
• Connect the nasogastric tube to the suction machine. Aspirate gastric contents by continuous low suction for 1½ hours. (Aspiration can also be performed manually, with a syringe.)
• Collect a specimen every 15 minutes, but discard the first two; this eliminates the specimen that could be influenced by the stress of the intubation.
• Record the color and odor of each specimen, and note the presence of food, mucus, bile, or blood. Label these specimens "Basal Contents," and number them 1 through 4.
• Remove the nasogastric tube or, if the nasogastric tube is to be left in place, clamp it or attach it to low intermittent suction, as ordered.

Special precautions

• During insertion, make sure the na-

The Hollander Test

I.V. injection of insulin in a patient with a normal blood glucose level causes hypoglycemia by promoting cellular absorption of glucose. In turn, hypoglycemia affects the vagus nerve, which stimulates acid secretion by the parietal and chief cells. A vagotomy—surgical transection of the vagus nerves—eliminates this neural stimulus for gastric acid secretion.

The Hollander test (insulin gastric analysis) evaluates the effectiveness of vagotomy and is best performed 3 to 6 months after surgery. In this test, gastric contents are aspirated under fasting conditions through a nasogastric tube, before and after a dose of insulin, and then compared; simultaneously, blood glucose levels are determined before and after the insulin injection. If the acid output after the insulin injection exceeds the preinjection acid output, the vagotomy is likely to be incomplete; if acid output fails to rise after the insulin injection, the vagotomy is considered complete. However, failure to increase acid output is significant only if achlorhydria persists after blood glucose falls below 50 mg/dl.

The Hollander test is contraindicated in patients with coronary artery or cerebrovascular disease, a predisposition to hypoglycemia, or other conditions that prohibit nasogastric intubation. It is not useful in patients with achlorhydria, as demonstrated by the gastric acid stimulation test, since such patients fail to respond to insulin injection.

sogastric tube enters the esophagus, and not the trachea; remove it immediately if the patient develops cyanosis or paroxysms of coughing.

• Monitor vital signs during intubation, and observe the patient carefully for dysrrhythmias.

• To prevent contamination of the specimens with saliva, instruct the patient to expectorate excess saliva.

Patient care checklist
Before the test

☑ Explain or clarify test purpose and procedure.

☑ Tell the patient that the test will take approximately 1½ hours (or 2½ hours if followed by the gastric acid stimulation test).

☑ Evaluate patient understanding.

☑ Restrict food for 12 hours prior to the test.

☑ Restrict fluids and smoking for 8 hours prior to the test.

☑ Withhold medications that may interfere with test results for 24 hours prior to the test, as ordered. If medications must be continued, note this on the laboratory slip.

☑ Just before the test, check the patient's pulse rate and blood pressure, then encourage the patient to relax.

After the test

☑ Observe the patient for complications—such as nausea, vomiting, or abdominal distention or pain—following removal of the nasogastric tube.

Interfering factors

• Failure to adhere to pretest restrictions increases basal secretion.

• Psychological stress can stimulate excessive basal secretion.

• Cholinergics, reserpine, alcohol, adrenergic blockers, and adrenocorticosteroids may increase basal secretion.

• Antacids, anticholinergics, and cimetidine may depress basal secretion. (See *The Hollander Test*.)

Cerebrospinal fluid analysis *(CSF)*

Purpose

• To measure CSF pressure as an aid in detecting obstruction of CSF circulation

• To aid in diagnosis of viral or bacterial meningitis, subarachnoid or intracranial hemorrhage, tumors, and brain abscesses

• To aid in diagnosis of neurosyphilis and chronic central nervous system (CNS) infections.

Normal and abnormal results

See *CSF Findings*, p. 288, for a summary of the findings in CSF analysis.

The basics

CSF, a clear substance that circulates in the subarachnoid space, has many vital functions. It protects the brain and spinal cord from injury and transports products of neurosecretion, cellular biosynthesis, and cellular metabolism through the CNS. For qualitative analysis, CSF is most commonly obtained by lumbar puncture (usually between the third and fourth lumbar vertebrae) and, occasionally, by cisternal or ventricular puncture. A sample of CSF for laboratory analysis is frequently obtained during other neurologic tests, including myelography and pneumoencephalography.

During the procedure, three tubes of CSF are normally collected. These are sent to the laboratory for analysis of protein, sugar, and cells, as well as for serologic testing, such as the Venereal Disease Research Laboratory (VDRL) test for neurosyphilis. A separate specimen is also sent to the laboratory for culture and sensitivity testing. Electrolyte analysis and Gram stain may be ordered as supplementary tests. CSF electrolyte levels are of special interest in patients with abnormal serum electrolyte levels or CSF infec-

CSF Findings

Test	Normal	Abnormal	Implications
Pressure	50 to 180 mm H_2O	Increase	Increased intracranial pressure due to hemorrhage, tumor, or edema caused by trauma
		Decrease	Spinal subarachnoid obstruction above puncture site
Appearance	Clear, colorless	Cloudy	Infection (elevated white blood cell [WBC] count and protein, or many microorganisms)
		Xanthochromic or bloody	Subarachnoid, intracerebral, or intraventricular hemorrhage; spinal cord obstruction; traumatic tap (usually noted only in initial specimen)
		Brown, orange, or yellow	Elevated protein, red blood cell (RBC) breakdown (blood present for at least 3 days)
Protein	15 to 45 mg/100 ml	Marked increase	Tumors, trauma, hemorrhage, diabetes mellitus, polyneuritis, blood in cerebrospinal fluid (CSF)
		Marked decrease	Rapid CSF production
Gamma globulin	3% to 12% of total protein	Increase	Demyelinating disease (such as multiple sclerosis), neurosyphilis, Guillain-Barré syndrome

tion, or in those receiving hyperosmolar agents.
Contraindications to this test include: infection at the puncture site, an uncooperative patient, and severe degenerative spinal joint disease.

In a patient with increased intracranial pressure, CSF should be removed with extreme caution, if at all, since the rapid reduction in pressure that follows withdrawal of fluid can cause cerebellar tonsillar herniation and medullary compression.

Procedure
• Position the patient on his side at the edge of the bed, with his knees drawn up to his abdomen and his chin on his chest.
• Provide pillows to support the patient's spine on a horizontal plane. (With the patient in this position, full flexion of the spine and easy access to the lumbar subarachnoid space are possible.)
• Help the patient maintain this position by placing one arm around his knees and the other arm around his neck. (If a sitting position is preferred, have the patient sit up and bend his chest and head toward his knees. Help him maintain this position throughout the procedure.)

Test	Normal	Abnormal	Implications
Glucose	50 to 80 mg/ 100 ml (⅔ of blood glucose)	Increase	Systemic hyperglycemia
		Decrease	Systemic hypoglycemia, bacterial or fungal infection, meningitis, mumps, postsubarachnoid hemorrhage
Cell count	0 to 5 WBCs	Increase	Active disease: meningitis, acute infection, onset of chronic illness, tumor, abscess, infarction, demyelinating disease (such as multiple sclerosis)
	No RBCs	RBCs	Hemorrhage or traumatic tap
VDRL and other serologic tests	Nonreactive	Positive	Neurosyphilis
Chloride	118 to 130 mEq/liter	Decrease	Infected meninges (as in tuberculosis or meningitis)
Gram stain	No organisms	Gram-positive or gram-negative organisms	Bacterial meningitis

• After the skin has been prepared for injection, the area will be draped. (During this time, warn the patient that he will probably experience a transient burning sensation when the local anesthetic is injected. Tell him that when the spinal needle is inserted, he may feel some local, transient pain. Ask him to report any pain or sensations that differ from or continue after this expected discomfort. These may indicate irritation or puncture of a nerve root, requiring repositioning of the needle.)
• Instruct the patient to remain still and breathe normally; movement and hyperventilation can alter pressure readings or cause injury.
• The anesthetic will be injected and the spinal needle inserted in the midline, between the spinous processes of the vertebrae (usually between the third and fourth lumbar vertebrae).
• The stylet will be removed from the needle. CSF will drip from the needle if it is properly positioned.
• A stopcock and manometer are attached to the needle to measure initial (or opening) CSF pressure. This pressure will be recorded.
• The physician will then check the appearance of the CSF.

Alternate Methods For Obtaining CSF

Cisternal Puncture

When lumbar puncture is contraindicated by infection at the puncture site, lumbar deformity, or some other problem, the physician may perform a cisternal puncture to obtain cerebrospinal fluid (CSF). A short-beveled, hollow needle is inserted into the cisterna cerebellomedullaris, below the occipital bone, between the first cervical vertebra and rim of the foramen magnum. Adverse effects are minimal; the severe headaches that often occur after lumbar puncture are uncommon with this procedure. Cisternal puncture is hazardous, however, because the needle is positioned close to the brain stem. Contraindications are the same as for lumbar puncture—infection or deformity at the puncture site, or increased intracranial pressure.

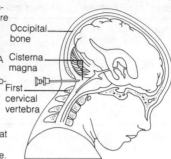

Prepare the patient as for lumbar puncture; a cisternal puncture tray contains the necessary equipment. The patient's neck should be flexed forward, so his chin touches his chest. Hold his head firmly in place to bring the brain stem and spinal cord forward and allow more space for the cisternal needle to enter. (If the physician prefers, the patient may assume a sitting position, with his neck flexed forward.)

Post-test care is the same as for lumbar puncture. If the procedure was performed on an outpatient, instruct a family member to check the puncture site for redness, swelling, and drainage and to observe the patient for signs of complications, such as neck rigidity, irritability, and decreased level of consciousness.

Ventricular Puncture

Although rarely performed, ventricular puncture is the procedure of choice when a spinal puncture may cause brain stem herniation or other complications. Ventricular puncture is usually done in the operating room. The physician makes a small incision in the parieto-occipital region of the scalp, then drills a hole in the skull. A short-beveled, hollow needle is inserted through the hole and into a lateral ventricle, and CSF is withdrawn. Complications—such as ventriculitis and hemorrhage from ruptured blood vessels—are rare. Post-test care is the same as for lumbar puncture, but do not elevate the head of the patient's bed more than 15° to

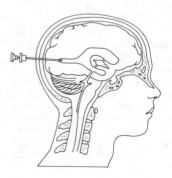

20°. Bed rest for 24 hours is usually prescribed.

• After the specimen has been collected, label the containers in the order in which they were filled, and ask the physician if he has any specific instructions for the laboratory. (See "The basics," p. 287, for more information.)

• A final pressure reading will be taken and the needle removed.

• Clean the puncture site with a local antiseptic, such as povidone-iodine solution, and apply a small adhesive bandage. (See *Alternate Methods for Obtaining CSF.*)

Special precautions

• Infection at the puncture site contraindicates removal of CSF.

CLINICAL ALERT: **During the procedure, observe the patient closely for signs of adverse reaction, such as elevated pulse rate, pallor, or clammy skin. Alert the physician immediately to any significant changes.**

• Record the collection time on the test request form.

Patient care checklist

Before the test

☑ Explain or clarify test purpose, procedure, and possible complications.

☑ Advise the patient that a headache is the most common adverse effect of a lumbar puncture. Reassure the patient that his cooperation during the test will minimize this effect.

☑ Evaluate patient understanding.

☑ Make sure the consent form is signed by the patient or a responsible family member.

☑ Assess vital signs, and notify the physician if the patient appears unusually anxious.

After the test

☑ Keep the patient lying flat, or elevate the head of his bed slightly, as ordered. (In most cases, you will be instructed to keep the patient lying flat for 8 hours after lumbar puncture. Some physicians, however, allow a 30° elevation at the head of the bed.) Re-

mind the patient that, although he must not raise his head, he can turn from side to side.

☑ Evaluate patient understanding.

☑ Encourage the patient to drink fluids. Provide a flexible straw.

☑ Check the puncture site for redness, swelling, and drainage every hour for the first 4 hours, then every 4 hours for the next 24 hours.

☑ If CSF pressure is elevated, assess neurologic status every 15 minutes for 4 hours. If the patient is stable, assess every hour for 2 hours, then every 4 hours or according to the pretest schedule.

Testing For Queckenstedt's Sign

If an obstruction in the spinal subarachnoid space is suspected, you may be asked to assist with testing for Queckenstedt's sign. After inserting the spinal needle, the physician will take an initial cerebral spinal fluid (CSF) pressure reading and then ask you to compress one or both of the patient's jugular veins with your fingers for 10 seconds. This obstructs blood flow from the cranium, increasing intracranial pressure and, in the absence of a subarachnoid block, causing CSF pressure to rise also. A partial subarachnoid block may cause CSF pressure to rise sluggishly; a complete block prevents it from rising at all.

Normally, the fluid column in the manometer should rise after 10 seconds of compression, then fall to the patient's initial pressure within 30 seconds. CSF pressure is recorded every 5 seconds from the time you begin compression until the pressure returns to baseline.

Because of the obvious danger of cerebellar tonsillar herniation and medullary compression, testing for Queckenstedt's sign is contraindicated in a patient with increased intracranial pressure.

CLINICAL ALERT: Observe the patient for complications of lumbar puncture, such as reaction to the anesthetic, bleeding into the spinal canal, and cerebellar tonsillar herniation and medullary compression. Signs of meningitis include fever, neck rigidity, and irritability; signs of herniation include decreased level of consciousness, changes in pupil size and equality, altered vital signs (including widened pulse pressure, decreased pulse rate, and irregular respirations), or respiratory failure.

Interfering factors
• The patient's position and activity can alter CSF pressure. Crying, coughing, or straining may increase pressure.
• Delay between collection time and laboratory testing can invalidate results, especially cell counts. (See *Testing for Queckenstedt's Sign*, p. 291.)

Gastric acid stimulation test

Purpose
To aid in diagnosis of duodenal ulcer, Zollinger-Ellison syndrome, pernicious anemia, and gastric carcinoma.

Normal results
Gastric secretion following stimulation ranges from 11 to 21 mEq/hour for females and from 18 to 28 mEq/hour for males.

Abnormal results
Markedly increased gastric secretion:
    Zollinger-Ellison syndrome.
Increased secretion:
    Duodenal ulcer.
Decreased secretion:
    Gastric carcinoma.
Achlorhydria:
    Pernicious anemia.

The basics
The gastric acid stimulation test mea-

sures the secretion of gastric acid for 1 hour after subcutaneous injection of pentagastrin or a similar drug that stimulates gastric acid output. It is indicated and usually immediately performed when the basal secretion test suggests abnormal gastric secretion.

Pentagastrin stimulates the parietal cells to secrete hydrochloric acid. If these cells are damaged or destroyed, acid secretion decreases or is absent; if the cells are hyperactive, acid secretion increases. Although this test detects abnormal gastric secretion, radiographic studies and endoscopy are necessary to determine the cause.

Contraindications to the test include: hypersensitivity to pentagastrin and conditions that prohibit nasogastric intubation.

Procedure
• Keep the nasogastric tube in place after basal gastric secretions have been collected.
• Record baseline vital signs.
• After subcutaneous injection of pentagastrin, observe the patient for adverse reactions to this substance during the test.
• Wait 15 minutes, and then collect a specimen every 15 minutes for 1 hour. Record the color and odor of each specimen, and note the presence of food, mucus, bile, or blood. Label all specimens "Stimulated Contents" and number them 1 through 4.
• If the nasogastric tube is to be left in place, clamp it or attach it to low intermittent suction, as ordered.

Special precautions
To prevent contamination of the specimens with saliva, instruct the patient to expectorate excess saliva.

Patient care checklist
Before the test
☑ Explain or clarify test purpose, procedure, and possible adverse effects such as abdominal pain, nausea, vomiting, flushing, transitory dizziness, faintness, and numbness of ex-

tremities. Instruct the patient to report such symptoms immediately.

☑ Evaluate patient understanding.

☑ Withhold medications that might interfere with test results. If they must be continued, note on laboratory slip.

After the test

☑ Observe the patient for complications such as nausea, vomiting, or abdominal distention or pain after removal of the nasogastric tube.

Interfering factors

• Failure to adhere to pretest restrictions may alter test results.

• Cholinergics, adrenergic blockers, and reserpine elevate gastric acid levels.

• Antacids, anticholinergics, and cimetidine depress gastric acid levels.

Pericardial fluid analysis
[Pericardiocentesis]

Purpose

To assist in identifying the cause of pericardial effusion and to help determine appropriate therapy.

Normal results

Pericardial fluid is clear and straw-colored, without evidence of pathogens, blood, or malignant cells. It contains less than 1,000 white blood cells/mm³. Its glucose concentration approximately equals the levels in whole blood.

Abnormal results

Pericardial effusions can be characteristic in:

Pericarditis
Neoplasms
Acute myocardial infarction
Tuberculosis
Rheumatoid disease
Systemic lupus erythematosus
Dissecting aortic aneurysm
Penetrating thoracic trauma
Dressler's syndrome

Closed chest trauma
Postcardiotomy syndrome.

The basics

Although this procedure is most useful as an emergency measure to relieve cardiac tamponade, pericardial fluid analysis provides a fluid sample to confirm diagnosis and identify the cause of pericardial effusion. However, pericardiocentesis, the needle aspiration of pericardial fluid, has both therapeutic and diagnostic purposes.

Normally, 10 to 50 ml of sterile fluid is present in the pericardium. Small amounts of plasma-derived fluid within the pericardium lubricate the heart, reducing friction during expansions and contractions. Excess pericardial fluid, pericardial effusion, may accumulate after inflammation, rupture, or penetrating trauma (gunshot or stab wounds) of the pericardium. Rapidly forming effusions, such as those after penetrating trauma, may induce cardiac tamponade—a potentially lethal syndrome marked by increased intrapericardial pressure that prevents complete ventricular filling and thus reduces cardiac output. Slowly forming effusions, such as those in pericarditis, generally pose less immediate danger since they allow the pericardium more time to adapt to the accumulating fluid.

Generally, pericardial effusions are classified as transudates or exudates. Transudates are protein-poor effusions that usually arise from mechanical factors altering fluid formation or resorption, such as increased hydrostatic pressure, decreased plasma oncotic pressure, or obstruction of the pericardial lymphatic drainage system by a tumor.

Most exudates result from inflammation and contain large amounts of protein. In these effusions, inflammation damages the capillary membrane, allowing protein molecules to leak into the pericardial fluid. Blood-tinged fluid may be caused by a traumatic tap. If so, it will clear as aspiration continues.

Pericardiocentesis should be performed cautiously because of the risk of potentially fatal complications, such as laceration of a coronary artery or of the myocardium; its other complications include ventricular fibrillation or vasovagal arrest, pleural infection, and accidental puncture of the lung, liver, or stomach. If possible, echocardiography should determine the effusion site before pericardiocentesis is performed, to minimize the risk of complications. Generally, surgical drainage and biopsy are safer procedures.

Procedure

• Start an I.V. line at a keep-vein-open rate (20 ml/hour).
• Administer premedication, as ordered.
• Assemble and prepare equipment, including the pericardiocentesis tray.
• Place the patient in a supine position with his thorax elevated 60°.
• When the patient is comfortable and well-supported, instruct him to remain still during the procedure.
• The patient's skin will be prepared with alcohol or povidone-iodine solution from the left costal margin to the xiphoid process.
• A local anesthetic will be administered at the insertion site.
• With the three-way stopcock open, a 50-ml syringe will be aseptically attached to one end and the cardiac needle to the other end.
• Using an alligator clip, the EKG lead wire will be attached to the hub of the needle.
• The EKG machine will be set to lead V, and turned on. (Or the patient will be connected to a bedside monitor.)
• The needle will be inserted through the chest wall into the pericardial sac, maintaining gentle aspiration until fluid appears in the syringe.
• The needle will be angled 35° to 45° toward the tip of the left costal margin and the xiphoid process; this subxiphoid approach minimizes the risk of lacerating the coronary vessels or the pleura.
• Once the needle has been properly positioned, a Kelly clamp will be attached to the needle at the skin surface so it will not advance further.
• While the fluid is being aspirated, the specimen tubes should be labeled and numbered.
• When the needle has been withdrawn, pressure should be applied to the site *immediately* with sterile gauze pads for 3 to 5 minutes, then a bandage should be applied.

Special precautions

CLINICAL ALERT: **Ensure that the EKG machine is properly grounded to prevent accidental ventricular fibrillation.**
• Carefully observe the EKG tracing during insertion of the cardiac needle: an ST segment elevation indicates that the needle has reached the epicardial surface and should be retracted slightly; an abnormally shaped QRS complex may indicate perforation of the myocardium. Premature ventricular contractions usually indicate that the needle has touched the ventricular wall.
• Watch for grossly bloody aspirate— a sign of inadvertent puncture of a cardiac chamber.
• Be sure to use specimen tubes with the proper additives. Although fibrin is not a normal component of pericardial fluid, it does appear in fluid in some pericardial diseases and in carcinoma, and clotting is possible.
• If bacterial culture and sensitivity tests are scheduled, record any antibiotic therapy on the laboratory slip. If anaerobic organisms are suspected, consult the laboratory concerning the proper collection technique to avoid exposing the aspirate to air. The aspirate may be placed in an anaerobic collection tube or the syringe may be filled completely, displacing all air, and the collection tube capped tightly with a sterile rubber tip.

Patient care checklist
Before the test

☑ Explain or clarify test purpose, preparation, procedure, and possible complications to the patient or a responsible family member if the patient is in shock.

☑ Tell the patient that the test will take 10 to 20 minutes.

☑ Tell the patient that, although fluid aspiration is not painful, he may experience pressure upon insertion of the needle into the pericardial sac.

☑ Advise the patient that he may be asked to briefly hold his breath to aid needle insertion and placement.

☑ Evaluate patient understanding.

☑ Make sure the consent form is signed by the patient or a responsible family member.

☑ Review the patient history for current antibiotic usage. Such usage should be recorded on the laboratory request form.

After the test

☑ Check the patient's blood pressure, pulse, respiration, and heart sounds every 15 minutes until stable, then every ½ hour for 2 hours, every hour for 4 hours, and every 4 hours thereafter. Reassure the patient that such monitoring is routine.

CLINICAL ALERT: **Observe the patient for respiratory or cardiac distress. Watch especially for signs of cardiac tamponade: muffled and distant heart sounds, distended neck veins, paradoxical pulse, and shock. Cardiac tamponade may result from rapid reaccumulation of pericardial fluid or puncture of a coronary vessel causing bleeding into the pericardial sac.**

Interfering factors

• Failure of aseptic technique can impair microbiologic analysis of the sample, since skin contaminants may be isolated and mistaken for causative organisms.

• Antibiotic therapy can prevent isolation of the causative organism.

• Failure to use the proper additives in test tubes may alter test results.

Peritoneal fluid analysis

Purpose

• To determine the cause of ascites
• To detect abdominal trauma.

Normal results

The accompanying chart gives normal values for peritoneal fluid. (See *Peritoneal Fluid Analysis,* p. 296.)

Abnormal results
Milk-colored peritoneal fluid
(may result from chyle escaping from a damaged or blocked thoracic duct):
Carcinoma
Lymphoma
Tuberculosis
Parasitic infection
Adhesion
Hepatic cirrhosis
Pseudochylous conditions that may result from the presence of leukocytes or tumor cells.
Cloudy or turbid fluid:
Peritonitis caused by primary bacterial infection
Ruptured bowel (after trauma)
Pancreatitis
Strangulated or infarcted intestine
Appendicitis.
Bloody fluid:
Benign or malignant tumor
Hemorrhagic pancreatitis
A traumatic tap (however, if the fluid fails to clear on continued aspiration, traumatic tap is not the cause).
Bile-stained green fluid:
Ruptured gallbladder
Acute pancreatitis
Perforated intestine
Duodenal ulcer.
Increased red blood cell count:
Over 100/μl:
Neoplasm
Tuberculosis.

Peritoneal Fluid Analysis

Element	Normal Value or Finding
Gross appearance	Sterile, odorless, clear to pale yellow color; scant amount (< 50 ml)
RBCs	None
WBCs	< 300/µl
Protein	0.3 to 4.1 g/dl (albumin, 50% to 70%; globulin, 30% to 45%; fibrinogen, 0.3% to 4.5%)
Glucose	70 to 100 mg/dl
Amylase	138 to 404 amylase units/liter
Ammonia	< 50 mcg/dl
Alkaline phosphatase	Male: > age 18—90 to 239 units/liter Female: < age 45—76 to 196 units/liter Female: > age 45—87 to 250 units/liter
LDH	Equal to serum level
Cytology	No malignant cells present
Bacteria	None
Fungi	None

Over 100,000/µl:
    Intraabdominal trauma.
White blood cell count over 300/µl:
    With 25% neutrophils:
        Spontaneous bacterial peritonitis
        Cirrhosis.
    With high percentage of lymphocytes:
        Tuberculous peritonitis
        Chylous ascites.
    With numerous mesothelial cells:
        Tuberculosis
        Peritonitis.
Glucose levels below 60 mg/dl:
    Tuberculous peritonitis (30% to 50% of affected patients)
    Peritoneal carcinomatosis.
Increased amylase levels:
    Pancreatic trauma (90% of patients)
    Pancreatic pseudocyst
    Acute pancreatitis

Intestinal necrosis
Intestinal strangulation.
Increased peritoneal alkaline phosphatase levels (more than twice normal):
    Ruptured or strangulated small intestine (90% of affected patients).
Increased peritoneal ammonia levels (twice normal):
    Ruptured or strangulated large and small intestines
    Ruptured ulcer or appendix.
Protein ascitic fluid/serum ratio of 0.5 or greater; lactate dehydrogenase (LDH) ascitic fluid/serum ratio over 0.6; ascitic fluid LDH level over 400 µ/ml:
    Malignant tuberculosis
    Pancreatic ascites.
    Any two of above findings:
        Indicates a nonhepatic cause.

None of the above findings:
Suggests uncomplicated hepatic disease.

Albumin gradient over 1 g/dl between ascitic fluid and serum:
Chronic hepatic disease.

A lesser albumin gradient suggests:
Malignancy.

Positive for bacteria:
Coliforms, anaerobes, and enterococci may indicate:
Ruptured organ or infections accompanying appendicitis, pancreatitis, tuberculosis, or ovarian disease.

Positive for Gram-positive cocci:
Primary peritonitis
Gram-negative organisms
Secondary peritonitis.

Positive for fungi:
Histoplasmosis
Candidiasis
Coccidioidomycosis.

The basics

Accumulation of fluid in the peritoneal space—ascites—can be caused by conditions such as hepatic, renal, or cardiovascular disorders; inflammation; infection; or neoplasm.

Peritoneal fluid analysis includes examination of gross appearance, erythrocyte and leukocyte counts, cytologic studies, microbiologic studies for bacteria and fungi, and determinations of protein, glucose, amylase, ammonia, and alkaline phosphatase levels.

This test assesses a sample of peritoneal fluid obtained by paracentesis, a procedure that entails inserting a trocar and cannula through the abdominal wall with the patient under a local anesthetic. If the sample of fluid is being removed for therapeutic purposes, the trocar can be connected to a drainage system. If only a small amount of fluid is being removed for diagnostic purposes, an 18G needle can be substituted for the trocar and cannula. In a four-quadrant tap, fluid is aspirated from each quadrant of the abdomen to verify abdominal trauma and confirm the need for surgery.

Complications associated with this test include shock and hypovolemia, perforation of abdominal organs, hemorrhage, and hepatic coma.

Procedure

• Obtain a paracentesis tray.

• Record baseline vital signs and weight for comparison with post-test readings; measure abdominal girth, as ordered.

• Position the patient, as ordered. Seat the patient on a bed or in a chair, with his feet flat on the floor and his back well supported. If he cannot tolerate being out of bed, place him in high Fowler's position. Make him as comfortable as you can. Except for the puncture site, keep him covered to prevent chilling.

• Provide a plastic sheet or absorbent pad to collect spillage and to protect the patient and bed linens.

• Shave the puncture site.

• Open the paracentesis tray, using sterile technique.

• The patient's skin is prepared and the area draped.

• A local anesthetic is injected, and the needle or trocar and cannula are usually inserted 1″ to 2″ (2.5 to 5 cm) below the umbilicus. (However, insertion may also be through the flank, the iliac fossa, the border of the rectus, or at each quadrant of the abdomen.) If a trocar and cannula are used, a small incision is made to facilitate insertion. When the needle pierces the peritoneum, it "gives" with an audible sound.

• The trocar is removed, and a sample of fluid is aspirated with a 50-ml Luer-Lok syringe and placed in the appropriate specimen and collection containers, usually found on the paracentesis tray.

• If additional fluid is to be drained, assist in attaching one end of an I.V. tube to the cannula and the other end to a collection bag.

• The fluid (no more than 1,500 ml) is then aspirated. If fluid aspiration is difficult, reposition the patient, as ordered.

• After aspiration, the trocar or needle is removed, and a pressure dressing is applied. Occasionally, the wound may be sutured first.

• Label the samples in the order they were drawn.

• If the patient has received antibiotic therapy, note this on the laboratory slip.

• Carefully dispose of needles and contaminated articles if the patient has a history of hepatitis; incinerate disposable items and return reusable ones to the central supply area.

Special precautions

• Use peritoneal fluid analysis cautiously in patients who are pregnant and in those with bleeding tendencies or unstable vital signs.

CLINICAL ALERT: **Check vital signs every 15 minutes during the procedure. Watch for deviations from baseline findings. Observe for dizziness, pallor, perspiration, and increased anxiety.**

• If rapid fluid aspiration induces hypovolemia and shock, reduce the vertical distance between the trocar and the collection bag to slow the drainage rate. If necessary, stop drainage by turning the stopcock off or by clamping the tubing.

• Avoid contamination of specimens, which alters their bacterial count.

Patient care checklist
Before the test

☑ Explain or clarify test purpose, procedure, and complications.

☑ Tell the patient that the procedure takes from 5 to 45 minutes to perform, and that blood may be drawn for laboratory analysis (hemoglobin, hematocrit, prothrombin time, activated partial prothrombin time, and platelet count).

☑ Inform the patient with severe ascites that the procedure will relieve his

discomfort and make breathing easier.

☑ Evaluate patient understanding.

☑ Provide psychological support and assurance as necessary to decrease patient anxiety.

☑ Make sure the consent form is signed by the patient or a responsible family member.

☑ Instruct the patient to void immediately prior to the start of the procedure. (This helps prevent accidental bladder injury during needle insertion.)

After the test

☑ Apply a gauze dressing to the puncture site. Check the dressing frequently (always when vital signs are taken), and reinforce as needed. Apply a pressure dressing, if needed.

☑ Monitor the patient's vital signs until stable. (If the patient's recovery is poor, vital signs should be checked every 15 minutes until stable.)

☑ Weigh the patient and measure his abdominal girth. Compare measurements with baseline measurements.

☑ Allow the patient to rest. Withhold treatments or procedures that might cause undue stress, when possible.

☑ Monitor urinary output for at least 24 hours. Observe for hematuria (may indicate bladder trauma).

CLINICAL ALERT: **If a large amount of fluid was aspirated, watch for signs of vascular collapse (color change, elevated pulse rate and respirations, decreased blood pressure and central venous pressure, mental changes, and dizziness).**

CLINICAL ALERT: **Watch for signs of hemorrhage and shock, or for increasing pain and abdominal tenderness. (These may indicate a perforated intestine or, depending on the site of the tap, puncture of the inferior epigastric artery, hematoma of the anterior cecal wall, or rupture of the iliac vein or bladder.)**

CLINICAL ALERT: **Observe the patient with severe hepatic disease for signs of hepatic coma, which may result from loss of sodium and po-**

tassium accompanying hypovolemia. Watch for mental changes, drowsiness, and stupor. Such a patient is also prone to uremia, infection, hemorrhage, and protein depletion.

☑ Administer I.V. infusions and albumin as ordered. Check the laboratory report for electrolyte (especially sodium) and serum protein levels.

Interfering factors

• Failure to send the sample to the laboratory immediately may alter test results.

• Unsterile collection technique may invalidate test results.

• Injury to underlying structures during paracentesis may contaminate the sample with bile, blood, urine, or feces.

Pleural fluid analysis
[Thoracentesis]

Purpose
To provide a fluid specimen to determine the cause and nature of pleural effusion.

Normal results
The pleural cavity maintains negative pressure and contains less than 20 ml of serous fluid.

Abnormal results

Transudate pleural fluid effusion can result from:
  Ascites
  Systemic and pulmonary venous hypertension
  Congestive heart failure
  Hepatic cirrhosis
  Nephritis.

Exudative effusion results from:
  Lymphatic drainage interference
  Infections
  Pulmonary infarctions
  Neoplasms
  Pleurisy associated with rheumatoid arthritis.

Culture studies of pleural effusions may reveal:
  Mycobacterium tuberculosis
  Staphylococcus aureus
  Streptococcus pneumoniae
  Other streptococci
  Hemophilus influenzae
  In ruptured pulmonary abscess, anaerobes.

Grossly purulent fluid may result from complications of:
  Pneumonia
  Pulmonary abscess
  Perforation of the esophagus
  Penetration from mediastinitis.

High percentage of neutrophils:
  Septic inflammation.

Predominating lymphocytes:
  Tuberculosis
  Fungal effusions
  Viral effusions.

Serosanguinous fluid:
  Pleural extension of a malignant tumor.

Increased lactic dehydrogenase (LDH):
  Malignancy (if effusion is nonpurulent, nonhemolyzed, and nonbloody).

Glucose levels 30 to 40 mg/dl lower than blood glucose levels:
  Malignancy
  Bacterial infection
  Nonseptic inflammation
  Metastases.

Increased amylase levels:
  Pleural effusion associated with pancreatitis.

The basics
The pleura, a two-layer membrane covering the lungs and lining the thoracic cavity, maintains a small amount of lubricating fluid between its layers to minimize friction during respiration. Increased fluid in this space—the result of diseases such as cancer or tuberculosis, or of blood or lymphatic disorders—can cause respiratory difficulty.

Pleural effusion results from the abnormal formation or reabsorption of pleural fluid. Certain characteristics classify pleural fluid as either a transudate (a low-protein fluid that has leaked from normal blood vessels) or an exudate (a protein-rich fluid that has leaked from blood vessels with increased permeability). (See *Characteristics of Pulmonary Transudate and Exudate*, p. 300.) Pleural fluid may contain blood (hemothorax), chyle (chylothorax), or pus and necrotic tissue. Blood-tinged fluid may indicate a traumatic tap; if so, the fluid should clear as aspiration progresses.

In pleural fluid aspiration (thoracentesis), the thoracic wall is punctured to obtain a specimen of pleural fluid for analysis or to relieve pulmonary compression and resultant respiratory distress. The specimen is examined for color, consistency, glucose and protein content, cellular composition, and the enzymes LDH and amylase; it is also examined cytologically for malignant cells and cultured for pathogens. Generally, cultures are positive during the early stages of infection; however, antibiotic therapy may produce a negative culture despite a positive Gram stain and grossly purulent fluid. Performing a physical examination and chest radiograph or ultrasound study to locate the fluid before performing thoracentesis lessens the risk of puncturing the lung, liver, or spleen. (See *Recognizing Complications of Thoracentesis*, p. 301.)

Contraindications to this test include: a history of bleeding disorders.

Procedure
• Record baseline vital signs.
• Shave the area around the needle insertion site, if necessary.
• Position the patient properly to widen intercostal spaces and to allow easier access to the pleural cavity; make sure he is well-supported and comfortable. Preferably, seat him at the edge of the bed, with a chair or stool supporting his feet and his head and arms resting on a padded overbed table. If he cannot sit up, position him on his unaffected side, with the arm on the affected side elevated above his head.
• Remind him not to cough, breathe deeply, or move suddenly during the procedure. (This will minimize the risk of injury to the lung.)
• After the patient has been properly

Characteristics of Pulmonary Transudate and Exudate

Characteristic	Transudate	Exudate
Appearance	Clear	Cloudy, turbid
Specific gravity	< 1.016	> 1.016
Clot (fibrinogen)	Absent	Present
Protein	< 3 g/dl	> 3 g/dl
White blood cells	Few lymphocytes	Many; may be purulent
Red blood cells	Few	Variable
Glucose	Equal to serum level	May be less than serum level
Lactic dehydrogenase	Low	High

positioned, the physician will disinfect the skin, drape the area, inject local anesthetic into the subcutaneous tissue, and insert the thoracentesis needle above the rib to avoid lacerating intercostal vessels.

• When the needle reaches the pocket of fluid, he will attach the 50-ml syringe and the stopcock and open the clamps on the tubing to aspirate fluid into the container.

• During aspiration, check the patient for signs of respiratory distress, such as weakness; dyspnea; pallor; cyanosis; changes in heart rate; tachypnea; diaphoresis; blood-tinged, frothy mucus; and hypotension.

• After the needle has been withdrawn, apply slight pressure and a small adhesive bandage to the puncture site.

• Label the specimen, and record the date and time of the test and the amount, color, and character of the fluid (clear, frothy, purulent, bloody) on the request slip. Note any signs of distress the patient exhibited during the procedure. Document the exact location where fluid was removed, since this information may aid diagnosis.

Patient care checklist
Before the test

☑ Explain or clarify test purpose, preparation, procedure, and possible complications.

☑ Tell the patient that a chest radiography or ultrasound study may precede the test to help locate fluid.

☑ Evaluate patient understanding.

☑ Review the patient history for contraindications to this procedure, such as bleeding disorders.

☑ Make sure the patient has signed a consent form.

After the test

☑ Reposition the patient comfortably on the affected side or as ordered by the physician. Tell the patient to remain on this side for at least 1 hour to seal the puncture site. Elevate the head of the bed to facilitate breathing.

☑ Monitor vital signs every 30 min-

Recognizing Complications of Thoracentesis

Identify the following possible complications of thoracentesis by watching for their characteristic signs and symptoms:

• *pneumothorax:* apprehension, increased restlessness, cyanosis, sudden breathlessness, tachycardia, chest pain

• *tension pneumothorax:* dyspnea, chest pain, tachycardia, hypotension, absent or diminished breath sounds on the affected side

• *fluid reaccumulation:* increasing and persistent cough, respiratory distress, hemoptysis, subcutaneous emphysema

• *mediastinal shift:* labored breathing, cardiac dysrhythmias, cardiac distress, pulmonary edema (pink, frothy sputum; paradoxical pulse).

---

utes for 2 hours, then every 4 hours until they are stable.

☑ Tell the patient to call a nurse immediately if he experiences difficulty breathing.

☑ Evaluate patient understanding.

CLINICAL ALERT: **Watch for signs of pneumothorax, tension pneumothorax, fluid reaccumulation, and if a large amount of fluid was withdrawn, pulmonary edema or cardiac distress caused by mediastinal shift. Usually, a post-test radiograph is ordered to detect these complications before clinical symptoms appear.**

☑ Check the puncture site for any fluid leakage. A large amount of leakage is abnormal.

Interfering factors
• Failure to use aseptic technique may contaminate the specimen.

• Antibiotic therapy before aspiration of fluid for culture may decrease the number of bacteria, making isolation of the infecting organism difficult.

• Failure to send the specimen to the

laboratory immediately may alter test results.

• Failure to add heparin to the container may alter test results.

Semen analysis

Purpose

• To evaluate male fertility in an infertile marriage (most common use)
• To substantiate the effectiveness of vasectomy.

For medicolegal purposes:

• To detect semen on the body or clothing of a suspected rape victim, or elsewhere at the crime scene
• To identify blood group substances to exonerate or incriminate a criminal suspect (rare)
• To rule out paternity on grounds of complete sterility (rare). (See *Semen Identification for Medicolegal Purposes.*)

Normal results

Normal semen volume ranges from 0.7 to 6.5 ml. Paradoxically, the semen volume of males in infertile marriages is frequently increased. Continence for 1 week or more results in progressively increased semen volume (sperm counts increase with abstinence up to 10 days; sperm motility progressively decreases; and sperm morphology remains the same). Liquefied semen is generally highly viscid, translucent, and gray-white, with a musty or acrid odor. After liquefaction, specimens of normal viscosity can be poured in drops. Normally, semen is slightly alkaline, with a pH of 7.3 to 7.9.

Other normal characteristics of semen include the following: it coagulates immediately and liquefies within 20 minutes; normal spermatozoa count ranges from 20 to 150 million/ml; at least 40% of spermatozoa have normal morphology; at least 20% of spermatozoa show progressive motility within 4 hours of collection.

The normal postcoital cervical mucus test shows at least 10 motile spermatozoa per microscopic high-power field and spinnbarkeit (a measurement of the tenacity of the mucus) of at least 4″ (10 cm). These findings indicate adequate spermatozoa and receptivity of the cervical mucus.

Abnormal results

Decreased sperm counts, decreased sperm motility, and abnormal morphology are usually associated with decreased fertility.

The basics

Inexpensive, technically simple, and reasonably definitive, semen analysis is usually the first test performed on the male to evaluate fertility. Fertility may also be determined by collecting semen postcoitally from the female, to assess the ability of the spermatozoa to penetrate the cervical mucus and remain active. The procedure for analyzing semen for infertility usually includes measuring the volume of seminal fluid, assessing sperm counts, and performing microscopic examination. Sperm are counted in much the same way that white blood cells, red blood cells, and platelets are counted on an anticoagulated blood sample. Staining and microscopic examination of a drop of semen permits the motility and morphology of the spermatozoa to be evaluated.

Abnormal semen is *not* synonymous with infertility. Only one viable spermatozoon is needed to fertilize an ovum. Although a normal sperm count is more than 20 million/ml, males with sperm counts below 1 million/ml have fathered normal children. Only males who cannot deliver *any* viable spermatozoa in their ejaculates during sexual intercourse are absolutely sterile.

Abnormal semen may require further testing (such as liver, thyroid, pituitary, and adrenal function tests) to identify its underlying cause and screening for metabolic abnormalities (such as diabetes mellitus). Significant

Semen Identification For Medicolegal Purposes

Spermatozoa (or their fragments) persist in the vagina for more than 72 hours after sexual intercourse. This allows detection and positive identification of semen from vaginal aspirates or smears, or from stains on clothing, other fabrics, skin, or hair, which is often necessary for medicolegal purposes—usually in connection with rape or homicide investigations. Spermatozoa taken from the vagina of an exhumed body that has been properly embalmed and remains reasonably intact can also be identified.

To determine which stains or fluids require further investigation, clothing or other fabrics can be scanned with ultraviolet light to detect the typical green-white fluorescence of semen. Soaking appropriate samples of clothing, fabric, or hair in physiologic saline solution elutes the semen and spermatozoa. Suspect deposits of dried semen can be gently sponged from the victim's skin.

The two most common tests to identify semen are the determination of *acid phosphatase concentration* (the more sensitive test) and *microscopic examination* for the presence of spermatozoa. Acid phosphatase appears in semen in significantly greater concentrations than in any other body fluid. In microscopic examination, spermatozoa or head fragments can be identified on stained smears prepared directly from vaginal scrapings or aspirates, or from the concentrated sediment of eluates or lavages.

Like other body fluids, semen contains the soluble A, B, and H blood group substances in the approximately 80% of males who are genetically determined secretors (males who have the dominant secretor gene in a homozygous or heterozygous state). Thus, the male who has group A blood and is a secretor has soluble blood group A substance in his seminal fluid and group A substance on the surface of his red blood cells. This fact may be of considerable medicolegal importance. Semen analysis can demonstrate that the semen of a suspect in a rape or homicide investigation is different from or consistent with semen found in or on the victim's body.

semen abnormalities—such as greatly decreased sperm count or motility, or marked increase in morphologically abnormal forms—may require testicular biopsy.

As described below, semen analysis has several purposes other than determining fertility. Some laboratories offer specialized semen tests, such as screening for antibodies to spermatozoa.

Procedure
For fertility studies:
  Males:
    Ask the patient to collect semen in a clean plastic specimen container.

Females (postcoital examination):
  • Place the patient in lithotomy position.
  • The examiner will insert a speculum into the vagina to collect the specimen.
  • The examiner will wipe any excess mucus from the external cervix and collect the specimen by direct aspiration of the cervical canal, using a 1-ml tuberculin syringe without a cannula or needle.
  From a rape victim:
  • Handle the victim's clothes as little as possible. If her clothes are moist, put them in a paper bag—not a plastic bag (which causes seminal stains and secretions to mold).

• Label the bag properly and send it to the laboratory immediately.

• Provide emotional support by speaking to the patient calmly and reassuringly. Encourage her to express her fears and anxieties. Listen sympathetically.

• Prepare her for insertion of the speculum as you would the patient scheduled for postcoital examination.

• If the rape victim is scheduled for vaginal lavage, tell her to expect a cold sensation when the saline solution is instilled to wash out the specimen. To help her relax during this procedure, instruct her to breathe deeply and slowly through her mouth.

• Just before the test, instruct the victim to urinate, but warn her not to wipe her vulva afterward, because this may remove semen.

• The physician will obtain a specimen from the vagina of a rape victim by direct aspiration, saline lavage, or a direct smear of vaginal contents using a Pap stick or, less desirably, a cotton applicator stick.

• Dried smears are usually collected from the suspected rape victim's skin by gently washing the skin with a small piece of gauze moistened with physiologic saline solution.

• Prepare direct smears on glass microscopic slides after labeling the frosted end.

• Immediately place smeared slides in Coplin jars containing 95% ethanol.

Special precautions
• *Do not* lubricate the vaginal speculum. Oil or grease hinders examination of spermatozoa by interfering with smear preparation and staining, and by inhibiting sperm motility through toxic ingredients. Instead, moisten the speculum with water or physiologic saline.

CLINICAL ALERT: **Use extreme caution in securing, labeling, and delivering all specimens to be used for medicolegal purposes. You may be asked to testify as to when, where, and from whom the specimen was obtained; the specimen's general appearance and identifying features; steps taken to ensure the specimen's integrity; and to whom the specimen was delivered for analysis. If your hospital or clinic uses routine slips for such specimens, fill them out carefully, and submit them to the permanent medicolegal file.**

Patient care checklist
Before the test

☑ Explain or clarify test purpose and procedure.

☑ Give a written list of instructions to the patient when possible.

☑ Tell the male patient to follow the physician's orders regarding the period of continence before the test, since it may increase his sperm count. (Some physicians specify a fixed number of days, usually between 2 and 5; others advise a period of continence equal to the usual interval between episodes of sexual intercourse.)

☑ For male specimen collection: Inform the patient that the most desirable specimen requires masturbation, ideally in a physician's office or a laboratory. Also tell the patient that alternatives to collection by masturbation include coitus interruptus or the use of a condom. For collection by coitus interruptus, instruct the patient to withdraw immediately before ejaculation and to deposit the ejaculate in a suitable specimen container. For collection by condom, tell the patient to wash the condom with soap and water, rinse it thoroughly, and allow it to dry completely. (Powders or lubricants applied to the condom may be spermicidal.) After collection, instruct the patient to tie the condom and place it in a glass jar.

☑ If the specimen is collected at home, instruct the patient to deliver the specimen to the laboratory within 3 hours of collection. Instruct the patient not to expose the specimen to extreme temperatures or to direct sunlight (which can also increase its temperature). Tell the patient that, ideally, the specimen should remain at body temperature until liquefaction is complete (about 20 minutes). To deliver a semen specimen to the laboratory in cold weather, suggest that the patient protect the specimen from exposure to cold by keeping the specimen container in a coat pocket on the way to the laboratory.

☑ For female specimen collection: Instruct the patient to report for examination during the ovulatory phase of her menstrual cycle, as determined by basal temperature records, and as soon as possible after sexual intercourse (within 8 hours) for the postcoital cervical mucus test. Explain to the patient scheduled for this test that the procedure takes only a few minutes.

☑ For the rape victim: Provide emotional support and reassurance.

After the test

☑ Inform the patient who is undergoing fertility studies that test results should be available in 24 hours.

☑ Refer the suspected rape victim to an appropriate specialist for counseling—a gynecologist, psychiatrist, clinical psychologist, nursing specialist, member of the clergy, or representative of a community support group, such as Women Organized Against Rape (WOAR).

☑ Evaluate patient understanding.

Interfering factors

• Delayed delivery of the specimen, exposure of the specimen to extremes of temperature or direct sunlight, or the presence of toxic chemicals in the specimen container or the condom can decrease the number of viable sperm.

• An incomplete specimen—from faulty collection by coitus interruptus, for example—diminishes the volume of the specimen.

Sweat test

Purpose

To confirm cystic fibrosis.

Normal results

Normal sodium values in sweat range from 10 to 30 mEq/liter. Normal chloride values range from 10 to 35 mEq/liter.

Abnormal results

Sodium and chloride (sweat electrolyte) levels > 80 mEq/liter:

Cystic fibrosis (only condition that raises levels this high).

Sweat electrolyte levels > 60 mEq/liter:

Confirm cystic fibrosis if typical clinical features can be identified.

Sweat electrolyte levels between 50 and 60 mEq/liter:

Strongly suggest cystic fibrosis.

Increased levels of sweat electrolytes also associated with:

Untreated adrenal insufficiency (Addison's disease)

Type I glycogen storage disease

Vasopressin-resistant diabetes insipidus

Meconium ileus

Renal failure.

The basics

The sweat test quantitatively measures electrolyte concentrations (primarily sodium and chloride) in sweat, usually through pilocarpine iontophoresis (pilocarpine is a sweat inducer). This test is used almost exclusively in children to confirm cystic fibrosis, a congenital condition that raises the sodium and chloride electrolyte levels in sweat.

Sweat glands are found over most body surfaces. When stimulated by the sympathetic nerves, these glands secrete a watery solution that contains sodium chloride, most plasma components (except proteins), urea, and lactate ions in greater amounts than in plasma. Elevated sodium and chloride sweat concentrations may also occur in persons predisposed to cystic fibrosis, such as those with family histories of the disease, or in those suspected of the disease because of malabsorption syndrome or failure to thrive.

In females, sweat electrolyte levels fluctuate cyclically: chloride concentrations usually peak 5 to 10 days before onset of menses, and most women retain fluid before menses. Men also show fluctuations (up to 70 mEq/liter).

Procedure

• With distilled water, wash the area to be iontophoresed, and dry it. (The flexor surface of the right forearm is commonly used, or when the patient's arm is too small to secure electrodes, as with an infant, the right thigh.)

• Place a gauze pad saturated with premeasured pilocarpine solution on the positive electrode; place the pad saturated with normal saline solution on the negative electrode.

• Apply both electrodes to the area to be iontophoresed, and secure them with straps.

• Lead wires to the analyzer—which are attached in a manner similar to that used for EKG electrodes—are given a current of 4 milliamperes in 15 to 20 seconds. This process (iontophoresis) is continued at 15- to 20-second intervals for 5 minutes.

• After iontophoresis, remove both electrodes. Discard the pads and cleanse the skin with distilled water, then dry it.

• Using forceps, place a dry gauze pad or filter paper (previously weighed on a gram scale) on the area where the pilocarpine was iontophoresed.

• Cover the pad or filter paper with a slightly larger piece of plastic, and seal the edges of the plastic with waterproof adhesive tape. Leave the gauze pad or filter paper in place for about 30 to 40 minutes. (The appearance of droplets on the plastic usually indicates induction of an adequate amount of sweat.)

• Remove the pad or filter paper with the forceps, place it immediately in the weighing bottle, and insert the stopper in the bottle. (The difference between the first and second weights indicates the weight of the sweat specimen collected.)

Special precautions

CLINICAL ALERT: **Always perform iontophoresis on the right arm (or right thigh) rather than on the left.** *Never* **perform iontophoresis on the chest, especially in a child, since the current can induce cardiac arrest.**

• To prevent electric shock, use battery-powered equipment, if possible.

CLINICAL ALERT: **Stop the test immediately if the patient complains of a burning sensation, which usually indicates that the positive electrode is exposed or positioned improperly. Adjust the electrode, and continue the test.**

• Make sure at least 100 mg of sweat is collected for analysis.

Patient care checklist
Before the test

☑ Explain or clarify test purpose and procedure. Since the patient is generally a child, explain the test to him as simply as possible (if he is old enough to understand). Explain the test thoroughly to his parents.

☑ Tell the child and his parents that the test takes from 20 to 45 minutes, depending on the equipment used. Tell the child that he may feel a slight tickling sensation during the procedure, but will not feel any pain.

☑ Evaluate patient/parent understanding.

☑ Encourage the parents to assist with preparations and to stay with their child during the test. Their presence will minimize the child's anxiety.

After the test

☑ Wash the iontophoresed area with soap and water, and dry thoroughly.

☑ If the iontophoresed area looks red, reassure the patient that this is normal and that the redness will disappear in a few hours.

Interfering factors

• Failure to obtain an adequate amount of sweat (common when testing newborns) may interfere with accurate determination of test results.

• Presence of pure salt depletion (common during hot weather) may cause false-normal test results.

• Failure to cleanse the skin thoroughly or to use sterile gauze pads may cause false elevations.

• Failure to seal the gauze pad or filter paper carefully may falsely elevate electrolyte levels through evaporation.

• Unstable clinical conditions allow erroneous interpretation of test results.

Synovial fluid analysis

Purpose

• To aid in differential diagnosis of arthritis, particularly septic or crystal-induced arthritis

• To identify the cause and nature of joint effusion

• To relieve the pain and distention resulting from accumulation of fluid within the joint

• To administer local drug therapy, usually corticosteroids.

Normal results

See *Normal Findings in Synovial Fluid*, p. 310.

Abnormal results

Noninflammatory disease:
  Traumatic arthritis
  Osteoarthritis.
Inflammatory disease:
  Systemic lupus erythematosus
  Rheumatic fever
  Pseudogout
  Gout
  Rheumatoid arthritis.

Septic disease:
  Tuberculosis
  Septic arthritis. (See *Synovial Fluid Analysis in Arthritis*, p. 308.)

The basics

Synovial fluid is found in small amounts in the diarthrodial (synovial) joints, bursae, and tendon sheaths. It is thought to be produced by the dialysis of plasma across the synovial membrane and by the secretion of hyaluronic acid, a mucopolysaccharide. Although its functions are not clearly understood, synovial fluid probably lubricates the joint space, nourishes the articular cartilage, and protects the cartilage from mechanical damage while stabilizing the joint.

In synovial fluid aspiration, or arthrocentesis, a sterile needle is inserted into a joint space—most commonly the knee—under strict aseptic conditions, to obtain a fluid specimen for analysis. Other joint sites used for synovial fluid aspiration include the shoulder, hip, elbow, wrist, and ankle.

Examination of synovial fluid in the laboratory can take many forms. Routine examination includes gross analysis for color, clarity, quantity, viscosity, pH, and the presence of a mucin clot, as well as microscopic analysis for white blood cell (WBC) count and differential. Special examination includes microbiologic analysis for formed elements (including crystals) and bacteria, serologic analysis, and chemical analysis for such components as glucose, protein, and enzymes.

This procedure is indicated in patients with undiagnosed articular disease and symptomatic joint effusion—the excessive accumulation of synovial fluid.

Although rare, complications associated with synovial fluid aspiration include joint infection and hemorrhage leading to hemarthrosis (accumulation of blood within the joint).

Synovial Fluid Analysis In Arthritis

Disease	Color	Clarity	Viscosity
Group I noninflammatory			
Traumatic arthritis	Straw to bloody to yellow	Transparent to cloudy	Variable
Group II inflammatory			
Osteoarthritis	Yellow	Transparent	Variable
Systemic lupus erythematosus	Straw	Clear to slightly cloudy	Variable
Rheumatic fever	Yellow	Slightly cloudy	Variable
Pseudogout	Yellow	Slightly cloudy (if acute)	Low (if acute)
Gout	Yellow to milky	Cloudy	Low
Rheumatoid arthritis	Yellow to green	Cloudy	Low
Tuberculous arthritis	Yellow	Cloudy	Low
Group III septic			
Septic arthritis	Gray or bloody	Turbid, purulent	Low

Adapted with permission from R. Jessar, "Synovianalysis in Arthritis," in Donald J. McCarty, *Arthritis and Allied Conditions: A Textbook of Rheumatology* (8th ed.; Philadelphia: Lea & Febiger, 1972).

Mucin Clot	WBC Count/ % Neutrophils	Cartilage Debris	Crystals	RA Cells	Bacteria
Good to fair	1,000; 25%	None	None	None	None
Good to fair	700; 15%	Usually present	None	None	None
Good to fair	2,000; 30%	None	None	LE cells	None
Good to fair	14,000; 50%	None	None	LE cells may be present	None
Fair to poor	15,000; 70%	Usually present	Calcium pyrophosphate	None	None
Fair to poor	20,000; 70%	None	Urate	None	None
Fair to poor	20,000; 70%	None	Occasionally, cholesterol	Usually present	None
Poor	20,000; 60%	None	None	None	Usually present
Poor	90,000; 90%	None	None	None	Usually present

Procedure

• Position the patient as ordered. Explain that he will need to maintain this position throughout the procedure. Tell him that, although he will receive a local anesthetic to minimize pain, he will probably feel some discomfort when the needle is inserted. (A sedative is sometimes ordered for a young child.)

• Clean the skin over the puncture site with surgical detergent and alcohol.

• Paint the site with tincture of povidone-iodine, and allow it to air dry for 2 minutes.

• After the local anesthetic has been administered, the physician will quickly insert the aspirating needle through the skin, subcutaneous tissue, and synovial membrane, into the joint space.

• As much fluid as possible will be aspirated into the syringe; a minimum of 10 to 15 ml should be obtained, although a lesser amount is usually adequate for analysis.

• The joint (except for the area around the puncture site) may be wrapped with an elastic bandage to compress the free fluid into this portion of the sac, en-

Normal Findings In Synovial Fluid

Analysis	Results	Analysis	Results
Gross		**Serologic**	
Color	Colorless to pale yellow	Complement	
Clarity	Clear	• for 10 mg protein/dl	3.7 to 33.7 units/ml
Quantity (in knee)	0.3 to 3.5 ml	• for 20 mg protein/dl	7.7 to 37.7 units/ml
Viscosity	5.7 to 1,160	Rheumatoid arthritis cells	None
pH	7.2 to 7.4	Lupus erythematosus cells	None
Mucin clot	Good		
Microscopic		**Chemical**	
White blood cell (WBC) count	0 to 200/μl	Total protein	10.7 to 21.3 mg/dl
WBC differential		Fibrinogen	None
• Lymphocytes	0 to 78/μl	Glucose	70 to 100 mg/dl
• Monocytes	0 to 71/μl	Uric acid	2 to 8 mg/dl (men)
• Clasmatocytes	0 to 26/μl		2 to 6 mg/dl (women)
• Polymorphonuclears	0 to 25/μl	Hyaluronate	0.3 to 0.4 g/dl
• Other phagocytes	0 to 21/μl	$PaCO_2$	40 to 60 mm Hg
• Synovial lining cells	0 to 12/μl	PaO_2	40 to 80 mm Hg
Microbiologic			
Formed elements	Absence of cartilage debris and crystals		
Bacteria	None		

suring maximal collection of fluid.
• Add anticoagulants to the specimen, according to which laboratory tests have been requested. Gently invert the tube several times to mix the specimen and anticoagulant adequately.

For cultures, obtain 2 to 5 ml of synovial fluid and, if possible, inoculate the medium immediately. Otherwise, add one or two drops of heparin to the specimen.

For cytologic analysis, add 5 mg of EDTA or one or two drops of heparin to 2 to 5 ml of synovial fluid.

For glucose analysis, add potassium oxalate, as specified by the laboratory, to 3 to 5 ml of fluid.

For crystal examination, add heparin, if specified by the laboratory.

For other studies, such as general appearance and clot evaluation, obtain 2 to 5 ml of synovial fluid, but do not add an anticoagulant.

• If a corticosteroid is to be injected, prepare the dosage, as ordered. For instillation, the physician will detach the syringe, leaving the needle in the joint, and attach the syringe containing the steroid to the needle instead.
• The physician will inject the steroid and withdraw the needle.
• Wipe the puncture site with alcohol.
• Apply pressure to the puncture site for about 2 minutes to prevent bleeding, then apply a sterile dressing.
• If synovial fluid glucose is to be measured, perform a venipuncture to obtain a specimen for blood glucose analysis.
• Send the properly labeled specimens to the laboratory immediately—gonococci are particularly labile. If a WBC count is to be performed, clearly label the specimen "Synovial Fluid" and "Caution—Do not use acid diluents."

Special precautions
Adhere to strict aseptic technique throughout aspiration to prevent contamination of the joint space or the synovial fluid specimen.

Patient care checklist
Before the test
☑ Explain or clarify test purpose and procedure.
☑ Tell the patient that, while he will receive a local anesthetic, he may still feel transient pain when the needle penetrates the joint capsule.
☑ Evaluate patient understanding.
☑ If glucose testing of synovial fluid is ordered, instruct the patient to fast for 6 to 12 hours before the test.
☑ Make sure the consent form has been signed.
☑ Review the patient's history for hypersensitivity to iodine compounds (such as povidone-iodine), procaine, lidocaine, or other local anesthetics.
After the test
☑ Apply ice or cold packs to the affected joint for 24 to 36 hours after aspiration to decrease pain and swelling.
☑ Use pillows to support the patient.
☑ If a large quantity of fluid was aspirated, apply an elastic bandage to stabilize the joint.
☑ If the patient's condition permits, tell him he may resume normal activity immediately after the procedure. However, warn him to avoid excessive use of the joint for a few days after the test, even though pain and swelling may have subsided. Excessive use may cause transient pain, swelling, and stiffness.
☑ Watch for increased pain or fever, which may indicate joint infection.
☑ Carefully handle the dressings and linens of patients with drainage from the joint space, especially if septic arthritis is confirmed or suspected.
☑ Advise the patient that he may resume his usual diet.

Interfering factors
• Acid diluents added to the specimen for WBC count precipitate the mucin and alter the cell count.
• Failure to mix the specimen and the

anticoagulant adequately may alter test results.
• Failure to send the specimen to the laboratory immediately may alter test results.

• Patient failure to adhere to dietary restrictions can affect glucose levels.
• Contamination of the specimen can invalidate test results.

Selected References

Brunner, Lillian S., and Suddarth, Doris S. *Textbook of Medical-Surgical Nursing*, 5th ed. Philadelphia: J.B. Lippincott Co., 1984.

Danforth, David N., ed. *Obstetrics and Gynecology*, 4th ed. Philadelphia: J.B. Lippincott Co., 1982.

Diagnostics, 2nd ed. Nurse's Reference Library. Springhouse, Pa.: Springhouse Corp., 1986.

Diseases, 2nd ed. Nurse's Reference Library. Springhouse, Pa.: Springhouse Corp., 1987.

Emergencies. Nurse's Reference Library. Springhouse, Pa.: Springhouse Corp., 1985.

Fischbach, Frances. *A Manual of Laboratory Diagnostic Tests*, 2nd ed. Philadelphia: J.B. Lippincott Co., 1984.

Glass, Robert H. *Office Gynecology*, 2nd ed. Baltimore: Williams & Wilkins Co., 1981.

Grossman, Zachary D., et al. *The Clinician's Guide to Diagnostic Imaging*. New York: Raven Press Pubs., 1983.

Henry, John Bernard, ed. *Todd-Sanford-Davidsohn Clinical Diagnosis and Management by Laboratory Methods*, vol. 1, 17th ed. Philadelphia: W.B. Saunders Co., 1984.

Kee, Joyce LeFever. *Laboratory and Diagnostic Tests with Nursing Implications*. East Norwalk, Conn.: Appleton-Century-Crofts, 1983.

Michaels, Davida, ed. *Diagnostic Procedures*. New York: John Wiley & Sons, 1983.

Neurologic Disorders. Nurse's Clinical Library. Springhouse, Pa.: Springhouse Corp., 1984.

Pagana, Kathleen D., and Pagana, Timothy James. *Diagnostic Testing and Nursing Implications*, 2nd ed. St. Louis: C.V. Mosby Co., 1986.

Procedures. Nurse's Reference Library. Springhouse, Pa.: Springhouse Corp., 1985.

Wallach, Jacques B. *Interpretation of Diagnostic Tests: A Handbook Synopsis of Laboratory Medicine*, 3rd ed. Boston: Little, Brown & Co., 1978.

6

FECAL TESTING

Introduction

The GI tract processes about 10 liters of chyme daily, of which 100 to 300 g are eventually expelled as feces. (See *Colon Physiology*, p. 314.) Normal defecation patterns—influenced by food and fluid intake, medications, exercise, and rate of digestion—vary from two or three times daily to two or three times weekly.

Fecal contents are normally 75% water and 25% solids, such as cellulose and other indigestible fiber, bacteria, unabsorbed minerals, fat and fat derivatives, desquamated epithelial cells, mucus, and small amounts of digestive enzymes and secretions.

Normal characteristics of stool are influenced by diet and metabolism. Feces are usually light-to-dark brown, soft, and slightly acidic. Their color depends on diet, drugs, absorption efficiency, and bilirubin concentration (See *Nonpathologic Causes of Variant Stool Color*, p. 315), their normal brown color, on metabolism of bile pigments to stercobilin. Fecal pH depends on dietary influences: acidic pH results from a high carbohydrate intake; alkaline pH results from a high protein intake. Fecal odor results from the presence of indole and skatole, end products of protein catabolism by bacterial action in the large intestine.

Stool is usually about 1″ (2.5 cm) in diameter and has the tubular shape of the colon, but may be larger or smaller, depending on the condition of the colon.

Variations in appearance of stool can result from a variety of GI changes. If the colon is partially obstructed or loses its elasticity, the passage of stool often traumatizes the colon and may cause bleeding; blood in the stool may also result from hemorrhoids. A black, tarry stool can result from bleeding high in the intestinal tract. A large, bulky, foul-smelling stool that floats on water may indicate malabsorption of fat (steatorrhea) or a large quantity of air or other gases in the stool. Diarrhea results from too-rapid passage of food through the GI tract, often spurred by viral infection. Mucus-containing stool can indicate colitis or a mucus-producing tumor. Pus, detected in microscopic analysis, can result from rectal abscesses or ulcerative colitis.

Fecal analysis begins with gross examination of color, consistency, odor, and other characteristics, and concludes with microscopic, chemical, or bacterial analysis. It includes examination for occult blood, lipids, leukocytes, bacteria, fecal urobilinogen, and parasites. (For information on bacteria and parasites, see "Stool culture," pp. 404 to 406, and "Stool examination for ova and parasites," pp. 406 and 407.) Fecal analysis is usually indicated with changed bowel habits, diarrhea, constipation, bleeding, or persistent abdominal pain, and is often required for diagnosis of infectious diseases, GI bleeding, and other GI tract disorders.

Patient-teaching guidelines

Patient-learner objectives:
- Define the test.
- State the specific purpose of the test.
- Explain the procedure.
- Discuss test preparation, procedure, and post-test care.

Teaching content:
- Define the test in terms the patient can understand.
- Explain the specific purpose of the test.
- Describe the procedure:

—To collect a random specimen, provide the hospitalized patient with a clean bedpan, and provide the home patient with a stool specimen container. Instruct him to avoid contaminating the stool with urine or toilet tissue, since urine will inhibit bacterial growth and toilet tissue contains bismuth, which interferes with test results. If the patient passes blood or

mucus with the stool, tell him to include it with the specimen. Tell the hospitalized patient to inform you as soon as he obtains the specimen, so you can transfer it to the stool specimen container and send it to the laboratory, properly labeled. Tell the home patient to tightly secure the lid of the container, carefully label it, and take it to the laboratory immediately, since a fresh specimen produces the most accurate results. If the specimen cannot be transported immediately, tell him to keep it refrigerated.

—To collect a timed specimen, provide the hospitalized patient with a clean bedpan, and provide the home patient with a large specimen container obtained from the laboratory. Tell the patient to consider the first stool passed as the start of the collection period. Instruct him to save *all* stools for the designated time period. Tell him to avoid contaminating the stool with urine or toilet tissue. Tell the home patient to keep specimens refrigerated or on ice during the collection period, and tell him where to take the specimen when the test is completed. Tell the hospitalized patient to inform you when he obtains each specimen, so that you can transfer it to the appropriate container. Tell the patient whether each specimen will be sent to the laboratory or if specimens will be kept refrigerated during the collection period.

- Itemize any dietary or medication restrictions or requirements for the test. Explain that these are necessary to provide more accurate test results.
- Provide written instructions for the home patient.

Evaluation:
After the patient-teaching session has been completed, evaluate whether or not the patient has satisfactorily met each patient-learner objective by obtaining necessary patient feedback. Refocus teaching as needed.

Colon physiology

When food reaches the ileocecal valve and enters the large intestine (3 to 10 hours after ingestion), all its nutritional value has been absorbed. The first half of the large intestine absorbs water, sodium, and chloride, reducing bulk; the second half stores and further dehydrates the digestive material until defecation. The second half of the large intestine may also excrete water, potassium, and bicarbonate. Bacterial action in the colon putrefies undigested foods; synthesizes vitamins K, B_{12}, B_2 (riboflavin), and B_1 (thiamine); and produces gas, which helps propel feces toward the anus. Intestinal gas may also result from swallowed air or diffusion of blood gases. Rectal distention by feces stimulates the defecation reflex, which is assisted by voluntary sphincter relaxation. Normal passage of feces through the large intestine takes 24 to 40 hours.

Nonpathologic Causes of Variant Stool Color

Stool Color	Food or Fluid	Drug
Red	Carrots, beets, tomatoes, red peppers	Pyrvinium
Black	Licorice, grape juice	Iron salts, phenylbutazone
Brown	Cocoa, high intake of meat protein (dark brown)	Anthraquinone
Green-blue or black	Spinach	Bismuth preparations
Yellow	Rhubarb; high intake of milk (yellow-brown)	Senna
White discoloration or speckling		Antacids (aluminum hydroxide types)

Leukocytes

Purpose
• To help distinguish between causes of diarrhea
• To assist in confirming active inflammatory bowel disease
• To identify the need for suitable antibiotic therapy to treat infections.

Normal results
Negative, or absence of leukocytes.

Abnormal results
The positive identification of leukocytes in a stool sample can result from:
  large-bowel pathogenic bacterial invasion of:
    Shigella
    Invasive *Escherichia coli*
    Campylobacter
    Entamoeba histolytica.
  The presence of (depending on the invasive properties of the strain and colonic involvement):
    Salmonella
    Yersinia
    Vibrio parahaemolyticus
    Clostridium difficile.
As a result of inflammatory processes, leukocytes from pus may occur with:
  Acute and chronic ulcerative colitis
  Colonic or rectal abscesses
  Diverticulitis
  Crohn's disease
  Rectal or anal fistulas.
Absence of leukocytes in the presence of diarrhea may occur with:
  Viral gastroenteritis
  Amebiasis
  Toxigenic organisms, such as *Vibrio cholerae* and enterotoxigenic *E. coli.*

The basics
This test is indicated whenever a patient presents with watery diarrhea of an unknown etiology. It is especially useful when differentiating diarrhea caused by invasive pathogens from diarrhea resulting from toxigenic or viral causes. It is also helpful in identifying medical problems, such as diverticulitis, that could be treated with appropriate antibiotic therapy.

Procedure

Collect a random stool specimen. Ideally, the specimen should be obtained prior to the administration of antibiotic therapy.

Special precautions

The presence of barium may obscure leukocyte identification, so the bowel should be cleaned if the test for leukocytes has been ordered following an upper barium swallow or a barium enema.

Patient care checklist

Before the test

☑ Explain or clarify test purpose, preparation, and procedure to the patient and to the parents, if the patient is a child.

☑ Explain how to obtain a random stool specimen and how to avoid contaminating the specimen with toilet tissue or urine.

☑ Tell parents of an infant or small child that the stool specimen can be obtained from the diaper.

☑ Evaluate understanding.

Interfering factors

• The presence of barium in the stool specimen may hinder identification of leukocytes.

• Urine in the stool specimen may dilute the sample, resulting in a lower-than-actual number of leukocytes.

• Recent, previous, or current antibiotic therapy may diminish the number of leukocytes found.

Lipids

Purpose

To confirm steatorrhea.

Normal results

Fecal lipids constitute less than 20% of excreted solids, with excretion of less than 7 g/24 hours.

Abnormal results

Increased fecal lipids:

Pancreatic insufficiency
Pancreatic resection
Cystic fibrosis
Chronic pancreatitis
Pancreatic ductal obstruction by stone or tumor
Hepatic disease
Biliary obstruction
Extensive small-bowel resection or bypass
Regional ileitis
Malnutrition
Celiac disease
Tropical sprue
Scleroderma
Radiation enteritis
Intestinal fistulas
Intestinal tuberculosis
Small-intestine diverticula
Altered intestinal flora
Whipple's disease
Lymphomas.

The basics

Normally, dietary lipids emulsified by bile are almost completely absorbed in the small intestine, provided biliary and pancreatic secretions are adequate. However, excessive excretion of fecal lipids—steatorrhea—may occur with various digestive and absorptive disorders. Digestive disorders may affect the production and release of pancreatic lipase or bile; absorptive disorders may affect the integrity of the intestine.

Both qualitative and quantitative tests can detect excessive excretion of lipids in patients with signs of malabsorption: weight loss, abdominal distention, and scaly skin. Only the quantitative test can confirm steatorrhea.

Procedure

Collect a 72-hour stool specimen.

Special precautions

• Do not use a waxed collection container, because the wax may become incorporated in the stool and interfere with accurate testing.

• Refrigerate the collection container between defecations, and keep it tightly covered.

Patient care checklist
Before the test

☑ Explain or clarify test purpose, preparation, and procedure.

☑ Instruct the patient on how to obtain a timed stool specimen, and tell him to avoid contaminating the specimen with toilet tissue or urine.

☑ Instruct the patient to abstain from alcohol and to maintain a high-fat diet (100 g/day) for 3 days before the test and during the collection period.

☑ Withhold medications that may interfere with test results, as ordered. If they must be continued, note this on the laboratory slip.

☑ Inform the patient that the laboratory requires 2 days to complete the analysis.

☑ Evaluate patient understanding.

Interfering factors

• The following substances may produce inaccurate test results by inhibiting absorption or affecting chemical digestion: azathioprine, bisacodyl, cholestyramine, kanamycin, neomycin, colchicine, aluminum hydroxide, calcium carbonate, alcohol, potassium chloride, and mineral oil.

• Failure to observe pretest instructions pertaining to diet and ingestion of alcohol, use of a waxed collection container, contamination of the sample, and incomplete stool specimen collection (total weight less than 300 g) interfere with accurate testing.

Occult blood tests

Purpose

• To detect GI bleeding
• To aid in early diagnosis of colorectal cancer.

Normal results

Less than 2.5 ml of blood is present, resulting in a green reaction.

Abnormal results

A positive test indicates GI bleeding. (See *Common Sites and Causes of Gastrointestinal Blood Loss*, p. 318.)

The basics

Fecal occult blood, invisible because of its minute quantity, can be detected by microscopic analysis or by chemical tests for hemoglobin, such as the guaiac or orthotolidin test. Because small amounts of blood (2 to 2.5 ml/ day) normally appear in the feces, tests for occult blood are designed to detect quantities larger than this. These tests are indicated in patients whose clinical symptoms and preliminary blood studies suggest GI bleeding. However, further tests are required to pinpoint the origin of the bleeding. Stool color correlates roughly with the site of bleeding: for example, melena usually results from hemorrhage in the esophagus or stomach. Gastric juices act to digest this blood, blackening it. Melena may also result from hemorrhage in the jejunum or ileum, provided its passage through the intestine is slow. Dark maroon stools result from hemorrhage beyond the ligament of Treitz.

This test is particularly important for early diagnosis of colorectal cancer, since 80% of persons with this type of cancer demonstrate positive results. Further tests are necessary to confirm the diagnosis. (Also see *Home Tests*, pp. 685 to 687.)

Procedure

• Collect three stool specimens or a random specimen, as ordered. Testing can take place in the laboratory or in a utility room on the nursing unit, depending on hospital policy.

• First, place a small amount of stool on a piece of filter paper.

• Then, add two drops each of tap water, glacial acetic acid, 1:60 solution of gum guaiac in 95% ethyl alcohol,

Common Sites and Causes of Gastrointestinal Blood Loss

Oral and pharyngeal
Hemangioma
Malignant tumor

Esophageal
Malignant and benign tumors
Aortic aneurysm
Eroding esophagus
Esophagitis
Varices
Peptic ulcer
Hiatal hernia

Hepatic
Liver cirrhosis (and other causes of portal hypertension)

Gastric
Varices
Diverticulum
Carcinoma
Benign tumor
Peptic ulcer
Gastritis
Erosions

Duodenal
Peptic ulcer
Duodenitis
Diverticulum
Ampullary tumor

Pancreatic
Pancreatitis
Eroding carcinoma

Jejunal and ileal
Peptic ulcer
Meckel's diverticulum
Mesenteric thrombosis
Intussusception
Benign tumor
Regional enteritis
Tuberculosis
Malignant tumor

Colonic and rectal
Polyps
Hemangioma
Malignant tumor
Diverticulitis or diverticulosis
Ulcerative colitis
Foreign body
Hemorrhoids
Fissure

Hemorrhagic conditions may also result in GI bleeding.

and 3% hydrogen peroxide, *or* two drops each of 0.2% orthotolidin and 0.3% hydrogen peroxide.
• Mix thoroughly with a tongue blade.
• Note the color immediately, and check it again after 5 minutes.
• When interpreting results, a dark blue reaction that appears within 5 minutes indicates that the test is positive for occult blood; a strongly positive reaction within 3 to 4 minutes is always abnormal. A faint blue reaction is weakly positive and is not necessarily abnormal.
• Be sure to obtain specimens from two different areas of each stool to

allow for variance in distribution of blood.

Patient care checklist
Before the test
☑ Explain or clarify test purpose, preparation, and procedure.
☑ Instruct the patient to collect three stool specimens or, if ordered, a random specimen.
☑ Instruct the patient to avoid contaminating the stool specimen with toilet tissue or urine.
☑ Instruct the patient to maintain a high-fiber diet and to refrain from eating red meats, poultry, fish, turnips,

and horseradish for 48 to 72 hours before the test, as well as throughout the collection period.

☑ Withhold medications that may interfere with test results, as ordered. If they must be continued, note this on the laboratory slip.

☑ Evaluate patient understanding.

Interfering factors

• Failure to adhere to dietary restrictions may alter test results.

• Failure to test the specimen immediately, or to send it to the laboratory immediately, may alter test results.

• Bleeding may result from use of iron preparations, bromides, rauwolfia derivatives, indomethacin, colchicine, phenylbutazone, or steroids.

• Ascorbic acid (vitamin C) can interfere with accurate testing by producing normal test results even in the presence of significant bleeding.

• Ingestion of 2 to 5 ml of blood, such as from bleeding gums, can cause abnormal results.

Urobilinogen

Purpose

To aid in diagnosis of hepatobiliary and hemolytic disorders.

Normal results

Fecal urobilinogen values range from 50 to 300 mg/24 hours.

Abnormal results

Decreased fecal urobilinogen levels:
may indicate obstructed bile flow, as in:

 Cirrhosis
 Hepatitis
 Tumor of the head of the pancreas, the ampulla of Vater, or the bile duct
 Choledocholithiasis.

may also occur due to depressed erythropoiesis in:

 Aplastic anemia.

Increased fecal urobilinogen levels:

 Hemolytic jaundice
 Thalassemia
 Hemolytic, sickle-cell, and pernicious anemia.

The basics

Urobilinogen, the end product of bilirubin metabolism, is a brown pigment formed by bacterial enzymes in the small intestine. It is excreted in feces or reabsorbed into portal blood, where it is returned to the liver and re-excreted in bile; a small amount of urobilinogen is also excreted in urine. Because bilirubin metabolism depends on a properly functioning hepatobiliary system and a normal erythrocyte life span, measurement of fecal urobilinogen is a useful indicator of hepatobiliary and hemolytic disorders. However, this test is rarely performed, since serum bilirubin and urine urobilinogen can be measured more easily.

Procedure

Collect a random stool specimen.

Special precautions

• Use a light-resistant collection container, since urobilinogen breaks down to urobilin on exposure to light.

• Send the specimen to the laboratory immediately. If transport or testing is delayed more than 30 minutes, refrigerate the specimen; if testing is being performed by an outside laboratory, freeze the specimen.

Patient care checklist

Before the test

☑ Explain or clarify test purpose, preparation, and procedure

☑ Instruct the patient on how to obtain a random stool specimen.

☑ Tell the patient to avoid contaminating the specimen with toilet tissue or urine.

☑ Withhold medications that may interfere with test results, as ordered, for 2 weeks before the test. If they must be continued, note this on the laboratory slip.

☑ Evaluate patient understanding.

Interfering factors
• Broad-spectrum antibiotics can depress fecal urobilinogen levels by inhibiting bacterial growth in the colon.
• Sulfonamides, which react with the reagent used by the laboratory in this test, and large doses of salicylates can raise fecal urobilinogen levels.
• Failure to use a light-resistant container may alter test results.
• Contamination of the specimen may alter test results.

Selected References

Diagnostics, 2nd ed. Nurse's Reference Library. Springhouse, Pa.: Springhouse Corp., 1986.

Diseases, 2nd ed. Nurse's Reference Library. Springhouse, Pa.: Springhouse Corp., 1987.

Fischbach, Frances. *A Manual of Laboratory Diagnostic Tests,* 2nd ed. Philadelphia: J.B. Lippincott Co., 1984.

Gastrointestinal Disorders. Nurse's Clinical Library. Springhouse, Pa.: Springhouse Corp., 1985.

Kee, Joyce LeFever. *Laboratory and Diagnostic Tests with Nursing Implications.* East Norwalk, Conn.: Appleton-Century-Crofts, 1983.

Leavelle, Dennis E., ed. *Mayo Medical Laboratories Test Catalog.* Rochester, Minn.: Mayo Medical Laboratories, 1984.

Pagana, Kathleen D., and Pagana, Timothy James. *Diagnostic Testing and Nursing Implications,* 2nd ed. St. Louis: C.V. Mosby Co., 1986.

DIAGNOSTIC TEST PROFILES FOR COMMON DISORDERS

Diagnostic Test Profiles for Common Disorders

The chart below lists diagnostic tests that may be performed for patients with medical disorders seen commonly in clinical practice today.

This quick-reference guide is intended to update you on the most recent tests available for the patient with a suspected disorder, to help you anticipate tests that may be performed and to help you understand the significance of test results for that patient.

In many instances, not all tests mentioned for each disorder will be performed. Many factors, such as the results of preliminary tests as well as test availability, are considered in ordering tests.

Although test results that typically occur with each disorder are identified, it is possible that an individual patient's response may vary.

Use of this chart: Information is presented in three columns. The first column, "Disorder," is arranged alphabetically for quick reference. Helpful comments are included when needed. The second column, "Test," lists the tests that may be performed for the disorder. Italicized information is often included for special or distinguishing details. The third column, "Results," provides the findings pertinent to the disorder. Bold type is used to indicate when results confirm the diagnosis.

Disorder	Test	Results
Acquired Immunodeficiency Syndrome (AIDS) (Screening tests for human T-cell lymphotropic virus, type III [HTLV-III] antibodies can only confirm the presence of antibodies to the AIDS virus. They do not confirm that the individual has AIDS. The Western Blot test is more reliable but technically more difficult. It is usually used to confirm positive results from the ELISA test.)	Enzyme-linked immunosorbent assay (ELISA) method (for detecting HTLV-III antibodies)	Color change indicates presence of HTLV-III antibodies.
	Western Blot test (for detecting HTLV-III antibodies)	**HTLV-III antibodies present**
	Tests performed to evaluate immunity and support the diagnosis:	
	Complete blood count (CBC)	Decreased lymphocytes ($< 1,500$ cells/mm^3)
	Total T cell and B cell numbers	Decreased T_4 (helper) lymphocytes; normal number of B lymphocytes
	$T_4 : T_8$ (helper:suppressor) lymphocyte ratio	Decreased (< 1.0)
	Skin testing with recall antigens	Diminished delayed hypersensitivity
Acute Lymphocytic Leukemia (ALL)	Bone marrow aspiration	Proliferation of immature lymphocytes; SBB stain negative; PAS stain positive

Diagnostic Test Profiles for Common Disorders (continued)

Disorder	Test	Results
Acute Lympho-cytic Leukemia (continued)	Bone marrow aspiration (continued)	**Bone marrow aspiration findings confirm diagnosis.**
	CBC	Typically, decreased red blood cell (RBC) count; increased white blood cell (WBC) count; decreased neutrophils
	Platelet count	Usually decreased
Adult Respiratory Distress Syn-drome (ARDS)	Arterial blood gas (ABG) analysis	On room air, ABGs initially show decreased P_{O_2} (< 60 mm Hg) and P_{CO_2} (< 35 mm Hg). The resulting pH usually reflects respiratory alkalosis. As ARDS becomes more severe, ABGs show respiratory acidosis (increasing P_{CO_2} [> 45 mm Hg]) and metabolic acidosis (decreasing HCO_3- [< 22 mEq/liter]) and a decreasing P_{O_2} despite oxygen therapy.
	Chest X-ray	Serial chest X-rays initially show bilateral infiltrates; in later stages, ground-glass appearance; and eventually (as hypoxia becomes irreversible), "white-outs" of both lung fields.
	Sputum culture	May be positive for gram-negative bacteria or other microorganisms with associated infection
	Blood cultures	May be positive for gram-negative bacteria if sepsis is associated with ARDS
Allergic Rhinitis, Seasonal (Hay-fever)	CBC	Increased eosinophils (4% to 8% or greater)

(continued)

Diagnostic Test Profiles for Common Disorders (continued)

Disorder	Test	Results
Allergic Rhinitis, Seasonal (continued)	Nasal smear	Increased eosinophils (3% to 10% or greater)
	Serum IgE level	Increased
	Allergy skin testing	Shows wheal and flare reaction to specific antigens **Results of skin testing confirm the diagnosis. Results also identify the cause.**
	Radioallergosorbent test (RAST)	Increased IgE levels to specific antigens
	Paranasal sinus X-ray	May show increased density over the maxillary and ethmoid sinuses
Alzheimer's Disease (Diagnosis is usually based on ruling out treatable causes of dementia and on clinical presentation.)	Positron emission tomography (PET) *(PET is a newer test, not in widespread use, that offers promise in the detection of this disorder.)*	Asymmetrical or reduced glucose metabolism in the temporoparietal cortex area
	Tests performed to rule out other disorders:	
	Intracranial computed tomography (CT) scan	Diffuse cortical atrophy
	EEG	Diffuse slowing in advanced disease
	Cerebrospinal fluid (CSF) analysis	Normal
	Magnetic resonance imaging (MRI)	Diffuse cortical atrophy
Amyotrophic Lateral Sclerosis (ALS) (ALS is usually diagnosed on the basis of clinical presentation.)	Creatine phosphokinase (CPK) levels	Increased; may be up to 10 times normal
	Electromyography (EMG)	Evidence of widespread acute and chronic denervation outside of a single anatomic distribution

Diagnostic Test Profiles for Common Disorders *(continued)*

Disorder	Test	Results
Amyotrophic Lateral Sclerosis *(continued)*	Muscle biopsy	Single-fiber hypertrophy, early in disease process; later, group atrophy and fiber-type grouping
	Tests performed to rule out other disorders:	
	Intracranial CT scan	Normal
	Spinal CT scan	Normal
	CSF analysis	Normal
	Myelography	Normal
	Serum calcium and phosphorus	Normal
Ankylosing Spondylitis	X-rays of the affected joints	X-rays show blurring of the bony margins of the joints, bilateral sacroiliac joint involvement, patchy sclerosis, squaring of vertebral bodies, "bamboo spine," and completely ankylosed sacroiliac joints. **X-ray findings confirm diagnosis.**
	Human leukocyte antigen (HLA) test	Shows positive HLA-B27 histocompatibility
Aortic Aneurysm, Abdominal	Abdominal X-ray (flat plate of the abdomen)	Aortic calcification; midline mass, if dissecting aneurysm
	Abdominal CT scan	Enlargement and calcification of the aorta
	Aortography	Opacification, dilation, and calcification of the aorta; false channel along the aortic lumen **Aortography can be a confirming test.**

(continued)

Diagnostic Test Profiles for Common Disorders *(continued)*

Disorder	Test	Results
Aortic Aneurysm, Abdominal *(continued)*	Abdominal aorta ultrasonography *(Ultrasonography is the most useful test for determining the size and position of the aorta.)*	Widened and abnormally shaped aorta; presence of a clot within the aorta; calcification and thickening of the aortic wall **Ultrasonography can be a confirming test.**
	Digital subtraction angiography (DSA)	Shows enhanced image of aneurysm
Aortic Aneurysm, Thoracic	Chest X-ray	Mass adjacent to thoracic aorta
	Thoracic CT scan	Calcification of the aorta; paraaortic mass; or widening of the aorta
	Aortography	Identifies the nature and relationship of aneurysm to surrounding structures
	DSA	Shows enhanced image of aneurysm
Arterial Occlusive Disease of the Lower Extremity	Doppler ultrasonography	Diminished blood velocity signal with no diastolic sound and a less prominent systolic component distal to the lesion
	Arteriography	Identifies the type of lesion, its location, the degree of obstruction, and the presence of collateral circulation **Arteriography results confirm the diagnosis.**
	DSA *(DSA uses less contrast media than arteriography does.)*	Shows enhanced image of the lesion, its location, the degree of obstruction, and the presence of any collateral circulation
Asbestosis	Chest X-ray	Shows fine, irregular, and linear diffuse infiltrates; extensive fibrosis results in a "honeycomb" or "ground-glass" appear-

Diagnostic Test Profiles for Common Disorders *(continued)*

Disorder	Test	Results
Asbestosis *(continued)*	Chest X-ray *(continued)*	ance. May also show pleural thickening and pleural calcification, with bilateral obliteration of costophrenic angles and, in later stages, an enlarged heart with a classic "shaggy" heart border. In extensive disease, it may be difficult to identify heart borders. Usually in early disease, pathology is found in the lower lobes; in later disease, it extends up from the bases, but usually not in the apices.
	Pulmonary function tests	Decreased vital capacity (VC); decreased forced vital capacity (FVC); decreased total lung capacity (TLC); decreased or normal forced expiratory volume 1 (FEV_1); decreasing diffusing capacity for carbon monoxide (DL_{CO}) as disease progresses
	ABG analysis	Decreased PaO_2; decreased $PaCO_2$ initially (as disease progresses, $PaCO_2$ increases)
	Sputum smear	When stained, may show an asbestos fiber
Asthma	CBC	Increased eosinophils (> 15%); increased WBCs with concurrent infection
	Sputum examination and culture	Increased eosinophils (> 5%); may show the presence of a bacterial organism (however, most concurrent infections are viral); may also show Charcot-Leyden

(continued)

Diagnostic Test Profiles for Common Disorders *(continued)*

Disorder	Test	Results
Asthma *(continued)*	Sputum examination and culture *(continued)*	crystals, Curschmann's spiral, and creola bodies. Sputum appears mucoid and tenacious.
	Chest X-ray	May be normal or show hyperlucent lungs, increased peribronchial markings, and atelectasis secondary to mucous plugging
	Pulmonary function tests	FVC, FEV_1, PFR (peak flow rate), and FEF 25% to 75% (forced expiratory flow during the middle 50% of vital capacity) are all decreased to < 75% of predicted values; following bronchodilator inhalation, improvements of > 20% may occur. **Pulmonary function test results confirm the diagnosis.**
	ABG analysis	Mild to moderately decreased PaO_2; decreased $PaCO_2$; with severe attack, greatly decreased PaO_2, severely increased $PaCO_2$, increased pH (acidosis)
	Allergy skin testing	Positive wheal and flare reaction in extrinsic asthma
	RAST	Elevated IgE levels to particular allergens in extrinsic asthma
	Serum IgE level	Increased; > 300 IU/ml in extrinsic asthma
	Nasal smear	Elevated eosinophils in extrinsic asthma

Diagnostic Test Profiles for Common Disorders *(continued)*

Disorder	Test	Results
Asthma *(continued)*	Exercise test	Decreased pulmonary function test of at least 15% below baseline following exercise
	EKG	During attack, sinus tachycardia is common but may reveal ventricular or atrial dysrhythmias. Changes may also include right axis deviation and ST- and T-wave abnormalities. EKG changes disappear as attack subsides.
Benign Prostatic Hypertrophy (BPH) (History and physical examination strongly suggest the diagnosis.)	Cystoscopy	Shows prostatic encroachment of the urethra, and may show evidence of obstruction, such as thickened muscle bundles of bladder (trabeculation) and possibly bladder diverticula and calculi.
	Tests performed to detect complications:	
	Intravenous pyelography (IVP) (excretory urography)	May show effects of urinary obstruction, such as hydronephrosis and bladder trabeculation
	Blood urea nitrogen (BUN)	Increased if renal impairment exists
	Serum creatinine	Increased if renal impairment exists
	Urine culture	Bacterial count > 100,000/mm^3 If infection is present
	Renal ultrasound *(Sometimes performed if IVP cannot be done)*	May show effects of urinary obstruction on kidneys

(continued)

Diagnostic Test Profiles for Common Disorders *(continued)*

Disorder	Test	Results
Bladder Cancer	Urinalysis	Increased RBC count; sometimes increased WBC count
	Urine cytology	May identify cancerous cells
	Cystoscopy	Bladder lesions or mucosal abnormalities are visualized.
	Biopsy (transurethral)	Histologic examination identifies cancerous cells. **Histologic examination of biopsy specimen confirms the diagnosis and identifies the cell type and grade of tumor.**
	Tests performed to determine the stage of the disease:	
	Abdominal CT scan	Usually identifies tumor extension beyond the bladder wall; may also detect enlarged retroperitoneal lymph nodes and liver metastasis
	Intravesicle ultrasound	May identify tumor extension beyond the bladder wall
	Bone scan	May show metastatic disease
Bone Metastasis	Bone scan	Reveals areas of increased uptake of radioactive tracer ("hot spots") in areas of increased bone metabolism
	Skeletal X-rays	Reveal areas of decreased density along affected bone(s)
	Serum alkaline phosphatase	Increased

Diagnostic Test Profiles for Common Disorders *(continued)*

Disorder	Test	Results
Bone Metastasis *(continued)*	Urine calcium	Increased
Brain Tumor	Intracranial CT scan *(Intracranial CT scan has become the preferred screening procedure for diagnosing and localizing brain tumors.)*	Reveals lesions of varying densities, edema, and structural displacement
	Cerebral angiography	May show neovascularization or vessel displacement
	Skull X-ray	Can detect tumors containing calcium, such as a meningioma or an oligodendroglioma. In a pituitary tumor, skull X-rays may show bone erosion of the sella turcica. In a tumor of the cerebral hemisphere, X-rays may show calcification and displacement of the pineal gland.
	MRI	Reveals altered tissue density and structural abnormality
	DSA	May show vessel displacement or vascular masses, but not fine details
	Biopsy (surgical)	Histologic examination identifies cancerous cells. **Biopsy results confirm diagnosis.**
	CSF cytology *(Lumbar puncture must be performed with extreme caution, if at all, with suspected brain tumor because of the possibility of brain stem herniation.)*	May show cancerous cells if meninges are involved **Results of CSF cytology may confirm the diagnosis.**

(continued)

Diagnostic Test Profiles for Common Disorders *(continued)*

Disorder	Test	Results
Breast Cancer (Breast self-examination (BSE) is often the first diagnostic clue.)	Mammography	Irregular, poorly outlined, and opaque areas suggest malignancy.
	Breast thermography	Asymmetrical appearance with "hot spots" (increased surface temperature) may suggest malignancy.
	Breast ultrasonography	Distinctive echo pattern suggests malignancy.
	Biopsy	Identifies cancerous cells **Biopsy confirms the diagnosis.**
	Hormonal receptor assay of the tumor *(Hormonal receptor assay is important when making therapy decisions.)*	Identifies if tumor is estrogen- or progesterone-dependent
Carpal Tunnel Syndrome (Diagnosis is largely dependent on the presence of Tinel's sign, a positive Phalen's wrist flexion test, and objective sensory tests.)	Hand X-ray	Palmar view and cross section of hand may reveal bony abnormalities, such as osteophytes.
	EMG	Detects a median nerve motor conduction delay of more than 5 msec
Cervical Cancer	Papanicolaou (Pap) test	Reveals atypical cells, suggesting malignancy
	Colposcopy with punch biopsy	Epithelial changes, keratinization, and atypical blood vessels may be visualized; biopsy may identify cervical intraepithelial neoplasia or microinvasive carcinoma. **Punch biopsy may confirm the diagnosis.**

Diagnostic Test Profiles for Common Disorders *(continued)*

Disorder	Test	Results
Cervical Cancer *(continued)*	Cervical conization for biopsy	Identifies specific type and extent of neoplasia **Conization may be needed to confirm the diagnosis.**
Chlamydial Infection (A Pap test may incidentally report apparent characteristics of *Chlamydia*; this is not diagnostic and can be unreliable.)	Tissue culture *(expensive test)*	Positive for presence of *Chlamydia trachomatis* **Tissue culture confirms diagnosis.**
	Direct smear fluorescent antibody test (urethral or cervical specimen) *(Direct smear fluorescent antibody test is used increasingly because it's less expensive and yields quicker results.)*	*Chlamydia* organisms stain green when visualized under the microscope. Positive findings may be reported as *C. trachomatis* detected by fluorescent antibody.
	ELISA (urethral or cervical specimen) *(The ELISA method is used in some centers and laboratories but is not yet widespread.)*	Color change indicates that an antigen-antibody reaction involving *C. trachomatis* has taken place. Results specify if infection is current or if an indication of past infection exists.
Cholecystitis, Acute	CBC	Increased WBC count
	Serum direct bilirubin	Increased with biliary obstruction
	Urine bilirubin	Increased with biliary obstruction
	Alkaline phosphatase	Increased with biliary obstruction
	Gallbladder and biliary system ultrasonography	Localizes the gallbladder; may demonstrate stones or a thickened wall
	Gallbladder scan *(Results of gallbladder scan can quickly rule out acute cholecystitis or strongly suggest the disorder.)*	Nonvisualization of gallbladder

(continued)

Diagnostic Test Profiles for Common Disorders *(continued)*

Disorder	Test	Results
Cholecystitis, Acute *(continued)*	Cholangiogram (operative or percutaneous)	May show stones in biliary ducts
Chronic Granulocytic Leukemia (CGL)	Bone marrow aspiration or biopsy	Reveals hypercellularity and infiltration by increased numbers of myeloid elements
	Chromosome analysis (from blood or bone marrow specimen)	Identifies Philadelphia chromosome **Presence of the Philadelphia chromosome and low leukocyte alkaline phosphatase levels confirm CGL.**
	Leukocyte alkaline phosphatase	Decreased
	Liver-spleen scan	Usually reveals splenomegaly
	CBC	Increased WBC count, usually to > 50,000/mm³; decreased hemoglobin level, often below 10 g/dl; decreased hematocrit level, < 30%; commonly, decreased platelets but may be normal or increased
Cirrhosis	Serum glutamic-oxaloacetic transaminase (SGOT)	Increased
	Serum glutamic-pyruvic transaminase (SGPT)	Increased
	Lactic dehydrogenase (LDH)	Increased
	Serum alkaline phosphatase	Normal to markedly increased
	Serum protein electrophoresis	Increased globulin

Diagnostic Test Profiles for Common Disorders *(continued)*

Disorder	Test	Results
Cirrhosis *(continued)*	Serum electrolytes	Decreased sodium, potassium, chlorides, and magnesium
	Total serum bilirubin	Increased
	Plasma ammonia	Increased
	CBC	Decreased hemoglobin, hematocrit, and WBC count
	Prothrombin time (PT)	Prolonged
	Partial thromboplastin time (PTT)	Prolonged
	Liver-spleen scan	Diffuse, patchy uptake over the liver; splenomegaly typical in cirrhosis
	Liver biopsy	Regenerative nodules or pseudolobules **Biopsy results confirm diagnosis.**
Colorectal Cancer	Proctosigmoidoscopy	Lesions or tumors of the anal canal, rectum, and distal sigmoid colon are visualized.
	Colonoscopy	Visual examination reveals the presence of lesions or tumors in the large intestine beyond the sigmoid colon, up to and including the cecum.
	Biopsy	Histologic examination identifies cancerous cells. **Biopsy results confirm diagnosis.**
	Barium enema *(Barium enema may not be sensitive enough for early diagnosis.)*	Carcinoma usually appears as a localized filling deficit, with a sharp transition between the normal and the necrotic mucosa.

(continued)

Diagnostic Test Profiles for Common Disorders *(continued)*

Disorder	Test	Results
Colorectal Cancer *(continued)*	Carcinoembryonic antigen (CEA)	Often increased; decreasing CEA levels suggest successful treatment
	Stool specimen for occult blood *(This is a good screening test.)*	Positive, but results are inconclusive
Congestive Heart Failure (CHF)	Chest X-ray	Shows increased pulmonary vascular markings, interstitial edema, or pleural effusion and cardiomegaly
	EKG	Reflects heart strain or enlargement, or ischemia; may also reveal atrial enlargement, tachycardia, and extrasystoles, suggesting CHF
	Pulmonary artery catheterization	Shows increased pulmonary artery and capillary wedge pressures, reflecting left ventricular end-diastolic pressure in left heart failure and increased right atrial pressure in right heart failure
	Central venous pressure monitoring	Shows increased readings as left heart failure progresses to right heart failure, or as hypervolemia results from increased retention of sodium and water
	Cardiac blood pool scanning	Shows decreased ejection fraction in left heart failure
	Echocardiography	May show ventricular hypertrophy, decreased contractility, and valvular disorders in both left and right heart failure

Diagnostic Test Profiles for Common Disorders *(continued)*

Disorder	Test	Results
Coronary Artery Disease (CAD)	Lipoprotein-cholesterol fractionation	Increased low-density lipoprotein (LDL) level
	Exercise EKG (stress test)	Patient experiences chest pain on exertion. Two findings on EKG tracing: a flat or downsloping ST segment depression of 1 mm or more for at least 0.08 second after the junction of the QRS and ST segments (J point); and a markedly depressed J point, with an upsloping but depressed ST segment of 1.5 mm below the baseline 0.08 second after the J point. Initial ST segment depression on the resting EKG must be further depressed by 1 mm during exercise to be considered abnormal. Hypotension resulting from exercise, ST segment depression of 3 mm or more, downsloping ST segments, and ischemic ST segments appearing within the first 3 minutes of exercise and lasting 8 minutes into the post-test recovery period may indicate multivessel or left CAD. ST segment elevation may indicate dyskinetic left ventricular wall motion or severe transmural ischemia.
	12-lead EKG	During angina, tracing shows ST segment depression. Dysrhythmias, such as premature ventricular contractions, may be present.

(continued)

Diagnostic Test Profiles for Common Disorders *(continued)*

Disorder	Test	Results
Coronary Artery Disease *(continued)*	Thallium myocardial imaging	Transient cold spots usually indicate ischemia due to CAD if present during peak exercise but not after a 3- to 6-hour rest.
	Cardiac catheterization	Constriction of the lumen of one or more coronary arteries **Cardiac catheterization findings confirm the diagnosis.**
Crohn's Disease (Regional Enteritis)	Sigmoidoscopy	Often, the rectum and sigmoid are normal. With involvement, the mucosa is thickened and nodular, giving a "cobblestone" appearance. Discrete ulcers are seen. Vascular pattern is normal.
	Colonoscopy *(Colonoscopy is contraindicated in fulminant disease.)*	Usually reveals patchy areas of inflammation, with some differentiating characteristics, as above
	Barium enema	Typically reveals segmental and patchy distribution of lesions. Barium study characteristically reveals deep ulcers, thickening of wall, and narrowed ileal lumen; air contrast study shows cobblestoning, longitudinal ulcers, and tiny aphthous ulcers; strictures are seen.
	Multiple biopsies	Show irregular distribution of inflammation; often reveal the presence of granuloma and show the lymphatic invasion of the epithelium **Presence of granuloma is the most specific histologic feature of Crohn's disease.**

Diagnostic Test Profiles for Common Disorders *(continued)*

Disorder	Test	Results
Cystic Fibrosis	Sweat test	Increased sodium and chloride values **Sodium and chloride concentrations > 60 mEq/liter, with typical clinical features, confirm the diagnosis. Concentrations of 50 to 60 mEq/liter strongly suggest cystic fibrosis.**
	Chest X-ray	May show thickening of the bronchial wall, segmental hyperinflation, and frequent hilar enlargement
	Examination of duodenal contents for pancreatic enzymes	Pancreatic enzymes are either completely absent or present in diminished quantities.
	Fecal lipids	Increased
	Fecal trypsin	Negative (in over 80% of children with cystic fibrosis)
	Pulmonary function tests	May be normal; may show decreased vital capacity (VC) and/or decreased peak flow rate (PFR); increased air flow resistance on inspiration and expiration
Cystitis	Urine culture	Bacterial count of a single microbe species of 100,000 or more/ml **Results of urine culture confirm a urinary tract infection. A lower bacterial count may indicate infection if urine is obtained by catheter or suprapubic tap.**
	Urinalysis	RBCs may be increased, especially in females; increased WBCs

(continued)

Diagnostic Test Profiles for Common Disorders *(continued)*

Disorder	Test	Results
Cystitis *(continued)*	Voiding cystourethrography *(Voiding cystourethrography is performed more commonly in children to identify treatable causes of infection.)*	May identify treatable causes of infection, such as ureteral reflux
	IVP (excretory urography) *(IVP is performed in children and sometimes in adults to look for treatable causes of infection.)*	May identify treatable causes of infection
Deep Vein Thrombophlebitis (DVT)	Doppler ultrasonography	Reduced or obstructed blood flow to a specific area
	Venography	Shows filling defects and diverted blood flow **Venography results confirm the diagnosis.**
	Impedance plethysmography	Shows reduced calf vein filling and venous outflow rate if significant thrombi are present in major deep vein
	Radionuclide venography, such as the ^{125}fibrinogen scan *(Radionuclide venography screens for DVT or attempts to detect the disorder in a patient who is too ill for venography or who is hypersensitive to the contrast medium.)*	An increase of > 20% in radioactivity between any adjacent sites on the same leg, from results of previous scans or from a corresponding scan on the opposite leg, suggests DVT. **Abnormal radionuclide results persisting for more than 24 hours confirm the diagnosis.**

Diagnostic Test Profiles for Common Disorders (continued)

Disorder	Test	Results
Diabetes Mellitus (Diagnosis in nonpregnant adults is restricted to those who meet one of the following three criteria:	*Tests performed on nonpregnant adults to diagnose diabetes mellitus:*	
	Random plasma glucose	200 mg/dl or greater
A random plasma glucose level of 200 mg/dl or greater must be accompanied by polydipsia, polyuria, and weight loss.	Fasting plasma glucose	140 mg/dl or greater
A fasting plasma glucose level of 140 mg/dl or greater must be obtained on at least two occasions.	Oral glucose tolerance test	Sustained increased plasma glucose levels during at least two oral glucose tolerance tests. The 2-hour sample and at least one other between 0 and 2 hours after the 75-g glucose dose should be 200 mg/dl or greater.
Oral glucose tolerance testing is necessary for patients with a fasting plasma glucose level of < 140 mg/dl. It is not necessary if the fasting plasma glucose level at the beginning of the test is 140 mg/dl or greater.)		

(continued)

Diagnostic Test Profiles for Common Disorders *(continued)*

Disorder	Test	Results
Diabetes Mellitus *(continued)* (Diagnosis in children is restricted to those who meet the following criteria: For diagnosis, a random plasma glucose level of 200 mg/dl or greater must be accompanied by polyuria, polydipsia, rapid weight loss, and ketonuria.)	*Tests performed on children to diagnose diabetes mellitus:*	
	Random plasma glucose	200 mg/dl or greater
	Fasting plasma glucose level and oral glucose tolerance tests	A fasting plasma glucose level of 140 mg/dl or greater on at least two occasions *and* sustained increased plasma glucose levels during at least two oral glucose tolerance tests. Both the 2-hour plasma glucose level and at least one other between 0 and 2 hours after the glucose dose (1.75 g/kg ideal body weight, up to 75 g) should be 200 mg/dl or greater.
	Test performed to monitor control of diabetes mellitus:	
	Glycosylated hemoglobin	Increased when diabetes is not under control
Disseminated Intravascular Coagulation (DIC)	PT	Prolonged (over 15 seconds)
	PTT	Prolonged (over 60 to 80 seconds)
	Plasma fibrinogen	Typically decreased below 160 mg/dl
	Platelet count	Decreased to < 100,000/ mm^3
	Fibrin split products	Increased, often to > 100 mcg/ml
Diverticulitis	Upper gastrointestinal (upper GI) and small-bowel series	Barium outlines and fills diverticulum(a) in the esophagus or small bowel.

Diagnostic Test Profiles for Common Disorders *(continued)*

Disorder	Test	Results
Diverticulitis *(continued)*	Barium enema	Barium outlines and fills diverticulum(a) in the large intestine.
	Erythrocyte sedimentation rate (ESR)	May be increased if diverticula are infected
	Abdominal CT scan	May show a paracolonic mass. A negative CT scan does not rule out the diagnosis.
	Proctosigmoidoscopy; colonoscopy	Diverticulum(a) may be visualized.
Ectopic Pregnancy	Serum human chorionic gonadotropin beta subunit (B-hCG)	Positive nearly 100% of the time with this diagnosis
	Urine hCG	Positive 75% of the time with this diagnosis
	Pelvic ultrasonography	May demonstrate the absence of an intrauterine pregnancy or the existence of a mass or gestational sac in the adnexa or fluid in the cul-de-sac
	Culdocentesis *(Culdocentesis is performed when ultrasonography is not immediately available, especially to decide whether emergency surgery is necessary.)*	Positive findings (blood in the cul-de-sac) occur with ruptured ectopic pregnancy.
	Laparoscopy	Reveals ectopic pregnancy **Laparoscopy confirms the diagnosis.**
Emphysema	Chest X-ray	In advanced disease, shows flattened diaphragm, reduced vascular markings at lung periphery, overaeration of lungs, enlarged antero-

(continued)

Diagnostic Test Profiles for Common Disorders *(continued)*

Disorder	Test	Results
Emphysema *(continued)*	Chest X-ray *(continued)*	posterior chest diameter, and large retrosternal air space
	Pulmonary function tests *(Characteristic physical findings and a decrease in DL_{CO} suggest the presence of emphysema.)*	VC, FEV_1, FEF, and diffusing capacity for DL_{CO} are all decreased. TLC and residual volume (RV) are increased.
	ABG analysis	Chronically decreased PaO_2, even at rest; normal $PaCO_2$ (until late in disease)
Endocarditis	CBC	Increased WBC count with a shift to the left; decreased hematocrit level; decreased platelets
	ESR	Increased
	Rheumatoid factor (RF)	Increased in > 50% of patients
	EKG	May show atrial fibrillation and other dysrhythmias accompanying valvular disease
	Blood cultures (three or more during a 24- to 48-hour period) *(Blood cultures are persistent and positive in most patients. Negative blood cultures may suggest fungal infection.)*	Usually ≤ 100 organisms/ml of blood; such organisms as staphylococci, streptococci, pneumococci, or gonococci may be identified
	Urinalysis	Commonly shows protein, RBCs, casts, and bacteria
	Two-dimensional echocardiography	May identify vegetations and valvular dysfunction
	Gallium scan	May show uptake in areas of infection

Diagnostic Test Profiles for Common Disorders (continued)

Disorder	Test	Results
Endometriosis	Laparoscopy	Dark powder burns on the peritoneum and serosa of pelvic and abdominal organs and varying degrees of fibrosis; biopsy reveals endometrial tissue **Laparoscopy with biopsy results confirm the diagnosis. However, biopsy is not always necessary if the pattern and appearance of implants are characteristic.**
	Cystoscopy; colonoscopy	Possibly, normal mucosa despite bleeding; however, mucosa can sometimes reveal implants or blue appearance with endometriosis
Epiglottitis, Acute	X-ray of the nasopharynx and upper airway	Enlarged epiglottis **X-ray findings confirm the diagnosis.**
	CBC	Increased WBC count; increased neutrophils
	Throat culture; blood cultures	Usually positive for *Hemophilus influenzae* type B, although other organisms may be identified
Fibrocystic Breast Disease	Mammography	Cysts usually appear as well-outlined, regular, and clear spots, often found bilaterally **Mammography often supplements physical findings to confirm the diagnosis.**
	Aspiration of cyst	Cysts of recent onset usually contain thin, yellow serous fluid. Cysts of longer duration usually contain darker fluid that is green, gray, dark brown, or black.

(continued)

Diagnostic Test Profiles for Common Disorders *(continued)*

Disorder	Test	Results
Gastrointestinal Bleeding, Acute	Hemoglobin and hematocrit	Decreased
	Stool specimen for occult blood	Positive. With upper GI bleeding: stool color is usually tarry black; with massive hemorrhage, may be red or maroon. With lower GI bleeding: stool color may be maroon or red.
	Gastric aspiration	Blood is present with esophageal, gastric, and possibly duodenal bleeding.
	Endoscopy (esophagogastroduodenoscopy; proctosigmoidoscopy; colonoscopy)	Site and cause of GI bleeding may be visualized.
	Barium X-ray studies (upper GI and small-bowel series; barium enema; air contrast of color) *(Because barium in the GI tract interferes with subsequent procedures, such as endoscopy, and because barium X-ray studies are not as sensitive, they are not generally used as initial studies with acute GI bleeding.)*	May demonstrate site and cause of GI bleeding
	Tagged RBCs (^{99m}Tc-tagged RBCs) *(Tagged RBCs, a noninvasive test, may be performed to demonstrate active bleeding prior to angiography or to localize bleeding when other techniques fail.)*	May identify the source of upper or lower GI bleeding

Diagnostic Test Profiles for Common Disorders *(continued)*

Disorder	Test	Results
Gastrointestinal Bleeding, Acute *(continued)*	Celiac and mesenteric arteriography *(Arteriography may be used for diagnosis as well as treatment [vasopressin infusion, embolization] of acute GI bleeding; however, the patient must be actively bleeding at the time of the test.)*	May reveal the site of GI bleeding
Gestational Diabetes	3-hour oral glucose tolerance test	Fasting: 105 mg/dl; 1 hour: 190 mg/dl; 2 hours: 165 mg/dl; 3 hours: 145 mg/dl. Following an oral glucose load of 100 g, gestational diabetes may be diagnosed if *two* plasma glucose values equal or exceed the results given here.
Glomerulonephritis, Acute (History of recent streptococcal infection is very important in establishing diagnosis.)	Urinalysis	Increased RBCs; casts present; protein present
	BUN	Increased
	Serum creatinine	Increased
	Creatinine clearance	Decreased
	Kidney-ureter-bladder (KUB) X-ray	Shows bilateral kidney enlargement
	Renal biopsy	Histologic examination shows characteristic changes of glomerulonephritis, such as deposition of complement and immune complexes along the basement membrane, increased cellularity of the glomeruli, infiltration of the glomeruli by WBCs, and widespread epithelial cell damage. **Renal biopsy results confirm the diagnosis.**

(continued)

Diagnostic Test Profiles for Common Disorders *(continued)*

Disorder	Test	Results
Glomerulonephritis, Acute *(continued)*	*Tests to verify recent streptococcal infection:*	
	Antistreptolysin 0 (ASO) titer	Increased
	Serum complement (C_3 and C_4)	Decreased
	Throat culture	Shows group A beta-hemolytic streptococcus organisms
Glomerulonephritis, Chronic	Urinalysis	Increased RBC count; RBC casts present; protein present
	BUN	Increased
	Serum creatinine	Increased
	Renal biopsy	Identifies histologic changes associated with the underlying cause
Gonorrhea	Gram stain of smear of genital exudate	Shows the presence of gram-negative diplococci **A positive Gram stain may confirm the diagnosis in males.**
	Culture (Possible sites include urethra, endocervix, anal canal, and oropharynx.) *(In disseminated disease, blood and synovial fluid cultures are also obtained.)*	Isolates the organism *Neisseria gonorrhoeae* **Culture confirms the diagnosis.**
Gout	Serum uric acid	Increased
	Urinary uric acid	Within normal limits or slightly increased
	Urinalysis	Protein present; decreased pH

Diagnostic Test Profiles for Common Disorders *(continued)*

Disorder	Test	Results
Gout *(continued)*	X-ray of affected joint	Shows clearly defined, punched-out areas of bone lysis with outward displacement of the overhanging margin from the bone contour
	Synovial fluid analysis	Examination of fluid from an acute gouty joint reveals needle-like urate crystals. **Results of synovial fluid analysis confirm the diagnosis, but this test is not always necessary.**
Guillain-Barré Syndrome (A history of preceding febrile illness [usually a respiratory tract infection] and typical clinical features [especially leg weakness that progresses upward] suggest Guillain-Barré syndrome; no confirming test exists.)	CSF analysis	Protein levels increase, peaking in 4 to 6 weeks. WBC count usually remains normal.
	CBC	Moderately increased WBC count and a shift to immature forms occur early in the illness, but blood studies soon return to normal.
	EMG	May show repeated firing of the same motor unit, instead of widespread sectional stimulation
	Nerve conduction time	Nerve conduction velocities are slowed soon after paralysis develops.
Hemophilia A	PTT	Prolonged
	Factor VIII assay	0 to 30% of normal
Hepatitis, Viral	SGOT	Increased
	SGPT	Increased
	LDH	Increased
	Alkaline phosphatase	Increased
	Serum albumin	Decreased

(continued)

Diagnostic Test Profiles for Common Disorders *(continued)*

Disorder	Test	Results
Hepatitis, Viral *(continued)*	Serum bilirubin	Increased
	Serum cholesterol	Decreased
	Urine bilirubin	Increased
	PT	Prolonged
	Serologic testing for antibody to hepatitis (anti-HAV)	Positive in recent acute hepatitis A **Presence of anti-HAV confirms hepatitis A.**
	Serologic testing for antibody (IgM) to hepatitis B core antigen (anti-HB_C IgM)	**Confirms recent hepatitis B**
	Serologic testing for antibody to hepatitis B e antigen (anti-HB_e)	Positive in early and late convalescence from hepatitis B
	Serologic testing for antibody to hepatitis B surface antigen (anti-HB_s)	Indicates clinical recovery and immunity to hepatitis B
Herniated Disk	Myelogram	Reveals spinal compression by herniated nucleus pulposus via a narrowing of the column of dye through the spinal canal **Myelography results confirm the diagnosis.**
	EMG	May show a decrease in the number of muscle fibers contracting (nerve root compression) in the area of herniation
	Spinal X-rays	May or may not show degenerative joint disease in the area of herniation
	Spinal CT scan	Shows obvious prolapse of nucleus pulposus with unilateral or bilateral nerve root compression. If the herniation is midline, spinal cord or cauda

Diagnostic Test Profiles for Common Disorders *(continued)*

Disorder	Test	Results
Herniated Disk *(continued)*	Spinal CT scan *(continued)*	equina compression will be seen, depending on the location of disk herniation.
Herpes Genitalis	Genital lesion smear	Shows multinucleated giant cells with intranuclear inclusions in a specimen prepared by Pap or other histochemical stain; or shows typical herpes simplex virus (HSV) morphology on electron microscopy; or detects herpes simplex virus antigen by radioisotope or enzyme assay **Results from smear are only presumptive for the disorder.**
	HSV viral tissue culture from cervix, urethra, or base of a genital lesion	Shows the characteristic cytopathogenic effect; serologic testing identifies type 1 or type 2 herpes simplex virus **Results of tissue culture confirm the diagnosis.**
Hodgkin's Disease	ESR	Usually increased with active disease
	Lymph node biopsy	May demonstrate Sternberg-Reed cells and can confirm the main histologic type: nodular sclerosis, mixed cellularity, lymphocyte predominance, or lymphocyte depletion **Sternberg-Reed cells are the characteristic malignant cells of Hodgkin's disease.**

(continued)

Diagnostic Test Profiles for Common Disorders *(continued)*

Disorder	Test	Results
Hodgkin's Disease *(continued)*	*Tests performed to demonstrate extent of disease or specific organ involvement:*	
	Alkaline phosphatase	Increased with bone or liver involvement
	BUN	Increased with renal involvement
	Serum creatinine	Increased with renal involvement
	Bone marrow biopsy	May demonstrate presence of Sternberg-Reed cells or bone marrow fibrosis with marrow involvement
	Liver-spleen scan	Shows splenic enlargement in generalized disease; may also show liver involvement
	Chest X-ray	May show hilar or mediastinal mass, if present
	Chest tomography	Shows extent of hilar or mediastinal adenopathy
	Bilateral lower extremity lymphangiogram	May show nodal involvement below level of the diaphragm, if present. Involvement of nodes on both sides of the diaphragm indicates at least Stage III disease
	Skeletal X-rays	May show bone involvement, if present
	Bone scan	More sensitive identification of bone lesions, if present
	Laparotomy with multiple biopsies	Identifies extent of abdominal disease

Diagnostic Test Profiles for Common Disorders *(continued)*

Disorder	Test	Results
Hyperthyroidism	Serum triiodothyronine (T_3)	Increased
	Serum thyroxine (T_4)	Increased. T_4 levels may be increased with other disorders.
	T_3 resin uptake (T_3RU)	High uptake percentage. High T_3RU, along with increased T_4 levels, indicates this disorder.
	Serum thyroid-stimulating hormone (TSH) *(Using improved assay techniques, TSH can be used as a quick screening test.)*	Below normal values
	Serum free thyroxine (FT_4) *(May replace the use of T_4 and T_3RU.)*	Usually increased; FT_4 is decreased in T_3 toxicosis
Hypothyroidism	Serum T_3	Characteristically decreased. T_3 radioimmunoassay may be normal in mild hypothyroidism.
	Serum T_4	Decreased
	T_3RU	Low uptake percentage. Low T_3RU, along with decreased T_4, indicates this disorder.
	Serum TSH	Increased in primary hypothyroidism (thyroid gland failure); decreased in secondary hypothyroidism (pituitary disease) and in tertiary hypothyroidism (hypothalamic disease)
	TSH challenge test	Increased response and increased TSH level in primary hypothyroidism; no response in secondary

(continued)

Diagnostic Test Profiles for Common Disorders *(continued)*

Disorder	Test	Results
Hypothyroidism *(continued)*	TSH challenge test *(continued)*	hypothyroidism; response often delayed in tertiary hypothyroidism
	Serum FT_4	Decreased
	Serum FT_3	Decreased
Impaired Glucose Tolerance (Borderline Diabetes) (Diagnosis is restricted to those with results of *both* tests, as identified here.)	Fasting plasma glucose	Less than 140 mg/dl in nonpregnant adults and children
	Oral glucose tolerance test	A 2-hour plasma glucose level of > 140 mg/dl in children; a 2-hour plasma glucose level between 140 and 200 mg/dl and an intervening plasma glucose level of 200 mg/dl or greater in nonpregnant adults
Infectious Mononucleosis (IM)	CBC	Leukocyte count increases 10,000 to 20,000/mm³ during the 2nd and 3rd weeks of illness. In the differential, lymphocytes and monocytes account for 50% to 70% of the total WBC count; at least 10% of the lymphocytes are atypical.
	Heterophil agglutination tests *(Slide tests have largely replaced the heterophil titer.)*	Heterophil antibody titer of 1:56 or greater
	Qualitative slide test, such as the Monospot, for IM	Positive for IM
	Indirect immunofluorescence studies for Epstein-Barr virus (EBV) antibodies *(Indirect immunofluorescence studies are more definitive, but their availability is somewhat limited.)*	Detects antibodies to EBV and cellular antigens

Diagnostic Test Profiles for Common Disorders *(continued)*

Disorder	Test	Results
Infectious Mono-nucleosis *(continued)*	*Tests done to check liver function:*	
	Serum bilirubin	Increased
	Alkaline phosphatase	Increased to high levels for a few days
Irritable Bowel Syndrome (Diagnosis requires a careful history, especially contributing psychological factors, and must rule out other disorders.)	Barium enema	Normal; may show narrowing of large bowel, indicating spasm
	Proctosigmoidoscopy	Essentially normal mucosa with the exception of mild hyperemia and evidence of increased mucous production; possibly increased sensitivity to rectal distention; lumen narrowing may be visualized
	Stool examination for blood, parasites, and bacteria	Negative
Iron Deficiency Anemia (Diagnosis may be obscured and values changed by superimposed conditions, such as chronic inflammation.)	CBC	Decreased hematocrit level; decreased hemoglobin level; increased RBC count, with microcytic and hypochromic cells
	RBC indices	Decreased mean corpuscular hemoglobin level in severe anemia
	Serum iron	Decreased
	Total iron-binding capacity	Increased
	Serum transferrin	Increased in severe iron deficiency
	Serum ferritin	Decreased
	Bone marrow aspiration *(Bone marrow aspiration is usually unnecessary.)*	Shows absent iron stores

(continued)

Diagnostic Test Profiles for Common Disorders *(continued)*

Disorder	Test	Results
Laryngeal Cancer	Laryngoscopy (direct or indirect)	Reveals presence and location of mass
	Laryngeal CT scan	Reveals extent of tumor, including involvement of cartilage and soft tissue
	Soft-tissue X-rays of neck	Demonstrates presence of a mass
	Barium swallow	Reveals exact anatomic and functional abnormalities associated with laryngeal mass
	Biopsy of the larynx	Histologic examination identifies cancerous cells. **Biopsy results confirm diagnosis.**
Liver Cancer (Primary Hepatic Carcinoma)	SGOT	Increased
	SGPT	Increased
	Alkaline phosphatase	Increased
	LDH	Increased
	Serum bilirubin	Increased only in later stages
	Serum alpha-fetoprotein	Increased
	Fasting plasma glucose	Decreased
	Total cholesterol	Decreased
	Liver CT scan	Usually reveals focal lesions of decreased density
	Liver ultrasonography	Reveals hypoechoic or echogenic areas that are either well defined or poorly defined
	Liver scan	Typically reveals focal defect

Diagnostic Test Profiles for Common Disorders *(continued)*

Disorder	Test	Results
Liver Cancer *(continued)*	Liver biopsy	Histologic examination reveals cancerous cells. **Biopsy results confirm diagnosis.**
	Peritoneal fluid cytology	May reveal malignant cells
	Celiac and mesenteric arteriography	Shows presence and distribution of hepatic tumor
Lung Cancer (Bronchogenic Carcinoma)	Chest X-ray	Identifies hilar or mediastinal mass or peripheral infiltrate or nodule; detects presence and location of most lesions at least 1 cm in diameter
	Sputum cytology *(Cells may be obtained from expectorated sputum sample or from bronchoscopic washing or brushing.)*	May detect atypical cells or lung cancer cells
	Bronchoscopy	Can visualize tumor mass in the bronchial tree
	Thoracic CT scan	Shows the exact dimension and internal composition of a pulmonary mass, revealing irregular borders in malignancy
	Biopsy (needle, transbronchial, or open lung)	Histologic examination identifies cancerous cells. **Biopsy results confirm diagnosis.**
	Chest tomography	Central calcification in a nodule suggests a benign lesion; an irregularly bordered tumor suggests malignancy; a sharply defined tumor suggests granuloma or nonmalignancy. Evaluation of the hilum can help differentiate blood vessels from nodes; identify bronchial

(continued)

Diagnostic Test Profiles for Common Disorders *(continued)*

Disorder	Test	Results
Lung Cancer *(continued)*	Chest tomography *(continued)*	dilation, stenosis, and endobronchial lesions; and detect tumor extension into the hilar lung area.
Malignant Melanoma	Skin biopsy	Histologic examination identifies cellular features of malignant melanoma. **Biopsy results confirm diagnosis.**
	Urine melanin	In the *presence* of a visible skin tumor, large quantities of melanin or melanogens in the urine indicate advanced internal metastasis; in the *absence* of a visible skin tumor, large quantities of melanin or melanogens in urine indicate an internal melanoma.
Meningitis	CSF analysis	In bacterial meningitis, CSF pressure may be elevated and color is cloudy; WBC count is elevated, protein level is elevated, and glucose level is decreased. In viral or septic meningitis, WBC count is elevated, and glucose and protein levels are usually normal. CSF culture may identify a causative organism, such as *Neisseria meningitidis* or *Hemophilus influenzae* in bacterial meningitis; or a virus, such as mumps virus or a coxsackie virus, by serologic methods.
	Blood cultures	May reveal causative bacterial organisms, such as *N. meningitidis* or *H. influenzae*
	CBC	Increased WBC count; differential shows increased neutrophils

Diagnostic Test Profiles for Common Disorders *(continued)*

Disorder	Test	Results
Meningitis *(continued)*	Intracranial CT scan	Normal, or may show meningeal enhancement
	MRI	Normal, or may show meningeal enhancement
Mitral stenosis	Chest X-ray	May show left atrial and ventricular enlargement, enlarged pulmonary arteries, and mitral valve calcification
	EKG	Shows left atrial hypertrophy; frequently, atrial fibrillation; with disease progression, right ventricular hypertrophy and right axis deviation
	Echocardiography	Identifies thickened mitral valve leaflets and left atrial enlargement
	Cardiac catheterization	Demonstrates diastolic pressure gradient across the mitral valve; elevated left atrial pressure and pulmonary capillary wedge pressure (PCWP > 15) with severe pulmonary hypertension and pulmonary arterial pressures; elevated right heart pressure; decreased cardiac output. Valve size may be less than 1 cm^2 in severe disease. Angiography may reveal abnormal contraction of the left ventricle.
Multiple Myeloma	CBC	Decreased RBC count; WBC differential may show 40% to 50% lymphocytes, but seldom more than 3% plasma cells. Differential smear shows rouleaux formation.

(continued)

Diagnostic Test Profiles for Common Disorders *(continued)*

Disorder	Test	Results
Multiple Myeloma *(continued)*	Serum protein electrophoresis	Shows an elevated globulin spike
	X-rays, such as skull, pelvic, spinal	Show multiple, sharply circumscribed osteolytic (punched-out) lesions, particularly on the skull, pelvis, and spine. May show vertebral compression fractures and demineralization
	Urine for Bence Jones protein	May be positive **Bence Jones protein confirms the diagnosis, but its absence does not rule it out.**
	Urine calcium	May be increased
	Bone marrow aspiration	Reveals an abnormal number of immature plasma cells **Bone marrow findings may be necessary to confirm the diagnosis.**
Multiple Sclerosis (MS) (A definite diagnosis of MS is rarely given unless there is neurologic evidence of *at least two* lesions—each one in a different area of the central nervous system [CNS]—and a course of exacerbation and remission, with the remissions separated by at least 1 month.)	Evoked potential studies	Delayed visual, auditory, and/or somatosensory evoked potentials may occur.
	CSF analysis	Increased WBC count ($>5/mm^3$); elevated IgG; the presence of oligoclonal IgG bonds; the presence of myelin basic protein
	Intracranial CT scan; MRI	May show lesions in the white matter of the brain, as well as more generalized atrophic changes and enlargement of the ventricles. Similar CT and MRI changes are seen in other CNS diseases.

Diagnostic Test Profiles for Common Disorders *(continued)*

Disorder	Test	Results
Muscular Dystrophy (MD) (Duchenne's) (Characteristic abnormalities of gait and other voluntary movements, with a typical medical and family history, suggest this diagnosis.)	Muscle biopsy	Increased connective tissue and fat deposits **Biopsy results confirm diagnosis.**
	EMG	Shows short, weak bursts of electrical activity in affected muscles
	CPK	Increased
	LDH	Increased
	SGOT	Increased
	DNA studies (on fluid from amniocentesis) *(This prenatal test using DNA probes is new and can detect Duchenne's MD in the fetus with 96% to 99% accuracy. It can also identify female carriers of the disease.)*	Identifies genetic variations called restriction fragment length polymorphisms on the short arm of the X chromosome.
Myasthenia Gravis	Tensilon test	2 to 10 mg of edrophonium chloride produces improved muscle function within 1 minute, or 2 mg of neostigmine bromide produces improved muscle function within 30 minutes. **The Tensilon test confirms the diagnosis.**
	EMG	Motor unit potentials may be normal initially but progressively diminish in amplitude with continuing contractions.
	Muscle biopsy	Postsynaptic membrane changes with a reduced number of acetylcholine receptor sites.
	Acetylcholine receptor antibody test	Titers may be elevated.

(continued)

Diagnostic Test Profiles for Common Disorders *(continued)*

Disorder	Test	Results
Myasthenia Gravis *(continued)*	Chest X-ray	May show abnormal mediastinal contour due to hyperplasia of thymus or a thymoma. An enlarged thymus is often associated with myasthenia gravis.
	Thoracic CT scan	May detect hyperplasia of thymus, or thymoma
Myocardial Infarction (MI)	Serial 12-lead EKG	EKG abnormalities may be absent or inconclusive during the first few hours after an MI. When present, characteristic abnormalities show serial ST-T segment changes in subendocardial MI, and Q waves representing transmural MI. An *inferior wall MI* will show typical pattern changes—a pathologic Q wave, ST segment elevation, and T-wave inversion—in leads II, III, and aVF. *Lateral wall involvement* will cause a reduced R wave, a T-wave inversion, and, in some cases, an elevation of the ST-T segment in the lateral leads V_5, V_6, aVL, and L_1. A *posterior wall infarction* causes a tall R wave and an upright T wave in V_1. An *anterior MI* will produce a typical infarction pattern in leads I, aVL, and V_2 to V_6. An *anteroseptal infarction* will cause the typical pattern in leads V_1 to V_4. An *anterolateral infarction* will produce the typical pattern in leads I, V_5, and V_6. An infarction within the anterolateral surface of the left ventricle—a *high antero-*

Diagnostic Test Profiles for Common Disorders *(continued)*

Disorder	Test	Results
Myocardial Infarction (MI) *(continued)*	Serial 12-lead EKG *(continued)*	*lateral infarction*—will produce typical changes in leads aVL, L_1, and V_6.
	Echocardiogram	Shows ventricular wall dyskinesia if the MI is transmural
	CPK	Increased
	CPK-MB (isoenzyme, the cardiac muscle fraction of CPK)	Increased. Typically, CPK-MB levels rise 4 to 8 hours after onset of acute MI, peak after 20 hours, and may remain elevated for up to 72 hours.
	LDH	Increased
	LDH_1 and LDH_2 (isoenzymes)	Increased. Typically, levels rise 8 to 12 hours after an acute MI, peak in 24 hours, and return to normal in 10 to 14 days. An LDH_1 level exceeding an LDH_2 level is indicative of an acute MI.
	SGOT	Increased
	Hydroxybutyric dehydrogenase	Increased
	ESR	Increased
	CBC	Increased WBC count
	Thallium myocardial imaging *(Test cannot differentiate old from new infarction.)*	Cold spots reveal acutely damaged myocardial tissue within the first few hours after an infarction.
	Technetium pyrophosphate scan *(Technetium scanning is particularly helpful when a patient presents a few days after the onset of symptoms, when EKGs*	Hot spots reveal acutely damaged myocardial tissue. A spot's size usually corresponds to the injury size.

(continued)

Diagnostic Test Profiles for Common Disorders *(continued)*

Disorder	Test	Results
Myocardial Infarction (MI) *(continued)*	Technetium pyrophosphate scan *(continued) may be stable and enzymes may have returned to normal. The greatest positivity occurs 4 to 7 days after MI.)*	
	PET *(PET is used to assess blood flow and metabolic activity in the myocardium. This test is not widely used because of limited availability.)*	Shows areas of damage or potential areas of underperfused but viable myocardium
Myocarditis	CPK	Increased
	CPK-MB (isoenzyme)	Increased
	LDH	Increased
	SGOT	Increased
	CBC	Increased WBC count
	ESR	Increased
	EKG	Typically shows diffuse ST segment and T-wave abnormalities, conduction defects (prolonged P-R interval), and other supraventricular ectopic dysrhythmias
	Cultures (throat and stool)	May identify causative bacteria
	Antibody titers, ASO titer	Increased in rheumatic fever
Osteoarthritis (Osteoarthritis is distinguished from rheumatoid arthritis by its clinical presentation and X-ray findings; no confirming laboratory test exists.)	X-rays of affected joint	X-rays characteristically reveal narrowing of joint space or margin, cystlike bony deposits in joint space and margins, joint deformity, and bony growths at weight-bearing areas.

Diagnostic Test Profiles for Common Disorders *(continued)*

Disorder	Test	Results
Osteoarthritis *(continued)*	ESR	May be mildly to moderately increased in some patients
Osteomyelitis	CBC	Increased WBC count
	ESR	Increased
	Blood cultures	May identify causative organisms; may be negative
	Plain X-rays	May show bone involvement but may not show bone involvement early in disease
	Bone scan	Shows hot spots in involved areas
	CT scan of involved site	Shows slight density shift where bone marrow is filled with pus and fluid; may show destruction of bony structure
	Gallium scan *(Gallium scanning is particularly helpful in diagnosing children, because hot spots on a bone scan may be normal during the growth period.)*	Abnormal concentration of gallium in infected area
Osteoporosis	Spinal X-rays	Show typical degeneration of the thoracic and lumbar vertebrae. As the spongy trabeculae become progressively fewer and more delicate, the cortical rims stand out by contrast. The involved bone has a ground-glass appearance. The vertebral bodies may appear flattened, with varying degrees of collapse and wedging, and may look denser than adjacent vertebrae.

(continued)

Diagnostic Test Profiles for Common Disorders *(continued)*

Disorder	Test	Results
Osteoporosis *(continued)*	*Tests performed to rule out other disorders:*	
	Serum calcium	Normal
	Serum phosphorus	Normal
	Alkaline phosphatase	Normal
	Serum protein electrophoresis	Normal
Ovarian Cancer	Abdominal X-ray	Findings range from nonspecific soft-tissue densities to discrete calcification on ovaries.
	IVP (excretory urography)	May show ureteral obstruction by ovarian tumor
	Pelvic ultrasonography	Reveals ovarian mass
	Exploratory laparotomy *(Exploratory laparotomy also allows for reductive surgery and biopsy sampling.)*	Permits direct visualization of the tumor and its extent **Exploratory laparotomy confirms the diagnosis.**
	Serum estrogen	Increased in some stromal hormone-producing tumors
	Serum testosterone	Increased in some stromal hormone-producing tumors
	24-hour urine for 17-ketosteroid excretion	Normal or slightly increased in some stromal hormone-producing tumors
	Serum alpha-fetoprotein	Increased in some germ-cell tumors
	Serum B-hCG	Increased in some germ-cell tumors
Ovarian Cysts	Pelvic ultrasonography	Typically identifies dimension and location of mass; may distinguish cyst from solid tumor

Diagnostic Test Profiles for Common Disorders *(continued)*

Disorder	Test	Results
Ovarian Cysts *(continued)*	Laparoscopy or laparotomy	Ovarian cyst is visualized. **Results of laparoscopy or laparotomy confirm the diagnosis.**
	Culdocentesis *(Culdocentesis is usually done only to determine whether emergency surgery is necessary.)*	May be positive (blood in cul-de-sac); positive results typically occur with ruptured corpus luteum cysts
Pancreatic Cancer	Pancreatic CT scan *(Pancreatic CT scan is usually preferred over ultrasonography for diagnosing this disorder.)*	May disclose a mass or, in the case of a small tumor, a change in pancreatic contour
	Pancreatic ultrasonography	May identify a pancreatic mass
	Endoscopic retrograde cholangiopancreatography	Typically shows encroachment of pancreatic tumor on the duodenal wall and blockage of the pancreatic ducts
	Pancreatic arteriography	Will identify major vessel encasement, if present
	Biopsy (CT-guided percutaneous needle biopsy, or laparotomy with biopsy)	Histologic examination identifies cancerous cells. **Biopsy results confirm the diagnosis.**
	Laboratory values supporting the diagnosis:	
	CEA	Often increased
	Serum bilirubin	Increased
	Serum amylase	Occasionally increased
	Serum lipase	Occasionally increased
	PT	May be prolonged
	Plasma insulin immunoassay	Measurable serum insulin in presence of islet cell tumors

(continued)

Diagnostic Test Profiles for Common Disorders *(continued)*

Disorder	Test	Results
Pancreatic Cancer *(continued)*	Alkaline phosphatase	Marked increase with biliary obstruction
Pancreatitis (Acute)	Serum amylase	Increased during first 24 to 72 hours; may be five or more times normal **Increased serum amylase levels usually confirm diagnosis.**
	Urine amylase	Increased for up to 2 weeks after acute episode
	Serum lipase	Increased. Serum lipase levels rise more slowly than serum amylase.
	Hematocrit; hemoglobin	Increased because of hemoconcentration.
	Serum calcium	Decreased
	WBC count	Increased
	Fasting plasma glucose	Sometimes increased
	Pancreatic ultrasonography	Shows enlarged pancreas with sonolucent texture
	Pancreatic CT scan	Shows enlarged pancreas
Parkinson's Disease (Diagnosis is usually based on clinical presentation and ruling out other disorders.)	PET *(PET is a promising new study not widely available yet.)*	Possible decrease in dopamine uptake in the basal ganglia
	Intracranial CT scan; MRI	Normal in primary Parkinson's disease
	EEG	Diffuse, nonspecific slowing of theta waves and abnormal sleep studies
	CSF analysis	Possible decrease in homovanillic acid (HVA), but HVA findings do not provide reliable confirmation of this disorder

Diagnostic Test Profiles for Common Disorders *(continued)*

Disorder	Test	Results
Pelvic Inflammatory Disease (PID)	CBC	Possibly increased WBC count; however, may not be increased in chronic disease
	Laparoscopy	Edema, hyperemia, and exudate of fallopian tube(s) can be visualized. **Results of laparoscopy confirm the diagnosis.**
	Cervical culture, or culture of tubal exudate done with laparoscopy or laparotomy	May identify causative organism, such as *Neisseria gonorrhoeae*
Peptic Ulcer	Upper GI and small-bowel series	May show abnormalities in the mucosa of the esophagus, stomach, or small bowel when an ulcer is present
	Basal gastric secretion test *(Results of basal gastric secretion test must be evaluated and interpreted with the results of the gastric acid stimulation test.)*	Increased gastric secretion
	Gastric acid stimulation test	Increased gastric secretion
	Esophagogastroduodenoscopy *(This test is typically the most accurate procedure for establishing the diagnosis.)*	Visualizes an ulcer in the esophagus, stomach, or small bowel
	Biopsy *(Biopsy may be performed to differentiate gastric ulcer from gastric carcinoma.)*	Absence of cancerous cells
	Fecal occult blood test	May be positive for GI bleeding

(continued)

Diagnostic Test Profiles for Common Disorders *(continued)*

Disorder	Test	Results
Pericarditis, Chronic Constrictive	EKG	May show low-voltage and nonspecific ST-T changes and intraatrial conduction defects
	Chest X-ray	Heart size varies. Pleural effusions are commonly seen.
	Cardiac fluoroscopy	May show pericardial calcifications and decreased cardiac pulsations.
	Echocardiography	No specific pattern; occasionally, abnormal ventricular septal motion and pericardial thickening are observed. Pericardial effusion, if present, is also readily recognized.
	Cardiac catheterization	Right atrial pressure is always greater than 9 mm Hg. Systolic pressure in the right ventricle is normal or slightly elevated. Right ventricular and left ventricular end-diastolic pressures, pulmonary artery diastolic pressure, and mean right atrial and left atrial pressures are usually equal. **Cardiac catheterization will usually confirm the diagnosis.**

Diagnostic Test Profiles for Common Disorders (continued)

Disorder	Test	Results
Pernicious Anemia	Serum vitamin B_{12}	Decreased
	Serum folate	Decreased or normal
	Bone marrow aspiration	Reveals erythroid hyperplasia (crowded red bone marrow), with increased numbers of megaloblasts but few normally developing RBCs
	RBC indices	Mean corpuscular volume and mean corpuscular hemoglobin increased
	Schilling test	Usually < 2% radioactive vitamin B_{12} excreted in urine in 24 hours; following administration of intrinsic factor with an oral tracer dose of vitamin B_{12}, urinary excretion of vitamin B_{12} becomes normal. **Schilling test results confirm the diagnosis.**
	Gastric acid stimulation test	Absence of free hydrochloric acid secretion following stimulation with pentagastrin
Pneumonia, Bacterial	Chest X-ray	Localized, well-defined, hazy shadow; airspace consolidation
	CBC	Increased WBC count, often to > 20,000/mm³
	Sputum culture and sensitivity	Abundant bacteria (most frequently pneumococci and staphylococci) and WBCs. Sputum specimen often shows contaminants from the oropharynx and mouth.
	Blood culture	Reveals pathogens in 25% to 40% of cases

(continued)

Diagnostic Test Profiles for Common Disorders *(continued)*

Disorder	Test	Results
Pneumonia, Bacterial *(continued)*	ABG analysis	PaO$_2$ may be decreased in varying degrees, depending on severity of disease.
Pneumonia, Post-influenza Viral	Chest X-ray	May be negative initially; as disease progresses, diffuse patchy consolidation appears. There may be minor infiltrates or any degree up to severe bilateral infiltrates.
	CBC	Normal WBC count
	Sputum culture and sensitivity	No bacteria; some epithelial debris; few WBCs. Sputum is usually minimal and clear, but can be purulent.
	Viral antibody titers	Increased
	ABG analysis	PaO$_2$ may be decreased in varying degrees, depending on severity of disease.
Prostatic Cancer (Diagnosis is suggested by prostatic mass felt on rectal examination.)	Biopsy	Histologic examination identifies cancerous cells. **Biopsy results confirm diagnosis.**
	Needle aspiration	Cytologic examination identifies cancerous cells.
	Acid phosphatase	May be increased if disease is disseminated or, if performed as a radioimmunoassay, may be increased with local disease
	IVP (excretory urography)	May show urethral, bladder neck, or ureteral obstruction

Diagnostic Test Profiles for Common Disorders (continued)

Disorder	Test	Results
Psoriasis (Diagnosis depends on patient history, appearance of the lesions, and, if needed, the results of skin biopsy.)	Skin biopsy	Psoriasiform histologic features
	Serum uric acid	Increased
	HLA test	HLA antigens 13 and 17 may be present.
Pulmonary Embolism (PE)	Chest X-ray	May or may not reveal the characteristic wedge-shaped infiltrate suggestive of PE; may show effusion
	Lung perfusion scan *(The lung perfusion scan and the ventilation scan are both needed to establish the diagnosis.)*	Cold spots indicate areas of poor perfusion.
	Ventilation scan	"Wash-in" phase reveals areas of hypoventilation, which fill slowly or not at all. "Wash-out" phase demonstrates air trapping.
	Pulmonary angiography	Shows interruption in the flow of contrast agent through the pulmonary circulation system **Pulmonary angiography is performed when scans are nondiagnostic and definitely confirms diagnosis.**
	ABG analysis	May or may not show a decreased PaO_2 and $PaCO_2$
	DSA *(DSA is sometimes performed before angiography and may eliminate the need for it. However, its results are not yet as good.)*	Interruption in flow of contrast media may be visualized.

(continued)

Diagnostic Test Profiles for Common Disorders (continued)

Disorder	Test	Results
Pyelonephritis, Acute (Diagnosis is suggested by history and physical findings of chills, fever, costovertebral tenderness, and urinary complaints.)	Urinalysis	RBCs may be increased; WBCs are increased; specific gravity is decreased; pH is slightly alkaline; protein may be present.
	Urine culture	Bacterial counts of more than 100,000/mm³
	IVP (excretory urography)	May show contributing cause as calculi or other obstructive lesions or anomalies
Renal Calculi	Urinalysis	May be normal or may show increased RBCs, increased WBCs, and presence of urate, calcium, or cystine crystals in sediment
	KUB radiography	May reveal opaque bodies, which reflect calculi
	IVP (excretory urography)	Identifies the size and location of calculi and detects obstruction to urine flow, if any **IVP results confirm the diagnosis.**
	Renal CT scan	Images calculi
	Renal ultrasonography	Shows hydronephrosis due to obstruction, if present. Hydronephrosis is indicated by a large, echo-free central mass that compresses the renal cortex.
Renovascular Hypertension	Rapid-sequence IVP	Delayed dye appearance on one side suggests unilateral stenosis of the renal artery.
	Saralasin test	Diastolic pressure drops by 7 to 10 mm Hg or more, or by more than 8%.

Diagnostic Test Profiles for Common Disorders (continued)

Disorder	Test	Results
Renovascular Hypertension (continued)	Radionuclide renography	When a renal artery is stenotic, the affected kidney takes up less of the isotope and does so more slowly than normal. It also excretes the isotope more slowly, and the vascular phase curve is shorter and less steep than normal. Similarly, the excretory phase curve returns to baseline more slowly than normal.
	Renal arteriography	Renal artery stenosis caused by arteriosclerosis produces a noticeable constriction in the blood vessels, usually within the proximal portion of its length. Renal artery dysplasia usually affects the middle and distal portions of the vessel. The characteristic lesions resemble a string of beads. **Results of renal arteriography confirm a diagnosis of renal artery stenosis.**
	Renal vein renin sampling	Severe stenosis is suggested by a renal vein specimen with a renin concentration of 50% more than the renin concentration in a vena cava specimen or 50% more than the average renin concentration in a mixed venous specimen, or a kidney-to-kidney ratio of 1.5 or more.

(continued)

Diagnostic Test Profiles for Common Disorders *(continued)*

Disorder	Test	Results
Renovascular Hypertension *(continued)*	DSA *(DSA is still being improved, but it may soon replace IVP and radionuclide renography as screening tests and may reduce the need for renal arteriography in some patients.)*	Image shows renal artery stenosis.
Reye's Syndrome	Plasma ammonia	Increased **Increased plasma ammonia levels and patient history of preceding viral disorder with characteristic clinical features strongly indicate Reye's syndrome.**
	SGOT	Increased
	SGPT	Increased
	CPK	Near normal or increased
	Serum bilirubin	Usually normal
	PT	Prolonged
	PTT	Prolonged
	Serum lactic acid	Increased. Serum lactic acid levels correlate with the degree of coma.
	Serum fatty acid	Increased
	Serum glucose	Normal or (in 15% of cases) decreased
	Intracranial CT scan	Nonfocal but may show cerebral edema
	CSF analysis	Protein and glucose levels normal; WBC count < 10/mm^3; normal or increased CSF pressure

Diagnostic Test Profiles for Common Disorders *(continued)*

Disorder	Test	Results
Reye's Syndrome *(continued)*	Liver biopsy	Reveals typical pattern of fatty droplets uniformly distributed throughout cells. While liver biopsy results may confirm the diagnosis, the test is usually not performed because of the risk of bleeding and the delay in obtaining test results.
Rheumatoid Arthritis (RA)	RF	Positive RF titers in 80% of patients with RA **RF titers above 1:80 are usually diagnostic of RA; titers between 1:20 and 1:80 may occur in other disorders.**
	Antinuclear antibodies (ANA)	May be increased
	Lupus erythematosus (LE) cell preparation	LE cells may or may not be present with RA.
	ESR	Increased in 85% to 90% of patients with RA. ESR decreases with positive response to therapy.
	C-reactive protein (CRP) test	Positive during acute phase of RA. CRP is absent when inflammation has decreased because of positive response to therapy.
	Serum protein electrophoresis	May show increased serum globulin levels
	CBC	Decreased hematocrit level; slightly increased WBC count
	Synovial fluid analysis of involved joint(s)	Increased volume and turbidity, but decreased viscosity and complement levels. WBC count is often > 10,000/mm^3.

(continued)

Diagnostic Test Profiles for Common Disorders *(continued)*

Disorder	Test	Results
Rheumatoid Arthritis (RA) *(continued)*	X-rays of involved area(s)	Show bone demineralization and soft-tissue swelling in early stages; later, loss of cartilage and narrowing of joint spaces; finally, cartilage and bone destruction, and erosion, subluxation, and deformities
Scoliosis	Spinal X-rays	A standing posterior-anterior view identifies and determines the degree of spinal curvature; a standing lateral view reveals the status of kyphosis or lordosis; standing posterior-anterior bending X-rays reveal the amount of flexibility of the curve. **Spinal X-rays confirm diagnosis, although the presence of scoliosis is often apparent on physical examination.**
Seizure Disorder	EEG *(EEG is still the cardinal test to document and classify a seizure disorder.)*	Paroxysmal dysrhythmias, such as high-voltage, fast spike waves in all leads in tonic-clonic seizures; generalized 3/second spike-wave discharges in absence seizures; and focal spike or sharp-wave discharges in a partial seizure disorder
	PET *(PET is a promising newer test not yet in widespread use; with refinement, it may uncover more about the etiology and neurochemical aspects of this disorder.)*	Abnormal isotope concentration may identify brain areas involved in seizure activity.

Diagnostic Test Profiles for Common Disorders *(continued)*

Disorder	Test	Results
Seizure Disorder *(continued)*	*Tests performed to determine the cause:*	
	Intracranial CT scan; MRI	May show pathology, such as edema, tumor, cerebral atrophy, cerebral hemorrhage, infarction, subdural hematoma, or A-V malformation
	Skull X-rays	Usually normal but may show pineal shifts, intracranial calcification, bony changes, and asymmetry due to underlying trauma or malignancy
	CSF analysis	Usually normal, unless underlying CNS disease, such as meningitis, is present
	Brain scan (radionuclide)	May show A-V malformation, vascular tumor, or subdural hematoma
	Plasma glucose	May be decreased if hypoglycemia is the cause
	Drug screen	May be positive if drugs were taken
Sickle-Cell Anemia	CBC	May show decreased RBC count, increased WBC count, increased platelets, increased reticulocytes, and elevated ESR
	Blood smear	Shows occasional sickled erythrocytes
	Sickle-cell test (hemoglobin S)	Positive for sickling phenomenon **A positive sickle-cell (hemoglobin S) test confirms the diagnosis.**
	Hemoglobin electrophoresis	Shows presence of hemoglobin S, variable hemoglobin F, absent hemoglobin A *(continued)*

Diagnostic Test Profiles for Common Disorders *(continued)*

Disorder	Test	Results
Sickle-Cell Anemia *(continued)*	DNA studies (parenteral venous blood and amniocentesis fluid) *(DNA studies are performed if parents are suspected carriers.)*	Detects whether fetus has sickle-cell trait or the disease
Small-Bowel Obstruction	Abdominal X-ray (flat plate of the abdomen)	A typical "stepladder" pattern emerges, with alternating fluid and gas levels apparent. Abnormal patterns of gas and fluid revealed on X-ray identify the presence and location of the obstruction.
	Tests performed to assess metabolic disturbance:	
	CBC	Increased WBC count and hematocrit level. Markedly increased WBC count usually indicates peritonitis from strangulation.
	Serum electrolytes	Typically decreased sodium, potassium, and chloride levels. Sodium values may appear normal because of hemoconcentration.
	Urinalysis	Increased specific gravity and osmolality
Stroke (Hemorrhagic or Ischemic)	Intracranial CT scan	Increased density in area of major cerebral vessel branch or subarachnoid area in a hemorrhagic stroke; localized hypodensity within several days following an ischemic stroke, eventually becoming cystic; distorted brain structures due to mass effect of edema. Aneurysm or A-V malformation may be evident if contrast medium is used.

Diagnostic Test Profiles for Common Disorders *(continued)*

Disorder	Test	Results
Stroke *(continued)*	DSA	Increased vascular opacity in a particular area, indicating a vascular filling defect
	Cerebral angiography	May show narrowed cerebral artery, such as the internal carotid or vertebral arteries; collateral circulation; occluded cerebral branches; retrograde filling of distal arteries; or aneurysm or A-V malformation
	EEG	Focal slowing or sharp waves or spikes in area of cortical infarction
	Lumbar puncture and CSF analysis *(Lumbar puncture is contraindicated when a large lesion has been identified by CT scan or when increased intracranial pressure is suspected, because of the danger of brain herniation)*	Bloody CSF and elevated pressure in subarachnoid hemorrhage or extensive intracranial hemorrhage
	MRI	May delineate edematous and necrotic areas
	Ophthalmoscopy	May show signs of hypertension and atherosclerotic changes in retinal arteries
	CBC	Hematocrit level may be increased; platelet count may be increased.
	Fibrinogen	May be increased
	Serum cholesterol and triglycerides	May be increased with atherosclerotic vascular disease

(continued)

Diagnostic Test Profiles for Common Disorders *(continued)*

Disorder	Test	Results
Syphilis	Dark field examination	Direct visualization of spirochetes *(Treponema pallidum)* from lesions of primary and secondary syphilis **Identifying *T. pallidum* on dark field examination confirms the diagnosis. Dark field examination of late secondary or tertiary syphilis is usually negative.**
	Veneral Disease Research Laboratory (VDRL) test *(VDRL test is typically an initial screening test; it's less sensitive on CSF.)*	Reactive in about 75% of patients with primary syphilis and nearly all with secondary syphilis
	Rapid plasma reagin (RPR) test *(RPR is also an initial screening test.)*	Reactive
	Fluorescent treponemal antibody absorption (FTA-ABS) test *(FTA-ABS test is more sensitive than the VDRL test in detecting all stages of untreated syphilis.)*	Reactive (in serum for primary and secondary stages; in CSF for tertiary stage)
	Microhemagglutination assay for *T. pallidum* (MHA-TP) *(MHA-TP, a newer test, is replacing the FTA-ABS test in many centers.)*	Positive
Systemic Lupus Erythematosus (SLE)	CBC	Decreased hematocrit level; decreased WBC count; possibly decreased platelet count
	ESR	Often increased
	Serum protein electrophoresis	May show increased gamma globulin levels
	ANA	Usually increased with active SLE

Diagnostic Test Profiles for Common Disorders (continued)

Disorder	Test	Results
Systemic Lupus Erythematosus (continued)	Anti-DNA antibodies (Anti-DNA is the most specific test for SLE since it is rarely positive in other disorders; however, the results may be decreased or absent if SLE is in remission. The test also helps monitor response to therapy.)	Usually increased with active SLE
	LE cell preparation	Presence of at least two LE cells may indicate SLE. LE cells may form in other disorders; some patients with SLE demonstrate no LE cells.
	Serum complement assays	Decreased C_3 and C_4 levels when disease is active
	Tests performed to assess effect of SLE on organs/systems:	
	Urinalysis	May show RBCs, WBCs, and casts
	24-hour urine protein	May show significant protein loss (> 3.5 g/24 hours)
	Kidney biopsy	May show focal to diffuse proliferative glomerulonephritis, membranous glomerulonephritis, or mesangial glomerulonephritis. Kidney biopsy results guide therapy and determine prognosis.
	Chest X-ray	Results may indicate pleurisy or lupus pneumonitis.
	EKG	May show conduction defect with cardiac involvement or pericarditis

(continued)

Diagnostic Test Profiles for Common Disorders *(continued)*

Disorder	Test	Results
Tay-Sachs Disease	Serum hexosaminidase A	Decreased **Serum hexosaminidase A findings confirm the diagnosis.**
	CSF analysis	May show increased levels of SGOT, SGPT, and LDH.
Testicular Cancer (Diagnosis is suggested by testicular mass felt on physical examination.)	Scrotal ultrasonography	Identifies a solid testicular mass. Ultrasonography can usually distinguish a tumor from other conditions, such as hydrocele.
	Inguinal exploration and biopsy or orchiectomy	Histologic examination identifies cancerous cells. **Biopsy results confirm the diagnosis.**
	Serum B-hCG	May be increased
	Serum alpha-fetoprotein	May be increased
	Total urine estrogen	Increased
	Tests performed to determine the stage of the disease:	
	Abdominal CT scan	May show retroperitoneal lymph nodes involved with metastatic cancer
	Chest CT scan; chest tomography	May identify chest metastasis
Ulcerative Colitis	Proctosigmoidoscopy	Typically shows diffuse erythema, mucosal friability, decreased mucosal detail, absence of discrete ulcers, and thick inflammatory exudate. In advanced stages, ulcerations are present.
	Colonoscopy *(Colonoscopy is contraindicated in fulminant disease.)*	Reveals the linear extent of disease, with same differentiating characteristics as above

Diagnostic Test Profiles for Common Disorders *(continued)*

Disorder	Test	Results
Ulcerative Colitis *(continued)*	Barium enema *(Barium enema is contra-indicated during acute phase.)*	Shows fine serrations, with superficial ulcerations that involve the entire mucosal surface. With progression, the pattern becomes more coarse. Pseudopolyps and strictures may also be seen.
	Multiple biopsies	Reveal diffuse, superficial inflammation and polymorphonuclear leukocyte invasion of epithelium; may show dysplasia associated with carcinoma with disease of long duration
	Serum potassium; hemoglobin	Decreased in severe disease
	ESR	Increased in severe disease

7 MICROBIOLOGICAL TESTING

Introduction

Diagnostic microbiology can provide rapid, reliable information concerning microorganisms that may be involved in infectious processes in the body. These living creatures—bacteria, fungi (yeasts and molds), protozoa, and viruses—are so small that single cells cannot be viewed with the unaided eye. (See *Microorganisms and Their Diagnostic Tests*.)

Microscopy is the most important tool in the study of microorganisms. Various techniques—bright-field, dark-field, phase-contrast, fluorescent, and electron microscopy—provide a wide range of magnifications and the ability to study various characteristics. Some microorganisms (for example, most parasites) are identified through microscopic examinations only, since cultural techniques are either unavailable or impractical.

Prepared specimens may include wet-mount films (material suspended in a liquid) or smears (thin films of material spread on a glass slide, dried, and stained). Wet mounts are useful when looking for parasites, yeasts, or mycelial elements in clinical specimens. Sometimes a stain is added to reveal greater cellular detail. For example, cryptococcal meningitis may be tentatively diagnosed by visualizing encapsulated yeast on an india-ink preparation of cerebrospinal fluid.

The most common and useful staining procedure in bacteriological exams is the Gram stain. This is a differential stain that divides bacteria into two physiological groups: gram-positive or gram-negative. Differences in cell-wall composition allow gram-positive organisms to retain a dye after decolorization, whereas gram-negative organisms cannot.

In addition to providing clues to the type of organisms present in a specimen, a Gram stain can give evidence of the inflammatory response of the patient and can help differentiate poorly collected material from that more representative of the infection site.

Identification of etiological agents based on Gram stain results should always be considered tentative, and must be confirmed by cultural isolation and identification.

Another staining procedure, the acid-fast method, helps identify organisms of the genus *Mycobacterium*. Use of this stain can be invaluable when examining a specimen containing many types of bacteria (for example, sputum) and for aiding in the diagnosis of tubercular infection. Recently, a newly recognized protozoan parasite, *Cryptosporidium*, has been found to possess this acid-fast quality, a valuable discovery since its small size allows it to be easily overlooked in routine parasitological examinations.

Other stains used in microscopy include trichrome, Giemsa, and Wright's stains, silver stains, and the periodic acid-Schiff (PAS) stain (used to identify certain protozoan parasites, fungi, *Pneumocystis carinii*, herpesvirus, and *Chlamydia*).

Microorganisms and Their Diagnostic Tests

Micro-organism	Description	Diagnostic tests
Bacteria	Ubiquitous, unicellular organisms; prokaryotic cell organization (few structures, primitive); few overt pathogens; mainly opportunistic	
Routine	Rapid-to-moderate growth; generally nonfastidious; aerobic, facultative, or anaerobic organisms	Gram stain: mainly used; presumptive Culture: mainly used; definitive Serology: sometimes used; presumptive Other immunology: sometimes used; presumptive
Mycobacteria	Slow-growing; fastidious; aerobic	Acid-fast stain: mainly used; preliminary Culture: mainly used; definitive Immunology: purified protein derivative (PPD) skin test; often used; preliminary
Legionella	Moderate-growing; fastidious	Smears: direct fluorescent antibody; often used; presumptive Gram, Gimenez and Dieterle stains: sometimes used; presumptive Culture: often used; definitive Serology: indirect fluorescent antibody; often used; presumptive
Spirochetes	Very slow-growing; some nonculturable; extremely fastidious	*Leptospira* Smears: dark-field, silver stains; sometimes used; preliminary Culture: often used; definitive Serology: mainly used; presumptive *Borrelia* Smears: dark-field exam; mainly used; Giemsa, Wright's, and silver stains; often used; presumptive Culture: animal host usually needed; rarely used; definitive

(continued)

Microorganisms and Their Diagnostic Tests *(continued)*

Micro-organism	Description	Diagnostic tests
Spirochetes *(continued)*		Serology: relapsing fever: sometimes used; presumptive Lyme disease: mainly used; presumptive *Treponema* Smears: dark-field; sometimes used; presumptive Culture: rarely used; unavailable for some species; definitive Serology: mainly used; presumptive
Viruses	Submicroscopic organisms with only one type of nucleic acid (RNA or DNA); depend on other living cells for their replication; very fastidious; slow-growing	Smears: electron microscopy; sometimes used for nonculturable agents; definitive Histological stains: sometimes used; presumptive Culture: often used; definitive Serology: mainly used; presumptive Other immunology: sometimes used; presumptive or definitive (depending upon specific agent and test methodology)
Chlamydia	Obligate intracellular bacteria; use host cells to replicate; very fastidious; slow-growing; often involved in sexually transmitted diseases	Smears: Giemsa; sometimes used; presumptive Culture: often used; definitive Serology: often used; presumptive Other immunology: often used; definitive
Mycoplasmas	Tiny prokaryotes lacking a cell wall; slow-growing; very fastidious; saprophytic to parasitic; cause respiratory or urogenital infections in humans; include the genera *Mycoplasma* and *Ureaplasma*	Smears: direct examination of clinical material unavailable Culture: sometimes used; definitive Serology: mainly used; presumptive
Fungi	Ubiquitous, mostly saprophytic eukaryotes (complex, structured cell organization); include yeast forms (unicellular; creamy colonies) and	Smears: often used; generally preliminary, but may be definitive in some instances Culture: mainly used; definitive

(continued)

Microorganisms and Their Diagnostic Tests *(continued)*

Micro-organism	Description	Diagnostic tests
Fungi *(continued)*	molds (filamentous; cottony, fluffy colonies with aerial extensions); some highly infectious species are dimorphous (a mold at room temperature, but yeastlike at body temperature)	Serology: often used; presumptive; usefulness as a diagnostic tool varies widely with individual agents and must be correlated with clinical presentation of patient. Other immunology: sometimes used; presumptive
Rickettsia	Obligate intracellular bacterial parasites; highly fastidious; infections geographically dependent; vectored by arthropods	Smears: histological stains; sometimes used; presumptive. Culture: rarely used; definitive. Serology: mainly used; presumptive. Other immunology: direct immunofluorescence; definitive
Protozoa	Microscopic, single-cell eukaryotic organisms; diverse group classified according to their morphology of locomotion: amebae, flagellates, ciliates, and sporozoans; various symbiotic relationships from commensal to blood and tissue parasitic	Smears: variety of wet and stained preparations; mainly used; definitive. Culture: unavailable for most species; definitive. Serology: use as diagnostic tool varies greatly with individual agents and disease state of patient; presumptive
Helminths	Include the flatworms (ribbon-like tapeworms and leaf-shaped flukes) and roundworms (cylindrical and elongated); adults visible to the naked eye; blood and tissue parasites	Smears: mainly used; although adults are macroscopic, microscopy is necessary for identification of infective eggs and larvae; definitive. Culture: unavailable for most species; definitive. Serology: use as diagnostic tool varies greatly with individual agents and disease state of patient; presumptive
Arthropods	Bilaterally symmetrical animals with paired appendices and stiff exoskeletons; important both as mechanical and biological vectors of parasitic diseases (ticks, flies, mosquitoes, beetles) and as ectoparasites themselves (lice, mites, maggots, ticks)	Microscopic examination: identification of eggs or adults can usually be made with the aid of a dissecting microscope alone; definitive

Cultural isolation and identification of microorganisms takes considerably longer than microscopic examination; nevertheless, identification of an infectious agent based on smear results usually must be confirmed by culture.

Specialized artificial media or tissue cell cultures provide the proper growth nutrients. In addition, specific environmental requirements (atmosphere, temperature, pH) must be met to ensure isolation of some pathogens. Cultures are incubated for a specified length of time, which varies according to the growth rate and nutritional requirements of the organism. Most common bacterial pathogens, such as Enterobacteriaceae, streptococci and staphylococci, can be isolated in 24 to 48 hours. Fungi and mycobacteria (including the causative agent of tuberculosis) may take several weeks to produce visible growth. Cultures for mycobacteria are held 8 weeks before reported as negative.

In addition to being slow-growing, some microorganisms (for example, *Mycoplasma* and *Chlamydia*) are extremely fastidious in their growth requirements. Only after obtaining a pure culture of the organisms can identification and any susceptibility studies begin. Depending upon the isolate in question, this may delay completion of the culture by an extra day to several weeks. After adequate culture growth has taken place, further microscopic and biochemical tests are done to provide definitive identification.

Sensitivity studies are performed on potentially pathogenic bacterial isolates whose susceptibility patterns are unpredictable. Qualitative susceptibility tests designate an organism as sensitive, moderately sensitive, intermediately sensitive, or resistant to a series of antibiotics. In serious clinical infections, or when qualitative test procedures are unreliable for the organism in question, quantitative susceptibility tests may be necessary to adequately correlate in vitro results with the clinically achievable levels of an antimicrobic. Neither qualitative nor quantitative tests can assess such variables as the inherent pharmacological properties of a drug, the efficacy of the antibiotic at the site of infection, or individual host factors, all of which impact on the appropriateness of the antibiotic selected. A specialized type of antimicrobial activity test is available to measure the inhibitory or lethal action of the patient's own serum against his infecting organism, thereby helping the clinician assess the adequacy of the therapeutic regime.

Recent trends in clinical microbiology have focused on instrumentation to speed up conventional testing procedures. Also, the expansion of noncultural identification techniques has produced more rapid results. For example, DNA probes identify pathogens by complexing directly with their nucleic acids. A variety of methodologies provide for the direct detection of antigens in clinical specimens. Immunofluorescent techniques identify an organism through the microscopic detection of a fluorescein-tagged antigen-antibody complex. Procedures are currently available for identifying several viral agents, *Bordetella pertussis*, *Legionella*, and a couple of chlamydial and rickettsial agents. Agglutination tests are commonly used to demonstrate certain bacterial, fungal, and viral antigens in body fluids. Recently, these techniques have been applied to the detection of Group A streptococci from throat swabs, and rotavirus in stool samples. Enzyme and radioimmunoassays are available for detecting a myriad of infectious antigens. They are especially valuable in identifying nonculturable agents. Although these methods are rapid (taking minutes to hours) and generally highly sensitive and specific, some tests are quite expensive and may require skilled personnel for proper interpretation. (For more information on immunological techniques, refer to Chapter 3.)

Whichever techniques are used for microbiological testing, accurate results always depend on careful and proper specimen collection. (See *Rules for Culturing*.)

Patient-teaching guidelines
Patient-learner objectives:
• Define the test.
• State the specific purpose of the test.
• Explain the procedure.
• Discuss test preparation, procedure, and post-test care.
Teaching content:
• Define the test in terms the patient can understand.
• Explain that the purpose of a culture

and sensitivity test is to determine if an infection is present and, if so, to identify the causative organism and the appropriate medication for treatment.
• Describe the procedure. Tell the patient what kind of specimen is needed, how it will be obtained, and who will obtain it. Explain whether any discomfort is expected. If the patient is primarily responsible for obtaining the specimen, such as for urine or sputum cultures, give the patient the appropriate sterile container and provide detailed instructions. Stress the need for him to wash his hands, and explain what other measures are necessary to avoid contaminating the specimen. Tell

---

Rules for Culturing

The quality of a culture specimen affects test validity. To produce reliable results, you must use proper culturing techniques.

Follow these guidelines to ensure quality specimens:
• Explain the procedure to the patient. Try to enlist his full cooperation.
• Wash your hands thoroughly before and after collecting the specimen.
• If possible, do not begin any antibiotic or antimicrobial therapy until after collecting the specimen.
• Use strict aseptic technique.
• Use the appropriate sterile container for the specimen. If you are unsure, check the hospital's procedure manual, or check with the laboratory.
• Make sure you have a representative specimen of the site. If the site is a large wound or there are multiple infection sites, take specimens from different sites. Use a separate sterile container for each specimen.
• Take a sufficient specimen quantity on the first culture. Repeating the procedure costs time and money, and may cause the patient unnecessary pain. Remember, if the physician ordered

more than one test, obtain a separate specimen for each test.
• Close all specimen containers tightly to prevent spillage and possible contamination. If a container does become soiled, or if the patient is in isolation, wipe it with a bactericide before sending it to the laboratory.
• Label the specimen container with the patient's name, room number, specimen type, wound location, diagnosis, date, and time collected. Number multiple containers in sequential order. Use an Addressograph unit to prepare a micro slip for each specimen, or write on the slip by hand. If the patient is on isolation precautions or antibiotic therapy, note this on the micro slip and the culture container
• Send the specimen to the laboratory as soon as possible to prevent organism destruction or overgrowth. If transport to the laboratory is delayed, some specimen types may be refrigerated for a short time. In the case of a viral culture, pack the specimen container in ice and take it to the laboratory as soon as possible.
• Be sure to document the procedure, date, and time.

the patient to inform you as soon as he obtains the specimen, so that you can send it to the laboratory immediately. Inform the patient when more than one specimen must be obtained.

• Explain whether any special preparation is needed before the test.

• Advise the patient not to begin antibiotic therapy until the specimen has been obtained, because it can interfere with accurate test results.

• If a culture is ordered, explain that sufficient growth must take place before the organism can be identified under the microscope or in other ways. Therefore, results may not be available for 24 to 72 hours. If the culture is being done to identify a fungus or virus or to confirm tuberculosis, results may take several weeks. If a smear is ordered, explain that this test permits more immediate laboratory examination and therefore quicker results; however, caution the patient that these results often provide the physician with a good lead, but that definite findings may await culture results.

Evaluation:

After the patient-teaching session has been completed, evaluate whether or not the patient has satisfactorily met each patient-learner objective by obtaining necessary patient feedback. Refocus teaching as needed.

Blood culture

Purpose

• To confirm bacteremia

• To identify the causative organism in bacteremia and septicemia.

Normal results

Blood cultures should be sterile; may be reported as negative or no growth.

Abnormal results

Positive blood cultures indicate:
  Bacteremia
  Septicemia

Contamination caused by skin bacteria (2% to 3% of blood samples).

Common blood pathogens include:
  Neisseria meningitidis
  Streptococcus pneumoniae
  Hemophilus influenzae
  Other *Streptococcus* species
  Staphylococcus aureus
  Pseudomonas aeruginosa
  Bacteroidaceae
  Brucella
  Enterobacteriaceae.

Common skin bacteria include:
  Staphylococcus epidermidis
  Diphtheroids
  Propionibacterium.

The basics

A blood culture is performed by inoculating a culture medium with a blood sample and incubating it for isolation and identification of the pathogens in bacteremia (bacterial invasion of the bloodstream) and septicemia (systemic spread of such infection). Blood culture can identify about 67% of pathogens within 24 hours and up to 90% within 72 hours.

Bacteria from local tissue infection usually invade the bloodstream through the lymphatic system by way of the thoracic duct. Occasionally, they enter the bloodstream directly through infusion lines, thrombophlebitis, or bacterial endocarditis from prosthetic heart valve replacements.

Positive blood cultures do not necessarily confirm pathologic septicemia, since many organisms may temporarily invade the bloodstream during the early stages of infection. Mild, transient bacteremia may occur during the course of many infectious diseases or may complicate other disorders. Persistent, continuous, or recurrent bacteremia reliably confirms the presence of serious infection. Although skin bacteria usually imply a contaminated blood sample, these organisms may be clinically significant when isolated from multiple cultures.

Timing of the specimens for blood cultures is somewhat debatable. Usually, it reflects the suspected type of bacteremia (intermittent or continuous) and the need to begin drug therapy.

Procedure

• After cleansing the venipuncture site with an alcohol sponge, clean it again with an iodine swab, starting at the site and working outward in a circular motion.

• Wait at least 1 minute for the skin to dry, and remove the residual iodine with an alcohol sponge. (Or you can remove the iodine after venipuncture.)

• Perform a venipuncture; draw 10 to 20 ml of blood for an adult, and one syringe of 2 to 6 ml of blood for a child.

• Clean the diaphragm tops of the culture bottles with alcohol or iodine, and change the needle on the syringe.

• If you are using broth, add blood to each bottle until you obtain a 1:5 or 1:10 dilution. For example, add 10 ml of blood to a 100-ml bottle. (Size of the bottle may vary depending on individual hospital protocol.)

• If you are using a special resin, such as Bactec resin medium or Antimicrobial Removal Device, add blood to the resin in the bottles and invert them gently to mix.

• If you are using the lysis-centrifugation technique (Isolator), draw the blood directly into a special collection/processing tube.

• Indicate the tentative diagnosis on the laboratory slip, and note any current or recent antibiotic therapy.

• Send each sample to the laboratory immediately after collection.

Patient care checklist
Before the test
☑ Explain or clarify test purpose and procedure.
☑ Evaluate patient understanding.

Interfering factors

• Improper collection technique may contaminate the sample.

• Previous or current antimicrobial therapy may result in negative cultures or delayed growth.

• Removal of culture bottle caps at bedside may prevent anaerobic growth.

• Use of incorrect bottle and media may prevent aerobic growth.

Duodenal contents culture

Purpose

• To detect bacterial infection of the biliary tract and duodenum; to differentiate between such infection and gallstones

• To rule out bacterial infection as the cause of persistent gastrointestinal symptoms (epigastric pain, nausea, vomiting, and diarrhea).

Normal results

A normal duodenal contents culture contains small amounts of polymorphonuclear leukocytes and epithelial cells with no pathogens. The bacterial count is usually less than 100,000.

Abnormal results

Bacterial counts of 100,000 or more indicate:
    Infection.
Pathogens, such as Salmonella, *in any number, indicate:*
    Infection.
Numerous polymorphonuclear leukocytes, copious mucous debris, and bile-stained epithelial cells in the bile fluid suggest:
    Inflammation of the biliary tract.
Many segmented neutrophils and exfoliated epithelial cells suggest:
    Inflammation of the pancreas, the duodenum, or bile ducts.
The presence of bile sand indicates:
    Cholelithiasis.

The basics

This test requires duodenal intubation, aspiration of duodenal contents, and cultivation of any microbes present to isolate and identify a duodenal or biliary pathogen. Occasionally, a specimen may be obtained during surgery, such as during a cholecystectomy. Duodenal contents (pancreatic and duodenal enzymes and bile) are normally almost sterile, but are subject to infection by many pathogens, such as *Escherichia coli, Staphylococcus aureus,* and *Salmonella.* Such microbial infection of the biliary tract and duodenum can result in duodenitis, cholecystitis, or cholangitis. Differential diagnosis requires further testing.

Contraindications to this test may include: pregnancy; acute pancreatitis; acute cholecystitis, esophageal varices, stenosis, diverticula or malignant neoplasms; recent severe gastric hemorrhage; aortic aneurysm; congestive heart failure; or myocardial infarction.

Procedure

• When possible, collect the specimen for culture before antibiotic therapy begins.
• After the nasoenteric tube is inserted, place the patient in a left lateral decubitus position, with his feet elevated, to allow peristalsis to move the tube into the duodenum. The pH of a small amount of aspirated fluid determines tube position: if the tube is in the stomach, pH is lower than 7.0; if the tube is in the duodenum, pH is higher than 7.0. Correct position of the tube can also be confirmed by fluoroscopy.
• After the tube position is confirmed, aspirate duodenal contents. Sometimes, a specimen for culture of duodenal contents can be obtained during duodenoscopy (see "Esophagogastroduodenoscopy," p. 424).
• Transfer the specimen to a sterile container, and label it with the patient's name and room number, physician's name, date, and time of collection. Note recent antibiotic therapy on the laboratory slip.
• Send the specimen to the laboratory immediately.

• Withdraw the tube slowly (6″ to 8″ [15 to 20 cm] every 10 minutes) until it reaches the esophagus; then clamp the tube and remove it quickly. Notify the physician if the tube cannot be withdrawn easily; *never* force the tube.

Patient care checklist

Before the test
☑ Explain or clarify test purpose, preparation, and procedure.
☑ Assure the patient that, although this procedure is uncomfortable, it is not dangerous. Explain that passage of the tube may make him gag, but following the examiner's instructions about proper positioning, breathing, swallowing, and relaxing will minimize discomfort.
☑ Suggest to the patient that he empty his bladder before the procedure to increase his general comfort.
☑ Evaluate patient understanding.
☑ Restrict the patient's food and fluids for 12 hours before the test.

After the test
☑ Observe the patient carefully for signs of perforation from tube passage, such as dysphagia, epigastric or shoulder pain, dyspnea, or fever.

Interfering factors

• Failure to observe a 12-hour fast can dilute the specimen, which decreases the bacterial count.
• Improper collection technique can contaminate the specimen.
• Recent antibiotic therapy decreases bacterial growth.

Duodenal test for parasites

Purpose

To detect parasitic infection when stool examinations are negative.

Normal results

No ova or parasites appear.

Abnormal results

The presence of **Giardia lamblia** *indicates:*

Giardiasis, possibly causing malabsorption syndrome.

The presence of **Strongyloides stercoralis** *suggests:*

Strongyloidiasis.

The presence of **Ancylostoma duodenale** *and* **Necator americanus** *implies:*

Hookworm disease.

The presence of **Clonorchis sinensis** *and* **Fasciola hepatica** *signifies:*

Histopathologic changes in the bile ducts.

The basics

This test evaluates duodenal contents for the presence of parasites in a specimen obtained by duodenal intubation and aspiration or by the string test (Entero test). Examination of duodenal contents for ova and parasites is performed only in a symptomatic patient with negative stool examinations.

Contraindications to this test may include: pregnancy; acute cholecystitis; acute pancreatitis; esophageal varices, stenosis, diverticula, or malignant neoplasms; recent severe gastric hemorrhage; aortic aneurysm; or congestive heart failure.

Procedure

• When possible, obtain the specimen before the start of drug therapy.

Using a nasoenteric tube:

• After the nasoenteric tube is inserted, place the patient in a left lateral decubitus position, with his feet elevated, to allow peristalsis to move the tube into the duodenum. The pH of a small amount of aspirated fluid determines tube position: if the tube is in the stomach, pH is lower than 7.0; if the tube is in the duodenum, pH is higher than 7.0. Correct positioning of the tube can also be determined by fluoroscopy.

• After position of the tube is confirmed, aspirate residual duodenal contents.

• Transfer the entire specimen to a sterile container; label it appropriately.

• Send the specimen to the laboratory immediately.

• Withdraw the tube slowly (6″ to 8″ [15 to 20 cm] every 10 minutes) to the esophagus; then clamp the tube and remove it quickly. *Never* force the tube.

Using an Entero test capsule with string:

• Tape the free end of the string to the patient's cheek.

• Then, instruct him to swallow the capsule (on the other end of the string) with water.

• Leave the string in place for 4 hours, then pull it out gently and place it in a sterile container.

• Label the container appropriately, and send the specimen to the laboratory immediately.

Patient care checklist

Before the test

☑ Explain or clarify test purpose, preparation, and procedure.

☑ If the test will be done with a nasoenteric tube, warn the patient that he may gag during the tube's passage, but assure him that following the examiner's instructions about positioning, breathing, and swallowing will minimize discomfort.

☑ Evaluate patient understanding.

☑ Restrict the patient's food and fluid for 12 hours before the test.

☑ Instruct the patient to empty his bladder just before the procedure.

After the test

☑ Observe the patient carefully for signs of perforation, such as dysphagia or fever.

Interfering factors

• Failure of the patient to observe the 12-hour fast can dilute the specimen.

• Delay in sending the specimen to the laboratory may interfere with test results, since detection may rest on observing the parasite's motility.

• Use of antiparasitic agents may decrease the amount of parasites in the specimen.

Gastric culture

Purpose
• To aid in diagnosis of mycobacterial infections
• To identify the infecting bacteria in neonatal septicemia.

Normal results
Culture specimen is negative for pathogenic mycobacteria.

Abnormal results
Isolation and identification of the organism M. tuberculosis *indicates:*
   Active tuberculosis.
Other species of mycobacterium may cause:
   Pulmonary disease that is clinically indistinguishable from tuberculosis.
   Pathogenic bacteria causing neonatal septicemia may also be identified through culture.

The basics
This test requires aspiration of gastric contents and cultivation of any microbes present to identify mycobacterial infection. It is performed in conjunction with a chest X-ray and a purified protein derivative skin test, and is especially useful when a sputum sample cannot be obtained by expectoration or nebulization. Gastric aspiration also provides a specimen for rapid presumptive identification of bacteria (by Gram stain) in neonatal septicemia.

Procedure
• If possible, obtain the specimens before the start of antibiotic therapy.
• Perform nasogastric intubation when the patient awakens and obtain gastric washings.

• Clamp the tube before removing it quickly.
• Note recent antibiotic therapy on the laboratory slip, along with the site and time of collection. Label the specimens with the patient's name and room number (if applicable) and the physician's name.
• Send the specimens to the laboratory immediately. Be sure the specimen container is tightly capped. Wipe the outside of the container with disinfectant, and send it to the laboratory upright in a plastic bag.

Special precautions
• Watch for signs that the tube has entered the trachea—coughing, cyanosis, or gasping.
• *Never* inject water into a nasogastric tube unless you are sure the tube is correctly placed in the patient's stomach. During lavage, use sterile, distilled water to decrease the risk of contamination with saprophytic mycobacteria.
• Since some patients develop dysrhythmias during this procedure, check the patient's pulse rate for irregularities.
• Handle the nasogastric tube with gloved hands, and dispose of all equipment carefully to prevent staff contamination.

Patient care checklist
Before the test
☑ Explain or clarify test purpose, preparation, and procedure to the patient (or parents if the patient is a child).
☑ Explain that the same procedure may be performed on three consecutive mornings. Advise the patient to remain in bed each morning until specimen collection has been completed, to prevent premature emptying of stomach contents.
☑ Inform the patient that the nasogastric tube may make him gag, but passes more easily if he relaxes and follows instructions about breathing and swallowing.

☑ Evaluate patient/parent understanding.

☑ Instruct the patient to fast for 8 hours before the test.

☑ Advise the patient (or parents) that the test results may take 2 months, since acid-fast bacteria generally grow slowly.

☑ Just before the procedure, obtain baseline heart rate and rhythm, and place the patient in high Fowler position.

Interfering factors

• Failure to observe an 8-hour fast before the test may decrease the amount of bacteria by diluting stomach contents or removing contents through digestion.

• Drugs such as tetracycline and aminoglycosides can weaken bacilli, causing false-negative culture results.

• The presence of saprophytic mycobacteria in gastric contents may cause false-positive acid-fast smears, since these bacteria cannot be microscopically distinguished from pathogenic mycobacteria.

Gonorrheal culture

Purpose

To confirm gonorrhea.

Normal results

No *Neisseria gonorrhoeae* appears in the culture.

Abnormal results

A positive culture confirms:
  Gonorrhea.

The basics

A stained smear of genital exudate can confirm gonorrhea in 90% of males with characteristic symptoms; nevertheless, a culture is often necessary, especially in asymptomatic females. Possible culture sites include the urethra (usual site in males), endocervix (usual site in females), anal canal, and oropharynx.

Gonorrhea almost exclusively results from sexual transmission of *Neisseria gonorrhoeae*. Its most common effect in females is a greenish yellow cervical discharge; but in many females, it produces no symptoms at all—a factor that contributes to the epidemic prevalence of this infection. In males, gonorrhea generally causes painful urination and a mucopurulent urethral discharge, symptoms of acute anterior urethritis.

Procedure

Endocervical culture:

• Place the patient in the lithotomy position, drape her, and instruct her to take deep breaths. Insert a vaginal speculum, lubricated only with warm water.

• Clean mucus from the cervix, using cotton balls in ring forceps.

• Then insert a dry, sterile cotton-tipped swab into the endocervical canal and rotate it from side to side. Leave the swab in place for several seconds for optimum absorption of organisms.

Urethral culture:

• Place the patient in supine position, and drape appropriately.

• Cleanse the urethral meatus with sterile gauze or a cotton swab, then insert a thin urogenital alginate swab or a wire bacteriologic loop ⅜″ to ¾″ (1 to 2 cm) into the urethra, and rotate the swab or loop from side to side. Leave it in place for several seconds for optimum absorption of organisms. If permitted, the patient may milk the urethra, bringing urethral secretions to the meatus for collection on a sterile cotton-tipped swab.

Rectal culture:

• After obtaining an endocervical or urethral specimen (and while the patient is still on the examining table), insert a sterile cotton-tipped swab into the anal canal about 1″ (2.5 cm), move the swab from side to side, and leave it in place for several seconds for optimum absorption. If the cotton-tipped swab is contaminated with feces, discard it and repeat the procedure with a clean swab.

Throat culture:
• Position the patient with his head tilted back and his eyes closed.
• Check his throat for inflamed areas, using a tongue depressor. Rub a sterile cotton-tipped swab from side to side over the tonsillar areas, including any inflamed or purulent sites. Be careful not to touch the teeth, cheeks, or tongue with the swab.

After collecting any of these specimens: Streaking of a Thayer-Martin plate or Transgrow medium is necessary. (See *Culturing for* Neisseria Gonorrhoeae below.)

Special precautions

CLINICAL ALERT: **Place the male patient in a supine position to prevent falling if vasovagal syncope occurs during introduction of the sterile urogenital alginate swab or wire loop into the urethra. Observe for pro-**

Culturing for *Neisseria Gonorrhoeae*

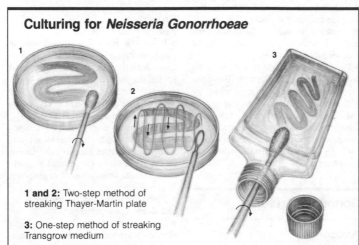

1 and 2: Two-step method of streaking Thayer-Martin plate

3: One-step method of streaking Transgrow medium

Modified Thayer-Martin (MTM) medium is a combination of hemoglobin, gonococcal growth-enhancing chemicals, and antimicrobial agents for culturing endocervical, urethral, or rectal specimens. To inoculate a culture plate treated with MTM medium and to spread organisms out of their associated mucus, roll the cotton-tipped swab in a Z pattern (1). Using the swab or a sterile wire loop, immediately cross-streak the plate (2). To demonstrate *Neisseria gonorrhoeae*, incubate within 15 minutes of streaking.

Transgrow, a modification of MTM medium, is available in a screw-cap bottle containing air and carbon dioxide. Transgrow bottles are used to transport suspect cultures when laboratory facilities are not available at the site of specimen collection. To prevent loss of carbon dioxide, inoculate the specimen bottle while it is in an upright position. After uncapping the bottle, immediately insert the cotton-tipped swab and soak up all excess moisture. Then, starting at the bottom of the bottle, roll the swab from side to side across the medium (3). Recap the bottle, and send it to the laboratory immediately. Subculturing should begin within 24 to 48 hours.

found hypotension, bradycardia, pallor, and sweating.
• Collect a urethral specimen at least 1 hour after the patient has voided to prevent loss of urethral secretions.
• After collecting the specimens, carefully dispose of gloves, swabs and wire bacteriologic loop (if the organism has been cultured), and speculum to prevent staff exposure to the organism.
• Send the specimen to the laboratory immediately, or arrange for immediate transport of the Transgrow bottle, since the specimen requires subculturing within 24 to 48 hours to obtain successful growths.

Patient care checklist
Before the test
☑ Explain or clarify test purpose, preparation, and procedure.
☑ Evaluate patient understanding.
☑ Instruct the female patient not to douche for 24 hours before the test.
☑ Instruct the male patient not to void during the hour before the test.
☑ Note any recent antibiotic therapy on the laboratory slip.
☑ Inform the patient that test results are usually available within 24 to 72 hours.
After the test
☑ Advise the patient to avoid intercourse and all sexual contact until test results are available. Explain that treatment usually begins after confirmation of a positive culture, except in a patient with symptoms of gonorrhea or a person who has had intercourse with someone known to have gonorrhea.
☑ Advise the patient that a repeat culture is required 1 week after completion of treatment to evaluate therapy.
☑ Inform the patient that positive culture findings must be reported to the local health department.

Interfering factors
• Improper collection technique may provide a nonrepresentative specimen or may contaminate the specimen.

• Fecal material may contaminate an anal culture.
• In males, voiding within 1 hour of specimen collection washes secretions out of the urethra, making fewer organisms available for culture.
• Recent antibiotic therapy may decrease bacterial growth.
• In females, douching within 24 hours of specimen collection washes out cervical secretions, making fewer organisms available for culture.

Nasopharyngeal culture

Purpose
• To identify pathogens causing upper respiratory tract symptoms
• To identify proliferation of normal nasopharyngeal flora, which may prove pathogenic in debilitated and other immunologically vulnerable persons
• To detect asymptomatic carriers of infectious organisms such as *N. meningitidis* and *B. pertussis*.

Normal results
Flora commonly found in the nasopharynx include nonhemolytic streptococci, alpha-hemolytic streptococci, *Neisseria* species (except *N. meningitidis* and *N. gonorrhoeae*), coagulase-negative staphylococci such as *Staphylococcus epidermidis,* and occasionally, the coagulase-positive *Staphylococcus aureus.*

Abnormal results
Pathogens include:
   Group A beta-hemolytic streptococci
   Groups B, C, and G beta-hemolytic streptococci
   Bordetella pertussis
   Corynebacterium diphtheriae
   Staphylococcus aureus
   Large amounts of *Hemophilus influenzae*, pneumococci, or *Candida albicans*.

The basics

This test evaluates nasopharyngeal secretions for the presence of pathogenic organisms. Direct microscopic inspection of a Gram-stained smear of the specimen provides preliminary identification of organisms that may guide clinical management, and determines the need for additional testing. Streaking a culture plate with the cotton-tipped swab containing the nasopharyngeal secretions and allowing any organisms present to grow permit isolation and identification of pathogens. Cultured pathogens may then require sensitivity testing to determine appropriate antibiotic therapy. Nasopharyngeal cultures are often useful for identifying *Bordetella pertussis* and *Neisseria meningitidis,* especially in very young, elderly, or debilitated patients.

Nasopharyngeal cultures can also be used to isolate viruses, especially to identify carriers of influenza virus A and B. However, the laboratory procedure required for such testing is complex, time-consuming, and costly, so such a culture is rarely performed.

Procedure

• Ask the patient to cough before you begin collection of the specimen.
• Then, position the patient with his head tilted back.
• Using a penlight and a tongue depressor, inspect the nasopharyngeal area.
• Next, gently pass the sterile cotton-tipped swab through the nostril and into the nasopharynx, keeping the swab near the septum and floor of the nose. Rotate the swab quickly, and remove it.
• Or, place the Pyrex tube in the patient's nostril, and carefully pass the sterile cotton-tipped swab through the tube into the nasopharynx. Rotate the swab for 5 seconds, and then place it in the culture tube with transport medium. Remove the Pyrex tube.
• Label the specimen appropriately, including the date and time of collection and the origin of the material. Also indicate the suspected organism and current or recent antibiotic therapy or chemotherapy.
• If the specimen is being collected for isolation of a virus, check with the laboratory for the recommended collection techniques.

Special precautions

• Maintain aseptic technique.
• Make sure the cotton-tipped swab does not touch the sides of the patient's nostril, or his tongue, to prevent any contamination of the specimen.
• Keep the container upright.
• Since certain organisms, such as *Corynebacterium diphtheriae* and *B. pertussis,* require special growth media, inform the laboratory if they are suspected.
• Refrigerate or freeze a viral specimen, according to your laboratory's procedure.

Patient care checklist

Before the test
☑ Explain or clarify test purpose and procedure.
☑ Tell the patient that he may experience slight discomfort and may gag, but reassure him that obtaining the specimen takes less than 15 seconds.
☑ Inform the patient that initial test results are generally available in 48 to 72 hours, but that viral test results take longer to obtain.
☑ Evaluate patient understanding.

Interfering factors

• Recent antibiotic therapy decreases bacterial growth.
• Improper collection technique may contaminate the specimen.
• Failure to place the specimen in a transport medium allows the specimen to dry out and the bacteria to deteriorate.
• Failure to send the specimen to the laboratory immediately after collection permits proliferation of organisms.

• Failure to keep a viral specimen cold allows the viruses to deteriorate.

Sputum culture

Purpose
To isolate and identify the cause of a pulmonary infection.

Normal results
Flora commonly found in the respiratory tract include alpha-hemolytic streptococci, *Neisseria* species, and diphtheroids. However, the presence of normal flora does not rule out infection.

Abnormal results
Sputum culture can aid in diagnosis of:
    Bronchitis
    Tuberculosis
    Lung abscess
    Pneumonia.
Pathogenic organisms commonly reported in sputum include:
    Streptococcus pneumoniae (pneumococcus)
    Mycobacterium tuberculosis
    Klebsiella pneumoniae
    Other Enterobacteriaceae
    Hemophilus influenzae
    Staphylococcus aureus
    Pseudomonas aeruginosa.

The basics
Bacteriologic examination of sputum—material raised from the lungs and bronchi during deep coughing—is an important aid to the management of lung disease. During passage through the throat and oropharynx, sputum specimens are commonly contaminated with indigenous bacterial flora, such as alpha-hemolytic streptococci, *Neisseria* species, diphtheroids, and some hemophili, pneumococci, staphylococci, and yeasts, such as *Candida*.

Besides the pathogens noted earlier, other agents, such as *Pneumocystis carinii,* the legionellae, *Mycoplasma pneumoniae,* and respiratory viruses, may exist in the sputum and can cause lung disease, but they usually require serologic or histologic diagnosis rather than diagnosis by sputum culture.

A Gram stain of expectorated sputum must be examined to ensure that it is a representative specimen of secretions from the lower respiratory tract (many white blood cells, few epithelial cells) rather than one contaminated by oral flora (few white blood cells, many epithelial cells).

Since cultures for tuberculosis take up to 2 months, diagnosis of this disorder generally depends on clinical symptoms, a smear for acid-fast bacilli, chest X-ray, and response to a purified protein derivative skin test.

Procedure
Expectoration:
• Instruct the patient to cough deeply and expectorate into the container. If the cough is nonproductive, use chest physiotherapy, heated aerosol spray (nebulization), or intermittent positive-pressure breathing with prescribed aerosol to induce sputum, as ordered.
• Using aseptic technique, close the container securely.
• Dispose of equipment properly; seal the container in a leakproof bag before sending it to the laboratory.
Tracheal suctioning:
• Administer oxygen to the patient before and after the procedure, as necessary.
• Attach the sputum trap to the suction catheter.
• Using sterile gloves, lubricate the catheter with normal saline solution, and pass the catheter through the patient's nostril, without suction. (The patient will cough when the catheter passes through the larynx.)
• Advance the catheter into the trachea. Apply suction for no longer than 15 seconds to obtain the specimen.
• Stop suction, and gently remove the catheter.

• Discard the catheter and gloves in the proper receptacle. Then, detach the in-line sputum trap from the suction apparatus and cap the opening.

Bronchoscopy:

• After a local anesthetic is sprayed into the patient's throat, or the patient gargles with a local anesthetic, the bronchoscope is inserted through the pharynx and trachea, into the bronchus.

• Secretions are then collected with a bronchial brush or aspirated through the inner channel of the scope, using an irrigating solution such as normal saline solution, if necessary.

• After the specimen is obtained, the bronchoscope is removed.

After obtaining a specimen by any of these methods:

• Label the container with the patient's name.

• Include on the test request form the nature and origin of the specimen, the date and time of collection, the initial diagnosis, and any current antibiotic therapy.

• Send the specimen to the laboratory immediately.

Special precautions

• Tracheal suctioning is contraindicated in patients with esophageal varices or cardiac disease.

CLINICAL ALERT: **In a patient with asthma or chronic bronchitis, watch for aggravated bronchospasms with use of more than 10% concentration of sodium chloride or acetylcysteine in an aerosol.**

CLINICAL ALERT: **During tracheal suctioning, suction for only 5 to 10 seconds at a time.** *Never* **suction longer than 15 seconds. If the patient becomes hypoxic or cyanotic, remove the catheter immediately, and administer oxygen.**

• Since the patient may cough violently during suctioning, wear a mask to avoid exposure to respiratory pathogens.

• *Do not* use more than 20% propylene glycol with water as an inducer for a

specimen scheduled for tuberculosis culturing, since higher concentrations inhibit the growth of *M. tuberculosis*. (If propylene glycol is not available, use 10% to 20% acetylcysteine with water or sodium chloride.)

Patient care checklist

Before the test

☑ Explain or clarify test purpose, preparation, and procedure.

☑ Evaluate patient understanding.

☑ Tell the patient that test results are usually available in 48 to 72 hours; however, culture results for tuberculosis may take up to 2 months.

☑ If the suspected organism is *M. tuberculosis*, tell the patient that at least three morning specimens may be required.

☑ If the specimen is to be collected by expectoration, encourage fluid intake the night before collection to help sputum production. Teach the patient how to expectorate by taking three deep breaths and forcing a deep cough. Emphasize that sputum is not the same as saliva, which will be rejected for culturing. Tell the patient not to brush his teeth or use mouthwash before the specimen collection, although he may rinse his mouth with water.

☑ If the specimen is to be collected by tracheal suctioning, tell the patient that he will experience discomfort as the catheter passes into the trachea.

☑ If the specimen is to be collected by bronchoscopy, instruct the patient to fast for 6 hours before the procedure. Tell the patient that he will receive a local anesthetic just before the test, to minimize discomfort during passage of the tube.

☑ Make sure the patient has signed a consent form.

After the test

☑ Provide good mouth care.

CLINICAL ALERT: **After bronchoscopy, observe the patient carefully for signs of hypoxemia (cyanosis), laryngospasm (laryngeal stridor), bronchospasm (paroxysms of coughing or wheezing), pneumothorax** (dyspnea, cyanosis, pleural pain, tachycardia), perforation of the trachea or bronchus (subcutaneous crepitus), or trauma to respiratory structures (bleeding). Also, check for difficulty in breathing or swallowing. Withhold liquids until the gag reflex returns.

Interfering factors
• Improper collection or handling of the specimen may invalidate test results.
• Failure to report current or recent antibiotic therapy does not allow the laboratory to correctly interpret decreased bacterial growth.
• Sputum collected over an extended period may allow pathogens to deteriorate or become overgrown by commensals, and will not be accepted as a valid specimen by most laboratories.

Sputum examination for ova and parasites

Purpose
To identify pulmonary parasites.

Normal results
Negative; no ova or parasites are present.

Abnormal results
The parasite identified indicates the type of pulmonary infection and the presence of adult-stage intestinal infection.

E. histolytica trophozoites:
Pulmonary amebiasis.
A. lumbricoides larvae and adults:
Pneumonitis.
E. granulosus cysts of larval stage:
Hydatid disease.
P. westermani ova:
Paragonimiasis.
S. stercoralis larvae:
Strongyloidiasis.
N. americanus larvae:
Hookworm disease.

The basics
This test evaluates a sputum specimen for parasites. Such infestation is rare in the United States. The specimen is obtained by expectoration or by tracheal suctioning.

Procedure
Expectoration:
• Instruct the patient to breathe deeply a few times and then to "deep-cough" and expectorate into the container. If the cough is nonproductive, use chest physiotherapy, heated aerosol spray (nebulization), or intermittent positive-pressure breathing with prescribed aerosol to induce sputum, as ordered.
• Close the container securely, and clean the outside of it.
• Dispose of equipment properly; take proper precautions in sending the specimen to the laboratory.
Tracheal suctioning:
• Administer oxygen before and after the procedure, if necessary.
• Attach a sputum trap to the suction catheter.
• While wearing a sterile glove, lubricate the tip of the catheter, and pass the catheter through the patient's nostril, without suction. (The patient will cough when the catheter passes into the larynx.)
• Advance the catheter into the trachea. Apply suction for no longer than 15 seconds to obtain the specimen.
• Stop suction, and gently remove the catheter.
• Discard the catheter and glove in a proper receptacle. Then, detach the sputum trap from the suction apparatus and cap the opening
After obtaining a specimen by either method:
• Label it carefully.
• Send the specimen to the laboratory immediately, or place it in preservative.

Special precautions
• Tracheal suctioning is contraindi-

cated in patients with esophageal varices or cardiac disease.

CLINICAL ALERT: **In a patient with asthma or chronic bronchitis, watch for aggravated bronchospasms with use of more than 10% concentration of sodium chloride or acetylcysteine in an aerosol.**

CLINICAL ALERT: **During tracheal suctioning, suction for only 5 to 10 seconds at a time. *Never* suction longer than 15 seconds. If the patient becomes hypoxic or cyanotic, remove the catheter immediately, and administer oxygen.**

Patient care checklist
Before the test
☑ Explain or clarify test purpose, preparation, and procedure.
☑ Evaluate patient understanding.
☑ Inform the patient that an early morning collection is preferred, because secretions accumulate overnight.
☑ If the specimen is to be collected by expectoration, encourage fluid intake the night before collection to help sputum production. Teach the patient how to expectorate by taking three deep breaths and forcing a deep cough.
☑ If the specimen is to be collected by tracheal suctioning, tell the patient that he will experience some discomfort from the catheter.
After the test
☑ Provide good mouth care.

Interfering factors
• Recent therapy with anthelmintics or amebicides may interfere with test results.
• Improper collection may produce a nonrepresentative specimen.

Stool culture

Purpose
• To identify pathogenic organisms causing gastrointestinal disease
• To identify carrier states.

Normal results
Approximately 96% to 99% of normal fecal flora consist of anaerobes, including non-spore-forming bacilli, clostridia, and anaerobic streptococci. The remaining 1% to 4% consist of aerobes, including gram-negative bacilli (predominantly *E. coli* and other Enterobacteriaceae, plus small amounts of *Pseudomonas*), gram-positive cocci (mostly enterococci), and a few yeasts.

Abnormal results
See *Pathogens of the Gastrointestinal Tract*.

The basics
Bacteriologic examination of feces is valuable for identifying pathogens that cause overt gastrointestinal disease—such as typhoid and dysentery—and carrier states. Identification of these organisms is vital not only to treatment and to prevention of possibly fatal complications—especially in a debilitated patient—but also to confinement of these severe infectious diseases. A sensitivity test may follow isolation of the pathogen. Isolation of some pathogens (such as *Salmonella, Shigella, Campylobacter, Yersinia,* and *Vibrio*) indicates bacterial infection in patients with acute diarrhea and may require antibiotic sensitivity tests. Since normal fecal flora may include *Clostridium difficile, E. coli,* and other organisms, isolation of these may require further tests to demonstrate invasiveness or toxin production. Isolation of pathogens such as *Clostridium botulinum* indicates food poisoning; however, the pathogens must also be isolated from the contaminated food. In a patient undergoing long-term antibiotic therapy, isolation of large numbers of *Staphylococcus aureus* or yeast, such as *Candida,* may indicate infection. (Asymptomatic carrier states are also indicated by these enteric pathogens.) Isolation of enteroviruses may indicate aseptic meningitis.

If a stool culture shows no unusual growth, detection of viruses such as rotavirus and paravirus by immunoassay or electron microscopy may diagnose nonbacterial gastroenteritis. Highly increased polymorphonuclear leukocytes in fecal material may indicate an invasive pathogen.

Procedure

• Collect a stool specimen directly into the container or, if the patient is not ambulatory, into a clean, dry bedpan.
• Then, using a tongue blade, transfer the specimen to the container.
• If you must collect the specimen by sterile rectal cotton-tipped swab, insert the swab past the anal sphincter, rotate it gently, and withdraw it. Then, place the swab in the appropriate container.
• Label the specimen with the patient's name and room number (if applicable), the physician's name, and the date and time of collection. Also indicate the suspected cause of enteritis and current antibiotic therapy on the laboratory slip.
• Send the specimen to the laboratory immediately.
• If the specimen is to be processed for a viral test, check with the laboratory for the proper collection procedure before obtaining a specimen.

Special precautions

• Be sure to include mucoid and bloody portions of the specimen. The specimen should always be representative of the first, middle, and last portions of the feces passed.
• Use aseptic technique when handling the specimen. Place the specimen container in a leakproof bag before transporting it to the laboratory.

Patient care checklist

Before the test
☑ Explain or clarify test purpose and procedure.
☑ Evaluate patient understanding.

Pathogens of the Gastrointestinal Tract

Presence of the following pathogens in a stool culture may indicate the disorders shown:
Shigella: shigellosis, bacillary dysentery
Salmonella: gastroenteritis, typhoid fever, nontyphoidal salmonellosis, paratyphoid fever
Campylobacter jejuni: gastroenteritis
Vibrio cholerae: cholera
Vibrio parahaemolyticus: food poisoning, especially from seafood
Toxin-producing *Clostridium difficile:* pseudomembranous enterocolitis
Yersinia enterocolitica: gastroenteritis, enterocolitis (resembles appendicitis), mesenteric adenitis, ileitis
Enterotoxigenic *Escherichia coli:* gastroenteritis (resembles cholera or shigellosis)
Staphylococcus aureus: food poisoning; suppression of normal bowel flora from antimicrobial therapy
Bacillus cereus: food poisoning, acute gastroenteritis (rare)
Clostridium perfringens: food poisoning
Clostridium botulinum: food poisoning and infant botulism, a possible cause of sudden infant death syndrome
Aeromonas hydrophila: gastroenteritis, which causes diarrhea, especially in children.

☑ Review patient history for dietary patterns and recent antibiotic therapy, and for recent travel that might suggest endemic infections or infestations.
☑ Tell the patient that the test may require the collection of a stool specimen on 3 consecutive days.
☑ Tell the patient to avoid contaminating the specimen with toilet tissue or urine.

Interfering factors

• Improper collection technique or the presence of urine may injure or destroy some enteric pathogens.

• Antibiotic therapy may decrease bacterial growth in the specimen.

• Failure to transport the specimen promptly or, if delivery is delayed, to use a transport medium that stabilizes pH (such as a buffered glycol medium) may result in loss of some enteric pathogens or overgrowth of nonpathologic organisms.

Stool examination for ova and parasites

Purpose

To confirm or rule out intestinal parasitic infection and disease.

Normal results

Negative; no parasites or ova appear in stool.

Abnormal results

The presence of E. histolytica:
  Confirms amebiasis.
The presence of G. lamblia:
  Confirms giardiasis.
The presence of the roundworms Ascaris lumbricoides *and* Necator americanus *(commonly called hookworm) or the tapeworms* Diphyllobothrium latum, Taenia saginata, *and rarely,* Taenia solium *indicates:*
  Helminthic infestation or helminthic disease.

The basics

Examination of a stool specimen can detect several types of intestinal parasites. Some of these parasites live in nonpathogenic symbiosis; others cause intestinal disease.

With amebiasis and giardiasis, the extent of infection depends on the degree of tissue invasion. If amebiasis is suspected but stool examinations are negative, specimen collection after saline cathartic using buffered sodium biphosphate or during sigmoidoscopy may be necessary. If giardiasis is suspected but stool examinations are negative, examination of duodenal contents may be necessary.

Since injury to the host is difficult to detect—even when helminth ova or larvae appear—the number of worms is usually correlated with the patient's clinical symptoms to distinguish between helminthic infestation and helminthic diseases. Eosinophilia may also indicate parasitic infection. Helminths may migrate from the intestinal tract, producing pathologic changes in other parts of the body. For example, the roundworm *Ascaris* may perforate the bowel wall, causing peritonitis, or may migrate to the lungs, causing pneumonitis. Hookworms can cause hypochromic microcytic anemia secondary to bloodsucking and hemorrhage, especially in patients with iron-deficient diets. The tapeworm *D. latum* may cause megaloblastic anemia by removing vitamin B_{12}.

Procedure

• Collect a stool specimen directly into the container. If the patient is bedridden, collect the specimen into a clean, dry bedpan; then, using a tongue depressor, transfer it into a properly labeled container.

• Note on the laboratory form the date and time of collection, specimen consistency, any recent or current antibiotic therapy, and any pertinent travel or dietary history.

• Send the specimen to the laboratory immediately. If a liquid or soft stool specimen cannot be examined within 30 minutes of passage, place some of it in a preservative; if a formed stool specimen cannot be examined immediately, refrigerate it or place it in preservative.

(See *Collection Procedure for Pinworms.*)

Special precautions

• Do not collect stool from a toilet bowl.

• If the entire stool cannot be sent to the laboratory, include macroscopic worms or worm segments and bloody and mucoid portions of the specimen.
• Observe aseptic precautions when handling the specimen, disposing of equipment, sealing the container, and transporting it. Wash hands thoroughly after specimen collection.

Patient care checklist
Before the test
☑ Explain or clarify test purpose, preparation, and procedure.
☑ Evaluate patient understanding.
☑ Instruct the patient to avoid treatments with castor or mineral oil, bismuth, magnesium or antidiarrheal compounds, barium enemas, and antibiotics for 7 to 10 days before the test.
☑ Inform the patient that the test requires three stool specimens—one every other day or every 3rd day. Up to six specimens may be required to confirm the presence of *E. histolytica*.
☑ Tell the patient to avoid contaminating the stool specimen with urine.

Interfering factors
• Improper collection technique or the presence of urine (which can destroy trophozoites) may cause false-negative results.
• Water is toxic to trophozoites and may contain organisms that interfere with test results.
• Collection of too few specimens may cause failure to detect the organism.
• Failure to transport the specimen promptly or to refrigerate or preserve it if transport is delayed may adversely affect test results.
• Excessive heat or excessive cold can destroy parasites.
• Failure to observe pre-test restrictions of castor or mineral oil, bismuth, magnesium or antidiarrheal compounds, barium enemas, or antibiotics may interfere with microscopic analysis or reduce the number of parasites.

Collection Procedure for Pinworms

The ova of the pinworm *Enterobius vermicularis* seldom appear in feces, because the female migrates to the anus and deposits her ova there. To collect them, place a piece of cellophane tape, sticky side out, on the end of a tongue depressor, and press it firmly on the anal area. Then transfer the tape, sticky side down, to a slide (kits with tape and a slide or a sticky paddle are available). Since the female usually deposits her ova at night, collect the specimen early in the morning, before the patient bathes or defecates.

• Use of antiparasitic agents, such as carbarsone, tetracycline, paromomycin, metronidazole, and diiodohydroxyquin, within 2 weeks before the test may alter test results.

Throat culture

Purpose
• To isolate and identify pathogens, particularly Group A beta-hemolytic streptococci
• To screen asymptomatic carriers of pathogens, especially *N. meningitidis*.

Normal results
Normal throat flora include nonhemolytic and alpha-hemolytic streptococci, *Neisseria* species, staphylococci, diphtheroids, some hemophilus, pneumococci, yeasts, and enteric gram-negative rods.

Abnormal results
The following pathogens may cause the disorders shown:
Group A beta-hemolytic streptococci **(S. pyogenes):**
   Scarlet fever
   Pharyngitis.

Candida albicans:
Thrush.
Corynebacterium diphtheriae:
Diphtheria.
B. pertussis:
Whooping cough.

The basics

A throat culture is used primarily to isolate and identify Group A beta-hemolytic streptococci (*Streptococcus pyogenes*)—allowing early treatment of pharyngitis—and to prevent sequelae, such as rheumatic heart disease or glomerulonephritis.

This test requires swabbing the throat, streaking a culture plate, and allowing the organisms to grow for isolation and identification of pathogens. A smear of the specimen is Gram-stained to provide preliminary identification, which may be helpful for clinical management and for determining the need for further examinations. Culture results necessitate correlation with clinical status, recent antibiotic therapy, and amount of normal flora.

Quick Diagnosis of Strep Pharyngitis

Tests such as the new Directogen Rapid Group A Strep Test Kit permit detection and identification of Group A streptococci directly from throat swabs in only 7 minutes. Using improved antibody-antigen technology, this test allows prompt diagnosis and treatment of streptococcal pharyngitis.

Other tests used to diagnose such infection depend on growing the organism in a culture, which can take from 24 to 48 hours.

This test will not identify the etiology of pharyngitis caused by microorganisms other than Group A streptococci. (Also see *Detecting Pathogens Quickly*, p. 169.)

Procedure

● When possible, obtain the specimen before the start of antibiotic therapy.
● Tell the patient to tilt his head back and close his eyes.
● With the throat well illuminated, check for inflamed areas, using a tongue depressor.
● Swab the tonsillar areas from side to side with the sterile cotton-tipped swab; include any inflamed or purulent sites. *Do not* touch the tongue, cheeks, or teeth with the cotton-tipped swab.
● Immediately place the swab in the culture tube. If a commercial sterile collection and transport system is used, crush the ampule and force the swab into the medium to keep the swab moist.
● Note recent antibiotic therapy on the laboratory slip. Label the specimen with the patient's name, the physician's name, the date and time of collection, and the origin of the specimen. Also indicate the suspected organism, especially *Corynebacterium diphtheriae* (requires two swabs and special growth medium), *B. pertussis* (requires a nasopharyngeal culture and a special growth medium), and *N. meningitidis* (requires enriched selective media).
● Send the specimen to the laboratory immediately.

Special precautions

To protect the specimen and prevent its exposure to pathogens, use aseptic technique during the procedure, and observe proper precautions when sending the specimen to the laboratory.

Patient care checklist

Before the test

☑ Explain or clarify test purpose and procedure.
☑ Evaluate patient understanding.
☑ Inform the patient that the test takes less than 30 seconds, and that test results should be available in 2 or 3 days.
☑ Obtain an immunization history, if pertinent to preliminary diagnosis.

Interfering factors

• Failure to report recent or current antibiotic therapy on the laboratory slip may cause erroneous evaluation of bacterial growth.

• Failure to send the specimen to the laboratory within 15 minutes may permit bacteria to grow or deteriorate.

• Failure to use the proper transport media may cause the specimen to dry out and the bacteria to die.

(See *Quick Diagnosis of Strep Pharyngitis.*)

Urine culture

Purpose

• To diagnose urinary tract infection

• To monitor microorganism colonization after urinary catheter insertion.

Normal results

No growth.

Abnormal results

Bacterial counts of 100,000 or more organisms/ml of a single microbe species:
   Probable urinary tract infection.
Bacterial counts under 100,000/ml:
   Possible urinary tract infection.
Bacterial counts under 10,000/ml:
   Probable contaminated specimen.
Isolation of M. tuberculosis:
   Tuberculosis of the urinary tract.
Isolation of more than two species of organisms:
   Probable contaminated specimen.
Isolation of vaginal or skin organisms:
   Probable contaminated specimen

The basics

Laboratory examination and culture of urine are necessary for evaluation of urinary tract infections, most commonly of bladder infections. Although urine in the kidneys and bladder is normally sterile, a small number of bacteria are usually present in the urethra. Consequently, urine may contain a variety of organisms. Nevertheless, bacteriuria generally results from the prevalence of a single type of bacteria. Indeed, the presence in a urine specimen of more than two distinct bacterial species strongly suggests contamination during collection. Polymicrobial infection may occur after prolonged catheterization or urinary diversion, such as via an ileal conduit.

A single negative culture does not always rule out infection, as in chronic, low-grade pyelonephritis. On the other hand, isolation of known pathogenic bacteria does not necessarily confirm urinary tract infection, since specimens are commonly contaminated by organisms from the urethra and external genitalia. Whenever contamination is suspected, a repeat culture is required.

Significant results of urine culture are possible only after quantitative examination. To distinguish between true bacteriuria and contamination, it is necessary to know the number of organisms in a milliliter of urine, estimated by a culture technique called a *colony count*. Although bacterial counts over 100,000/ml usually indicate an infection, those under 100,000 may be significant depending on the patient's age, sex, history, and other individual factors.

Clean-voided midstream collection is now considered the method of choice rather than collection by suprapubic aspiration or catheterization. (See "Clean-catch midstream collection," p. xviii.)

Procedure

• When possible, obtain the specimen before the start of antibiotic therapy.

• Collect a urine specimen, as ordered.

• Seal the cup with a sterile lid.

• Record the suspected diagnosis, the collection time and method, current antibiotic therapy, and fluid- or drug-induced diuresis on the laboratory slip.

• Send the specimen to the laboratory

immediately. If transport is delayed longer than 30 minutes, store the specimen at 39.2° F. (4° C.) or place it on ice.

• Collect at least 3 ml of urine, but do not fill the specimen cup more than halfway.

Patient care checklist
Before the test
☑ Explain or clarify test purpose and procedure.
☑ Instruct the patient on how to collect a clean-voided midstream specimen, or, if appropriate, explain catheterization or suprapubic aspiration procedures.
☑ Evaluate patient understanding.
☑ Inform the patient with suspected tuberculosis that specimen collection may be necessary on three consecutive mornings.

Interfering factors
• Improper collection technique may contaminate the specimen.
• Fluid- or drug-induced diuresis and antibiotic therapy may lower bacterial counts.
• Failure to refrigerate the specimen may alter test results.
• Failure to send the specimen to the laboratory immediately may invalidate test results.
(See *Quick Centrifugation Test.*)

Quick Centrifugation Test

A new test for determining whether the source of urinary tract infection is in the lower tract (bladder) or the upper tract (kidneys) is centrifugation of urine in a test tube, after which the sediment is stained with fluorescein. Viewed under a fluorescent microscope, the sediment fluoresces in upper tract infection; it does not fluoresce in lower tract infection.

Urogenital secretion examination for trichomonads

Purpose
To confirm trichomoniasis.

Normal results
Trichomonads are normally absent from the urogenital tract.

Abnormal results
The presence of trichomonads confirms:
  Trichomoniasis.

The basics
Microscopic examination of urine or vaginal, urethral, or prostatic secretions can detect urogenital infection by *Trichomonas vaginalis*—a parasitic, flagellate protozoan, usually transmitted sexually. This test is performed more often on females than on males, since females more often exhibit symptoms. Males with trichomoniasis may have symptoms of urethritis or prostatitis. However, in approximately 25% of women and most infected males, trichomonads may be present without associated pathology.

Procedure
If possible, obtain the urogenital specimen before treatment with a trichomonacide begins.
Vaginal secretion:
• With the patient in lithotomy position, an unlubricated vaginal speculum is inserted, and discharge is collected with a sterile cotton-tipped swab.
• The swab is then placed in the tube containing normal saline solution, and the speculum is removed.
Prostatic material:
After prostatic massage, collect secretions with a sterile cotton-tipped swab, and place the swab in normal saline solution.

Urethral discharge:
Collect the discharge with a sterile cotton-tipped swab, and place the swab in normal saline solution.
Urine:
Include the first portion of a voided random (not midstream) specimen.
After collecting any of these specimens:
• Label the specimen appropriately, including the date and time of collection.
• Send the specimen to the laboratory immediately.

Patient care checklist
Before the test
☑ Explain or clarify test purpose and procedure.
☑ Tell the female patient that the test requires a specimen of vaginal secretion or urethral discharge; tell the male patient that the test requires a specimen of urethral or prostatic secretion.
☑ Evaluate patient understanding.
☑ Instruct the female patient not to douche before the test.
After the test
☑ Provide perineal care.

Interfering factors
• Failure to send the specimen to the laboratory immediately causes trichomonads to lose their motility.
• Improper collection technique may interfere with detection.
• Collection of the specimen after trichomonacide therapy begins decreases the number of parasites in the specimen.

Wound culture

Purpose
To identify an infectious microbe in a wound.

Normal results
No pathogens are present in a clean wound.

Abnormal results
Presence of pathogens indicates:
Wound infection.
The most common aerobic pathogens include:
   Staphylococcus aureus
   Group A beta-hemolytic streptococci
   Escherichia coli and other Enterobacteriaceae
   Group D streptococci, including enterococci and *Streptococcus bovis,* and some *Pseudomonas* species.
The most common anaerobic pathogens include:
   Some *Clostridium, Proteus,* and *Bacteroides* species.

The basics
A wound culture consists of microscopic analysis of a specimen from a lesion to confirm infection. Wound cultures may be aerobic (for detection of organisms that usually require oxygen to grow and usually appear in a superficial wound) or anaerobic (for organisms that need little or no oxygen and appear in areas of poor tissue perfusion, such as postoperative wounds, ulcers, or compound fractures). Indications for wound culture include fever, and inflammation and drainage in damaged tissue.

Procedure
• Prepare a sterile field and cleanse the area around the wound with antiseptic solution.
For an aerobic culture:
• Express the wound and—using a sterile cotton-tipped swab—collect as much exudate as possible, or insert the swab deeply into the wound and gently rotate it.
• Immediately place the swab in the aerobic culture tube.
For an anaerobic culture:
Insert a sterile cotton-tipped swab deeply into the wound, gently rotate it, and immediately place the swab in the anaerobic culture tube; or insert a needle into the wound, aspirate 1 to 5

ml of exudate into the syringe, and immediately inject the exudate into the anaerobic culture tube. If the needle is covered with a rubber stopper, the aspirate may be sent to the laboratory in the syringe.

After collection by one of the previous methods:

• Record on the laboratory slip recent antibiotic therapy, the source of the specimen, and the suspected organism. Also, label the specimen container appropriately with the patient's name and room number, the physician's name, the wound site, and the time of specimen collection.

• Keep the specimen container upright, and send it to the laboratory within 15 minutes.

Special precautions

• Cleanse the area around the wound thoroughly to limit contamination of the culture by normal skin flora, such as diphtheroids, *Staphylococcus epidermidis,* and alpha-hemolytic streptococcus. However, *do not* cleanse the area around a perineal wound.

• Make sure no antiseptic enters the wound.

• Obtain exudate from the entire wound, using more than one sterile cotton-tipped swab.

• Since some anaerobes die in the presence of even a small amount of oxygen, place the specimen in the culture tube quickly, take care that no air enters the tube, and check that double stoppers are secure.

• Use aseptic technique during the procedure, and use necessary isolation precautions when sending the specimen to the laboratory.

Patient care checklist

Before the test

☑ Explain or clarify test purpose and procedure.

☑ Evaluate patient understanding.

After the test

☑ Dress the wound, as ordered.

Interfering factors

• Failure to report recent or current antibiotic therapy may cause erroneous evaluation of bacterial growth.

• Poor collection technique may contaminate or invalidate the specimen.

• Failure to use the proper transport media may cause the specimen to dry up and the bacteria to die.

• Failure to send the specimen to the laboratory within 15 minutes may permit growth or deterioration of microbes.

Selected References

Diagnostics, 2nd ed. Nurse's Reference Library. Springhouse, Pa.: Springhouse Corp., 1986.

Diseases, 2nd ed. Nurse's Reference Library. Springhouse, Pa.: Springhouse Corp., 1987.

Finegold, Sidney M., and Martin, William J. *Bailey and Scott's Diagnostic Microbiology,* 6th ed. St. Louis: C.V. Mosby Co., 1982.

Lennette, E.H., et al., eds. *Manual of Clinical Microbiology,* 3rd ed. Washington, D.C.: American Society for Microbiology, 1980.

Volk, Wesley A. *Essentials of Medical Microbiology,* 2nd ed. Philadelphia: J.B. Lippincott Co., 1982.

8 ENDOSCOPIC TESTING

Introduction

In endoscopic tests, a rigid or flexible tube called an endoscope is inserted into a viscus of the body to allow visualization of the internal structure. Endoscopic procedures can sometimes eliminate the need for open surgery. All endoscopes contain a light source and channels that can accommodate biopsy forceps, a cytology brush, suction, lavage, an anesthetic, or oxygen. Most types of endoscopes also allow use of a microscope, camera, and implements for performing minor surgery, such as cauterization of a bleeding point or removal of polyps or foreign bodies.

Rigid endoscopes have a larger internal diameter than flexible endoscopes and allow removal of larger specimens and secretions or excretions that obliterate the view. Rigid endoscopes, however, cannot be passed beyond strictures, and a general anesthetic is usually required.

Flexible endoscopes are tolerated with a minimum of discomfort, and carry less risk of trauma from intubation than rigid endoscopes. Flexible endoscopes allow visualization of distant structures (such as the bronchial tree and colon) and out-of-the-way structures (such as the larynx and the nasopharynx).

Endoscopic procedures may be performed at the bedside or in a treatment room, an operating room, or the radiology department.

Patient-teaching guidelines

Patient-learner objectives:
- Define the test.
- State the specific purpose of the test.
- Explain the procedure.
- Discuss test preparation, procedure, and post-test care.
- Identify possible risks or adverse effects.

Teaching content:
- Define the test in terms the patient can understand.
- Explain the specific purpose of the test.
- Describe the procedure. Explain where the test will be performed and who will be performing it. Describe the equipment, what sensations or discomfort (if any) to expect, and what positions the patient will be placed in, since unfamiliarity with the test may provoke extreme anxiety.
- If a local anesthetic will be used, explain that it will alleviate some discomfort, but that the patient will remain alert. If a general anesthetic will be used, explain that the patient will not be conscious during the procedure.
- If a sedative will be administered before the test, explain that this will make the patient drowsy and will help alleviate anxiety. Advise the outpatient to arrange transportation home, since it is not safe to drive for about 12 hours after sedation.
- Inform the patient of any special preparations for the test. Be sure to specify dietary restrictions and indicate the applicable time period.
- Tell the patient if discomfort or any other problem is a normal consequence of the test. Reassure him that

it is only temporary and, when possible, explain what will be done to alleviate the problem.

• Describe any other special care or restrictions following the test. Be sure to explain why they are necessary. If assessment measures will be implemented frequently, alleviate undue patient anxiety by explaining this as a routine precaution.

• Answer any questions the patient may still have after the physician explains the risks associated with the test.

• Inform the patient (especially the outpatient) of signs or symptoms of complications; tell him whom to contact if these should occur and to do so at once.

• Provide the outpatient with written instructions.

Evaluation:
After the patient-teaching session is completed, evaluate whether the patient has satisfactorily met each patient-learner objective by obtaining necessary patient feedback. Refocus teaching as needed.

Arthroscopy

Purpose
• To detect and diagnose meniscal, patellar, condylar, extrasynovial, and synovial diseases
• To monitor the progression of disease
• To perform joint surgery.

Normal results
The knee joint is surrounded by muscles, ligaments, cartilage, and tendons, and is lined with synovial membrane. In children, the menisci are smooth and opaque, with their thick outer edges attached to the joint capsule and their inner edges lying snugly against the condylar surfaces, unattached. Articular cartilage appears smooth and white; ligaments and tendons appear cablelike and silvery. The synovium is smooth and marked by a fine vascular network. Degenerative changes begin during adolescence.

Abnormal results
Arthroscopy of the knee may reveal:
Meniscus injury
Chondromalacia patellae
Patellar dislocation, subluxation, fracture
Degenerative articular cartilage
Osteochondritis dissecans
Loose bodies from osteochondral and chondral fractures
Torn ligaments
Baker's cyst
Ganglion cyst
Synovitis
Rheumatoid and degenerative arthritis
Foreign bodies associated with gout.

The basics
Arthroscopy is the visual examination of the interior of a joint with a specially designed fiberoptic endoscope. It is most commonly used to examine the knee. In evaluating a patient with suspected or confirmed joint disease, arthroscopy is usually considered a secondary tool; the initial diagnostic approach consists of a complete history and physical examination, plain X-ray films, and arthrography. However, the diagnostic accuracy of arthroscopy (about 98%) surpasses that of arthrography and radiographs, and it may prove to be the definitive diagnostic procedure.

Unlike radiographic studies, arthroscopy permits concurrent surgery or biopsy using a technique called triangulation, in which instruments are passed through a separate cannula. Thus, arthroscopy provides a safe, convenient alternative to open surgery (arthrotomy) or separate biopsy. Although arthroscopy is commonly performed under a local anesthetic, it may also be performed under a spinal or general anesthetic, particularly when surgery is anticipated.

Contraindications to this test include: fibrous ankylosis with flexion of less than 50° and local skin or wound infection.

Complications associated with arthroscopy rarely occur but may include infection, hemarthrosis, swelling, synovial rupture, thrombophlebitis, infrapatellar anesthesia, and joint injury.

Procedure
• A tourniquet is applied to the upper thigh. (Some physicians prefer not to inflate the tourniquet for the procedure, unless excessive bleeding occurs.)
• The patient's knee is flexed at a 90° angle.
• The skin is cleansed, and a waterproof stockinette is applied to the lower leg and foot.
• The joint is injected with about 50 ml of sterile saline solution to distend the knee and provide better visualization.
• A small incision, 5 to 6 mm long, is made.
• The arthroscope is inserted. A common insertion point is the anterior joint line, below the patella's apex, either medial or lateral to the patellar tendon.
• The arthroscope is connected to a light system for viewing, and an irrigating system is set up to flush the joint.
• All parts of the knee are carefully visualized.
• A synovial biopsy or appropriate surgery may be performed, or treatment applied, as indicated.
• The arthroscope is removed, and gentle manual pressure is applied to the knee to help remove the saline solution.
• The incision is closed with a suture. An adhesive strip is applied, and an elastic roller bandage is wrapped around the knee.

Patient care checklist
Before the test
☑ Explain or clarify test purpose, preparation, procedure, and post-test care.

☑ If a local anesthetic will be used, tell the patient that he may experience transient discomfort from its injection and from the pressure of the tourniquet.
☑ Evaluate patient understanding.
☑ Restrict food and fluids after midnight before the test.
☑ Make sure that the patient or a responsible member of the family has signed a consent form.
☑ Check the patient's history for hypersensitivity to the anesthetic. Report any hypersensitivity to the physician.
☑ Review the patient's history and use assessment skills to detect local skin or wound infections. Notify the physician, as needed.
☑ Shave the area 5″ (13 cm) above and below the joint.
☑ Administer a sedative, as ordered, just before the procedure.

After the test
☑ Watch for fever, and for swelling, increased pain, and localized inflammation at the incision site. If the patient reports discomfort, administer aspirin, as ordered.
☑ Tell the patient that he may walk as soon as he is fully awake, but he should avoid excessive use of the joint for a few days.

Bronchoscopy

Purpose
• To visually examine a possible tumor, obstruction, secretion, or foreign body in the tracheobronchial tree, as demonstrated on radiograph
• To help diagnose bronchogenic carcinoma, tuberculosis, interstitial pulmonary disease, or fungal or parasitic pulmonary infection, by obtaining a specimen for bacteriologic and cytologic examination
• To locate a bleeding site in the tracheobronchial tree
• To remove foreign bodies, malignant or benign tumors, mucous plugs, or

excessive secretions from the tracheo-bronchial tree.

Normal results

The trachea, a 4½" (11.3-cm) tube extending from the larynx to the bronchi, normally consists of smooth muscle containing C-shaped rings of cartilage at regular intervals, and is lined with ciliated mucosa. The bronchi appear structurally similar to the trachea; the right bronchus is slightly larger and more vertical than the left. Smaller secondary bronchi, bronchioles, alveolar ducts, and eventually alveolar sacs and alveoli branch off from the main bronchi.

Abnormal results

Bronchoscopy may reveal:
   Inflammation
   Tumors
   Abscesses
   Enlarged submucosal lymph nodes
   Stenosis
   Ulceration
   Blood, secretions, calculi, foreign bodies in bronchial lumen
   Irregular bronchial branching and abnormal bifurcation due to diverticulum.

Results of tissue and cell studies may reveal:
   Bronchogenic cancer
   Interstitial pulmonary disease
   Tuberculosis
   Other pulmonary infection.

The basics

Bronchoscopy is the direct visualization of the trachea and tracheobronchial tree through a standard metal bronchoscope or a fiberoptic bronchoscope.

A flexible fiberoptic bronchoscope is used most often since it is smaller, allows a greater range of view of the segmental and subsegmental bronchi, and carries less risk of trauma than the rigid bronchoscope. A large rigid bronchoscope, however, is necessary to remove foreign objects, excise en-dobronchial lesions, and control massive hemoptysis.

Correlation of radiographic, bronchoscopic, and cytologic findings with clinical signs and symptoms is essential.

Complications resulting from bronchoscopy may include bronchial or tracheal perforation, infection, and pneumothorax.

Procedure

• Place the patient in a supine position on a table or bed, or have him sit upright in a chair.
• Tell him to remain relaxed, with his arms at his sides, and to breathe through his nose.
• After the local anesthetic is sprayed into the patient's throat and takes effect (usually 1 to 2 minutes), the doctor introduces the bronchoscope (possibly tipped with lidocaine jelly) through the patient's mouth or nose. When the bronchoscope is just above the vocal cords, approximately 3 to 4 ml of 2% to 4% lidocaine is flushed through the inner channel of the scope to the vocal cords, to anesthetize deeper areas.
• The physician inspects the anatomic structure of the trachea and bronchi, observes the color of the mucosal lining, and notes unusual masses or inflamed areas.
• Biopsy forceps may be used to remove a tissue specimen from a suspect area, a bronchial brush to obtain cells from the surface of a lesion, or suction apparatus to remove foreign bodies or mucous plugs.
• Send specimens in their properly labeled containers to the laboratory immediately.
• This test takes 45 to 60 minutes to perform.

Special precautions

CLINICAL ALERT: **A patient with severe respiratory failure who cannot breathe adequately by himself should be placed on a ventilator before bronchoscopy.**

Patient care checklist

Before the test

☑ Explain test purpose, preparation, procedure, and post-test care.

☑ Inform the patient that the room will be darkened.

☑ Warn him that he may experience some discomfort during the procedure.

☑ Reassure the patient that his airway will not be blocked during the procedure, and that oxygen will be administered through the bronchoscope.

☑ Reassure the patient that hoarseness, loss of voice, and sore throat occurring after the procedure are only temporary.

☑ Evaluate patient understanding.

☑ Restrict food and fluids for 6 to 12 hours before the test.

☑ Make sure that the patient or a responsible family member has signed the consent form.

☑ Check the patient's history for hypersensitivity to the anesthetic. Report any hypersensitivity to the physician.

☑ Obtain baseline vital signs.

☑ Administer the preoperative sedative, as ordered.

☑ If the patient is wearing dentures, instruct him to remove them just before the test.

After the test

☑ Monitor vital signs. Immediately notify the physician of any adverse reaction to the anesthetic or sedative.

☑ As ordered, place the conscious patient in semi-Fowler's position; place the unconscious patient on his side with the head of the bed slightly elevated to prevent aspiration.

☑ Provide an emesis basin, and instruct the patient to spit out saliva rather than swallow it. Observe sputum for blood, and notify the physician immediately if excessive bleeding occurs.

☑ If ordered, collect all sputum for 24 hours after bronchoscopy for cytologic examination, since irritation produced during bronchial brushing often results in delayed shedding of malignant cells.

☑ Tell the patient who had a biopsy to refrain from clearing his throat and coughing, which may dislodge the clot at the biopsy site and cause hemorrhaging.

CLINICAL ALERT: **Immediately report any subcutaneous crepitus around the patient's face and neck—a possible indication of tracheal or bronchial perforation.**

CLINICAL ALERT: **Watch for and immediately report symptoms of respiratory difficulty, such as laryngeal stridor and dyspnea, resulting from laryngeal edema or laryngospasm. Observe for signs of hypoxemia (cyanosis), pneumothorax (dyspnea, cyanosis, diminished breath sounds on affected side), bronchospasm (dyspnea, wheezing), or bleeding (hemoptysis). Keep resuscitative equipment and a tracheotomy tray available for 24 hours after the test.**

☑ Restrict food and fluids until the gag reflex returns (usually in 2 hours). Then the patient may resume his usual diet, beginning with sips of clear liquid or ice chips.

☑ Provide lozenges or a soothing liquid gargle to ease throat discomfort when his gag reflex returns.

Interfering factors

Failure to place the specimens in the appropriate containers and to send the specimens to the laboratory immediately may affect the test results.

Colonoscopy

Purpose

• To detect or evaluate inflammatory and ulcerative bowel disease

• To locate the origin of lower gastrointestinal bleeding

• To aid in diagnosis of colonic strictures and benign or malignant lesions

• To evaluate the colon postoperatively for recurrence of polyps or malignant lesions.

Normal results

The mucosa of the large intestine beyond the sigmoid colon appears light pink-orange and is marked by semilunar folds and deep tubular pits. Blood vessels are visible beneath the intestinal mucosa, which glistens from mucous secretions.

Abnormal results

Colonoscopy may reveal:

Site of lower gastrointestinal bleeding

Diverticula

Polyps

Stricture

Tumor

Site of suspected ulcerated colitis or Crohn's disease.

The basics

Colonoscopy is the visual examination of the lining of the large intestine with a flexible fiberoptic endoscope. This test is indicated for patients with histories of constipation and diarrhea, persistent rectal bleeding, or lower abdominal pain when results of proctosigmoidoscopy and the barium enema test prove negative or inconclusive. Histologic and cytologic tests of specimens obtained are often needed to confirm the diagnosis. Colonoscopy is usually a safe procedure but can cause perforation of the large intestine, excessive bleeding, and retroperitoneal emphysema.

Contraindications to this test include: ischemic bowel disease, acute diverticulitis, peritonitis, fulminant granulomatous colitis, or fulminant ulcerative colitis.

Procedure

• Place the patient on his left side, with his knees flexed, and drape him.

• Instruct him to breathe deeply and slowly through his mouth as the physician inserts his gloved, lubricated index finger into the anus and rectum, and palpates the mucosa.

• After a water-soluble lubricant has been applied to the patient's anus and to the tip of the colonoscope, tell the patient that the colonoscope is about to be inserted.

• The physician advances the colonoscope through the twists and bends of the colon.

• Air is insufflated through the colonoscope to distend the bowel lumen and provide better visualization.

• A thorough examination is performed, especially during withdrawal.

• During the examination, suction may be used to remove blood or excessive secretions that obscure vision.

• Biopsy forceps or a cytology brush may be passed through a channel in the colonoscope to obtain specimens for histologic and cytologic examinations, respectively; an electrocautery snare may be used to remove polyps.

• Send any specimens in their properly labeled containers to the laboratory immediately.

• The test usually takes about 30 to 60 minutes to perform.

Special precautions

CLINICAL ALERT: **Watch closely for side effects of the sedative, such as respiratory depression, hypotension, excessive diaphoresis, bradycardia, and confusion. Have available emergency resuscitation equipment and a narcotic antagonist, such as naloxone, for intravenous use, if necessary.**

• If a polyp is removed but not retrieved during the examination, give enemas and strain stools, as ordered, to retrieve it.

Patient care checklist

Before the test

☑ Explain or clarify test purpose, preparation, procedure, and post-test care.

☑ Inform the patient that he may receive a sedative I.M. or I.V. to help him relax.

☑ Assure him that the colonoscope is well lubricated to ease its insertion, and that he may feel an urge to defecate when it is inserted and advanced. Instruct him to breathe deeply and slowly through his mouth to relax his abdominal muscles.

☑ Evaluate patient understanding.

☑ Provide the patient with a clear liquid diet for 48 hours before the test.

☑ Tell the patient that the large intestine must be thoroughly cleansed to be clearly visible. Give him a laxative, such as 10 oz (300 ml) of magnesium citrate or 3 tbsp (45 ml) of castor oil, in the evening, and a warm tap-water or sodium biphosphate enema 3 to 4 hours before the test, as ordered, until the return is clear. Do not administer a soapsuds enema, since this irritates the mucosa and stimulates mucous secretions that may hinder the examination.

☑ Make sure that the patient or a responsible family member has signed the consent form.

☑ Check the patient's vital signs 30 minutes before the test; if they are stable, administer the sedative, as ordered.

After the test

CLINICAL ALERT: **Observe the patient closely for signs of bowel perforation: malaise, rectal bleeding, abdominal pain and distention, fever, and mucopurulent drainage. Notify the physician immediately if such signs develop.**

☑ Check vital signs until stable.

☑ After the patient has recovered from sedation, he may resume his usual diet.

☑ Tell the patient that he may pass large amounts of flatus, resulting from the air insufflated to distend the colon. Provide privacy in order to minimize embarrassment.

☑ If a polyp has been removed, inform the patient that there may be some blood in his stool.

Interfering factors

• Barium retained in the intestine from previous diagnostic studies makes accurate visual examination impossible.

• Blood from acute colonic hemorrhage interferes with the examination.

• Fixation of the sigmoid colon from inflammatory bowel disease, surgery, or irradiation may inhibit passage of the colonoscope.

• Failure to place histologic or cytologic specimens in the appropriate preservative or to send the specimens to the laboratory immediately may affect test results.

Colposcopy

Purpose

• To help confirm cervical intraepithelial neoplasia or invasive carcinoma after a positive Papanicolaou (Pap) test

• To evaluate vaginal or cervical lesions

• To monitor conservatively treated cervical intraepithelial neoplasia

• To monitor patients whose mothers received diethylstilbestrol during pregnancy.

Normal results

Cervical vessels show a network and hairpin capillary pattern. Surface contour is smooth and pink; columnar epithelium appears grapelike. Different tissue types are sharply demarcated.

Abnormal results

Colposcopy may reveal:

Cervical intraepithelial neoplasia
Invasive carcinoma
Inflammatory changes (usually from infection)
Atrophic changes (usually from aging or, less often, the use of oral contraceptives)
Erosion (probably from increased pathogenicity of vaginal flora, due to changes in vaginal pH)
Papilloma and condyloma (possibly from viruses).

The basics

In colposcopy, the cervix and vagina are visually examined by means of an instrument containing a magnifying lens and a light (colposcope). Although originally used as a screening test for cancer, colposcopy is now used primarily to evaluate abnormal cytology or grossly suspicious lesions, and to examine the cervix and vagina after a positive Pap test. During the examination, a biopsy may be performed and photographs taken with the colposcope and its attachments of suspicious lesions. Histologic study of the biopsy specimen confirms colposcopic findings. However, if the results of the examination and biopsy are inconsistent with the results of the Pap test and biopsy of the squamocolumnar junction, conization of the cervix for biopsy may be indicated. Risks of biopsy include bleeding (especially during pregnancy) and infection.

Procedure
• With the patient in lithotomy position, the examiner inserts the speculum and, if indicated, performs a Pap test.
• The cervix is swabbed with acetic acid solution to remove mucus.
• After the cervix and vagina are examined, using the colposcope, a biopsy is performed on areas that appear abnormal.
• Finally, the bleeding is stopped by applying pressure or hemostatic solutions, or by cautery.
• Send any specimens in their properly labeled containers to the laboratory immediately.
• This test takes 10 to 15 minutes to perform.

Patient care checklist
Before the test
☑ Explain or clarify test purpose, preparation, and procedure.
☑ Inform the patient that the procedure is safe and painless.
☑ Tell the patient that a biopsy may be performed at the time of examination, and that this may cause minimal, but easily controlled, bleeding.
☑ Evaluate patient understanding.

After the test
☑ After biopsy, instruct the patient to abstain from intercourse, and tell her not to insert anything in her vagina (except a tampon) until healing of the biopsy site is confirmed.

Interfering factors
Failure to cleanse the cervix of foreign materials, such as creams and medications, may impair visualization.

Cystoscopy
[Cystourethroscopy]

Purpose
To diagnose and evaluate urinary tract disorders.

Normal results
The urethra, bladder, and ureteral orifices appear normal in size, shape, and position. The mucosa lining the lower urinary tract should appear smooth and shiny, with no evidence of erythema, cysts, or other abnormalities. The bladder should be free of obstructions, tumors, and calculi.

Abnormal results
Cystoscopy may reveal:
  Prostatic hypertrophy
  Urethral stricture
  Vesical neck contracture
  Bladder calculi
  Bladder tumors
  Bladder diverticula
  Bladder polyps
  Trabeculated bladder wall
  Congenital anomalies, such as ureteroceles, duplicate ureteral orifices, or urethral valves.

The basics
Cystoscopy allows direct visual examination of the bladder and the urethra. It also permits a readily available channel for additional procedures, such as biopsy, dilation of a constricted urethra, lesion resection, col-

lection of calculi, or passage of a ureteral catheter to the renal pelvis for pyelography.

Kidney-ureter-bladder (KUB) radiography and excretory urography usually precede cystoscopy.

Contraindications to this test include: acute forms of urethritis, prostatitis, or cystitis, since instrumentation can lead to sepsis.

Procedure
• After a general or regional anesthetic (as required) has been administered, the patient is placed in lithotomy position on a cystoscopic table.
• The genitalia are cleansed with an antiseptic solution, and the patient is draped. (A local anesthetic is instilled at this point.)
• As the first step in cystoscopy, most urologists prefer to visually examine the urethra as they move the instrument toward the bladder. To do this, a urethroscope is inserted into the well-lubricated sheath (instead of an obturator), and both are passed gently through the urethra into the bladder. The urethroscope is removed, and a cystoscope inserted through the sheath into the bladder.
• After the bladder is filled with irrigating solution, the scope is rotated to inspect the entire surface of the bladder wall and ureteral orifices.
• The cystoscope is removed, the urethroscope is reinserted, and both the urethroscope and the sheath are slowly withdrawn, permitting examination of the bladder neck and the various portions of the urethra, including the internal and external sphincters.
• During cystoscopy, a urine specimen is routinely taken from the bladder for culture and sensitivity testing, and residual urine is measured.
• More invasive procedures may be performed, if needed.
• The test takes about 20 to 30 minutes to perform.

Patient care checklist
Before the test
☑ Explain or clarify test purpose, preparation, procedure, and post-test care.
☑ If the patient will receive a local anesthetic, inform him that he may experience a burning sensation when the instrument is passed through the urethra. He may also feel an urgent need to urinate as the bladder is filled with irrigating solution. Reassure him that these sensations are common and generally transient.
☑ Inform the patient that he may experience some discomfort after the procedure, including a slight burning when he urinates.
☑ Evaluate patient understanding.
☑ If a general anesthetic will be administered, restrict food and fluids for 8 hours before the test (fasting is not required if a local anesthetic will be given).
☑ Check the patient's history for hypersensitivity to anesthetic. Report any hypersensitivity to the physician.
☑ Make sure that the patient or a responsible member of the family has signed a consent form.
☑ Ask the patient to urinate just before the procedure.
☑ Administer a sedative, as ordered, just before the procedure.
After the test
☑ Monitor vital signs, as ordered, until they stabilize.
☑ Instruct the patient to drink fluids freely and to take the prescribed analgesic. Reassure him that burning and frequency will soon subside.
☑ Administer antibiotics, as ordered, to prevent bacterial sepsis due to urethral tissue trauma.
☑ Report flank or abdominal pain, chills, fever, or low urinary output to the physician immediately.
☑ Record intake and output for 24 hours, and observe the patient for distention. If the patient does not void within 8 hours after the test, or if bright red blood continues to appear after three voidings, notify the physician.

☑ Instruct the patient to abstain from alcohol for 48 hours.

Endoscopic retrograde cholangiopancreatography (ERCP)

Purpose
• To evaluate obstructive jaundice
• To help diagnose cancer of the duodenal papilla, the pancreas, and the biliary ducts
• To locate calculi and stenosis in the pancreatic ducts and hepatobiliary tree.

Normal results
The duodenal papilla appears as a small red or sometimes pale erosion protruding into the lumen. Its orifice is commonly bordered by a fringe of white mucosa, and a longitudinal fold running perpendicular to the deep circular folds of the duodenum helps mark its location. The pancreatic and hepatobiliary ducts are patent and, although they usually unite in the ampulla of Vater and empty through the duodenal papilla, separate orifices are sometimes present. The contrast medium uniformly fills the pancreatic duct, the hepatobiliary tree, and the gallbladder.

Abnormal results
Examination may reveal:
  Stones
  Strictures.
Examination may suggest:
  Biliary cirrhosis
  Primary sclerosing cholangitis
  Carcinoma of the bile ducts
  Pancreatic cysts
  Pancreatic pseudocysts
  Pancreatic tumor
  Carcinoma of the head of the pancreas
  Chronic pancreatitis
  Pancreatic fibrosis
  Carcinoma of the duodenal papilla
  Papillary stenosis.

The basics
ERCP is the radiographic examination of the pancreatic ducts and hepatobiliary tree after injection of a contrast medium into the duodenal papilla. ERCP is indicated in patients with confirmed or suspected pancreatic disease, or obstructive jaundice of unknown etiology. With the development of smaller, side-viewing endoscopes, ERCP is being performed more frequently, especially when abdominal ultrasonography, computerized tomography, liver scanning, hypotonic duodenography, and biliary tract X-ray studies (including percutaneous transhepatic cholangiography) prove diagnostically inadequate.
Contraindications to this test include: infectious disease, stricture or obstruction of the esophagus or duodenum, and acute pancreatitis, cholangitis, or cardiorespiratory disease. Complications may include cholangitis and pancreatitis.

Procedure
• An I.V. is started with 150 ml of normal saline solution.
• A local anesthetic is administered.
• The patient is placed in the left lateral position.
• 5 to 20 mg of diazepam is administered I.V.
• The endoscope is inserted through the patient's mouth and advanced through the esophagus and stomach.
• When the endoscope reaches the duodenum, the patient is assisted to the prone position.
• An anticholinergic or glucagon I.V. is administered to induce duodenal atony and to relax the ampullary sphincter.
• A cannula is passed through the endoscope and a contrast medium is instilled to visualize the pancreatic and common bile ducts.
• Rapid-sequence X-rays are taken after each instillation of the dye.

• Before the endoscope is withdrawn, a tissue specimen may be obtained or fluid aspirated for histologic and cytologic examination, respectively.

• Send any specimens in their properly labeled containers to the laboratory immediately.

• The test takes 30 to 60 minutes to perform.

Special precautions

CLINICAL ALERT: **Vital signs are monitored, and the airway is kept patent throughout the procedure. If you assist with this procedure, watch for signs of respiratory depression, apnea, hypotension, excessive diaphoresis, bradycardia, and laryngospasm. Be sure to have available emergency resuscitation equipment and a narcotic antagonist, such as naloxone.**

Patient care checklist

Before the test

☑ Explain or clarify test purpose, preparation, procedure, and post-test care.

☑ Inform the patient that a local anesthetic will be sprayed into his mouth to calm the gag reflex. Warn him that the spray has an unpleasant taste and makes the tongue and throat feel swollen, causing difficulty in swallowing. Instruct him to let saliva drain from the side of his mouth, and tell him that suction may be used to remove saliva.

☑ If the patient has teeth, tell him that a mouth guard will be inserted to protect them and the endoscope; assure him that the mouth guard will not obstruct his breathing.

☑ Assure the patient that he will receive a sedative before insertion of the endoscope, to help him relax, but that he will remain conscious.

☑ Warn him that he may experience transient flushing on injection of the contrast medium.

☑ Advise him that he may have a sore throat for 3 or 4 days after the examination.

☑ Evaluate patient understanding.

☑ Restrict food and fluids after midnight before the test.

☑ Make sure that the patient or a responsible family member has signed the consent form.

☑ Check the patient's history for hypersensitivity to iodine, seafood, or contrast media used for other diagnostic procedures. Report hypersensitivity to the physician.

☑ Just before the procedure, obtain baseline vital signs.

☑ Ask the patient to remove dentures, all metal or other radiopaque objects, and constricting undergarments, right before the procedure.

☑ Ask the patient to void before the procedure, to minimize the discomfort of urinary retention that may follow the procedure.

After the test

CLINICAL ALERT: **Observe the patient closely for signs of cholangitis and pancreatitis. Hyperbilirubinemia, fever, and chills are the immediate signs of cholangitis; hypotension associated with gram-negative septicemia may develop later. Upper left quadrant pain and tenderness, elevated serum amylase levels, and transient hyperbilirubinemia are the usual signs of pancreatitis. Draw blood samples for amylase and bilirubin determinations, if ordered, but remember that these levels usually rise after ERCP.**

☑ Continue to watch for signs of respiratory depression, apnea, hypotension, excessive diaphoresis, bradycardia, and laryngospasm. Monitor vital signs, as ordered.

☑ Withhold food and fluids until the gag reflex returns. When it does return, allow fluids and a light meal.

☑ Check for signs of urinary retention. Notify the physician if the patient has not voided within 8 hours.

☑ If the patient has a sore throat, provide soothing lozenges and warm saline gargles to ease discomfort.

Esophagogastro-duodenoscopy

Purpose
• To determine the site and cause of upper GI bleeding
• To diagnose structural abnormalities and upper GI disease
• To obtain a biopsy specimen
• To evaluate the stomach and duodenum postoperatively
• To obtain emergency diagnosis, such as esophageal injury, caused by ingestion of chemicals.

Normal results
The smooth mucosa of the esophagus is normally yellow-pink and is marked by a fine vascular network. A pulsation on the anterior wall of the esophagus between 8″ to 10″ (20 to 25 cm) from the incisor teeth represents the aortic arch. The orange-red mucosa of the stomach begins at the Z line, an irregular transition line slightly above the esophagogastric junction. Unlike the esophagus, the stomach has rugal folds, and its blood vessels are not visible beneath the gastric mucosa. The reddish mucosa of the duodenal bulb is marked by a few shallow longitudinal folds. However, the mucosa of the distal duodenum has prominent circular folds, is lined with villi, and appears velvety.

Abnormal results
Esophagogastroduodenoscopy may indicate:
  Site of upper gastrointestinal bleeding
  Peptic ulcer
  Tumor
  Esophagitis
  Gastritis
  Duodenitis
  Diverticula
  Varices
  Esophageal rings
  Esophageal and pyloric stenoses
  Hiatal hernia
  Mallory-Weiss syndrome.

The basics
Esophagogastroduodenoscopy is the visual examination of the lining of the esophagus, the stomach, and the upper duodenum, using an endoscope. Depending on the purpose of the test, the physician may order only an esophagoscopy, gastroscopy, duodenoscopy, or esophagogastroscopy.

This test is indicated in patients with hematemesis, melena, or substernal or epigastric pain, and in postoperative patients with recurrent or new symptoms. This procedure is generally safe, but can cause perforation of the esophagus, stomach, or duodenum, especially if the patient is restless or uncooperative. During the procedure, specimens may be obtained for histologic or cytologic testing, which may be needed to confirm the diagnosis.
Contraindications to this test usually include: Zenker's diverticulum, large aortic aneurysm, or recent ulcer perforation.

Procedure
• A local anesthetic is administered.
• The physician may inject diazepam (Valium) intravenously before the procedure.
• The patient is placed in the left lateral position.
• The endoscope is inserted through the patient's mouth and slowly advanced through the esophagus, stomach, and duodenum.
• During the examination, air may be instilled into the gastrointestinal tract to open the bowel lumen and flatten tissue folds, water instilled to rinse material or fluid from the lens, and suction applied to remove unnecessary insufflated air or secretions. A camera may be attached to the endoscope to photograph areas for later study, or a measuring tube passed through the endoscope to determine the size of a lesion. Biopsy forceps to obtain a tissue specimen, or a cytology brush to ob-

tain cells, may also be passed through the scope.

• Following this, the endoscope is slowly withdrawn, and suspicious areas are reexamined.

• Send any specimens in their properly labeled containers to the laboratory immediately.

• This test takes about 30 minutes to perform.

Special precautions

CLINICAL ALERT: **Observe the patient closely for medication side effects: respiratory depression, apnea, hypotension, excessive diaphoresis, bradycardia, and laryngospasm. Have available emergency resuscitation equipment and a narcotic antagonist, such as naloxone or levorphanol tartrate. Be prepared to intervene, as necessary.**

Patient care checklist

Before the test

☑ Explain or clarify test purpose, preparation, procedure, and post-test care.

☑ Inform the patient that a bitter-tasting local anesthetic will be sprayed into his mouth and throat to calm the gag reflex, and that his tongue and throat may feel swollen, making swallowing seem difficult. Advise him to let the saliva drain from the side of his mouth; a suction machine may be used to remove saliva, if necessary.

☑ If the patient has teeth, tell him that a mouth guard will be inserted to protect his teeth and the endoscope; assure him that the mouth guard will not obstruct his breathing.

☑ Tell the patient that he will receive a sedative to help him relax before the endoscope is inserted, but that he will remain conscious. If the procedure is being done on an outpatient basis, advise the patient to arrange for transportation home, since he may feel drowsy from the sedative.

☑ Tell the patient that he may experience pressure in his stomach as the endoscope is moved about, and a feeling of fullness when air or carbon dioxide is insufflated. However, there will be no pain.

☑ Evaluate patient understanding.

☑ Review the patient's history for hypersensitivity to the medications and anesthetic ordered for the test. Report any hypersensitivity to the physician.

☑ Restrict food and fluids for 6 to 12 hours before the test.

☑ Make sure that the patient or a responsible family member has signed a consent form.

☑ Administer medications, such as atropine sulfate, as ordered, about 30 minutes before the test.

☑ Just before the procedure, instruct the patient to remove dentures, eyeglasses, necklaces, hairpins, combs, and constricting undergarments.

☑ Obtain baseline vital signs just before the procedure.

After the test

CLINICAL ALERT: **Observe the patient for possible perforation. Perforation in the cervical area of the esophagus produces pain on swallowing and with neck movement; thoracic perforation causes substernal or epigastric pain that increases with breathing or with movement of the trunk; diaphragmatic perforation produces shoulder pain and dyspnea; gastric perforation causes abdominal or back pain, cyanosis, fever, or pleural effusion.**

☑ Monitor vital signs, as ordered.

☑ Withhold food and fluids until the gag reflex returns. When it does return, usually in 1 hour, allow fluids and a light meal, as ordered.

☑ Keep the side rails up until the sedative has worn off.

☑ Tell the patient that he may burp some insufflated air and may have a sore throat for 3 or 4 days. Provide throat lozenges and warm saline gargles to ease his discomfort.

☑ Be sure the outpatient has transportation home, since he should not drive for 12 hours due to drowsiness from sedation. Instruct him to watch for persistent difficulty in swallowing,

and for pain, fever, black stools, or
vomiting blood. Tell him to notify the
physician immediately if any of these
complications develop.

Interfering factors
• Failure to adhere to dietary restrictions may affect test results.
• Scheduling an esophagogastroduodenoscopy within 2 days after an upper
gastrointestinal series hinders visual
examination because of barium retention.
• Failure to place histologic or cytologic specimens in the appropriate preservative and to send the specimens to
the laboratory immediately could
cause improper test results.

Laparoscopy

Purpose
• To identify the cause of pelvic pain
• To help detect endometriosis, ec-
topic pregnancy, or pelvic inflamma-
tory disease (PID)
• To evaluate pelvic masses or the fal-
lopian tubes of infertile patients
• To stage carcinoma
• To view the liver and to obtain a liver
biopsy.

Normal results
The uterus and fallopian tubes are of
normal size and shape, free of adhesions, and mobile. The ovaries are of
normal size and shape; cysts and endometriosis are absent. Dye injected
through the cervix flows freely from
the fimbria. The liver is of normal size
and shape.

Abnormal results
Laparoscopy may reveal:
  Ovarian cysts
  Adhesions
  Endometriosis
  Uterine fibroids
  Hydrosalpinx
  Tubal pregnancy
  PID

  Cirrhosis
  Ascites
  Tumors.

The basics
Laparoscopy permits visualization of
the peritoneal cavity by the insertion
of a laparoscope through the anterior
abdominal wall. This surgical technique may be used diagnostically as
well as therapeutically to perform procedures such as lysis of adhesions,
ovarian or liver biopsy, tubal steril-
ization, removal of foreign bodies, and
fulguration of endometriotic implants.
Since laparoscopy requires a smaller
incision, it can be completed in less
time, causes less physiologic stress and
therefore allows faster recovery, reduces the risk of postoperative adhesions, and is less costly than other
procedures. For all of these reasons,
laparoscopy has often replaced laparotomy; nevertheless, laparotomy is
usually preferred when extensive surgery is indicated.
   A potential risk of laparoscopy is a
punctured visceral organ, which could
cause bleeding or spilling of intestinal
contents into the peritoneum.
Contraindications to this test include:
advanced abdominal wall malignancy,
advanced respiratory or cardiovascular
disease, intestinal obstruction, palpable abdominal mass, large abdominal
hernia, chronic tuberculosis, or a history of peritonitis.

Procedure
• The patient is positioned on her
back.
• She then receives a local or general
anesthetic.
• The skin is cleansed.
• An incision is made at the inferior
rim of the umbilicus.
• A Verees needle is inserted into the
peritoneal cavity, and approximately 2
to 3 liters of carbon dioxide or nitrous
oxide are insufflated to distend the abdominal wall and provide an organ-
free space for insertion of the trocar.

• The needle is removed and a trocar and sheath are inserted into the peritoneal cavity.

• After removal of the trocar, the laparoscope is inserted through the sheath to examine the pelvis and abdomen.

• If the examiner wants to evaluate tubal patency, he infuses a dye through the cervix and observes the fimbria of the tubes for spillage.

• Following the examination, minor surgical procedures, such as ovarian biopsy, may be performed. A second trocar may be inserted at the pubic hairline to provide a channel for the insertion of other instruments.

• The laparoscope is removed. The site is closed with two sutures, and small adhesive bandages are applied.

Patient care checklist
Before the test

☑ Explain or clarify test purpose, preparation, procedure, and post-test care.

☑ Warn the patient that she may experience pain at the puncture site and in the shoulder.

☑ Evaluate patient understanding.

☑ Restrict food and fluids after midnight before the test.

☑ Tell the patient whether the procedure will require an outpatient visit or overnight hospitalization.

☑ Make sure that the patient or a responsible family member has signed a consent form.

☑ Check the patient's history for hypersensitivity to the anesthetic. Report any hypersensitivity to the physician.

☑ Obtain baseline vital signs.

After the test

☑ Monitor vital signs and urinary output. Report sudden changes immediately; they may indicate complications.

☑ Provide usual precautions if a general anesthetic was given.

☑ Administer analgesics, as ordered, for abdominal and shoulder pain.

Interfering factors
Adhesions or marked obesity may obstruct the field of vision.

Laryngoscopy (direct)

Purpose
• To detect lesions, strictures, or foreign bodies in the larynx
• To aid in diagnosis of laryngeal cancer
• To remove benign lesions or foreign bodies from the larynx
• To examine the larynx when the view provided by indirect laryngoscopy is inadequate.

Normal results
The larynx shows no evidence of inflammation, lesions, strictures, or foreign bodies.

Abnormal results
Direct laryngoscopy may reveal:
    Lesions
    Strictures
    Foreign bodies.
Combined results of direct laryngoscopy, biopsy, and possibly radiography may:
    Indicate laryngeal carcinoma
    Distinguish laryngeal edema from radiation reaction or tumor.

The basics
Direct laryngoscopy, the visualization of the larynx by the use of a fiberoptic endoscope or laryngoscope passed through the mouth and pharynx to the larynx, usually follows indirect laryngoscopy, the more common procedure. (See *Indirect Laryngoscopy*, p. 428.) Direct laryngoscopy permits visualization of areas that are inaccessible through indirect laryngoscopy, and is indicated for children; for patients with strong gag reflexes due to anatomic abnormalities; for those with symptoms of pharyngeal or laryngeal disease, such as stridor or hemoptysis; or for those who have had no response

Indirect Laryngoscopy

Indirect laryngoscopy, normally an office procedure, allows visualization of the larynx, using a warm laryngeal mirror positioned at the back of the throat, a head mirror held in front of the mouth, and a light source.

The patient sits erect in a chair and sticks his tongue out as far as possible. The tongue is grasped with a piece of gauze and held in place with a tongue depressor. If the patient's gag reflex is sensitive, a local anesthetic may be sprayed on the pharyngeal wall. The larynx is observed at rest and during phonation. A simple excision of polyps may also be performed during this procedure.

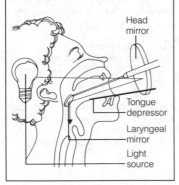

Head mirror

Tongue depressor

Laryngeal mirror

Light source

to short-term symptomatic therapy. The procedure may include the collection of secretions or tissue for further studies and the removal of foreign bodies.

Contraindications to this test may include: epiglottitis, since trauma can quickly cause edema and airway obstruction; however, when this test is absolutely necessary in such patients, it may be performed in the operating room, with resuscitative equipment available.

Procedure
• Place the patient in a supine position, or have him sit upright in a chair.
• Encourage him to relax with his arms at his sides and to breathe through his nose.
• A general anesthetic is administered or the patient's mouth and throat are sprayed with a local anesthetic.
• The patient's head is positioned and held, while the physician introduces the laryngoscope through the patient's mouth.
• The larynx is examined for abnormalities, and a specimen or secretions may be removed for further study.
• Minor surgery, such as removal of polyps or nodules, may be performed at this time.

Patient care checklist
Before the test
☑ Explain or clarify test purpose, preparation, procedure, and post-test care.
☑ Reassure the patient that this procedure will not obstruct his airway.
☑ Instruct the patient to refrain from clearing his throat and coughing after the procedure, since this may dislodge the clot at the biopsy site and cause hemorrhaging.
☑ Advise the patient to avoid smoking after the procedure until vital signs are stable and there is no evidence of complications.
☑ Inform the patient that voice loss, hoarseness, and sore throat may occur temporarily after the procedure.
☑ Evaluate patient understanding.
☑ Make sure that the patient or a responsible family member has signed a consent form.
☑ Restrict food and fluids for 6 to 8 hours before the test.
☑ Check the patient's history for hypersensitivity to the anesthetic. Report any hypersensitivity to the physician.
☑ Obtain baseline vital signs.
☑ Administer the sedative and atropine to the patient, as ordered (usually 30 minutes to 1 hour before the test).

☑ Just before the test, instruct the patient to remove dentures, contact lenses, and jewelry, and tell him to void.

After the test

☑ As ordered, place the conscious patient in semi-Fowler's position; place the unconscious patient on his side with his head slightly elevated to prevent aspiration.

☑ Monitor vital signs, as ordered.

☑ Immediately report any adverse reaction to the anesthetic or sedative (tachycardia, palpitations, hypertension, euphoria, excitation, and rapid, deep respirations).

☑ Apply an ice collar to prevent or minimize laryngeal edema.

☑ Provide an emesis basin, and instruct the patient to spit out saliva rather than swallow it. Observe sputum for blood, and notify the physician immediately if excessive bleeding occurs.

CLINICAL ALERT: **Immediately report any subcutaneous crepitus around the patient's face and neck— a possible indication of tracheal perforation.**

CLINICAL ALERT: **Observe the patient with epiglottitis for signs of airway obstruction. Immediately report signs of respiratory difficulty, such as laryngeal stridor and dyspnea, resulting from laryngeal edema or laryngospasm. Keep emergency resuscitative equipment available; keep a tracheotomy tray nearby for 24 hours.**

☑ Restrict food and fluids until the gag reflex returns (usually 2 hours). Then the patient may resume his usual diet, beginning with sips of water.

☑ Provide throat lozenges or a soothing liquid gargle to ease throat discomfort when his gag reflex returns.

Interfering factors

Failure to place specimens in the appropriate containers and to send the specimens to the laboratory immediately may affect test results.

Mediastinoscopy

Purpose

To biopsy lymph nodes in the mediastinum.

Normal results

Lymph nodes appear as small, smooth, flat oval bodies of lymphoid tissue.

Abnormal results

Mediastinoscopy, along with biopsy, may aid in diagnosis of:

Lung cancer

Sarcoidosis

Lymphomas (such as Hodgkin's disease).

The basics

Mediastinoscopy allows direct visualization of mediastinal structures— through an exploring speculum with built-in fiber light and side slit—and palpation and biopsy of paratracheal and carinal lymph nodes. The mediastinum is the mass of tissues and organs behind the sternum, separating the lungs. Its major contents include the heart and its vessels, the trachea, esophagus, thymus, and lymph nodes. Examination of the nodes, which receive lymphatic drainage from the lungs, can detect lymphoma (including Hodgkin's disease) and sarcoidosis, and aids in staging lung cancer, which helps determine a therapeutic regimen.

A surgical procedure, mediastinoscopy is indicated when tests such as sputum cytology, lung scans, radiography, and bronchoscopic biopsy fail to confirm diagnosis.

The right side of the mediastinum allows easy exploration, and since mediastinoscopy can diagnose bronchogenic carcinoma at an early stage, this procedure is now replacing the scalene fat pad biopsy. Exploring the left side, however, is less satisfactory and more hazardous, due to the close proximity of the aorta. Although rare, complications of the test may include pneumothorax, perforation of the esophagus, infection, hemorrhage, and left recurrent laryngeal nerve damage.

If laboratory analysis confirms malignancy of a resectable tumor, a thoracotomy and pneumonectomy may follow immediately.
Contraindications to this test include: scarring of the area as a result of a previous mediastinoscopy.

Procedure

• After the patient has an endotracheal tube in place, the surgeon makes a small transverse suprasternal incision.
• Using finger dissection, a channel is formed and the lymph nodes are palpated.
• A mediastinoscope is inserted into the mediastinum, and tissue specimens are collected and sent to the laboratory for frozen section examination.
• Send any specimens in their properly labeled containers to the laboratory immediately.
• The test takes about 1 hour to perform.

Patient care checklist
Before the test
☑ Explain or clarify test purpose, preparation, procedure, and post-test care.
☑ Inform the patient that a general anesthetic will be administered.
☑ Tell the patient that he may temporarily experience chest pain, tenderness at the incision site, or a sore throat (from intubation).
☑ Reassure him that, although complications are possible with this procedure, they rarely occur.
☑ Evaluate patient understanding.
☑ Restrict food and fluids after midnight before the procedure.
☑ Make sure that the patient or a responsible family member has signed the consent form.
☑ Check the patient's history for hypersensitivity to the anesthetic. Report any hypersensitivity to the physician.
☑ Obtain baseline vital signs.

☑ As ordered, administer a sedative the night before the test and before the procedure is performed.
After the test
☑ Monitor vital signs, and check the dressing for bleeding or fluid drainage.
CLINICAL ALERT: **Observe for signs of the following complications: fever (mediastinitis); crepitus (subcutaneous emphysema); dyspnea, cyanosis, and diminished breath sounds on the affected side (pneumothorax); tachycardia and hypotension (hemorrhage).**
☑ Administer the prescribed analgesic, as needed.

Ophthalmoscopy

Purpose
To detect and evaluate eye disorders and ocular manifestations of systemic disease.

Normal results
The red reflex should be visible through the aperture. The slightly oval optic disk, measuring approximately 1.5 mm vertically, lies to the nasal side of the fundus center. Although its color varies widely, it is usually pink, with darker edges at its nasal border. The physiologic cup, a pale depression in the center of the disk, varies widely in size; it tends to be larger in patients with myopia and smaller in those with hyperopia.

The semitransparent retina surrounds the optic disk. Branching out from the disk are the retinal vessels, including venules and the slightly smaller arterioles. Vessel diameter progressively decreases with distance from the optic disk. Retinal arterioles generally have a medium red color; venules appear dark red or blue.

The macula, a small avascular area that appears darker than the surrounding retina, is located approximately 2½ disk diameters temporal from the optic disk and slightly behind the horizontal

Abnormal Ophthalmoscopic Findings

Disorder	Typical ophthalmoscopic finding
Cataract	Lens opacification
Central retinal artery occlusion	A milky-white retina characterizes the acute phase; the fovea, in contrast to the ischemic macula, appears as a bright red spot.
Central retinal vein occlusion	Widespread retinal hemorrhaging, patches of white exudate, and disk elevation
Diabetic retinopathy	Retinal changes, such as venous dilation and twisting, patches of white exudate, microaneurysms, hemorrhages, or edema
Glaucoma (acute closed angle)	Pale optic disk
Glaucoma (chronic closed angle)	Cupping and atrophy of optic disk late in disease
Glaucoma (chronic open angle)	Cupping and atrophy of optic disk
Hypertensive retinopathy	Hard, shiny deposits (in early stages); tiny hemorrhages; elevated arterial blood pressure; cotton-wool patches (in late stages); exudates; retinal edema; papilledema; hemorrhages and microaneurysms
Keratoconus	High plus lens reveals round, shadowlike reflex in central cornea
Optic atrophy	Pallor of optic disk
Optic neuritis	Elevated, more vascular disk with small hemorrhages possible
Papilledema (from increased intracranial pressure)	Abnormal elevation of the disk, blurring of disk margins, engorged vessels, and hemorrhages
Retinal detachment	Gray, opaque retina, with an indefinite margin, possibly with areas of red vascular choroid exposed by retinal tears; in severe detachment, inward-bulging, gently rippled or folded retina; almost black arteriole and venules
Uveitis	Active choroid and retina lesions appearing yellow-white through a cloudy vitreous
Vitreous hemorrhage	Loss of fundus detail and floating red debris

meridian. In its center lies a small, even darker spot—the fovea. A tiny light reflex can be seen at the center of the fovea, caused by reflection of the ophthalmoscopic light from the concave inner surface of the area.

Abnormal results

See *Abnormal Ophthalmoscopic Findings,* p. 431.

The basics

Ophthalmoscopy—an important part of routine physical examinations and eye evaluations—allows magnified examination of living vascular and nerve tissue of the fundus, including the optic disk, retinal vessels, macula, and retina. The instrument used in this test—either the direct or the indirect ophthalmoscope—is considered one of the most important diagnostic tools in ophthalmology. Generally, examiners use the direct ophthalmoscope—a small, hand-held instrument consisting of a light source, viewing device, reflecting device to channel light into the patient's eyes, and spherical lenses to correct refractive error of the patient or examiner. This direct model is easier to use than the indirect model. If a slit lamp is not available, the examiner may also use the ophthalmoscope to examine the patient's cornea, iris, and lens. After an ophthalmologic evaluation, referral for complete medical evaluation may be necessary. (See also *Indirect Ophthalmoscopy.*)

Procedure

• Administer mydriatic eye drops, as ordered, if needed.
• Have the patient sit upright in the examination chair, and darken the room.
• To examine the patient's right eye first, hold the ophthalmoscope in your right hand and in front of your right eye. Position your right index finger on the lens selection dial to facilitate rapid lens changes, and sit slightly to the patient's right.
• Set the illuminated dial to zero, and tell the patient to look straight ahead at a specific object 20′ (6 m) away—a large symbol on a standardized vision chart, for example. Tell him to maintain fixation throughout the examination.
• Remaining on the patient's right side, move forward slightly, until you are about 6″ (15 cm) from him.
• Direct the light beam into the pupil; select the proper lens aperture on the ophthalmoscope, and look through it for the red reflex. The red reflex can be seen without magnification and represents a red reflection from the fundus. Keeping this reflection in view and reminding the patient to maintain fixation, move slowly toward the patient until you are 1½″ to 2″ from him. Rotate the lenses on the scope to focus on the optic disk, and note its size, shape, and color.
• Next, look for a white, central depression in the disk—the physiologic cup. Observe the retinal vessels that emerge from the optic disk. Follow each vessel as far as possible to the periphery.

Indirect Ophthalmoscopy

A more expensive and more sophisticated instrument than the direct ophthalmoscope, the indirect ophthalmoscope is used with a convex lens, which the ophthalmologist holds a few inches from the patient's eye, and a headlamp, which provides a strong source of illumination. The lens focuses light reflected from the retina, producing an image that is rotated 180° but is unaffected by refractive errors or opacities in the media. Since the indirect ophthalmoscope provides a wide-angle, stereoscopic view of the peripheral retina, many surgeons depend on it for preoperative diagnosis and during retinal detachment surgery.

• Examine the macula—a yellowish depression lying approximately two disk diameters away from and slightly below the center of the optic disk—and its center, the fovea. To examine the extreme periphery, tell the patient to look up, down, and to each side. Examine the superior, inferior, temporal, and nasal portions of the retina, respectively.

• Repeat the procedure to examine the patient's left eye, moving slightly to the patient's left side and holding the ophthalmoscope in your left hand and in front of your left eye. Adjust the lens selection dial to account for a different refractive state, if necessary.

Special precautions

CLINICAL ALERT: **Do not administer dilating eye drops to a patient who has a history of hypersensitive reaction to them or who has narrow-angle glaucoma.**

Patient care checklist

Before the test

☑ Explain or clarify test purpose, preparation, and procedure.

☑ Advise the patient that eye drops may be instilled to dilate the pupils for a clearer examination, but reassure him that he will feel no discomfort during the test.

☑ Evaluate patient understanding.

☑ Check the patient's history for previous use of dilating eye drops, possible hypersensitivity to the eye drops, and narrow angle glaucoma. Consult with the physician as needed.

Interfering factors

• Poor patient cooperation or conditions that prohibit a good view of the fundus, such as insufficient dilation, dense cataracts, cloudy media, or gross nystagmus, may affect test results.

• Improper examination conditions (an insufficiently darkened room or an inadequate light source on the ophthalmoscope, for instance) may interfere with accurate diagnosis.

Otoscopy

Purpose

• To detect foreign bodies, cerumen, or stenosis in the ear canal

• To detect external or middle ear pathology, such as infection or tympanic membrane perforation.

Normal results

The tympanic membrane is thin, translucent, shiny, and slightly concave. It appears as a pearl gray or pale pink disk that reflects light in its inferior portion. The short process, manubrium mallei, and umbo should be visible but not prominent.

Abnormal results

See *Common Abnormalities of the Tympanic Membrane,* p. 434, and *External Ear Disorders,* p. 435.

The basics

Otoscopy is the direct visualization of the external auditory canal and the tympanic membrane through an otoscope. It is the basic element of any physical examination of the ear and should be performed before other auditory or vestibular tests. Otoscopy indirectly provides information about the eustachian tube and the middle ear cavity.

Procedure

• When assembling the otoscope, test the lamp and be sure to attach the largest speculum that fits comfortably into the patient's ear.

• With the patient seated, tilt his head slightly away from you, so that the ear to be examined is pointed upward.

• Pull the auricle upward and backward (pull downward if the patient is under age 3); insert the otoscope gently into the ear canal, with a downward and forward motion.

• Look through the lens and gently advance the speculum until the eardrum becomes visible. Obtain as full a view as possible, and note redness, swelling, lesions, or scaling in the canal.

• Check the eardrum for a cone of light that appears at the 5 o'clock position in the right ear, and at the 7 o'clock position in the left ear; this is a reflection of the otoscope lamp.

• Locate the malleus, which should be partially visible through the translucent tympanic membrane. The malleus—comprised of the short process, manubrium mallei, and umbo—extends downward to the center of the tympanic membrane.

• Examine the membrane itself and the surrounding fibrous rim (annulus).

Special precautions

• The otoscope should be advanced slowly and gently through the medial portion of the ear canal to avoid irritation of the canal lining, especially if an infection is suspected.

• Continuing to insert an otoscope against resistance may cause a perforation or other damage.

Patient care checklist

Before the test

☑ Explain or clarify test purpose and procedure.

☑ Reassure the patient that the examination is usually painless and takes less than 5 minutes to perform.

☑ Evaluate patient understanding.

Interfering factors

• Obstruction of the ear canal by cerumen or foreign matter obscures the tympanic membrane.

• Recumbent positioning of a patient during otoscopy can mask serious otitis media.

Common Abnormalities of the Tympanic Membrane

Abnormal findings	Usual cause
Bright red	Inflammation (otitis media)
Yellowish	Pus or serum behind the tympanic membrane (acute or chronic otitis media)
Bubble behind tympanic membrane	Serous fluid in middle ear (serous otitis media)
Absent light reflection	Bulging tympanic membrane (acute otitis media)
Absent or diminishing landmarks	Thickened tympanic membrane (chronic otitis media, otitis externa, or tympanosclerosis)
Oval dark areas	Perforated or scarred tympanic membrane (otitis media or trauma)
Very prominent malleus	Retracted tympanic membrane (nonfunctional eustachian tube)
Reduced mobility	Stiffened middle ear system (serous otitis media or, more rarely, middle ear adhesions)

External Ear Disorders

Disorder	Typical otoscopic finding
Acute otitis externa	• Edematous canal • Pain obvious with procedure
Chronic otitis externa	• Eardrum normal • Auricle and canal red, thick, excoriated; often crusted • Canal and tympanic membrane insensitive
Otomycosis	• Eardrum whitish gray with black dots; may be cottony • Canal edema and debris
Furunculosis	• Eardrum normal unless otitis media present • Furuncles visible in canal

Proctosigmoidoscopy

Purpose
To aid in diagnosis of disorders in the rectosigmoid area.

Normal results
The mucosa of the sigmoid colon appears light pink-orange and is marked by semilunar folds and deep tubular pits. The rectal mucosa appears redder because of its rich vascular network, deepens to a purple hue at the pectinate line (the anatomic division between the rectum and anus), and has three distinct valves. The lower two thirds of the anus (anoderm) is lined with smooth gray-tan skin and joins with the hair-fringed perianal skin.

Abnormal results
Proctosigmoidoscopy may detect:
Anorectal abscess
Anal fissures
Hemorrhoids
Anal fistulas
Tumors in rectosigmoid area
Inflammation in rectosigmoid area
Ulcerative colitis
Polyps.

The basics
Proctosigmoidoscopy is the endoscopic examination of the lining of the distal sigmoid colon, the rectum, and the anal canal. If a flexible sigmoidoscope is used, the descending colon can also be seen. It is indicated in patients with recent changes in bowel habits, lower abdominal and perineal pain, prolapse on defecation, pruritus, or the passage of mucus, blood, or pus in the stool. It is mainly used to detect and diagnose cancer. Biopsy is needed to confirm the diagnosis.

Procedure
• Place the patient in a knee-chest or left lateral position, with knees flexed, and drape him.
• After inspection and digital examination, the sigmoidoscope is lubricated and inserted into the anus, and advanced, eventually reaching the sigmoid colon.
• During the procedure, air is carefully insufflated to open the bowel lumen and permit thorough examination of all areas.
• If fecal matter obscures vision, the eyepiece on the scope is removed, a cotton swab is inserted through the scope, and the bowel lumen is

swabbed. (A suction machine may remove blood, excessive secretions, or liquid feces.)
• Specimens may be obtained from suspicious areas. An electrocautery snare may be used to remove polyps.
• The sigmoidoscope is then withdrawn.

Proctoscopy:
• After the sigmoidoscope is withdrawn, the proctoscope is lubricated and inserted into the anus, and gently advanced.
• After insertion to its full length, the instrument is slowly withdrawn, and the rectal and anal mucosa are carefully examined. Specimens may also be obtained.

Patient care checklist

Before the test

☑ Explain or clarify test purpose, preparation, and procedure.

☑ Inform the patient that he may experience the urge to defecate when the instrument is inserted and advanced. Instruct him to breathe deeply and slowly through his mouth during the procedure and to relax his abdominal muscles.

☑ Evaluate patient understanding.

☑ As ordered, instruct the patient concerning dietary restrictions and bowel preparation. If ordered, provide a clear liquid diet for 48 hours before the test, and restrict food and fluids the morning of the procedure.

☑ If ordered, administer a warm tap-water or sodium biphosphate enema 3 to 4 hours before the procedure.

☑ Make sure that the patient or a responsible family member has signed the consent form.

☑ If the patient has rectal inflammation, provide a local anesthetic, if ordered, to minimize discomfort, about 15 to 20 minutes before the procedure.

After the test

CLINICAL ALERT: **Observe the patient closely for signs of bowel perforation (malaise, rectal bleeding, abdominal distention and pain, mucopurulent drainage, and fever) and for vasovagal attack due to emotional stress (depressed blood pressure, pallor, diaphoresis, and bradycardia). Notify the physician immediately if such signs develop.**

☑ If air was introduced into the intestine, tell the patient that he may pass a large amount of flatus. Provide privacy while he rests after the test.

☑ If a biopsy or polypectomy was performed, inform the patient that blood may appear in his stool.

Interfering factors

• Barium retained in the intestine from diagnostic studies within the preceding week makes accurate visual examination impossible.
• Large amounts of stool in the intestine hinder visual examination and the advancement of the endoscope.
• Failure to place histologic or cytologic specimens in the appropriate preservative or to send the specimens to the laboratory immediately may affect test results.

Selected References

Diagnostics, 2nd ed. Nurse's Reference Library. Springhouse, Pa.: Springhouse Corp., 1986.

Fischbach, Frances. *A Manual of Laboratory Diagnostic Tests*, 2nd ed. Philadelphia: J.B. Lippincott Co., 1984.

Given, Barbara A., and Simmons, Sandra J. *Gastroenterology in Clinical Nursing*, 4th ed. St. Louis: C.V. Mosby Co., 1983.

Northern, J., and Downs, M.P. *Hearing in Children*, 3rd ed. Baltimore: Williams & Wilkins Co., 1984.

Pagana, Kathleen D., and Pagana, Timothy James. *Diagnostic Testing and Nursing Implications*, 2nd ed. St. Louis: C.V. Mosby Co., 1986.

Procedures. Nurse's Reference Library. Springhouse, Pa.: Springhouse Corp., 1983.

Surgeon
460 - 6200

$250.00 ACLS
$250.00 Car
$40.00 Alberta Health
$50.00 Blue Cross
$625.00 Car Insurance
$200.00 RRSP
$50.00 Gas
$125.00 MasterCard [50]
$100.00 Leisure
$250.00 AARN

431 - 8878 $1342 - Sept 27

478 - 9666.   Elizabeth Seton
                Catholic Elem/Jr
Library Renewal   High School
496 - 7047

                3711 - 135 Ave
                478 - 7754

9 HISTOLOGIC, CYTOLOGIC, AND CYTOGENIC TESTING

Introduction

Improved technology in histologic, cytologic, and cytogenic testing has greatly aided identification of abnormal cells. This has special significance in the detection of malignancy and genetic abnormalities.

Histology

Histology, the study of the microscopic structure of tissues and cells, is vital to confirm malignant disease and has made biopsy—extraction of a living tissue specimen—a common procedure. New tissue preparation techniques and needle designs allow rapid specimen removal from even deep tissues without surgery.

Biopsies may be incisional or excisional. In *incisional* biopsy, a scalpel, cutting or aspiration needle, or punch is used to remove a portion of tissue from large, multiple, hidden lesions. Fine-needle aspiration differs slightly from traditional needle biopsy. Although the procedure is the same, it provides a smaller specimen, requires cytologic (not histologic) studies, and is usually performed on outpatients for breast biopsies. Incision of a hidden lesion is called a closed, or blind, biopsy. In *excisional* biopsy, a scalpel is used to remove abnormal tissue from the skin or subcutaneous tissue. When such tissue can be easily and completely removed, excisional biopsy is preferred, because it combines diagnosis and treatment.

Biopsies commonly take place in the hospital, but they may also take place in clinics and physicians' offices. Open biopsy, performed in the operating room, usually requires general anesthesia. Open biopsy is required when the results of a closed biopsy or other diagnostic tests (such as a CT scan) suggest the need for complete excision of a tissue mass.

Routine **tissue preparation** involves several time-consuming steps. These include fixation—placing the tissue in fluid (generally, 10% buffered formaldehyde) to kill and harden it; initial examination of the tissue by a pathologist; sectioning and encapsulating the tissue for processing through fixing, dehydrating, and clearing fluids and then into melted paraffin, which infiltrates the tissue; and, finally, cutting and staining the tissue specimen for examination by the pathologist. Because of these preparations, a stat tissue report generally takes 24 hours.

Frozen sections, an alternative method of preparing tissue for study, permit rapid, accurate analysis of potentially malignant tissue during surgery. This technique allows pathologic diagnosis within 10 to 15 minutes after excision. Results from frozen section analysis are usually reliable, but standard analysis on tissue from the same specimen must verify the diagnosis.

After standard analysis, **classification of tissue** takes place. The pathologist's report provides both gross and microscopic descriptions, which result in histopathologic classification of the tumor. Typically, results of this analysis are expressed on a scale of four grades: G1—well differentiated; G2—moderately well differentiated; G3—poorly differentiated; G4—anaplastic. A staging system is then used to direct treatment and predict prog-

---

TNM System of Staging Cancer

The internationally recognized TNM staging system allows an accurate tumor description that can be adjusted as the disease progresses. This system helps direct treatment, predict prognosis, and contribute to cancer research by ensuring reliable comparison of patients in various hospitals.

T for primary tumor
T—the anatomic extent of the primary tumor—depends on its size, depth of invasion, and surface spread.
T_0 No evidence of primary tumor
T_1 A mobile, often superficial tumor (<2 cm in diameter) confined to the organ of origin
T_2 A localized tumor (2 to 5 cm in diameter) with some loss of mobility and deep extension into adjacent tissues
T_3 An advanced tumor (>5 cm in diameter) with complete loss of mobility, involving a region
T_4 A massive tumor (>10 cm in diameter) with extension into another organ (causing a fistula or sinus), major nerves, arteries and veins, or bone

N for nodal involvement
N depends on the size, mobility, and firmness of the tumor; capsular invasion and the depth of invasion; the number of nodes involved; and ipsilateral, contralateral, bilateral, and distant node involvement.
N_0 No evidence of lymph node involvement
N_1 Palpable, mobile lymph nodes, limited to the first station. Involved nodes are usually solitary, larger (2 to 3 cm in diameter), and firmer than normal nodes.

N_2 Palpable, partially mobile, firm-to-hard nodes (3 to 5 cm in diameter), limited to the first station. Involved nodes may show capsular and partial matted muscle invasion, and contralateral or bilateral involvement.
N_3 A node (>5 cm in diameter) with extension beyond the capsule and fixation to bone, large blood vessels, skin, or nerves
N_4 Fixed and destructive nodes (>10 cm in diameter) with extension to second or distant stations
Nx Nodes inaccessible to evaluation

M for metastasis
M refers to the presence or absence of metastasis.
M_0 No evidence of metastasis
M_1 Solitary metastasis
M_2 Multiple metastasis in one organ with no or minimal functional impairment
M_3 Metastasis to multiple organs with no or minimal-to-moderate functional impairment
M_4 Metastasis to multiple organs with moderate-to-severe functional impairment
Mx No metastatic workup done

Stages and survival
Stage I
$T_1 N_0 M_0$
70% to 90% 5-year survival
Stage II
$T_2 N_1 M_0$
50% to 70% 5-year survival
Stage III
$T_3 N_0 M_0$
$T_{1-3} N_1 M_0$
25% to 45% 5-year survival
Stage IV
$T_4 N_{0-1} M_0$
$T_{0-4} N_{2-3} M_0$
$T_{0-4} N_{0-4} M_1$
5% to 20% 5-year survival

nosis when biopsy results confirm malignancy. (See *TNM System of Staging Cancer*.)

Cytology

Cytology is the study of cells, including their formation, origin, structure, function, biochemical activities, and pathology. Cytologic tests are inexpensive, useful screening tests that help detect suspected malignant or premalignant conditions and assess the effectiveness of therapy. However, they fail to determine the location and size of a malignancy and may require further histologic confirmation.

Tissue scraping is one type of cytologic test. One of the most common is the Papanicolaou (Pap) test, in which cervical scrapings are evaluated.

Cytology specimens may also be obtained by aspiration or by cell washing. (See *Common Cytologic Specimens*.) **Fine-needle** (19G to 23G) **aspiration** of body fluids permits evaluation of a palpable mass, a lymph node, or a lesion that has been localized by X-rays. **Cell washing** is performed by instilling a solution into the bronchial tree, esophagus, stomach, or uterine cavity and subsequently aspirating it out. This procedure loosens exfoliated cells from crevices and suspends them in the solution, thereby increasing the number of cells collected for cytologic examination. The procedure also increases the probability of finding recently exfoliated cells.

Cytogenics

Cytogenics is the branch of genetics that studies cellular components concerned with heredity, primarily the structure, function, and origin of the chromosomes. Cytogenic tests identify abnormal genetic factors or patterns seen in conditions such as Down's syndrome and Turner's syndrome.

Common Cytologic Specimens

Sputum	Pleural fluid
Bronchial washings	Ascitic fluid
	Spinal fluid
Lung aspirate	
	Bladder urine
Breast mass aspirate	
	Vaginal pool scrapings
Bone marrow aspirate	
	Cervical scrapings
Cul-de-sac of Douglas aspirate	
	Endometrial scrapings
Solid tumor aspirate	

Patient-teaching guidelines
Patient-learner objectives:
• Define the test.
• State the specific purpose of the test.
• Explain the procedure.
• Discuss test preparation, procedure, and post-test care.
• Identify possible risks or adverse effects.
Teaching content:
• Define the test in terms the patient can understand.
• Explain the specific purpose of the test.
• Describe the procedure. Explain where the procedure will be performed and who will be performing it. Tell the patient how the specimen will be obtained.
• Describe what discomfort, if any, to expect during the procedure.
• If a local anesthetic will be used, explain that it may alleviate some discomfort, but that the patient will remain alert. If a general anesthetic is used, explain that the patient will not be conscious for the procedure, and that food and fluids are not permitted after midnight before the test.

• Answer any questions the patient may still have after the physician's explanation, if there are any risks associated with the test.

• Tell the patient if discomfort or any other problem is a normal consequence of the test. Reassure the patient that it is only temporary and, when possible, explain what will be done to alleviate the problem.

• Describe any other special care, positioning, or restrictions following the test, and explain why these are necessary.

• If applicable, tell the patient to report tenderness, redness, swelling or bleeding at the site, and tell him whom to contact.

• If sutures are needed, instruct the patient to keep them clean and dry. Tell him when and where to report to have them removed.

• Provide the outpatient with written instructions and, if sedation will be used, advise him to have someone accompany him for transportation.

• Inform the patient when test results will be available, since this patient may be especially anxious.

Evaluation:
After the patient-teaching session is completed, evaluate whether or not the patient has satisfactorily met each patient-learner objective, by obtaining necessary patient feedback. Refocus teaching as needed.

Breast biopsy

Purpose
To differentiate between benign and malignant breast tumors.

Normal results
Healthy breast tissue consists of cellular and noncellular connective tissue, fat lobules, and various lactiferous ducts. It is pink, more fatty than fibrous, and shows no abnormal development of cells or tissue elements.

Abnormal results
Benign tumors include:
  Fibrocystic disease
  Adenofibroma
  Intraductal papilloma
  Mammary fat necrosis
  Plasma cell mastitis.
Malignant tumors include:
  Adenocarcinoma
  Cystosarcoma
  Intraductal carcinoma
  Infiltrating carcinoma
  Inflammatory carcinoma
  Medullary or circumscribed carcinoma
  Colloid carcinoma
  Lobular carcinoma
  Sarcoma
  Paget's disease.

The basics
Breast tumors are common in women and account for 27% of female cancers; such tumors are rare in men (0.2% of male cancers). Eighty percent of breast lumps are benign. Although mammography, thermography, and X-rays aid diagnosis of breast masses, only histologic examination of breast tissue obtained by biopsy can confirm or rule out cancer.

Needle biopsy or fine-needle biopsy can provide a core of tissue or a fluid aspirate, but needle biopsy should be restricted to fluid-filled cysts and advanced malignant lesions. Both methods have limited diagnostic value because of the small and perhaps unrepresentative specimens they provide. If the aspirate is clear yellow and the mass disappears, the aspiration procedure is both diagnostic and therapeutic, and the aspirate is discarded. If aspiration yields no fluid, or if the lesion recurs two or three times, an open biopsy is then considered appropriate. Open biopsy provides a complete tissue specimen, which can be sectioned to allow more accurate evaluation. All three techniques require only a local anesthetic and can often be performed on outpatients; however, open biopsy may require a general anesthetic if the patient is fearful or uncooperative.

Breast biopsy is indicated in patients with palpable masses, suspicious areas in mammography, or persistently encrusted, inflamed, or eczematoid breast lesions or bloody discharge from the nipples. (See *Nipple Discharge Cytology*.) Breast tissue analysis often includes an estrogen and progesterone receptor assay to help select therapy if the mass proves malignant. (See *Measurement of Hormone Receptors in Breast Biopsy*, p. 442.) This assay measures quick-frozen tumor tissue to determine the binding capacity of its estrogen and progesterone receptors.

Procedure
Needle biopsy
• Instruct the patient to undress to the waist.
• Guide her to a sitting or recumbent position, with her hands at her sides, and tell her to remain still.
• The biopsy site is prepared, a local anesthetic is administered, and the syringe (Luer-Lok syringe for aspiration, Vim-Silverman needle for tissue specimen) is introduced into the lesion.
• Fluid aspirated from the breast is expelled into a properly labeled, heparinized tube; the tissue specimen is placed in a labeled specimen bottle containing normal saline solution or formaldehyde. (With fine-needle aspiration, a slide is made for cytologic study and viewed immediately under a microscope.)
• Pressure is exerted on the biopsy site, and after bleeding stops, an adhesive bandage is applied.
Open biopsy
• After the patient receives a general or local anesthetic, an incision is made in the breast, to expose the mass.
• The examiner may then incise a portion of tissue or excise the entire mass. If the mass is smaller than ¾″ (2 cm) and appears benign, it is usually excised; if it is larger or appears malig-

Nipple Discharge Cytology

Nipple discharge occurs normally only during lactation. However, when this discharge cannot be attributed to lactation or occurs without breast masses or other signs of breast cancer, cytologic study of the discharge can help determine its cause. (The presence of signs of breast cancer necessitates breast biopsy and other tests.) For example, cytologic study of discharge can differentiate between malignant conditions, such as intraductal papillary carcinoma and intracystic infiltrating carcinoma, and benign conditions, such as mastitis and intraductal papilloma.

Before obtaining a discharge specimen, wash the patient's nipple and pat it dry. Then show the patient how to "milk" the breast to express the fluid. Discard the first drop and collect the next drop by moving a labeled glass slide across the nipple. (If a larger specimen is required, you will need to collect it with a breast pump.) Fix the specimen immediately with cytology spray, or place it in 95% ethanol solution. Label the specimen and send it to the laboratory immediately for staining. Note which breast was used to obtain the specimen. Also note if the patient is pregnant, perimenopausal, or taking drugs that alter hormonal balance, such as oral contraceptives, phenothiazines, digitalis, diuretics, or steroids.

nant, a specimen is usually incised before the mass is excised. (Incisional biopsy generally provides an adequate specimen for histologic analysis.)
• The specimen is placed in a properly labeled specimen bottle containing 10% formaldehyde solution. Tissue that appears malignant is sent for frozen section and receptor assays. (Re-

Measurement of Hormone Receptors in Breast Biopsy

In breast cancer, measurement of hormone receptors helps predict patient response to hormonal therapy. The test measures estrogen receptor (ER) and, frequently, progesterone receptor (PR) levels in biopsy specimens. ER levels of less than 3 femtomoles (a femtomole equals 10^{-15} moles of receptor protein per milligram of cytosol protein) are considered negative; levels of 3 to 10 femtomoles/mg are intermediate; and levels greater than 10 femtomoles/mg are positive.

About 50% of ER-positive patients show a favorable response to hormonal therapy. In contrast, less than 10% of ER-negative patients show a favorable response. Also, the presence of PR improves the chances of successful hormonal therapy. Some investigational studies demonstrate that the PR level is more important as a prognostic indicator than the ER level.

ceptor assay specimens must not be placed in formaldehyde.)
• The wound is sutured, and an adhesive bandage is applied.

Patient care checklist
Before the test
☑ Explain or clarify test purpose and procedure.
☑ Evaluate patient understanding.
☑ Offer emotional support.
☑ If the patient is to receive a general anesthetic, restrict food and fluids from midnight before the test.
☑ Make sure that the patient or a responsible family member has signed the consent form.
☑ Administer preoperative medication, if ordered.

After the test
☑ Monitor vital signs, as ordered.
☑ Check dressing at biopsy site.
☑ Administer an analgesic, as ordered.
☑ Watch for and report redness or increased tenderness at the biopsy site.
☑ Provide emotional support to the patient who is awaiting diagnosis. If the biopsy confirms cancer, the patient will require follow-up tests, including radiographic tests, blood studies, bone scans, and urinalysis, to determine appropriate treatment.

Interfering factors
• Failure to obtain an adequate tissue specimen.
• Failure to place the specimen in the proper solution container.

Bone biopsy

Purpose
To distinguish between benign and malignant bone tumors.

Normal results
Healthy bone tissue consists of fibers of collagen, osteocytes, and osteoblasts. Normal bone is of two histologic types: compact and cancellous. Compact bone has dense, concentric layers of mineral deposits, or lamellae. Cancellous bone has widely spaced lamellae, with osteocytes and red and yellow marrow lying between them.

Abnormal results
Benign tumors, generally well circumscribed and nonmetastasizing, include:
   Osteoid osteoma
   Osteoblastoma
   Osteochondroma
   Unicameral bone cyst
   Benign giant-cell tumor
   Fibroma.

Malignant tumors, which spread irregularly and rapidly, most commonly include:

Multiple myeloma
Osteosarcoma
Ewing's sarcoma.

The basics

Bone biopsy is the removal of a piece or a core of bone for histologic examination. It is performed either by using a special drill needle, under local anesthesia, or by surgical excision, under general anesthesia. Bone biopsy is indicated in patients with bone pain and tenderness or after a bone scan, computed tomography scan, X-ray, or arteriography reveals a mass or deformity. Excision provides a larger specimen than drill biopsy and permits immediate surgical treatment if quick histologic analysis of the specimen reveals malignancy.

Most malignant tumors spread to bone through the blood and lymph systems from the breast, lungs, prostate, thyroid, or kidneys. In the presence of tumors, the bone bows slightly, thickens, and sometimes fractures—the result of increased osteoblastic or osteoclastic activity, or both.

Possible complications of bone biopsy include bone fracture, damage to surrounding tissue, and infection (osteomyelitis). Bone biopsy should be performed cautiously in patients with coagulopathy.

Procedure

Drill biopsy

• After the local anesthetic is injected, the physician makes a small incision (usually about ⅛" [3 mm]) and pushes the biopsy needle with pointed trocar into the bone.

• When the bone core is obtained, the trocar is withdrawn by reversing the drilling motion, and the specimen is placed in a properly labeled bottle containing 10% formaldehyde solution.

• Pressure is applied to the site with a sterile gauze pad.

• When bleeding stops, the gauze is removed and a topical antiseptic (povidone-iodine ointment) and an adhesive bandage or other sterile covering are applied, to close the wound and prevent infection.

Open biopsy

• The patient is anesthetized, and the biopsy site is prepared by shaving the area, cleansing it with surgical soap, then disinfecting it with an iodine wash and alcohol.

• The physician makes an incision and removes a piece of bone.

• The specimen is sent to the histology laboratory immediately for analysis. Further surgery can then be performed, depending on bone specimen findings.

Patient care checklist

Before the test

☑ Explain or clarify test purpose and procedure.

☑ If the patient is to receive local anesthesia, tell him that he will still experience discomfort and pressure when the biopsy needle enters the bone. Stress the importance of his cooperation during the biopsy.

☑ Evaluate patient understanding.

☑ If the patient is to receive general anesthesia, restrict food and fluids from midnight before the test.

☑ If the patient is to receive a local anesthetic, prepare the biopsy site and position the patient as ordered.

☑ Make sure that the patient or a responsible family member has signed the consent form.

☑ Administer preoperative medication, as ordered.

After the test

☑ Monitor vital signs, as ordered.

☑ Check dressing of biopsy site.

☑ Administer an analgesic, as ordered.

CLINICAL ALERT: For several days after the biopsy, watch for indications of bone infection: fever, headache, pain on movement, and tissue red-

ness or abscess at or near the biopsy site. Notify the physician if these symptoms develop.

Interfering factors
• Failure to obtain a representative bone specimen.
• Failure to use the proper fixative.
• Failure to send the specimen to the laboratory immediately.

Bone marrow aspiration and biopsy

Purpose
• To diagnose thrombocytopenia, leukemias, granulomas, and aplastic, hypoplastic, and pernicious anemias
• To diagnose primary and metastatic tumors
• To determine the cause of infection
• To aid staging of disease, such as Hodgkin's disease
• To evaluate the effectiveness of chemotherapy and help monitor myelosuppression.

Normal results
Yellow marrow contains fat cells and connective tissue; red marrow contains hematopoietic cells, fat cells, and connective tissue. (See *Bone Marrow: Normal Values and Implications of Abnormal Findings*, pp. 446 to 447.)

In addition, special stains that detect hematologic disorders produce these normal findings: the iron stain, which measures hemosiderin (storage iron), has a +2 level; the Sudan Black B (SBB) stain, which shows granulocytes, is negative; and the periodic acid-Schiff (PAS) stain, which detects glycogen reactions, is negative.

Abnormal results
Histologic examination of a bone marrow specimen can help detect myelofibrosis, granulomas, lymphoma, or cancer. Hematologic analysis, including the differential count and myeloid-erythroid ratio, can implicate a wide

range of disorders. (See *Bone Marrow: Normal Values and Implications of Abnormal Findings*, pp. 446 to 447.)

In an iron stain, decreased hemosiderin levels may indicate a true iron deficiency. Increased levels may accompany other types of anemias or blood disorders. A positive SBB stain can differentiate acute granulocytic leukemia from acute lymphocytic leukemia (SBB negative) or may indicate granulation in myeloblasts. A positive PAS stain may indicate acute or chronic lymphocytic leukemia, amyloidosis, thalassemia, lymphomas, infectious mononucleosis, iron-deficiency anemia, or sideroblastic anemia.

The basics
Bone marrow, the soft tissue contained in the medullary canals of long bone and in the interstices of cancellous bone, may be removed by aspiration or needle biopsy, under local anesthetic. In aspiration biopsy, a fluid specimen in which pustula of marrow are suspended is removed from the bone marrow. In needle biopsy, a core of marrow—cells, not fluid—is removed. These methods are often used concurrently to obtain the best possible marrow specimens. Because bone marrow is the major site of hematopoiesis, the histologic and hematologic examination of its contents provides reliable diagnostic information about blood disorders. Marrow removed from the bone may be red or yellow. Red marrow, which comprises about 50% of an adult's marrow, actively produces red blood cells; yellow marrow contains fat cells and connective tissue and is inactive. Because yellow marrow can become active in response to the body's needs, an adult has a large hematopoietic capacity. An infant's marrow is mainly red and, consequently, reflects a small hematopoietic capacity.

Bleeding and infection may result from bone marrow biopsy at any site, but the most serious complications occur at the sternum. Such complications

Positioning for Bone Marrow Aspiration and Biopsy

Posterior superior iliac spine is the preferred site, since no vital organs or vessels are located nearby. With the patient in a lateral position with one leg flexed, the doctor inserts the needle several centimeters lateral to the iliosacral junction, entering the bone plane crest with the needle directed downward and toward the anterior inferior spine, or entering a few centimeters below the crest at a right angle to the surface of the bone.

Sternum involves the greatest risks but is commonly used for marrow aspiration, because it is near the surface, the cortical bone is thin, and the marrow cavity contains numerous cells and relatively little fat or supporting bone. For this procedure, the patient is supine on a firm bed or examining table with a small pillow beneath the shoulders to elevate the chest and lower the head. The doctor secures the needle guard 3 to 4 mm from the tip of the needle to avoid accidental puncture of the heart or a major vessel. Then he inserts the needle at the midline of the sternum at the second intercostal space.

Spinous process is preferred if multiple punctures are necessary, marrow is absent at other sites, or the patient objects to sternal puncture. In this procedure, the patient sits on the edge of the bed, leaning over the bedside stand; or, if the patient is uncooperative, he may be placed in the prone position with restraints. The doctor selects the spinous process of the third or fourth lumbar vertebrae and inserts the needle at the crest or slightly to one side, advancing the needle in the direction of the bone plane.

Tibia is the site of choice for infants younger than age 1. The infant is placed in a prone position on a bed or examining table with a sandbag beneath the leg. The foot is taped to the surface of the table, or an assistant holds the leg stationary by placing a hand under it. The doctor inserts the needle about ⅜" (1 cm) below the tibial tuberosity and slightly toward the medial side, being careful to angle the needle point toward the foot to avoid epiphyseal injury.

are rare but include puncture of the heart and major vessels—causing severe hemorrhage—and puncture of the mediastinum—causing mediastinitis or pneumomediastinum.

Contraindications to this test include: severe bleeding disorders.

Procedure

• Position the patient according to biopsy site (see *Positioning for Bone Marrow Aspiration and Biopsy*) and instruct him to remain as still as possible.

• Offer emotional support during the biopsy by talking quietly to the patient,

describing what is being done, and answering any questions.

• The test takes 5 to 10 minutes to perform, and results are generally available in 1 day.

For aspiration biopsy:

• After the skin over the biopsy site is prepared and the area is draped, the local anesthetic is injected.

• With a twisting motion, the marrow aspiration needle is inserted through the skin, the subcutaneous tissue, and the cortex of the bone.

• The stylet is removed from the needle, and a 10- to 20-ml syringe is attached.

Bone Marrow: Normal Values and Implications of Abnormal Findings

Cell types	Normal mean values		
	Adults	Children	Infants
Normoblasts, total	25.6%	23.1%	8.0%
Pronormoblasts	0.2% to 1.3%	0.5%	0.1%
Basophilic	0.5% to 2.4%	1.7%	0.34%
Polychromatic	17.9% to 29.2%	18.2%	6.9%
Orthochromatic	0.4% to 4.6%	2.7%	0.54%
Neutrophils, total	56.5%	57.1%	32.4%
Myeloblasts	0.2% to 1.5%	1.2%	0.62%
Promyelocytes	2.1% to 4.1%	1.4%	0.76%
Myelocytes	8.2% to 15.7%	18.3%	2.5%
Metamyelocytes	9.6% to 24.6%	23.3%	11.3%
Bands	9.5% to 15.3%	0	14.1%
Segmented	6.0% to 12.0%	12.9%	3.6%
Eosinophils	3.1%	3.6%	2.6%
Basophils	0.01%	0.06%	0.07%
Lymphocytes	16.2%	16.0%	49.0%
Plasma cells	1.3%	0.4%	0.02%
Megakaryocytes	0.1%	0.1%	0.05%
Myeloid: Erythroid ratio	2.3	2.9	4.4

Clinical implications	
Elevated values	**Depressed values**
Polycythemia vera	Vitamin B_{12} or folic acid deficiency; hypoplastic or aplastic anemia
Acute myeloblastic or chronic myeloid leukemia	Lymphoblastic, lymphatic, or monocytic leukemia; aplastic anemia
Bone marrow carcinoma, lymphadenoma, myeloid leukemia, eosinophilic leukemia, pernicious anemia (in relapse)	
No relationship between basophil count and symptoms	No relationship between basophil count and symptoms
B- and T-cell chronic lymphocytic leukemia, other lymphatic leukemias, lymphoma, mononucleosis, aplastic anemia, macroglobulinemia	
Myeloma, collagen disease, infection, antigen sensitivity, malignancy	
Old age, chronic myeloid leukemia, polycythemia vera, megakaryocytic myelosis, infection, idiopathic thrombocytopenic purpura, thrombocytopenia	Pernicious anemia
Myeloid leukemia, infection, leukemoid reactions, depressed hematopoiesis	Agranulocytosis, hematopoiesis after hemorrhage or hemolysis, iron deficiency anemia, polycythemia

Adapted with permission from *Pediatric Hematology*, by A.M. Mauer, © 1969, McGraw-Hill Book Company, and from *Clinical Hematology*, by M.M. Wintrobe, © 1981, Lea & Febiger.

Preparing Children for Bone Marrow Biopsy

To prepare a child for a bone marrow biopsy, give him his own biopsy kit: a syringe without a needle, cotton balls, and adhesive bandages. Illustrate the procedure by using a doll or a stuffed animal as a model. In this way, you can gain the child's confidence and answer any questions he may have. Be sure to prepare him by describing the kinds of pressure and discomfort he will feel during the procedure.

Before the biopsy, explain the equipment on the tray to the child. Ask the parents to get involved: they can help you hold the child still and reassure him. Tell the child he will feel some pain when the doctor aspirates the bone marrow, and it's OK to cry or yell if he wants to, but the pain will go away quickly.

• The examiner aspirates 0.2 to 0.5 ml of marrow, then withdraws the needle.
• Pressure is applied to the site for 5 minutes, while marrow slides are being prepared. (If the patient has thrombocytopenia, pressure should be applied to the site for 10 to 15 minutes.)
• The biopsy site is cleansed again, and a sterile adhesive bandage is applied.

For needle biopsy:
• After preparing the biopsy site and draping the area, the examiner marks the skin at the site with an indelible pencil or marking pen.
• A local anesthetic is then injected intradermally, subcutaneously, and at the surface of the bone.
• The biopsy needle is inserted into the periosteum, and the needle guard is set, as indicated.
• The needle is advanced with a steady boring motion, until the outer needle passes through the cortex of the bone.

• The inner needle with trephine tip is inserted into the outer needle, and the stylet is removed. By alternately rotating the inner needle clockwise and counterclockwise, the examiner directs the needle into the marrow cavity and then removes a tissue plug.
• The needle assembly is withdrawn, and the marrow is expelled into a labeled bottle containing Zenker's acetic acid solution.
• After the biopsy site is cleansed, a sterile adhesive bandage or a pressure dressing is applied.

Patient care checklist
Before the test
☑ Explain or clarify test purpose and procedure. (See *Preparing Children for Bone Marrow Biopsy* for special instructions on preparing a child for this procedure.)
☑ Inform the patient or parents that more than one bone marrow specimen may be required and that a blood sample will be collected before biopsy, for laboratory testing.
☑ Inform the patient or parents that a local anesthetic will be administered, but that the patient will feel pressure on insertion of the biopsy needle and a brief, pulling pain on removal of the marrow.
☑ Evaluate patient/parent understanding.
☑ Make sure that the patient or a responsible family member has signed a consent form.
☑ As ordered, administer a mild sedative one hour before the test.
After the test
☑ Check dressing at biopsy site.

Interfering factors
• Failure to obtain a representative specimen.
• Failure to use a fixative (for histologic analysis).
• Failure to send the specimen to the laboratory immediately.

Cervical punch biopsy

Purpose
• To evaluate suspicious cervical lesions
• To diagnose cervical cancer.

Normal results
Cervical tissue is composed of columnar and squamous epithelial cells, loose connective tissue, and smooth-muscle fibers, with no dysplasia or abnormal cell growth.

Abnormal results
Histologic examination of a cervical tissue specimen identifies abnormal cells and differentiates the tissue as intraepithelial neoplasia or invasive cancer.

The basics
Cervical punch biopsy is the excision by sharp forceps of a tissue specimen from the cervix for histologic examination. Generally, multiple biopsies are done to obtain specimens from all areas with abnormal tissue, or from the squamocolumnar junction and other sites around the cervical circumference. This procedure is indicated in women with suspicious cervical lesions and should be performed when the cervix is least vascular (usually one week after menses). Biopsy sites are selected by direct visualization of

Endometrial and Ovarian Biopsies

Method	Purpose	Special considerations
Endometrial Biopsy • Dilatation and curettage (D&C) • Endometrial washing (by jet irrigation, aspiration, or brushing)	• To evaluate uterine bleeding • To diagnose suspected endometrial carcinoma • To diagnose a missed abortion	• Time of menstrual cycle affects accuracy of biopsy results • Type of specimen obtained depends on patient's age and disorder • Endometrial washing requires no anesthesia and can be done in a doctor's office • D&C may follow negative biopsy by endometrial washing • Specimens obtained by D&C may be processed as frozen sections
Ovarian Biopsy • Transrectal or transvaginal fine-needle biopsy • Aspiration biopsy during laparoscopy	• To detect an ovarian tumor • To determine the spread of malignancy	• Fine needle biopsy may follow palpation, laparoscopy, or computed tomography that detects an abnormal ovary • Aspiration during laparoscopy is particularly useful for young women who are infertile or who have lesions that appear benign

the cervix with a colposcope—the most accurate method—or by Schiller's test, which stains normal squamous epithelium a dark mahogany but fails to color abnormal tissue.

If the cause of an abnormal Pap test is not demonstrated by cervical biopsy, or if the specimen shows advanced dysplasia or carcinoma in situ, a cone biopsy is performed in the operating room, under general anesthesia. Cone biopsy garners a larger tissue specimen and allows a more accurate evaluation of dysplasia. (For information on biopsies involving other areas of the reproductive system, see *Endometrial and Ovarian Biopsies*, p. 449.)

Procedure
• Place the patient in the lithotomy position, and tell her to relax as the unlubricated speculum is inserted.
Direct visualization:
• The colposcope is inserted through the speculum, the biopsy site is located, and the cervix is cleansed with a swab soaked in 3% acetic acid solution.
• The biopsy forceps are then inserted through the speculum or the colposcope, and tissue is removed from any lesion or from selected sites, starting from the posterior lip to avoid obscuring other sites with blood.
• Each specimen is immediately put in 10% formaldehyde solution in a labeled bottle.
• To control bleeding after biopsy, the cervix is swabbed with 5% silver nitrate solution (cautery or sutures may be used instead). If bleeding persists, the examiner may insert a tampon.
• The patient's and physician's names and the biopsy sites should be recorded on the laboratory slip.
Schiller's test:
• An applicator stick saturated with iodine solution is inserted through the speculum. This stains the cervix to identify lesions for biopsy.

• Tissue for biopsy is removed using biopsy forceps, and the procedure continues as described under "Direct visualization."

Patient care checklist
Before the test
☑ Explain or clarify test purpose and procedure.
☑ Tell the patient that she may experience mild discomfort during and after the biopsy. Advise the outpatient to have someone accompany her home after the biopsy.
☑ Evaluate patient understanding.
☑ Make sure that the patient or a responsible family member has signed a consent form.
☑ Just before the biopsy, ask the patient to void.
After the test
☑ Instruct the patient to avoid strenuous exercise for 8 to 24 hours after the biopsy. Encourage the outpatient to rest briefly before leaving the office.
☑ If a tampon was inserted after the biopsy, tell the patient to leave it in place for as long as ordered. Inform her that some bleeding may occur after its removal, but tell her to report heavy bleeding (heavier than menstrual) to the physician. Warn the patient to avoid using tampons, which can irritate the cervix and provoke bleeding, according to her physician's directions.
☑ Tell the patient to avoid douching and intercourse for 2 weeks, or as directed.
☑ Inform the patient that a foul-smelling, gray-green vaginal discharge is normal for several days after biopsy and may persist for three weeks. This occurs as a result of the natural healing process.

Interfering factors
• Failure to obtain representative specimens.
• Failure to place specimens in the preservative immediately.

Chromosome analysis

Purpose
To identify chromosomal abnormalities as the underlying cause of malformation, maldevelopment, or disease.

Normal results
The normal somatic cell contains 46 chromosomes.
Females: 44 autosomes and 2 sex chromosomes (XX).
Males: 44 autosomes and 2 sex chromosomes (XY).

Abnormal results
Whole chromosome abnormalities:
  Down's syndrome
  Trisomy 1315
  Trisomy 18.
Sex chromosome abnormalities:
  See *Sex Chromosome Anomalies,* pp. 452 to 453.
Philadelphia chromosome (Ph¹):
  Present in 85% of patients with chronic granulocytic leukemia.

The basics
Chromosomes—threadlike bodies in the cellular nucleus—each contain thousands of genes with biochemical programs for cell function that are stored in deoxyribonucleic acid (DNA), the basic genetic material. Chromosome analysis, an integral facet of cytogenetics, studies the relationship between the microscopic appearance of chromosomes and the person's phenotype—the expression of the genes in physical, biochemical, or physiologic traits.

Light microscopy can visualize the chromosomes but is not yet capable of showing individual genes. Ideally, chromosomes should be studied during metaphase, the middle phase of mitosis, when new cell poles appear. Only rapidly dividing cell lines, such as bone marrow or neoplastic cells, permit direct, immediate study. Most other cell types require stimulation of mitosis by addition of phytohemagglutinin to the culture. Subsequently, the addition of colchicine (a cell poison) arrests the cell division in metaphase. Harvested, stained, and viewed under

Chromosome Analysis: Specimen and Indications

Blood
• To evaluate abnormal appearance or development suggesting chromosomal irregularity
• To evaluate couple with history of miscarriages, or to identify balanced translocation carriers having unbalanced offspring
• To detect chromosomal rearrangements in rare genetic diseases predisposing patient to malignant neoplasms

Blood or bone marrow
• To identify Philadelphia chromosome and confirm chronic myelogenous leukemia

Skin
• To evaluate abnormal appearance or development suggesting chromosomal irregularity

Amniotic fluid
• To evaluate developing fetus with possible chromosomal abnormality

Placental tissue
• To evaluate products of conception after a miscarriage to determine if abnormality is fetal or placental in origin

Tumor tissue
• For research purposes only

Sex Chromosome Anomalies

Disorder and chromosomal aneuploidy	Cause and incidence	Phenotypic features
Klinefelter's syndrome • 47,XXY • 48,XXXY • 49,XXXXY • 48,XX,YY • 49,XXX,YY • Mosaics: XXY, XXXY, or XXXXY/XX or XY	Nondisjunction or improper chromatid separation during anaphase I or II of oogenesis or spermatogenesis results in abnormal gamete 1/500 to 600 male births	• Syndrome usually inapparent until puberty • Small penis and testes • Sparse facial and abdominal hair; feminine distribution of pubic hair • Somewhat enlarged breasts (gynecomastia) • Sexual dysfunction • Sterility • Possible mental retardation (greater incidence with increased X chromosomes)
Polysomy Y • 47,XYY	Nondisjunction during anaphase II of spermatogenesis causes both Y chromosomes to pass to the same pole and results in a YY sperm 1/1,000 male births	• Above average stature (often over 72" [180 cm]) • May display aggressive, psychopathic, or criminal behavior • Normal fertility
Turner's syndrome (ovarian dysgenesis) • 45,XO • Mosaics: XO/XX or XO/XXX • Aberrations of X chromosomes, including deletion of short arm of one X chromosome, presence of a ring chromosome, or presence of an isochromosome on the long arm of an X chromosome	Nondisjunction during anaphase I or II of spermatogenesis results in sperm without any sex chromosomes 1/3,500 female births (most common chromosome complement in first trimester abortions)	• Short stature (usually under 57" [145 cm]) • Webbed neck • Low hairline • Broad chest with widely spaced nipples • Underdeveloped breasts • Juvenile external genitalia • Primary amenorrhea common • Sterility due to underdeveloped internal reproductive organs (ovaries are merely strands of connective tissue) • No mental retardation, but possible problems with space perception and orientation
Other X polysomes	Nondisjunction at anaphase I or II of oogenesis	

(continued)

Sex Chromosome Anomalies *(continued)*

Disorder and chromosomal aneuploidy	Cause and incidence	Phenotypic features
Other X polysomes *(continued)*		
• 47,XXX	1/1,400 female births	• Often, no obvious anatomical abnormalities • Normal fertility
• 48,XXXX	Rare	• Mental retardation • Ocular hypertelorism • Reduced fertility
• 49,XXXXX	Rare	• Severe mental retardation • Ocular hypertelorism, with uncoordinated eye movement • Abnormal development of sexual organs • Various skeletal anomalies

a microscope, the cells are finally photographed to provide a karyotype, the systematic arrangement of chromosomes in groupings according to size and shape.

Indications for the test determine the type of specimen required (blood, bone marrow, amniotic fluid, skin, or placental tissue) and the procedure performed. Test results on a blood sample are generally available 72 to 96 hours after stimulation. Analysis of skin biopsy specimens or amniotic fluid cells may take several weeks.

Procedure
Follow the procedure for obtaining a specimen from the blood, bone marrow, skin, amniotic fluid, placental tissue, or tumor tissue. (See *Chromosome Analysis: Specimen and Indications,* p. 451.)

Special precautions
• Keep all specimens sterile, especially those requiring a tissue culture.

• If transport to the laboratory must be delayed, refrigerate the specimen, but *never* freeze it.

CLINICAL ALERT: **Before skin biopsy, make sure that the povidone-iodine solution is thoroughly removed with alcohol. This solution may prevent cell growth in tissue culture.**

Patient care checklist
Before the test
☑ Explain or clarify test purpose and procedure.
☑ Evaluate patient understanding.
After the test
☑ Provide appropriate post-test care, depending on the procedure used to collect the specimen.
☑ If necessary, recommend appropriate genetic or other counseling and follow-up care, such as an infant stimulation program for Down's syndrome.

Interfering factors
• Chemotherapy may cause abnormal results, such as chromosome breaks.

• Contamination of tissue with bacteria, fungus, or a virus may inhibit growth of the culture.

• Inclusion of maternal cells in a specimen obtained by amniocentesis, with subsequent culturing, may cause false results.

Liver biopsy (percutaneous)

Purpose

To diagnose hepatic parenchymal disease, malignancy, and granulomatous infections.

Normal results

The healthy liver consists of sheets of hepatocytes supported by a reticulin framework.

Abnormal results

Examination of the hepatic tissue may reveal diffuse hepatic disease, such as cirrhosis or hepatitis, or granulomatous infections, such as tuberculosis. Primary malignant tumors include hepatocellular carcinoma, cholangiocellular carcinoma, and angiosarcoma, but hepatic metastases are more common.

The basics

Percutaneous biopsy of the liver is the needle aspiration of a core of tissue for histologic analysis. This procedure is performed under local or general anesthesia. Such analysis can identify hepatic disorders after ultrasonography, computed tomography, and radionuclide studies have failed to detect them.

Because many patients with hepatic disorders have clotting defects, testing for hemostasis should precede liver biopsy.

Contraindications to this test include: presence of empyema of the lungs, pleurae, peritoneum, biliary tract, or liver; vascular tumor; hepatic angiomas; hydatid cyst; or tense ascites.

If extrahepatic obstruction is suspected, ultrasonography or subcutaneous transhepatic cholangiography should rule out this condition before the biopsy is considered.

Procedure

• For aspiration biopsy using the Menghini needle, place the patient in a supine position, with his right hand under his head.

• Instruct him to maintain this position and to remain as still as possible during the procedure.

• The liver is palpated, the biopsy site is selected and marked, and the anesthetic is then injected.

• The needle flange is set to control the depth of penetration, and 2 ml of sterile normal saline solution are drawn into the syringe.

• The syringe is attached to the biopsy needle, and the needle is introduced into the subcutaneous tissue, through the right eighth or ninth intercostal space, between the anterior and posterior axillary lines.

• One ml of normal saline solution is injected to clear the needle and the plunger, then the plunger is drawn back to the 4-ml mark to create negative pressure.

• At this point in the procedure, ask the patient to take a deep breath, exhale, and hold his breath at the end of expiration to prevent any movement of the chest wall.

• As the patient holds his breath, the biopsy needle is quickly inserted into the liver and withdrawn in one second.

• After the needle is withdrawn, tell the patient to resume normal respirations.

• The tissue specimen is then placed in a properly labeled specimen cup containing 10% formalin solution.

• Apply pressure to the biopsy site to halt bleeding.

Special precautions

CLINICAL ALERT: **Instruct the patient to hold his breath while the needle is in place, to prevent acci-**

dental puncture of the pleural cavity or diaphragm.

Patient care checklist

Before the test

☑ Explain or clarify test purpose, preparation, and procedure.

☑ Inform the patient that he will receive a local anesthetic, but may experience momentary pain as the biopsy needle is inserted.

☑ Evaluate patient understanding.

☑ Check blood studies for a platelet count below 100,000 or prothrombin time longer than 15 seconds. Notify the doctor of the above results.

☑ Check patient history for hypersensitivity to local anesthetic.

☑ Make sure that the patient or a responsible family member has signed the consent form.

☑ Restrict food and fluids for 4 to 8 hours before the test, as ordered.

☑ Just before the biopsy, tell the patient to void, and take his vital signs.

After the test

☑ Position the patient on his right side for 2 hours, with a small pillow or sandbag under the costal margin to provide extra pressure. Advise bed rest for 24 hours.

☑ Monitor vital signs, as ordered, and observe patient for signs of shock.

CLINICAL ALERT: Watch for bleeding or signs of bile peritonitis—tenderness and rigidity around the biopsy site. Be alert for symptoms of pneumothorax —rising respiration rate, depressed breath sounds, dyspnea, persistent shoulder pain, and pleuritic chest pain. Report such complications promptly.

☑ If the patient experiences pain, which may persist for several hours after the test, administer analgesic medication, as ordered.

Interfering factors

• Failure to obtain a representative specimen.

• Failure to place the specimen in the proper preservative.

• Delayed transport of the specimen to the laboratory.

Lung biopsy

Purpose

To confirm diagnosis of diffuse parenchymal pulmonary disease and pulmonary lesions.

Normal results

Healthy pulmonary tissue shows uniform texture of the alveolar ducts, alveolar walls, bronchioles, and small vessels.

Abnormal results

Histologic examination may reveal:

Squamous cell carcinoma

Oat cell carcinoma

Adenocarcinoma.

The basics

In biopsy of the lung, a specimen of pulmonary tissue is excised by closed or open technique for histologic examination. Closed technique, performed under local anesthesia, includes both needle and transbronchial biopsies; open technique, performed under general anesthesia in the operating room, includes both limited and standard thoracotomies. Needle biopsy is appropriate when the lesion is readily accessible, or when it originates in the lung parenchyma, is confined to it, or is affixed to the chest wall; it provides a much smaller specimen than the open technique. Transbronchial biopsy, the removal of multiple tissue specimens through a fibroptic bronchoscope, is appropriate for diffuse infiltrative pulmonary disease or tumors, or when severe debilitation contraindicates open biopsy. Open biopsy is appropriate for the study of a well-circumscribed lesion that may require resection.

Generally, a biopsy of the lung is recommended after chest X-ray, computed tomography scan, bronchoscopy, and sputum for cytology (see *Sputum Cytology Collection*) and microbiology have failed to identify the cause of diffuse parenchymal pulmonary disease or of a pulmonary lesion.

Complications of lung biopsy include bleeding, infection, and pneumothorax.

Contraindications: the presence of a lesion that has separated from the chest wall or that is accompanied by emphysematous bullae, cysts, or gross emphysema, and patients with coagulopathy, hypoxia, pulmonary hypertension, or cardiac disease with cor pulmonale.

Procedure
• After the biopsy site is selected, lead markers are placed on the patient's skin and X-rays are ordered to verify their correct placement.
• Place the patient in a sitting position, with arms folded on a table in front of him, and instruct him to maintain this position, remaining as still as possible, and to refrain from coughing.
• The skin over the biopsy site is prepared, and the area is draped.
• After a local anesthetic is administered, a small incision is made and the biopsy needle is introduced into the tumor or pulmonary tissue.
• The specimen is obtained and the needle is withdrawn. The specimen is divided immediately: the tissue for histology is placed in a properly labeled bottle containing 10% neutral buffered formaldehyde solution; the tissue for microbiology is placed in a sterile container.
• Pressure is exerted on the biopsy site to stop the bleeding, and then a small bandage is applied.
• A chest X-ray is repeated immediately after the biopsy.
• The procedure takes 30 to 60 minutes, and test results should be available in a few days.

Special precautions
CLINICAL ALERT: **During biopsy, observe for signs of respiratory distress—shortness of breath, elevated pulse, and cyanosis (late sign)—and if they develop, report them immediately.**
• Since coughing or movement during biopsy can cause tearing of the lung by the biopsy needle, keep the patient calm and still.

Patient care checklist
Before the test
☑ Explain or clarify test purpose, preparation, and procedure.
☑ Tell the patient that he will receive a local anesthetic, but may experience a sharp, transient pain when the biopsy needle touches the lung.
☑ Evaluate patient understanding.
☑ Restrict food and fluids after midnight before the test.
☑ Make sure that the patient or a responsible family member has signed the consent form.
☑ Check patient history for hypersensitivity to the local anesthetic.

Sputum Cytology Collection

Cytologic examination of sputum helps detect lung cancer. Examination of early morning specimens collected over several days (usually 3) increases test sensitivity because of an overnight accumulation of sputum containing cells exfoliated from the bronchi and lung parenchyma.

Before the test, the patient brushes his teeth or rinses with saline solution to reduce specimen contamination with oral bacteria and food particles; then, he inhales repeatedly to full capacity, and finally exhales with an expulsive cough. In the hospital, if the patient is unable to raise a sputum sample, he may require aerosol inhalation of a saline solution via nebulizer or endotracheal suction with a sputum trap.

☑ Administer a mild sedative, as ordered, 30 minutes before the biopsy, to help the patient relax.

☑ Just before the procedure, take vital signs.

After the test

☑ Monitor vital signs, as ordered, and observe the patient for signs of respiratory distress.

Interfering factors

• Failure to obtain a representative tissue specimen.

• Failure to store the specimens for histology and microbiology in the appropriate containers.

Lymph node biopsy

Purpose

• To determine the cause of lymph node enlargement

• To distinguish between benign and malignant lymph node tumors

• To stage metastatic carcinoma.

Normal results

A lymph node is encapsulated by collagenous connective tissue, and is divided into smaller lobes by tissue strands called *trabeculae*. It has an outer *cortex*, composed of lymphoid cells and nodules or follicles containing lymphocytes, and an inner *medulla* composed of reticular phagocytic cells that collect and drain fluid.

Abnormal results

Histologic examination of the tissue specimen distinguishes between malignant and nonmalignant causes of lymph node enlargement.

The basics

Lymph node biopsy is the surgical excision of an active lymph node, or the needle aspiration of a nodal specimen, for histologic examination. Both techniques usually employ local anesthesia and sample the superficial nodes in the cervical, supraclavicular, axillary, or inguinal region. Excision is the preferred technique, because it provides a larger specimen.

Lymph nodes swell from their usually flat, bean shape during infection, but return to normal size as infection clears. When nodal enlargement is prolonged and is accompanied by backache, leg edema, breathing and swallowing difficulties and, later, weight loss, weakness, severe itching, fever, night sweats, cough, hemoptysis, or hoarseness, biopsy is indicated. Generalized or localized lymph node enlargement is typical of diseases such as chronic lymphatic leukemia, Hodgkin's disease, infectious mononucleosis, and rheumatoid arthritis.

Complete blood count, liver function studies, liver and spleen scans, and X-rays should precede this test.

Procedure

Excisional biopsy:

• The skin over the biopsy site is prepared, then draped for privacy.

• A local anesthetic is administered.

• The examiner makes an incision, removes an entire node, and places it in a properly labeled bottle containing normal saline solution.

• The wound is sutured, and a sterile dressing is applied.

Needle biopsy:

• After preparing the biopsy site and administering a local anesthetic, the examiner grasps the node between his thumb and forefinger.

• A biopsy needle is inserted directly into the node, and a small core specimen is obtained.

• The needle is then removed, and the specimen is placed in a properly labeled bottle containing normal saline solution.

• Pressure is exerted on the biopsy site to control bleeding, and an adhesive bandage is applied.

• The procedure takes 15 to 30 minutes, and the analysis takes 1 day to complete.

Special precautions

Storing the tissue specimen in normal saline solution instead of in 10% formaldehyde solution allows part of the specimen to be used for cytologic impression smears, which are studied along with the biopsy specimen.

Patient care checklist

Before the test

☑ Explain or clarify test purpose, preparation, and procedure.

☑ Evaluate patient understanding.

☑ For excisional biopsy, restrict food and fluids as ordered.

☑ Make sure that the patient or a responsible family member has signed the consent form.

☑ Check patient history for hypersensitivity to the anesthetic.

☑ Just before the biopsy, take vital signs.

After the test

☑ Monitor vital signs, as ordered.

☑ Watch for bleeding, tenderness, and redness at the biopsy site.

Interfering factors

• Improper specimen storage.

• Failure to obtain a representative tissue specimen.

Papanicolaou test of the female genital tract
[Pap test]

Purpose

• To detect malignant cells

• To detect inflammatory tissue changes

• To assess response to chemotherapy and radiation therapy

• To detect viral, fungal, and occasionally parasitic invasion.

Normal results

No malignant, abnormal, or atypical cells are present.

Abnormal results

A Pap test may be graded in different ways. The following system is the traditional classification method:

Class I:

Normal pattern; absence of atypical or abnormal cells.

Class II:

Benign abnormality; atypical, but nonmalignant, cells present.

Class III:

Atypical cells consistent with dysplasia.

Class IV:

Suggestive of, but inconclusive for, malignancy.

Class V:

Conclusive for malignancy.

The basics

The Pap test, a cytologic test, is widely known for its use in early detection of cervical cancer. To perform this test, a physician or specially trained nurse scrapes secretions from the patient's cervix and spreads them on a slide. After the slide is immersed in a fixative, it is sent to the laboratory for cytologic analysis. This test relies on the ready exfoliation of malignant cells from the cervix. Although cervical scrapings are the most common test specimen, this test also permits cytologic examination of the vaginal pool, prostatic secretions, urine, gastric secretions, cavity fluids, bronchial aspirations, sputum, and solid tumor cells obtained by fine-needle aspiration. It also shows cell maturity, metabolic activity, and morphology variations.

The American Cancer Society recommends a Pap test every 3 years for women between ages 20 and 40 who are not in a high-risk category and who have had negative results from two previous Pap tests. Yearly tests (or at intervals dictated by the patient's physician) are advisable for women over age 40, for those in a high-risk category, and for those who have had a positive test. If a Pap test is positive or suggests malignancy, cervical biopsy can confirm diagnosis. A vaginal smear specimen for detection of vaginitis may also be obtained at the time the Pap test specimen is obtained (see *Vaginal Smears*).

The test should not be scheduled during the menstrual period; the best time is mid-cycle. The woman should not douche or insert vaginal medications for 24 hours before the test, since doing so can wash away cellular deposits and change the vaginal pH, thus altering test results. Test results should be available within a few days.

Procedure
See *Performing a Pap Test,* p. 460.

Special precautions
- Preserve the slides *immediately*.
- Be sure the cervical specimen is aspirated and scraped from the cervix. Aspiration of the posterior fornix of the vagina can supplement a cervical specimen, but should not replace it.
- If vaginal or vulval lesions are present, scrapings taken directly from the lesion are preferred.
- In a patient whose uterus is involuting or atrophying from age, use a small pipette, if necessary, to aspirate cells from the squamocolumnar junction and the cervical canal.

Patient care checklist
Before the test

☑ Explain or clarify test purpose and procedure.

☑ Tell the patient she may experience slight discomfort when the cervix is scraped.

☑ Evaluate patient understanding.

☑ Just before the test, ask the patient to empty her bladder.

☑ Fill out the laboratory slip and label the slides appropriately, including the date; the patient's name, age, and date of her last menstrual period; and the collection site and method.

☑ Ask the patient to undress from the waist down, assist her to the lithotomy position, and drape her appropriately.

Vaginal Smears

Although the Pap test was not developed to detect vaginitis, a cytologist can usually identify cells associated with vaginitis while examining the stained cells for cancer. The most reliably detected cells are *Trichomonas vaginalis, Candida,* and herpes progenitalis. If such cells are present, the Pap test indicates Class II findings—atypical cells, but no evidence of malignancy.

The most conventional way to detect vaginitis is the vaginal smear. Using a cotton-tipped applicator or wooden spatula, the examiner collects vaginal secretions and places them at opposite ends of a slide. After adding a drop of normal saline solution to one end of the slide and a drop of 10% to 20% potassium hydroxide (KOH) to the other end (wet mount preparation), he examines the slide immediately. Trichomonads, white cells, epithelial cells, "clue" cells, and bacteria readily appear at the saline-treated end; *Candida,* at the KOH-treated end.

In the vaginal pool smear, secretions are aspirated through a pipette attached to a bulb for suction. Part of the secretion is smeared on a slide and fixed. Vaginal pool smears are more sensitive to uterine cancer than cervical smears. However, the latter are better detectors of cervical cancer.

Scrapings for cytohormonal evaluation can also be taken from the vaginal pool. In this procedure, the lateral vaginal wall is gently scraped, and the scrapings spread on a glass slide and fixed. Using the pyknotic index, the estrogenic effect is assessed by determining the percentage of superficial and intermediate squamous cells with a fatty pyknotic nucleus.

Performing a Pap Test

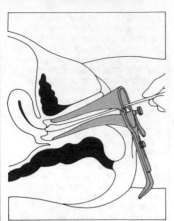

Figure 1
An unlubricated speculum is inserted into the vagina. To make insertion easier and more comfortable, the speculum is held under warm running water before insertion.

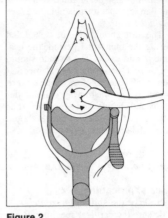

Figure 2
The cervix is exposed by opening the speculum blades. A saline-moistened Pap stick is inserted through the speculum and secretions are scraped from the cervical canal.

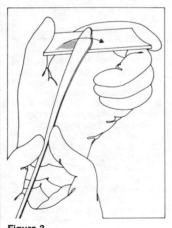

Figure 3
The specimen is spread on a slide.

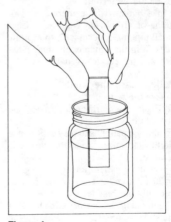

Figure 4
Immediately, the slide is placed in a fixative solution or sprayed with a commercial fixative.

Interfering factors

• Delay in fixing a specimen allows the cells to dry, destroys the effectiveness of the nuclear stain, and makes cytologic interpretation difficult.

• Collecting the specimen during menstruation, using lubricating jelly on the speculum, douching, or applying vaginal medications 24 hours before the test can affect test results.

Pleural biopsy

Purpose

• To differentiate between nonmalignant and malignant disease

• To diagnose viral, fungal, or parasitic disease, and collagen vascular disease of the pleura.

Normal results

The pleura consists primarily of mesothelial cells, flattened in a uniform layer. Layers of areolar connective tissue—containing blood vessels, nerves, and lymphatics—lie below.

Abnormal results

Histologic examination of the tissue specimen can reveal:

    Malignant disease
    Tuberculosis
    Viral disease
    Fungal disease
    Parasitic disease
    Collagen vascular disease.

The basics

Pleural biopsy is the removal of pleural tissue, by needle biopsy or open biopsy, for histologic examination. Needle pleural biopsy is performed under local anesthesia. It generally follows thoracentesis—aspiration of pleural fluid—which is performed when the etiology of the effusion is unknown, but it can be performed separately.

Open pleural biopsy, performed in the absence of pleural effusion, permits direct visualization of the pleura and the underlying lung. It is performed in the operating room.

Contraindications to this test include: severe bleeding disorders.

Procedure

• Seat the patient on the side of the bed, with his feet resting on a stool and his arms supported by the overbed table or upper body.

• Tell him to hold this position and remain still during the procedure.

• Prepare the skin and drape the area.

Vim-Silverman needle biopsy:

• After a local anesthetic is administered, the needle is inserted through the appropriate intercostal space into the biopsy site.

• The entire assembly is rotated 360 degrees, and the needle and tissue specimen are withdrawn.

Cope's needle biopsy:

• After a local anesthetic is administered, the trocar is introduced through the appropriate intercostal space into the biopsy site.

• While the outer tube is held stationary, the inner tube is twisted to cut off the tissue specimen, and the assembly is withdrawn.

• The specimen from either type of needle biopsy is immediately put in 10% neutral buffered formaldehyde solution in a labeled specimen bottle.

• Cleanse the skin around the biopsy site, and apply an adhesive bandage.

Patient care checklist

Before the test

☑ Explain or clarify test purpose, preparation, and procedure.

☑ Tell the patient that blood studies will precede the biopsy, and that chest X-rays will be taken before and after the biopsy.

☑ Tell him that he will receive a local anesthetic and should experience little pain.

☑ Evaluate patient understanding.

☑ Review patient history for hypersensitivity to the local anesthetic.

☑ Make sure that the patient or a responsible family member has signed the consent form.

☑ Just before the procedure, take vital signs.

After the test

CLINICAL ALERT: **Monitor vital signs as ordered, and observe the patient for signs of complications such as pneumothorax (immediate) and pneumonia (delayed).**

☑ Make sure that the chest X-ray is repeated immediately after the biopsy.

Interfering factors
• Failure to use proper fixative.
• Failure to obtain adequate specimens.

Prostate gland biopsy

Purpose
• To confirm prostatic cancer
• To determine the cause of prostatic hypertrophy.

Normal results
The prostate gland consists of a thin, fibrous capsule surrounding the stroma, which is made up of elastic and connective tissues and smooth-muscle fibers. The epithelial glands, found in these tissues and muscle fibers, drain into the chief excreting ducts.

Abnormal results
Histologic examination can detect:
   Prostatic carcinoma
   Benign prostatic hyperplasia
   Prostatitis
   Tuberculosis
   Lymphoma
   Rectal and bladder carcinoma.

The basics
Prostate gland biopsy is the needle excision of a prostate tissue specimen for histologic examination. A perineal, transrectal, or transurethral approach may be used; the transrectal approach

is usually used for high prostatic lesions. Indications include potentially malignant prostatic hypertrophy and prostatic nodules. The procedure takes less than 30 minutes. Complications include transient, painless hematuria and bleeding into the prostatic urethra and bladder.

Procedure
Perineal approach:
• Place the patient in the proper position (left lateral, knee-chest, or lithotomy), and cleanse the perineal skin.
• After the local anesthetic is administered, a ⅛″ (2-mm) incision may be made into the perineum.
• The examiner immobilizes the prostate by inserting a finger into the rectum, and introduces the biopsy needle into a prostate lobe.
• The needle is rotated gently, pulled out about ¼″ (5 mm), and reinserted at another angle.
• The procedure is repeated at several areas.
• Specimens are placed immediately in a labeled specimen bottle containing 10% formaldehyde solution.
• Pressure is exerted on the puncture site, which is then bandaged.

Transrectal approach (this approach may be performed on outpatients without an anesthetic):
• Place the patient in a left lateral position.
• A curved needle guide is attached to the finger palpating the rectum.
• The biopsy needle is pushed along the guide, into the prostate. As the needle enters the prostate, the patient may experience pain.
• The needle is rotated to cut off the tissue, and then is withdrawn.
• The specimen is placed immediately in a labeled specimen bottle containing 10% formaldehyde solution.

Transurethral approach:
• An endoscopic instrument is passed through the urethra, permitting direct viewing of the prostate and passage of a cutting loop.

• The loop is rotated to chip away pieces of tissue, and is then withdrawn.

• The specimen is placed immediately in a labeled specimen bottle containing 10% formaldehyde solution.

Patient care checklist

Before the test

☑ Explain or clarify test purpose and procedure.

☑ Tell the patient that he will receive a local anesthetic (unless the transrectal approach is used) and that he must remain still during the procedure and follow instructions.

☑ Evaluate patient understanding.

☑ For a transrectal approach, prepare the bowel by administering enemas until the return is clear. As ordered, administer an antibacterial to minimize the risk of infection.

☑ Check patient history for hypersensitivity to the anesthetic.

☑ Make sure that the patient or a responsible family member has signed the consent form.

☑ Just before the biopsy, check vital signs and administer a sedative, as ordered.

After the test

☑ Monitor vital signs, as ordered.

☑ Observe the biopsy site for a hematoma and for signs of infection, such as redness, swelling, and pain.

☑ Watch for complications of urinary retention or frequency, or hematuria.

Interfering factors

• Failure to obtain an adequate tissue specimen.

• Failure to place the specimen in formaldehyde solution.

Renal biopsy (percutaneous)

Purpose

• To aid diagnosis of renal parenchymal disease

• To monitor progression of renal disease and to assess the effectiveness of treatment.

Normal results

A section of kidney tissue shows Bowman's capsule (the area between two layers of flat epithelial cells), the glomerular tuft, and the capillary lumen. The tubule sections differ depending on the area of tubule involved. The proximal tubule is one layer of epithelial cells with microvilli that form a brush border. The descending Henle's loop has flat squamous epithelial cells, unlike the ascending, distal convoluted, and collecting tubules, which are lined with squamous epithelial cells.

Abnormal results

Histologic examination can reveal:
  Wilms' tumor
  Renal cell carcinoma
  Disseminated lupus erythematosus
  Amyloid infiltration
  Acute and chronic glomerulonephritis
  Renal vein thrombosis
  Pyelonephritis.

The basics

Percutaneous renal biopsy is the needle excision of a core of kidney tissue to obtain a specimen for histologic examination, using light, electron, and immunofluorescent microscopy. Such examination provides valuable information about glomerular and tubular function. Acute and chronic glomerulonephritis, pyelonephritis, renal vein thrombosis, amyloid infiltration, and systemic lupus erythematosus produce characteristic histologic changes in the kidneys.

Complications of percutaneous biopsy include bleeding, hematoma, arteriovenous fistula, and infection. Despite the risk of these complications, this procedure is considered safer than open biopsy, which is usually the preferred method for removing a tissue specimen from a solid lesion. However, more recent noninvasive procedures, especially renal ultrasonography and computed tomography scan, have replaced percutaneous renal biopsy in many hospitals. Urine cytology (see below) and urinary tract brush biopsies (see next page) are also performed to evaluate urinary tract pathology.

Contraindications to this test include: renal tumors, severe bleeding disorders, markedly reduced plasma or blood volume, severe hypertension, hydronephrosis, perinephric abscess, advanced renal failure with uremia, or the presence of only one kidney.

Procedure

• Place the patient in a prone position on a firm surface, with a sandbag beneath his abdomen.

• Tell him to take deep breaths while his kidney is being palpated.

• Instruct the patient to hold his breath

Urine Cytology

Epithelial cells line the urinary tract and exfoliate easily into the urine, so a simple cytologic examination of these cells can aid diagnosis of urinary tract disease. Although urine cytology is not done routinely, it is particularly useful for detecting cancer and inflammatory diseases of the renal pelvis, ureters, bladder, and urethra. In fact, it is especially useful for detecting bladder cancer in high-risk groups, such as smokers, people who work with aniline dyes, and patients who have received treatment for bladder cancer. Urine cytology can also determine whether bladder lesions that appear on X-rays are benign or malignant. This test can also detect cytomegalovirus infection and other viral diseases.

To perform the test, the patient must collect a 100 to 300 ml clean-catch urine specimen 3 hours after his last voiding. (He should not use the first-voided specimen of the morning.) Then the urine specimen is sent to the cytology laboratory immediately so that it can be examined before the cells begin to degenerate.

The specimen is prepared in one of the following ways and stained with Papanicolaou stain:

• *Centrifuge:* After the urine is spun down, sediment is smeared on a slide and stained for examination.

• *Filter:* Urine is poured through a filter, which traps the cells so that they can be stained and examined directly.

• *Cytocentrifuge:* After the urine is centrifuged, the sediment is resuspended and placed on slides, which are spun in a cytocentrifuge and stained for examination.

Normal urine is relatively free of cellular debris but should have some epithelial and squamous cells that appear normal under a microscope. Identification of malignant cells or any other signs of malignancy may indicate cancer of the kidney, renal pelvis, ureters, bladder, or urethra. It could also indicate a metastatic tumor. An overgrowth of epithelial cells, an excess of red blood cells, or the presence of leukocytes or atypical cells may indicate a lower urinary tract inflammation, which can result from prostatic hyperplasia, urinary calculi, bladder diverticula, strictures, or malformations. Large intranuclear inclusions may indicate a cytomegalovirus infection, which usually affects the renal tubular epithelium. This viral infection generally occurs in cancer patients undergoing chemotherapy and transplant patients receiving immunosupressive drugs. Cytoplasmic inclusion bodies may also indicate measles and may precede the characteristic Koplik's spots.

Urinary Tract Brush Biopsy

Retrograde brush biopsy of the urinary tract may be used to obtain a renal tissue specimen when X-rays show a lesion in the renal pelvis or calyx. It can also be used to obtain specimens from other areas of the urinary tract. However, retrograde brush biopsy is contra-indicated in patients with acute urinary tract infection or an obstruction at or below the biopsy site.

To prepare the patient for brush biopsy, describe the procedure and tell him he may feel some discomfort. Inform him who will perform the biopsy and when. The procedure will take 30 to 60 minutes.

Make sure the patient or a responsible family member has signed an appropriate consent form. Because this procedure requires use of a contrast agent and general, local, or spinal anesthesia, check the patient's history for hypersensitivity to anesthetics, contrast media, or iodine-containing foods, such as shellfish. Just before the biopsy procedure, administer a sedative to the patient, as ordered.

After the patient has received a sedative and an anesthetic, place him in the lithotomy position. Using a cystoscope, the physician passes a guide wire up the ureter and passes a urethral catheter over the guide wire. Contrast medium is instilled through the catheter, which is positioned next to the lesion under fluoroscopic guidance. The contrast medium is washed out with normal saline solution to prevent cell distortions from the dye. A nylon or steel brush is passed up the catheter and the lesion is brushed. This procedure is repeated at least six times, using a new brush each time.

As each brush is removed from the catheter, a smear is made for Papanicolaou staining and the brush tip is cut off and placed in formalin for 1 hour. The biopsy material is then removed from the brush tip for histologic examination. When the last brush is withdrawn, the catheter is irrigated with normal saline solution to remove additional cells. These cells are also sent for histologic examination.

Results differentiate between malignant and benign lesions, which may appear the same on X-rays.

Because brush biopsy may cause such complications as perforation, hemorrhage, sepsis, or contrast medium extravasation, carefully monitor the patient's vital signs. Be sure to record the time, color, and amount of voiding, being alert for hematuria and abdominal or flank pain. Report any abnormal findings to the physician immediately, and administer analgesics and antibiotics, as ordered.

and remain immobile as the 7″ 20G needle is inserted into the skin and down to the kidney capsule.
• After the needle is inserted, tell the patient to take several deep breaths. If the needle swings smoothly during deep breathing, it has penetrated the kidney capsule.
• After the penetration depth is marked on the needle shaft, instruct the patient to hold his breath and re-

main as still as possible while the needle is withdrawn, injecting the local anesthetic into the back tissues.
• After a small incision is made in the anesthetized skin, instruct the patient to hold his breath and remain immobile while the Vim-Silverman needle with stylet is inserted through the incision, down the tract of the infiltrating needle, to the measured depth.

• Tell the patient to breathe deeply. If the characteristic needle swing occurs, instruct the patient to hold his breath and remain still while the tissue specimen is obtained.
• After the tissue is examined immediately under a hand lens to ensure that the specimen contains tissue from both cortex and medulla, the tissue is placed on a saline-soaked gauze pad and placed in a properly labeled container.
• If an inadequate tissue specimen has been obtained, the procedure is repeated immediately.
• After an adequate specimen is secured, pressure is applied to the biopsy site for 3 to 5 minutes to stop superficial bleeding. Then a pressure dressing is applied.

Special precautions
CLINICAL ALERT: **The patient must hold his breath and remain still whenever the needle or prongs are advanced into or retracted from the kidney.**

Patient care checklist
Before the test
☑ Explain or clarify test purpose, preparation, and procedure.
☑ Tell the patient that he will receive a local anesthetic but may experience a pinching pain when the needle is inserted through his back into his kidney.
☑ Evaluate patient understanding.
☑ Make sure that the patient or a responsible family member has signed a consent form.
☑ Check patient history for hypersensitivity to the local anesthetic.
☑ As ordered, 30 minutes to 1 hour before the biopsy administer a mild sedative to help the patient relax.
☑ Check vital signs and tell the patient to void just before the test.
After the test
☑ Monitor vital signs, as ordered.
☑ Instruct the patient to lie flat on his back without moving for at least 12 hours to prevent bleeding.

☑ Examine all urine for blood; small amounts may be present after biopsy but should disappear within 8 hours. Occasionally, hematocrit may be monitored after the procedure, to screen for internal bleeding.
☑ Encourage fluids, to initiate mild diuresis, which minimizes colic and obstruction from blood clotting within the renal pelvis.

Interfering factors
• Failure to obtain an adequate tissue specimen.
• Failure to store the specimen properly.
• Failure to send the specimen to the laboratory immediately.

Sex chromatin tests

Purpose
• To screen quickly for abnormal sexual development (both X and Y chromatin tests)
• To aid assessment of an infant with ambiguous genitalia (X chromatin test only)
• To determine the number of Y chromosomes in an individual (Y chromatin test only).

Normal results
A normal female (XX) has only one X chromatin mass (the number of X chromatin masses discernible is one less than the number of X chromosomes in the cells examined). For various reasons, an X chromatin mass is ordinarily discernible in only 20% to 50% of the buccal mucosal cells of a normal female. A normal male (XY) has only one Y chromatin mass (the number of Y chromatin masses equals the number of Y chromosomes in the cells examined).

Abnormal results
See *Sex Chromosome Anomalies*, pp. 452 to 453.

The basics

Although sex chromatin tests can screen for abnormalities in the number of sex chromosomes, they have been largely replaced by the full karyotype (chromosome analysis) test, which is faster, simpler, and more accurate. Sex chromatin tests are usually indicated for abnormal sexual development, ambiguous genitalia, amenorrhea, and suspected chromosomal abnormalities.

After the cause of chromosomal abnormal sexual development has been identified, the patient or his parents require genetic counseling. If a child is phenotypically of one sex and genotypically of the other, a team of doctors, psychologists, psychiatrists, and possibly educators must decide the child's sex. This careful evaluation should be made early to prevent developmental problems related to incorrect gender identification. The laboratory usually requires as long as 4 weeks to complete the analysis.

Procedure

• Scrape the buccal mucosa firmly with a wooden or metal spatula at least twice to obtain an adequate specimen. (Vaginal mucosa is occasionally used in young women.)
• Rub the spatula over the glass slide, making sure the cells are evenly distributed.
• Spray the slide with cell fixative, or place it in a container with a preservative, and send the slide to the laboratory with a brief patient history and indications for the test.

Special precautions

Make sure that the buccal mucosa is scraped firmly to ensure a sufficient number of cells. Check that the specimen is not saliva, which contains no cells.

Patient care checklist

Before the test
☑ Explain or clarify test purpose and procedure.

☑ Evaluate patient/parent understanding.

Interfering factors

• Obtaining saliva instead of buccal cells provides a false specimen.
• Failure to apply cell fixative to the slide allows cells to deteriorate.

Skin biopsy

Purpose

• To provide differential diagnosis among basal cell carcinoma, squamous cell carcinoma, malignant melanoma, and benign growths
• To diagnose chronic bacterial or fungal skin infections
• To aid in the diagnosis or treatment of systemic lupus erythematosus
• To aid in the diagnosis of blistering skin disorders and vasculitis.

Normal results

Healthy skin consists of squamous epithelium (epidermis) and fibrous connective tissue (dermis).

Abnormal results

Benign lesions include:
 Cysts
 Seborrheic keratoses
 Warts
 Pigmented nevi (moles)
 Keloids
 Dermatofibromas
 Multiple neurofibromas.
Malignant lesions include:
 Basal cell carcinoma
 Squamous cell carcinoma
 Malignant melanoma.
Cutaneous immunofluorescence testing may reveal:
 Lupus erythematosus lesions
 Pemphigus
 Pemphigoid
 Vasculitis.
Cultures can detect:
 Chronic bacterial infections
 Chronic fungal infections.

The basics

Skin biopsy is the removal of a small piece of tissue, under local anesthesia, from a lesion suspected of malignancy or other dermatoses. A specimen for histologic examination may be secured by one of three techniques—shave, punch, or excision. A shave biopsy cuts the lesion at the skin line and, since it leaves the lower layers of dermis intact, permits further biopsy at the site. The punch biopsy removes an oval core from the center of a lesion. Excision biopsy, the procedure of choice, removes the entire lesion and is indicated for rapidly expanding lesions; for sclerotic, bullous, or atrophic lesions; and for examination of the border of a lesion and the surrounding skin.

Lesions suspected of harboring malignancy usually have changed color, size, or appearance, or have failed to heal properly after injury. Since fully developed lesions provide more diagnostic information than those that are resolving or in early developing stages, whenever possible such full-blown lesions should be selected for biopsy. For example, if the skin shows blisters, biopsy should include the most mature ones. Test results are usually available in 1 day.

Procedure

• Position the patient comfortably, and cleanse the biopsy site. The local anesthetic is then administered.

Shave biopsy:
• The protruding growth is cut off at the skin line.
• The tissue is placed immediately in a properly labeled specimen bottle containing 10% formaldehyde solution.
• Pressure is applied to the area to stop the bleeding.

Punch biopsy:
• The skin surrounding the lesion is pulled taut, and the punch is firmly introduced into the lesion and is rotated to obtain a tissue specimen.
• The plug is lifted with forceps or a needle and is severed as deeply into the fat layer as possible.
• The specimen is placed in a properly labeled specimen bottle containing 10% formaldehyde solution, or in a sterile container, if indicated.
• The wound is closed with sutures if necessary, and a dressing is applied.

Excision biopsy:
• An incision is made as wide and as deep as necessary.
• The tissue specimen is removed and placed immediately in a properly labeled specimen bottle containing 10% formaldehyde solution.
• Pressure is applied to the site to stop the bleeding.
• The wound is sutured closed, and a dressing is applied.

Patient care checklist

Before the test
☑ Explain or clarify test purpose and procedure.
☑ Tell the patient that he will receive a local anesthetic to minimize pain during the procedure.
☑ Evaluate patient understanding.
☑ Check patient history for hypersensitivity to the local anesthetic.
☑ Make sure that the patient or a responsible family member has signed a consent form.

After the test
☑ Check the biopsy site for bleeding.
☑ If the patient experiences pain at the biopsy site, administer medication, as ordered.
☑ Advise the patient with sutures to keep the area clean and as dry as possible. Tell him that facial sutures will be removed in 3 to 5 days; trunk sutures, in 7 to 14 days. Instruct the patient with adhesive strips to leave them in place for 14 to 21 days.

Interfering factors

• Failure to use the appropriate fixative.
• Failure to use a sterile container when it is indicated.

Small-bowel biopsy

Purpose
To help diagnose diseases of the small bowel.

Normal results
A normal small-bowel biopsy sample consists of fingerlike villi, crypts, columnar epithelial cells, and round cells.

Abnormal results
Histologic changes may indicate:
   Whipple's disease
   Abetalipoproteinemia
   Lymphoma
   Lymphangiectasia
   Eosinophilic enteritis
   Giardiasis
   Coccidiosis.
Histologic changes may suggest:
   Celiac sprue
   Tropical sprue
   Infectious gastroenteritis
   Intraluminal bacterial overgrowth
   Folate and B_{12} deficiency
   Radiation enteritis
   Malnutrition.

The basics
Small-bowel biopsy helps evaluate diseases of the intestinal mucosa, which may cause malabsorption or diarrhea. Using a capsule, it produces larger specimens than does endoscopic biopsy (see *Endoscopic Biopsy of the GI Tract*, p. 470) and allows removal of tissue from those areas beyond an endoscope's reach.

The biopsy sample verifies diagnosis of some diseases, such as Whipple's disease; it may help confirm others, such as tropical sprue. Capsule biopsy is an invasive procedure, but it causes little pain and complications are rare.

Contraindications to this test include: uncooperative patients, those taking aspirin or anticoagulants, and those with uncontrolled coagulation disorders.

Procedure
• Check the tubing and the mercury bag for leaks.
• Lightly lubricate the tube and the capsule with a water-soluble lubricant, and moisten the mercury bag with water.
• The back of the patient's throat is sprayed with a local anesthetic to decrease gagging during passage of the tube.
• Assist the patient to a sitting position.
• The capsule is placed in the patient's pharynx, and he is asked to flex his neck and swallow as the doctor advances the tube about 20″ (50 cm).
• Assist the patient onto his right side, after which the tube is advanced into his stomach, through the pylorus, and into the small bowel.
• Assist the patient to a supine position.
• The capsule is used to obtain a tissue specimen, and is then removed.
• The capsule is opened and the specimen is gently removed with forceps, placed mucosal side up on a piece of mesh, and placed in a biopsy bottle with required fixative.

Special precautions
• Keep suction equipment nearby to prevent aspiration if the patient vomits.
• Tell the patient not to bite down on the tubing. This creates a suction, which closes the capsule. When the capsule closes, tissue is grabbed.

Patient care checklist
Before the test
☑ Explain or clarify test purpose, preparation, and procedure.
☑ Evaluate patient understanding.
☑ Restrict food and fluids for at least 8 hours before the test.
☑ Ensure that coagulation tests have been performed and that the results are recorded on the patient's chart.
☑ Make sure that the patient or a responsible family member has signed the consent form.

Endoscopic Biopsy of the GI Tract

Endoscopy allows direct visualization of the GI tract and any site that requires biopsy of tissue samples for histologic analysis. This relatively painless procedure helps detect, support diagnosis of, or monitor GI tract disorders. Its complications, notably hemorrhage, perforation, and aspiration, are rare.

Careful patient preparation is vital for this procedure. Describe the procedure to the patient and reassure him that he will be able to breathe with the endoscope in place. Tell him to fast for at least 8 hours before the procedure. (For lower GI biopsy, cleanse the bowel, as ordered.) Make sure the patient or a responsible family member has signed a consent form.

Just before the procedure, sedate the patient, as ordered. He should be relaxed but not asleep, because his cooperation promotes smooth passage of the endoscope. Spray the back of his throat with a local anesthetic, to suppress his gag reflex. Have suction equipment and bipolar cauterizing electrodes available, to prevent aspiration and excessive bleeding.

After the physician passes the endoscope into the upper or lower GI tract and visualizes a lesion, node, or other abnormal area, he pushes a biopsy forceps through a channel in the endoscope until this, too, can be seen. Then he opens the forceps, positions them at the biopsy site, and closes them on the tissue. The closed forceps and tissue sample are removed from the endoscope, and the tissue is taken from the forceps. The specimen is placed mucosal side up on fine mesh gauze or filter paper and then placed in a labeled biopsy bottle containing fixative. When all samples have been collected, the endoscope is removed. Samples are sent to the laboratory immediately.

Endoscopic biopsy of the GI tract can diagnose cancer, lymphoma, amyloidosis, candidiasis, and gastric ulcers; support diagnosis of Crohn's disease, chronic ulcerative colitis, gastritis, esophagitis, and melanosis coli in laxative abuse; and monitor progression of Barrett's esophagus, multiple gastric polyps, colon cancer and polyps, and chronic ulcerative colitis.

After the test
☑ Diet may be resumed after gag reflex returns.

☑ Complications are rare. However, watch for signs of hemorrhage, bacteremia with transient fever and pain, and bowel perforation. Tell the patient to report abdominal pain or bleeding.

Interfering factors
• Incorrect handling or positioning of the specimen can alter test results.
• Failure to fast before the biopsy may yield a poor specimen or cause vomiting and aspiration.
• Failure to place the specimen in fixative will affect test results.

• Delay in transport of the specimen will affect test results.

Synovial membrane biopsy

Purpose
• To diagnose gout, pseudogout, bacterial infections and lesions, and granulomatous infections
• To aid diagnosis of rheumatoid arthritis, systemic lupus erythematosus (SLE), or Reiter's disease, and to monitor joint pathology.

Normal results

The synovial membrane contains cells identical to those found in other connective tissue. The membrane surface is relatively smooth, except for villi, folds, and fat pads that project into the joint cavity. The membrane tissue produces synovial fluid, and contains a capillary network, lymphatic vessels, and a few nerve fibers. Pathology of the synovial membrane also affects the cellular composition of the synovial fluid.

Abnormal results

Histologic examination of synovial tissue can diagnose:

Coccidioidomycosis
Gout
Pseudogout
Hemochromatosis
Tuberculosis
Sarcoidosis
Amyloidosis
Pigmented villonodular synovitis
Synovial tumors
Synovial malignancy.

Histologic examination can aid diagnosis of:

Rheumatoid arthritis
SLE
Reiter's disease.

The basics

Biopsy of the synovial membrane is the needle excision of a tissue specimen for histologic examination of the thin epithelium lining the diarthrodial joint capsules. In a large joint, such as the knee, preliminary arthroscopy can aid selection of the biopsy site. Synovial membrane biopsy is performed when analysis of synovial fluid proves nondiagnostic or when the fluid itself is absent.

Test results are usually available in 1 or 2 days. Complications include infection and bleeding into the joint, but these are rare.

Procedure

• Assist the patient to a comfortable position, and provide support for the joint to be biopsied.

• After the local anesthetic is injected into the joint space, a trocar is forcefully thrust into the joint space.

• The biopsy needle is inserted through a trocar and is twisted to cut off a tissue segment.

• The biopsy needle is withdrawn, and the specimen is placed in a properly labeled sterile container or a specimen bottle containing absolute ethyl alcohol, as indicated.

• By changing the angle of the biopsy needle, several specimens can be obtained without reinserting the trocar.

• The trocar is then removed, the biopsy site is cleaned, and a pressure bandage is applied.

Patient care checklist

Before the test

☑ Explain or clarify test purpose and procedure.

☑ Tell the patient that he will receive a local anesthetic to minimize discomfort, but he will experience transient pain when the needle enters the joint.

☑ Tell him which site—knee (most common), shoulder, elbow, wrist, or ankle—has been chosen for this biopsy (usually, the most symptomatic joint is selected).

☑ Evaluate patient understanding.

☑ Make sure that the patient or a responsible family member has signed the consent form.

☑ Check patient history for hypersensitivity to the local anesthetic.

After the test

☑ Observe the joint for swelling and tenderness, which are signs of bleeding into the joint.

☑ Administer analgesics, as ordered, if the patient experiences pain at the biopsy site.

☑ Instruct the patient to rest the joint from which the tissue specimen was removed for 1 day before resuming normal activity.

Interfering factors
• Failure to obtain several biopsy specimens.
• Failure to obtain these specimens away from the infiltration site of the anesthetic.
• Failure to store the specimens in the appropriate solution.
• Failure to send the tissue specimen to the laboratory immediately.

Thyroid biopsy

Purpose
• To differentiate between benign and malignant thyroid disease
• To help diagnose Hashimoto's thyroiditis, subacute granulomatous thyroiditis, hyperthyroidism, and nontoxic nodular goiter.

Normal results
Histologic examination of healthy tissue shows fibrous networks dividing the gland into pseudolobules that include follicles and capillaries. Cuboidal epithelium lines the follicle walls and contains the protein thyroglobulin, which stores serum triiodothyronine (T_3) and serum thyroxine (T_4).

Abnormal results
Malignant tumors appear as well-encapsulated, solitary nodules of uniform but not abnormal structure. Papillary carcinoma is the most common thyroid malignancy. Follicular carcinoma, a less common form, strongly resembles normal cells.

Benign tumors—such as nontoxic nodular goiter—demonstrate hypertrophy, hyperplasia, and hypervascularity. Distinct histologic patterns characterize subacute granulomatous thyroiditis, Hashimoto's thyroiditis, and hyperthyroidism.

Since thyroid malignancies are frequently multicentric and small, a negative histologic report does not rule out malignancy.

The basics
Thyroid biopsy is the excision of a thyroid tissue specimen for histologic examination. This procedure is indicated in patients with thyroid enlargement (even if T_3 and T_4 levels are normal), breathing and swallowing difficulties, vocal cord paralysis, weight loss, hemoptysis, and a sensation of fullness in the neck. It is commonly performed when noninvasive tests, such as thyroid ultrasonography and scans, are abnormal or inconclusive.

Thyroid tissue may be obtained with a hollow needle, under local anesthesia, or during open (surgical) biopsy, under general anesthesia. Open biopsy, performed in the operating room, is obviously more complex and provides more accurate information than needle biopsy. In open biopsy, the surgeon obtains a tissue specimen from the exposed thyroid and sends it to the histology laboratory for rapid analysis. This method also permits direct examination and immediate excision of suspicious thyroid tissue.

Coagulation studies should always precede thyroid biopsy, since bleeding may persist in a patient with abnormal prothrombin time or abnormal activated partial thromboplastin time.

Procedure
• For needle biopsy, place the patient in a supine position, with a pillow under his shoulder blades. (This position pushes the trachea and thyroid forward and allows the neck veins to fall backward.)
• Prepare the skin over the biopsy site.
• As the examiner prepares to inject the local anesthetic, warn the patient not to swallow.
• After the anesthetic is injected, the biopsy needle is inserted into the thyroid gland.
• After the specimen is obtained, the needle is removed and the specimen is placed immediately in formaldehyde.
• Apply pressure to the biopsy site to stop bleeding. If bleeding continues for

more than a few minutes, press on the site for up to an additional 15 minutes.
• Apply an adhesive bandage.

Patient care checklist
Before the test

☑ Explain or clarify test purpose and procedure.

☑ Tell the patient that he will receive a local anesthetic to minimize pain during the procedure, but that he may experience some pressure when the tissue specimen is procured.

☑ Advise him that he may have a sore throat the day after the test.

☑ Evaluate patient understanding.

☑ If the patient is to receive general anesthesia, restrict food and fluids as ordered.

☑ Make sure that the patient or a responsible family member has signed the consent form.

☑ Check patient history for hypersensitivity to the local anesthetic.

☑ Administer a sedative to the patient

15 minutes before the biopsy, as ordered.

After the test

☑ To make the patient more comfortable, place him in semi-Fowler's position. Tell him that he may avoid undue strain on the biopsy site by putting both hands behind his neck when he sits up.

CLINICAL ALERT: Watch for signs of bleeding, tenderness, or redness at the biopsy site. Observe for difficult breathing due to edema or hematoma, with resultant tracheal collapse. Also check the back of the neck and the patient's pillow for bleeding, every hour for 8 hours. Report bleeding immediately.

Interfering factors
• Failure to obtain a representative tissue specimen.
• Failure to place the specimen in formaldehyde solution.

Selected References

Arndt, Kenneth A. *Manual of Dermatologic Therapeutics,* 2nd ed. Boston: Little, Brown and Co., 1978.

Berkow, Robert, ed. *The Merck Manual of Diagnosis and Therapy,* 14th ed. Rahway, N.J.: Merck Sharp & Dohme, 1982.

Brunner, Lillian S., and Suddarth, Doris S. *Textbook of Medical-Surgical Nursing,* 5th ed. Philadelphia, J.B. Lippincott Co., 1984.

Conn, Rex B., ed. *Current Diagnosis,* 7th ed. Philadelphia: W.B. Saunders Co., 1985.

Diagnostics, 2nd ed. Nurse's Reference Library. Springhouse, Pa.: Springhouse Corp., 1986.

Diseases, 2nd ed. Nurse's Reference Library. Springhouse, Pa.: Springhouse Corp., 1987.

Fischbach, Frances. *A Manual of Laboratory Diagnostic Tests,* 2nd ed. Philadelphia: J.B. Lippincott Co., 1984.

Harvey, A. McGehee, ed. *The Principles and Practice of Medicine,* 21st ed. East Norwalk, Conn.: Appleton-Century-Crofts, 1984.

Henry, John Bernard, ed. *Todd-Sanford-Davidsohn Clinical Diagnosis and Management by Laboratory Methods,* 17th ed. Philadelphia: W.B. Saunders Co., 1984.

Kee, Joyce LeFever. *Laboratory and Diagnostic Tests with Nursing Implications.* East Norwalk, Conn.: Appleton-Century-Crofts, 1983.

Markus, Susan. "Taking the Fear Out of Bone Marrow Examinations," *Nursing81* 11:64-67, April 1981.

Neoplastic Disorders. Nurse's Clinical Library. Springhouse, Pa.: Springhouse Corp., 1985.

Pagana, Kathleen D., and Pagana, Timothy James. *Diagnostic Testing and Nursing Implications,* 2nd ed. St. Louis: C.V. Mosby Co., 1986.

Petersdorf, Robert G., and Adams, Raymond D., eds. *Harrison's Principles of Internal Medicine,* 10th ed. New York: McGraw-Hill Book Co., 1983.

Price, Sylvia, and Wilson, Lorraine. *Pathophysiology: Clinical Concepts of Disease Processes,* 2nd ed. New

York: McGraw-Hill Book Co., 1982.

Sabiston, D.C., Jr., ed. *Davis-Christopher Textbook of Surgery: The Biological Basis of Modern Surgical Practice,* 12th ed. Philadelphia: W.B. Saunders Co., 1981.

Sheehan, Dezna C., and Hrapchak, Barbara B. *Theory and Practice of Histotechnology,* 2nd ed. St. Louis: C.V. Mosby Co., 1980.

Tannebaum, Myron, ed. *Urologic Pathology: The Prostate.* Philadelphia: Lea & Febiger, 1977.

Tilkian, Sarko M., et al. *Clinical Implications of Laboratory Tests,* 3rd ed. St. Louis: C.V. Mosby Co., 1983.

Wyngaarden, James, and Smith, Lloyd. *Cecil Textbook of Medicine,* 16th ed. Philadelphia: W.B. Saunders Co., 1982.

10 RADIOGRAPHIC TESTING

Introduction

A means of visualizing bony and soft tissues of the body, radiographic (X-ray) testing is one of the best aids to diagnosis available today. X-rays are produced when high-voltage electrons strike a tungsten or molybdenum target in an X-ray tube. When these X-rays pass through a patient's body, they are attenuated (partially absorbed) before exposing the underlying X-ray film. For example, bone is dense and absorbs more X-rays than bowel gas. Therefore, the part of the film underneath bone will be less exposed and, thus, will appear *white*. In contradistinction, the parts of the film underneath the bowel gas will be relatively more exposed and will appear *black*. Those body parts (such as muscle) of intermediate density will appear as shades of *gray*. After the exposure is made, the film is developed and then interpreted by the radiologist. Barium and iodinated contrast materials are used in various diagnostic radiologic procedures to show anatomic detail of certain structures. (See *General Types of Radiographic Procedures*, pp. 476 to 477, and *Lixi Imaging Scope*, p. 478.)

Use of contrast media

Contrast media are necessary when diagnosis requires visualization of details of body cavities not visible on plain X-ray films. They include materials that change the radiopacity of one body part in comparison with surrounding parts, thus permitting better visualization.

Barium, an inert material, is used to fill and examine all parts of the GI tract. It is contraindicated when bowel perforation is present or suspected, since it may cause peritonitis if extravasation occurs.

Gastrografin is a liquid, water-soluble, iodinated contrast material used to examine the GI tract when bowel perforation is suspected, since it will not result in peritonitis. Another use of Gastrografin is to fill the GI tract during body CT scans, in order to clearly demarcate its position. Gastrografin is contraindicated in patients who may aspirate, since it causes pulmonary edema when it comes in contact with the lower respiratory tree.

Telepaque (iopanoic acid) is ingested in order to opacify the gallbladder for oral cholecystography. This iodinated contrast agent is absorbed through the bowel, processed by the liver, and excreted into the biliary tree. Some patients may develop transient nausea and vomiting after ingestion.

Myelographic contrast, either iophendylate (Pantopaque), which is oil-based, or metrizamide, which is water-soluble, is injected into the subarachnoid cerebrospinal fluid space bathing the spinal cord and nerve roots (within the thecal sac) in order to define abnormalities of these structures: examples include herniated intervertebral disks, metastatic disease in and around the spinal cord, and primary

General Types of Radiographic Procedures

Type	Explanation
Plain films	Radiographs of bones and soft tissue structures without the use of contrast materials
Fluoroscopy	Continuous X-ray visualization of body parts
Tomography	Thin section radiography produced by moving the film and X-ray tube simultaneously and in opposite directions in order to blur out structures anterior and posterior to the area of interest
Computed Tomography	Thin section axial tomography performed with computer assistance. 1) Cranial CT—examination of skull and brain, 2) Spinal CT—examination of disorders of spine and spinal cord, 3) Body CT—examination of neck, thorax, abdomen, and extremities
Cineradiography	Continuous moving picture X-ray filming of structures
Angiography	Study of blood vessels of the body
Digital subtraction angiography	Computer assisted angiography

Contrast Agents Used	Uses & Advantages	Disadvantages
None	For routine and general survey purposes	
All types may be employed during various fluoroscopy procedures	Allows dynamic visualization of body parts and contrast agents within them during procedures	Higher radiation dose than plain films
Only during intravenous pyelography	Permits clearer visualization of thin sections of certain structures by blurring out interfering structural shadows. (Examples: evaluates complex facial and spinal fractures, bone tumors or osteomyelitis, and masses and calculi during IVU in renal tomography)	Higher radiation dose than plain films
Intravenous contrast may be used to examine vasculature. Gastrografin or dilute barium may be used to delineate GI tract.	Excellent for examining soft tissues and bones of body	Possibility of contrast reaction
Intravascular contrast	Dynamic visualization of structural and functional abnormalities of a structure. Example: Coronary artery catherization.	Higher radiation dose than plain films. Possibility of contrast reaction.
Intraarterial or intravenous contrast	Demonstrates tumors, infarcts, aneurysms, vascular injury, thrombosis, stenoses, arteriovenous malformations, arteriovenous fistula	Radiation dose during fluoroscopy. Possibility of contrast reaction.
Intraarterial or intravenous contrast	Generally, lower amount of contrast given to patient	Increased radiation dose during fluoroscopy. Possibility of contrast reaction. Generally lower resolution and more artifacts than in conventional angiography.

Lixi Imaging Scope

The first completely portable X-ray machine, called the Lixi Imaging Scope, can provide X-rays on the spot. It is hand-held, emits less than one millirad (mrad) of radiation per second, and can X-ray a 2″ area of the body.

It helps diagnose athletic injuries, such as fractured wrists or ankles, right on the field. It can also help surgeons insert catheters and position pins, and screen auto accident victims, helping to ensure that they are safely removed from their vehicles. A camera can be attached to permanently record each X-ray.

spinal cord tumors. Arachnoiditis (an inflammation of the meninges) can occur following myelography.

Cystografin is used to distend the bladder and examine it and the urethra during full and voiding states.

Sinografin (diatrizoate meglumine and iodipamide meglumine) is used during hysterosalpingography to fill and examine the female genital tract.

Intravenous/intraarterial contrast (includes different concentrations of diatrizoate meglumine, diatrizoate sodium, iothalamate meglumine, ioxaglate meglumine, and ioxaglate sodium) is used during angiography to examine arteriovenous anatomy for abnormalities. Allergic reactions, cardiotoxicity, and nephrotoxicity may occur following administration.

Intravenous contrast during intravenous urography (IVU) is filtered by the kidneys and excreted into the urinary collecting system, thus defining its anatomy and abnormalities. Diatrizoate meglumine and/or diatrizoate sodium are commonly used agents. Adverse reactions include allergic reactions, cardiotoxicity, and nephrotoxicity.

Contrast reactions

A contrast reaction refers to any allergic or cytotoxic reaction following administration of iodinated contrast agents. The risk is greatest with intravenous and intraarterial injections, and in patients with an allergic history.

Anaphylaxis is a systemic hypersensitivity reaction to a sensitizing substance—in this case, contrast media. The reaction may be mild to severe and can quickly become a medical emergency leading to respiratory failure, hypovolemic shock, and sudden death. Therefore, prompt recognition of signs and symptoms, and immediate treatment, are essential. (See *Pathway of Anaphylaxis,* and *Drugs Used to Reverse Anaphylaxis,* pp. 480 to 481.)

If the patient has a history of known hypersensitivity to contrast, and its use is essential, prophylaxis is carried out. Measures include:

—*hydrocortisone* (Solu-Cortef), or its equivalent in other forms of corticosteroids, 100 mg P.O. or I.V. at least 12 hours prior to contrast injection

—*diphenhydramine* (Benadryl), antihistamine, 25 mg P.O. approximately 1 hour before contrast injection (There is controversy as to whether this premedication is efficacious.)

—*resuscitative equipment* available in case significant contrast reaction occurs.

Organ toxicity refers to direct cytotoxicity resulting from the use of iodinated contrast agents:

In *nephrotoxicity,* contrast-induced acute tubular necrosis and/or acute tubular obstruction can result in oliguria or anuria with or without azotemia. Patients with multiple myeloma, diabetic nephropathy, or preexisting renal failure are at greatest risk. Adequate hydration is the best preventative measure in patients of this type. Hemodialysis or peritoneal dialysis may be required as an adjunctive therapy to clear contrast from the blood in patients with poor renal function.

In *cardiotoxicity,* high doses and bolus injections of contrast are most likely to induce myocardial ischemia, cardiac arrhythmias, and conduction abnormalities. Patients at risk include those with preexisting myocardial and valvular disease, atherosclerosis, and conduction disturbances. Signs and symptoms include chest pain, syncope, arrhythmias, and cardiac arrest.

In *pulmonary toxicity,* sludging of red cells can occur in the pulmonary capillary bed, resulting in increased pulmonary artery pressure (which could lead to right heart failure) and decreased gas exchange at the alveolar level.

Radiation hazard

All ionizing radiation can be harmful. There are two broad categories of harmful effects:

—*Somatic,* which involves cellular damage to the person irradiated

—*Genetic,* which describes effects harmful to future generations.

The maximum permissible dose for an occupationally exposed individual (e.g., radiologist) is 5 rem/year; the dose limit for the occasionally exposed (e.g., nurse) is 0.5 rem/year; and the dose limit for the general population is 0.17 rem/year. This does not include radiation required for medical purposes for the individual.

The effects of high acute radiation exposure may vary according to the total dose and include immediate cell death (especially GI tract epithelium, white blood cells, and bone marrow), induction of cancer, and death of the individual. Cumulative effects of lower doses of radiation may include genetic mutations, carcinogenesis, and organ dysfunction due to cell death.

Fluoroscopy delivers a higher radiation dose than plain X-ray films, since the radiation output for fluoros-

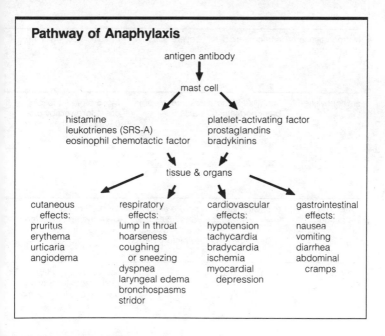

Pathway of Anaphylaxis

antigen antibody

mast cell

histamine
leukotrienes (SRS-A)
eosinophil chemotactic factor

platelet-activating factor
prostaglandins
bradykinins

tissue & organs

cutaneous
effects:
pruritus
erythema
urticaria
angiodema

respiratory
effects:
lump in throat
hoarseness
coughing
or sneezing
dyspnea
laryngeal edema
bronchospasms
stridor

cardiovascular
effects:
hypotension
tachycardia
bradycardia
ischemia
myocardial
depression

gastrointestinal
effects:
nausea
vomiting
diarrhea
abdominal
cramps

Drugs Used To Reverse Anaphylaxis

Drug	Classification	Indication	Dosage
diphenhydra-mine (Benadryl)	antihistamine	mild anaphylaxis	*P.O.:* 25-100 mg t.i.d. *I.M./I.V.:* 25-50 mg q.i.d.
epinephrine (Adrenalin Chloride solution)	adrenergic	*severe anaphylaxis* (drug of choice)	*initial infusion:* 0.2-0.5 mg of epinephrine (0.2-0.5 ml of 1:1,000 strength diluted in 10 ml normal saline) given I.V. slowly over 5-10 min., followed by continuous infusion. *continuous infusion:* 1-4 μg/min. (Mix 1 ml of 1:1,000 epinephrine in 250 ml of D_5W to get concentration of 4 μg/ml.)
hydrocortisone (Solu-Cortef)	corticosteroid	*severe anaphylaxis*	*I.V.:* 100-200 mg q 4-6 hrs.
aminophylline	methylxanthine bronchodilator	*severe anaphylaxis*	*I.V.:* 5-6 mg/kg loading dose, followed by 0.4-0.9 mg/kg/min. infusion
cimetidine (Tagamet)	antihistamine	*severe anaphylaxis* (experimental use in refractory cases)	*I.V.:* 600 mg diluted in D_5W and administered over 20 min.
atropine sulfate	antiarrhythmic		*I.V.:* 0.5 to 1 mg I.V. push; repeat q 5 minutes, to maximum 2 mg.

Action	Special Considerations
• competes with histamine for H_1-receptor sites • prevents laryngeal edema • controls localized itching	• Administer I.V. doses slowly to avoid hypotension. • Monitor patient for hypotension. • Drug causes drowsiness and slows reflexes. • Offer fluids for dry mouth.
alpha-adrenergic effects: • increases blood pressure • reverses peripheral vasodilation and systemic hypotension • decreases angioedema and urticaria • improves coronary blood flow by raising diastolic pressure • causes peripheral vasoconstriction *beta-adrenergic effects:* • causes bronchodilation • causes positive inotropic and chronotropic cardiac activity • decreases synthesis and release of chemical mediator	• Select large vein for infusion. • Use infusion controller to regulate drip. • Check blood pressure and monitor patient for dysrhythmias. • Check solution strength, dosage, and label before administering. • Watch for signs of extravasation at infusion site. • Monitor intake and output. • Assess color and temperature of extremities.
• prevents neutrophil and platelet aggregation • inhibits synthesis of mediators • decreases capillary permeability	• Monitor fluid and electrolyte balance, intake and output, and blood pressure closely. • Maintain patient on ulcer regimen and antacid prophylactically.
• causes bronchodilation • stimulates respiratory drive • dilates constricted pulmonary arteries • causes diuresis • strengthens cardiac contractions • increases vital capacity • causes coronary vasodilation	• Monitor vital signs carefully. • Monitor intake and output, hydration status, and aminophylline and electrolyte levels. • Monitor patient for dysrhythmias. • Use I.V. controller to reduce risk of overdose. • Maintain serum levels at 10-20 µg/ml.
• competes for H_2 histamine receptors • prevents laryngeal edema	• Tagamet is incompatible with aminophylline. • Dose may be reduced for patients with impaired renal or hepatic function.
• blocks the vagal effects on the SA node, relieving nodal or sinus bradycardia and associated hypotension.	• Watch for tachycardia in cardiac patients. • Watch closely for side effects, especially in elderly or debilitated patients. • Monitor urinary output.

copy is continuous and the duration is determined by the operator. Federal and state regulations are strictly imposed upon the radiation output per hour of fluoroscopy units in order to keep doses to acceptable levels and to lower risks to patients.

Any staff member or other person not required to be in immediate attendance to the patient during radiographic testing should leave the area during the exposure. A staff member who must be present during the exposure should wear a protective lead apron and possibly protective lead gloves (if hands would be in or near the radiation field). Lead-impregnated glasses are sometimes used to protect the lenses of the operator's eyes during fluoroscopy.

Radiography should be used judiciously for children, since they are at relatively higher risk. Radiography should not be used for pregnant women unless absolutely necessary, since it places the fetus at risk. If radiography is used for a pregnant woman, her uterine region should be shielded. Fetal risk for death and malformation is greatest during the first trimester of pregnancy.

With any radiographic procedure, the doctor must weigh the possible benefits against the potential risks.

Patient-teaching guidelines
Patient-learner objectives:
• Define the test.
• State the specific purpose of the test.
• Explain the procedure.
• Discuss test preparation, procedure, and post-test care.
• Identify possible risks or adverse effects.
Teaching content:
• Define the test in terms the patient can understand.
• Explain the specific purpose of the test.
• Describe the procedure. Be sure to describe the equipment, which may be large, unfamiliar, and anxiety-producing.

• Inform the patient where the X-ray will be taken. Most will be performed in an X-ray department, but bedside testing may be warranted for some patients.
• Explain that X-rays are not painful; however, if contrast material will be injected, this may cause some discomfort.
• Caution the patient to follow directions carefully. For example, he may be told not to move when the X-ray is taken; this is to prevent blurring of images on the X-ray. Failure to follow directions may necessitate a repeat test.
• Assure the patient that he will receive only a small amount of radiation. If fluoroscopy is ordered, the patient is exposed to more radiation than for a plain X-ray, but the additional amount is not considered harmful in itself.
• If the patient is pregnant (or even if there is a chance she may be) and an X-ray is necessary, advise her that a special shield will be used to prevent the rays from reaching her uterus and placing the fetus at risk.
• Inform the patient of any special preparation for the specific test. For any X-ray, explain that he will have to remove any jewelry or metal objects in the X-ray field, because these could block the rays.
• Describe any special care or restrictions following the test. Be sure to explain why these are necessary. If assessment measures will be implemented frequently, alleviate undue patient anxiety by explaining these as a routine precaution.
• Provide the outpatient with written instructions.
Evaluation:
After the patient-teaching session is completed, evaluate whether or not the patient has satisfactorily met each patient-learner objective, by obtaining necessary patient feedback. Refocus teaching as needed.

Antegrade pyelography

Purpose
• To evaluate the upper collecting system for obstruction by stricture, stone, clot, or tumor
• To evaluate hydronephrosis revealed during intravenous pyelography or ultrasonography, and to enable placement of a percutaneous nephrostomy tube
• To evaluate the function of the upper collecting system after ureteral surgery or urinary diversion.

Normal results
The upper collecting system fills uniformly and appears normal in size and course. Normal structures are outlined clearly.

Abnormal results
Enlargements of the upper collecting system and parts of the ureteropelvic junction:
Obstruction.
Marked distention of the ureteropelvic junction:
Hydronephrosis.

The basics
This radiographic procedure allows examination of the upper collecting system when ureteral obstruction rules out retrograde pyelography or when cystoscopy is contraindicated. It depends on percutaneous needle puncture for injection of contrast medium into the renal pelvis or calyces. Antegrade pyelography is also indicated when intravenous pyelography or renal ultrasonography demonstrates hydronephrosis and the need for therapeutic nephrostomy.

Antegrade pyelography shows the degree of dilatation, clearly defines obstructions, and demonstrates intrarenal reflux. Results of recent surgery or urinary diversion will be obvious; for example, a dilated stenotic area will be clearly visualized. Renal pressure

can be measured during the procedure. Intrarenal pressures that exceed 20 cmH_2O indicate obstruction. Also, urine can be collected for cultures and cytologic studies (to confirm antegrade pyonephrosis or malignancy, respectively).
Contraindications to this test include:
bleeding disorders.

Procedure
• The patient is placed prone on the X-ray table. The skin over the kidney is cleansed, and a local anesthetic is injected.
• Exercising proper precautions, the radiologist inserts a percutaneous needle into the renal collecting system and connects it to flexible tubing.
• If intrarenal pressure is to be measured, the manometer is connected to the tubing as soon as it is in place. Urine specimens are taken if needed.
• Contrast medium is injected, under fluoroscopic guidance.
• X-rays are taken.
• A nephrostomy tube may be inserted, if drainage is needed.
• If drainage is not needed, the catheter is withdrawn and a sterile dressing is applied.
• The test takes approximately 1 hour to perform.

Special precautions
The patient should be assessed for hypersensitivity to the contrast medium.

Patient care checklist
Before the test
☑ Explain or clarify test purpose, preparation, procedure, and post-test care.
☑ Tell the patient that he may feel mild discomfort during injection of the local anesthetic and contrast medium, and that he may also feel transient burning and flushing from the contrast medium.
☑ Explain that, if necessary, a tube will be left in the kidney for drainage.
☑ Evaluate patient understanding.

☑ If ordered, restrict food for 4 hours before the test, but encourage the patient to continue to drink fluids.

☑ Check the patient's history for hypersensitivity to local anesthetics, iodine, shellfish, or the contrast media used in other diagnostic tests. Report any hypersensitivity to the physician.

☑ Also check the history and recent coagulation studies for indications of bleeding disorders. Consult with the physician, as needed.

☑ Make sure that the patient or a responsible family member has signed an appropriate consent form.

☑ Just before the procedure, administer a sedative, as ordered.

After the test

☑ Monitor vital signs, as ordered.

☑ Check dressings for bleeding or urine leakage at the puncture site, at each check of vital signs. For bleeding, apply pressure. Report urine leakage to the physician.

☑ Monitor fluid intake and urine output for 24 hours. Notify the physician if the patient does not void within 8 hours. Observe each specimen for hematuria. Report hematuria if it persists after the third voiding.

CLINICAL ALERT: **Watch for and report signs of sepsis or extravasation of contrast medium (chills, fever, rapid pulse or respirations, hypotension). Also watch for and report signs that adjacent organs have been punctured: pain in the abdomen or flank, or pneumothorax (sudden onset of pleuritic chest pain, dyspnea, tachypnea, decreased breath sounds on the affected side, tachycardia).**

☑ If a nephrostomy tube is inserted, check to be sure that it is patent and functioning well.

☑ Administer antibiotics for several days after the procedure, as ordered, to prevent infection. Administer analgesics, as ordered.

Interfering factors

• Recently performed barium procedures, or the presence of feces or gas in the bowel, can impair the visualization of the kidney, inhibiting accurate results.

• Failure to remove radiopaque objects from the X-ray field interferes with radiologic interpretation.

Arthrography

Purpose

To detect abnormalities of encapsulated joints.

Normal results

Normal bursae, menisci, ligaments, and articular cartilage.

Abnormal results

Arthrography may reveal:

Medial meniscus tears and lacerations
Osteochondritis dissecans
Chondromalacia patellae
Osteochondral fractures
Tears of ligaments
Synovial abnormalities
Cartilaginous abnormalities
Tenosynovitis
Rupture of rotator cuff
Arthritis
Dislocation.

The basics

Arthrography is the radiographic examination of a joint—usually the knee or shoulder—following the injection of air (pneumoarthrography), a radiopaque contrast medium, or both, into the joint space, using strict asepsis. Arthrography outlines soft tissue not usually visualized by standard radiographs such as the meniscus, cartilage, or ligaments of the knee, and structures of the joint capsule, rotator cuff, and subacromial bursa.

Arthrography, performed as an outpatient procedure under a local anesthetic, is indicated in a patient with persistent unexplained knee or shoulder discomfort. Complications may include occasional infection at the puncture site or in the joint or, rarely, allergic reactions to the contrast medium.

Contraindications to this test include: active arthritis or joint infection, and possibly previous sensitivity to radiopaque media.

Procedure

• The skin over the joint is cleansed.

• A local anesthetic is injected around the puncture site. It is not usually necessary to anesthetize the joint space itself.

• A needle is inserted into the joint space, and any effusion is aspirated. (See "Synovial Fluid Analysis," p. 307.) Then, under fluoroscopic guidance, contrast medium is injected.

• When the needle is removed, the joint may be moved through range of motion, or the patient may be asked to walk a few steps, to distribute the dye in the joint space.

• A film series is quickly taken with the joint held in various positions.

• A bandage is applied.

Special precautions

The patient should be assessed for signs of a hypersensitivity reaction.

Patient care checklist

Before the test

☑ Explain or clarify test purpose, procedure, and post-test care.

☑ Tell the patient that, while the joint area will be anesthetized, he may experience a tingling sensation or pressure in the joint on injection of the contrast medium. Instruct him to remain as still as possible during the procedure, except when following instructions to change position.

☑ Evaluate patient understanding.

☑ Check the patient's history for hypersensitivity to shellfish, iodine, or contrast media, or to the local anesthetic. Notify the physician of any hypersensitivity.

After the test

☑ Tell the patient to rest the joint for at least 12 hours after the procedure.

☑ If knee arthrography was performed, wrap the knee in an elastic bandage, if ordered. Tell the patient to keep the bandage in place for several days, and teach him how to wrap it.

☑ Inform the patient that he may experience some swelling or discomfort, or may hear crepitant noises in the joint after the test, but that these symptoms usually disappear after 1 or 2 days; tell him to contact the physician if symptoms persist. Advise him to apply ice to the joint if swelling occurs and to take a mild analgesic for pain.

Interfering factors

• Incomplete aspiration of the joint fluid dilutes the contrast medium, diminishing the quality of the film.

• Improper injection technique may cause misplacement of contrast medium.

• Failure to remove radiopaque objects from the X-ray field interferes with radiologic interpretation.

Barium enema
[Lower gastrointestinal examination]

Purpose

• To aid diagnosis of colorectal cancer and inflammatory disease

• To detect polyps, diverticula, and structural changes in the large intestine.

Normal results

Uniform filling and normal passage of barium throughout the colon; normal colon contour, patency, position, and mucosal pattern.

Abnormal results

Barium enema may reveal:

　Carcinoma

　Diverticulitis

　Chronic ulcerative colitis

　Granulomatous colitis

　Polyps

Intussusception
Gastroenteritis
Stenosis
Irritable colon
Vascular injury from arterial occlusion
Selected cases of acute appendicitis.

The basics
Barium enema is the radiographic examination of the large intestine after rectal instillation of barium sulfate (single-contrast technique) or barium sulfate and air (double-contrast technique). It is indicated in patients with histories of altered bowel habits, lower abdominal pain, or the passage of blood, mucus, or pus in the stool. It may also be indicated after colostomy or ileostomy; in such patients, barium (or barium and air) is instilled through the stoma. The double-contrast technique best detects small intraluminal tumors (especially polyps), the early mucosal changes of inflammatory disease, and the subtle intestinal bleeding caused by ulcerated polyps or shallow ulcerations of inflammatory disease.

Although barium enema clearly outlines most of the large intestine, proctosigmoidoscopy provides the best view of the rectosigmoid region. Endoscopic biopsy may be needed to confirm a diagnosis. Barium enema should precede the barium swallow and upper gastrointestinal and small bowel series, since barium ingested in the latter procedure may take several days to pass through the gastrointestinal tract and thus may interfere with subsequent X-ray studies.

Contraindications to this test include: patients with tachycardia, fulminant ulcerative colitis associated with systemic toxicity and megacolon, toxic megacolon, or suspected perforation.

It should be performed cautiously in patients with obstruction, acute inflammatory conditions (such as ulcerative colitis, diverticulitis), acute vascular insufficiency of the bowel, acute fulminant bloody diarrhea, and suspected pneumatosis cystoides intestinalis.

Procedure
• After the patient is in a supine position on a tilting radiographic table, scout films of the abdomen are taken.
• The patient is then assisted to Sims' position, and a well-lubricated rectal tube is inserted through the anus.
• The barium is then administered slowly, and the filling process is monitored fluoroscopically.
• To aid filling, the patient assumes various positions.
• Spot films are taken during the flow of barium, and overhead films are taken when the intestine is filled with barium.
• The rectal tube is withdrawn, and the patient is escorted to the toilet or provided with a bedpan and is instructed to expel as much barium as possible.
• After evacuation, an additional overhead film is usually taken to record the mucosal pattern of the intestine and to evaluate the efficiency of colonic emptying.
• The test takes 30 to 45 minutes to perform.

Patient care checklist
Before the test
☑ Explain or clarify test purpose, preparation, and procedure.
☑ Stress to the patient that accurate results depend on his cooperation in the prescribed dietary restrictions and bowel preparation.
☑ Inform the patient that he may experience cramping or the urge to defecate as the barium or air is introduced into the intestine. Instruct him to breathe deeply and slowly through his mouth to ease this discomfort. Tell him to keep his anal sphincter tightly contracted against the rectal tube; this holds the tube in position and helps prevent leakage of barium. Stress the importance of retaining the barium enema; if the intestinal walls are not adequately coated with

barium, test results may be inaccurate. Assure the patient that the barium enema is fairly easy to retain because of its cool temperature.

☑ Evaluate patient understanding.

CLINICAL ALERT: Certain conditions, such as ulcerative colitis and active gastrointestinal bleeding, may prohibit the use of laxatives and enemas. Consult with the physician, as needed.

☑ Follow specific instructions from the X-ray department regarding patient preparation, since this varies considerably.

☑ If ordered, provide a low-residue diet for 1 to 3 days before the test.

☑ If ordered, restrict intake to clear liquids the day before the test or for the evening meal.

☑ Encourage the patient to drink water or clear liquids for 12 to 24 hours before the test.

☑ Administer the ordered laxatives the afternoon or evening before the test.

☑ Administer the suppository and/or enemas as ordered, in the evening or early morning of the test.

☑ If ordered, provide a light breakfast of toast and black coffee or clear tea.

After the test

☑ Be sure further X-ray studies have not been ordered before allowing the patient food and fluids. Encourage extra intake of fluids, as ordered, since bowel preparation and the test itself can cause dehydration.

☑ Since retention of barium after this test can cause intestinal obstruction or fecal impaction, administer a mild cathartic or a cleansing enema, as ordered. Tell the patient that his stool will be lightly colored for 24 to 72 hours. Record and describe any stool passed by the patient in the hospital.

Interfering factors

• Inadequate bowel preparation impairs the quality of the X-ray films.

• Barium swallow performed within several days before barium enema impairs the quality of subsequent X-ray films.

• The patient's inability to retain the barium enema causes an incomplete test.

• Failure to remove radiopaque objects from the X-ray field interferes with radiologic interpretation.

Barium swallow
[Esophagography]

Purpose

To detect pharyngeal and esophageal abnormalities.

Normal results

The barium sulfate bolus evenly fills and distends the lumen of the pharynx and esophagus, and the mucosa appears smooth and regular. Esophageal size, contour, and peristalsis are normal.

Abnormal results

Barium swallow may reveal:
   Hiatus hernia
   Esophageal diverticula
   Esophageal varices.

Barium swallow may help detect:
   Strictures
   Tumors
   Polyps
   Ulcers
   Pharyngeal muscular disorders
   Esophageal spasms
   Achalasia.

The basics

Barium swallow is the cineradiographic examination of the pharynx and the fluoroscopic examination of the esophagus after ingestion of thick and thin mixtures of barium sulfate. This test, most commonly performed as part of the upper gastrointestinal series, is indicated in patients with histories of dysphagia and regurgitation. Definitive diagnosis commonly necessitates endoscopic biopsy or, for motility disorders, manometric studies.

Contraindications to this test usually include: intestinal obstructions. (Also see *Gastroesophageal Reflux Scanning,* p. 571.)

Procedure

• The patient is placed in an upright position behind the fluoroscopic screen, and his heart, lungs, and abdomen are examined.

• He is then instructed to take one swallow of the thick barium mixture, and the pharyngeal action is recorded, using cineradiography.

• The patient is then told to take several swallows of the thin barium mixture. The passage of the barium is examined fluoroscopically, and spot films of the esophageal region are taken.

• The patient is placed in other positions and instructed to swallow barium. Additional fluoroscopic observation and spot films are taken.

• During fluoroscopic examination of the esophagus, the cardia and fundus of the patient's stomach are also carefully studied, because neoplasms in these areas may invade the esophagus and cause obstruction.

• The test takes approximately 30 minutes to perform.

Patient care checklist

Before the test

☑ Explain or clarify test purpose, preparation, procedure, and post-test care.

☑ Describe to the patient the milk-shake consistency and chalky taste of the barium preparation he will be required to ingest. Although it is flavored, he may find it unpleasant to swallow. Tell him that he will first receive a thick mixture, then a thin one, and that he must drink 12 to 14 oz (350 to 425 ml) during the examination.

☑ Evaluate patient understanding.

☑ Restrict food and fluids after midnight before the test. (If the patient is an infant, delay feeding to ensure complete digestion of barium.)

☑ Withhold antacids, as ordered, if gastric reflux is suspected.

After the test

☑ Check that additional spot films and repeat fluoroscopic evaluation have not been ordered before allowing the patient to resume his usual diet.

☑ Administer a cathartic, if ordered.

☑ Inform the patient that his stools will be chalky and light-colored for 24 to 72 hours. Record description of all stools passed by the patient in the hospital. Barium retained in the intestine may harden, causing obstruction or fecal impaction. Notify the physician if the patient has not expelled the barium in 2 or 3 days.

Biliary tract and liver computed tomography *(CT)*

Purpose

• To detect intrahepatic tumors and abscesses, subphrenic and subhepatic abscesses, cysts, and hematomas

• To distinguish between obstructive and nonobstructive jaundice.

Normal results

The liver and bile ducts appear normal. The liver has a uniform density that is slightly greater than that of the pancreas, kidneys, and spleen. Biliary ducts appear as low-density structures.

Abnormal results

Biliary tract and liver computed tomography may reveal:

   Primary hepatic neoplasms
   Metastatic hepatic neoplasms
   Hepatic abscesses
   Hepatic cysts
   Hepatic hematomas
   Dilated biliary ducts (which indicate obstructive rather than nonobstructive jaundice)
   The cause of biliary obstruction, such as calculi or pancreatic cancer.

The basics

In CT of the biliary tract and liver, multiple X-rays pass through the upper abdomen and are measured while detectors record differences in tissue attenuation. A computer reconstructs this data as a three-dimensional image on a television screen. Since soft tissue appearance varies with tissue attenuation, CT accurately distinguishes the biliary tract and the liver if the ducts are large.

CT images can specify focal defects detected by liver-spleen scanning as solid, cystic, inflammatory, and vascular lesions; however, biopsy may be necessary to rule out malignancy or to distinguish between metastatic and primary tumors. Most focal hepatic defects appear less dense than the normal parenchyma. Use of rapid-sequence scanning with I.V. contrast medium helps distinguish between the two, since the normal parenchyma shows greater enhancement than focal defects.

Although both CT and ultrasonography detect biliary tract and liver disease, the latter technique is performed more often. CT is more expensive than ultrasonography and involves patient exposure to moderate amounts of radiation. However, it is the test of choice in patients who are obese and in those with livers positioned high under the rib cage, since bone and excessive fat hinder ultrasound transmission. It is also the preferred test to determine the cause of sonographically confirmed dilated ducts. If results are inconclusive, percutaneous transhepatic cholangiography or, less commonly, endoscopic retrograde cholangiopancreatography may be performed.

Barium studies should precede this test by at least 4 days, since barium may hinder visualization.

Procedure

• The patient is placed in supine position on a radiographic table, and the table is positioned within the opening in the scanning gantry.

• A series of transverse X-ray films are taken and recorded on magnetic tape.
• This information is reconstructed by a computer and appears as images on a television screen.
• These images are studied, and selected ones are photographed.
• Contrast enhancement may be ordered. After the contrast medium is injected, a second series of films is taken, and the patient is carefully observed for allergic reaction.
• The test usually takes about 1½ hours to perform.

Special precautions

If I.V. contrast medium is being used, the patient should be assessed for signs of a hypersensitivity reaction.

Patient care checklist

Before the test

☑ Explain or clarify test purpose, preparation, and procedure.

☑ Assure the patient that the test is painless.

☑ Stress the importance of remaining still during the test, because movement can cause artifacts, thereby prolonging the test and limiting its accuracy.

☑ If I.V. contrast medium is being used, inform the patient that he may experience transient discomfort from the needle puncture and a localized feeling of warmth on injection.

☑ Evaluate patient understanding.

☑ Restrict food and fluids after midnight.

☑ Make sure that the patient or a responsible family member has signed a consent form.

☑ Check the patient's history for hypersensitivity to iodine, seafood, or the contrast media used in other diagnostic tests. Report any hypersensitivity to the physician.

☑ If ordered, give the patient 300 to 400 ml of gastrografin about 10 minutes before the test.

Interfering factors
• Use of P.O. or I.V. contrast media that are excreted in the bile in previous diagnostic studies can interfere with detection of biliary dilatation, since they may cause the biliary tract to appear as dense as the surrounding parenchyma.
• Barium studies performed within 4 days before CT may obscure the test results.
• Failure to remove radiopaque objects from the X-ray field interferes with radiologic interpretation.

Bronchography

Purpose
• To help detect bronchiectasis, bronchial obstruction, pulmonary tumors, cysts, and cavities, and indirectly, to pinpoint the cause of hemoptysis
• To provide permanent films of pathologic findings
• To provide guidance while performing a bronchoscopy.

Normal results
The bronchi are free of obstruction or lesions.

Abnormal results
Bronchography may reveal:
   Bronchiectasis
   Pulmonary tumors
   Pulmonary cysts
   Pulmonary cavities
   Foreign objects.

The basics
Bronchography is X-ray examination of the tracheobronchial tree after instillation of a radiopaque iodine contrast agent. Bronchography has been performed infrequently since the development of tomography and the flexible bronchoscope. Currently, it is used primarily for guidance during a bronchoscopy or to provide permanent films of pathologic findings. Findings require correlation with physical ex-

amination, patient history, and possibly other pulmonary diagnostic studies.

Bronchography may be performed using a local anesthetic instilled through a catheter or bronchoscope, although a general anesthetic may be necessary for children or during a concurrent bronchoscopy (see "Bronchoscopy," p. 415).
Contraindications to this test include: respiratory insufficiency and hypersensitivity to the contrast medium.

Procedure
• After a local anesthetic is sprayed into the patient's mouth and throat, a bronchoscope or catheter is passed into the trachea, and the anesthetic and contrast agent are instilled.
• The patient is placed in various positions during the test, to promote movement of the contrast agent into different areas of the bronchial tree.
• After radiographs are taken, the dye is removed through postural drainage or nebulization.

Special precautions
CLINICAL ALERT: **Observe the patient with asthma for laryngeal spasm secondary to the instillation of the contrast agent.**
CLINICAL ALERT: **Observe the patient with chronic obstructive pulmonary disease for airway occlusion secondary to the instillation of the contrast agent.**
CLINICAL ALERT: **Observe the patient for a hypersensitivity reaction to the dye.**

Patient care checklist
Before the test
☑ Explain or clarify test purpose, preparation, procedure, and post-test care.
☑ Instruct the patient to perform good oral hygiene the night before and the morning of the test.
☑ If the procedure is to be performed under a local anesthetic, tell the pa-

tient that he will receive a sedative to help him relax and to suppress the gag reflex. Prepare him for the unpleasant taste of the anesthetic spray. Warn him that he may experience some difficulty breathing during the procedure, but reassure him that his airway will not be blocked and that he will receive enough oxygen. Tell him that the catheter or bronchoscope will pass more easily if he relaxes.

☑ If bronchography is to be performed under a general anesthetic, inform the patient that he will receive a sedative before the test, to help him relax.

☑ Evaluate patient understanding.

☑ Restrict food and fluids for 12 hours before the test.

☑ Make sure that the patient or a responsible family member has signed a consent form.

☑ Check the patient's history for hypersensitivity to anesthetics, iodine, shellfish, or contrast media used in other diagnostic tests. Report any hypersensitivity to the physician.

☑ If the patient has a productive cough, administer an expectorant and perform postural drainage 1 to 3 days before the test is performed, as ordered.

After the test

CLINICAL ALERT: **Watch for signs of laryngeal spasms (dyspnea) or edema (hoarseness, dyspnea, laryngeal stridor) secondary to traumatic intubation.**

☑ Withhold food, fluid, and oral medications until gag reflex returns (usually 2 hours).

☑ Watch for signs of chemical or secondary bacterial pneumonia—fever, dyspnea, rales, or rhonchi—the result of incomplete expectoration of the contrast agent.

☑ If the patient has a sore throat, reassure him that it is only temporary, and provide throat lozenges or a liquid gargle when his gag reflex returns.

☑ Advise the outpatient to postpone resuming his usual activities until the following day.

Interfering factors

The presence of secretions or failure to position the patient properly may inhibit the contrast agent from adequately filling the bronchial tree.

Cardiac radiography

Purpose

• To help detect cardiac disease and abnormalities that change the size, shape, or appearance of the heart and lungs

• To ensure correct positioning of pulmonary artery and cardiac catheters, and of pacemaker wires.

Normal results

Cardiac silhouette is of normal size, shape, and appearance. Pulmonary vasculature appears normal.

Abnormal results

Cardiac radiography may reveal:

  Left or right ventricular enlargement
  Left atrial enlargement
  Pulmonary vascular congestion
  Chronic pulmonary venous hypertension
  Acute alveolar edema
  Interstitial pulmonary edema.

The basics

Among the most frequently used tests for evaluating cardiac disease and its effects on the pulmonary vasculature, cardiac radiography provides images of the thorax, mediastinum, heart, and lungs. In a routine evaluation, posteroanterior and left lateral views are taken. The posteroanterior view is preferable to the anteroposterior view because it places the heart slightly closer to the plane of the film, giving a sharper, less distorted image. Using portable equipment, cardiac radiographs may be taken of bedridden patients, but such equipment can provide only anteroposterior views.

The Cardiac Series

Now superseded by echocardiography for most diagnostic purposes, the cardiac series remains useful for comprehensive examination of heart action. Using X-rays, it provides a constant image of the heart in motion on a fluoroscope. By examining the beating heart from four directions, the test permits observation of cardiac pulsations, assessment of heart chamber structural abnormalities (such as aneurysm and congenital heart disease), detection of aortic and mitral valve calcification, and evaluation of prosthetic valve function. When performed with a barium swallow, the cardiac series highlights abnormal deviation of esophageal contours (possibly caused by left atrial enlargement) or makes abnormalities of the aortic arch more visible. Views may be preserved for later study on spot films or motion pictures.

Since the cardiac series entails exposure to 15 to 20 times more radiation than the cardiac X-ray films, it may be contraindicated in some patients, especially pregnant women. If this test is necessary during pregnancy, the patient's pelvic and abdominal areas must be adequately shielded during the test.

Cardiac X-ray films must be evaluated in light of the patient's history, physical examination, electrocardiography results, and results of previous radiographic tests for cardiac abnormalities. (See also *The Cardiac Series*.)

Procedure

• The patient stands for the procedure and is positioned for the posteroanterior view and then for the left lateral view.
• With each view, the patient is asked to take a deep breath and hold it during the X-ray film exposure.
• To obtain an anteroposterior view of a bedridden patient, the head of the bed is elevated as much as possible, and the patient is assisted to an upright position. The film cassette is centered under the patient's back. The patient is instructed to take a deep breath and hold it during the X-ray film exposure.

Special precautions

When testing a bedridden patient, be sure anyone else in the room is protected from X-rays by a lead shield, a room divider, or sufficient distance.

Patient care checklist

Before the test
☑ Explain or clarify test purpose and procedure.
☑ Evaluate patient understanding.

Interfering factors

• Patient failure to maintain inspiration or to remain motionless during the test interferes with the clarity of the image.
• If the patient's chest is not centered on the film cassette, the costophrenic angle may not be visible on the X-ray film.
• Thoracic deformity, such as scoliosis, affects radiographic interpretation.
• Failure to remove radiopaque objects from the X-ray field interferes with radiologic interpretation.

Celiac and mesenteric arteriography

Purpose

• To locate the source of gastrointestinal (GI) bleeding
• To help distinguish between benign and malignant neoplasms
• To evaluate cirrhosis and portal hypertension
• To evaluate vascular damage after abdominal trauma
• To detect vascular abnormalities.

Normal results

X-ray films show the three phases of perfusion—arterial, capillary, and venous. The arteries normally taper regularly, becoming gradually smaller with subsequent divisions. The contrast medium then spreads evenly within the sinusoids. The portal vein appears 10 to 20 seconds after the injection.

Abnormal results

Celiac and mesenteric arteriography may reveal:

Upper GI hemorrhage, usually excluding esophageal hemorrhage

Lower GI hemorrhage

Abdominal neoplasms, both benign and malignant

Progressing and advanced cirrhosis

Splenic rupture from trauma

Intrahepatic and subcapsular hematomas from trauma.

The basics

Celiac and mesenteric arteriography is the radiographic examination of the abdominal vasculature after intraarterial injection of contrast medium through a catheter. As the contrast medium flows through the abdominal vasculature, serial radiographs outline abdominal vessels in the arterial, capillary, and venous phases of perfusion. Celiac and mesenteric arteriography is performed (among other indications) when endoscopy is unable to locate the source of GI bleeding or when barium studies, ultrasonography, and nuclear medicine or computed tomography scanning prove inconclusive in evaluating neoplasms.

Complications associated with this test include hemorrhage, venous and intracardiac thrombosis, cardiac arrhythmia, and emboli caused by dislodging atherosclerotic plaques.

Procedure

• After placing the patient in supine position on the radiographic table, an I.V. infusion of 5% dextrose in water is started.

• Scout films of the patient's abdomen are taken, and the peripheral pulses are palpated and marked.

• The puncture site is cleansed, and a local anesthetic is injected.

• A needle is gently inserted into the femoral artery, then a guide wire is passed through the needle into the aorta.

• The needle is then removed.

• After the angiographic catheter is inserted over the guide wire, catheter placement is checked, and the guide wire is withdrawn.

• The catheter is advanced into one of the major arteries—celiac, superior mesenteric, or inferior mesenteric—under fluoroscopic guidance. After correct placement of the catheter is verified, the contrast medium is injected, and a series of films is taken in rapid sequence.

• After injecting one or more major arteries, superselective catheterization may be performed. The catheter is repositioned in a specific branch of a major artery, contrast medium is injected, and rapid-sequence films are ordered. If necessary, several specific branches may be catheterized.

• After filming, the catheter is withdrawn, and firm pressure is applied to the puncture site for about 15 minutes.

• The site is observed for hematoma formation, a pressure dressing is applied, and peripheral pulses are checked.

• The test takes 30 minutes to 3 hours, depending on the number of vessels studied.

Special precautions

CLINICAL ALERT: **Celiac and mesenteric arteriography should be performed cautiously in patients with coagulopathy.**

• The patient should be assessed for signs of a hypersensitivity reaction.

Patient care checklist

Before the test

☑ Explain or clarify purpose, preparation, procedure, and post-test care.

☑ Inform the patient that he may feel pressure when the femoral artery is palpated, but the local anesthetic will minimize the pain when the needle is introduced into the artery. Tell him that he may feel a transient burning as the contrast medium is injected, and that he may experience a transient headache and salty taste.

☑ Instruct the patient to lie still during the test to avoid blurring the films.

☑ Evaluate patient understanding.

☑ Restrict food and fluids for 8 hours before the test.

☑ Administer a cathartic the day before the test, as ordered.

☑ Make sure that the patient or a responsible family member has signed the consent form.

☑ Check the patient's history for hypersensitivity to iodine, shellfish, or the contrast medium used in other diagnostic tests. Report any hypersensitivity to the physician.

☑ Make sure blood studies (hemoglobin, hematocrit, clotting time, prothrombin time, activated partial thromboplastin time, and platelet count) have been completed.

☑ Obtain baseline vital signs and tell the patient to void immediately just before the procedure.

☑ Administer a sedative, if ordered.

After the test

☑ Instruct the patient to lie flat, and enforce bed rest for at least 12 hours after the test.

☑ Monitor vital signs, as ordered, until stable, and check peripheral pulses. Note the color and temperature of the leg that was used for the test.

☑ Check the puncture site for bleeding and hematoma. (A sandbag may be placed over the site for the first 2 to 4 hours to prevent bleeding.) If bleeding develops, apply pressure to the site; if bleeding continues or is excessive, notify the physician. If a hematoma develops, apply warm soaks.

☑ Ask the physician if the patient can resume his usual diet. If the patient is not receiving I.V. infusions, encourage intake of fluids, to speed excretion of the contrast medium.

Cerebral angiography

Purpose

• To detect cerebrovascular abnormalities

• To study vascular displacement

• To locate clips applied to blood vessels during surgery and to evaluate the postoperative status of such vessels.

Normal results

Blood flow to the brain is normal. Cerebral vasculature appears normal (symmetrical).

Abnormal results

Cerebral angiography commonly confirms the presence of:

   Aneurysm
   Arteriovenous malformation
   Thrombosis
   Stenosis
   Occlusion.

It may also identify vascular changes caused by:

   Tumor
   Hematoma
   Cyst
   Edema
   Herniation
   Arterial spasm
   Hydrocephalus.

The basics

Cerebral angiography allows radiographic examination of the cerebral vasculature after injection of a contrast medium. Possible injection sites include the femoral, carotid, or brachial arteries; the femoral artery is used most often because it allows visualization of four vessels (the carotid and the vertebral arteries). The usual clinical indication for this test is a suspected abnormality of the cerebral vasculature, often as suggested by intracranial computed tomography or a radionuclide scan of the brain.

Contraindications to this test include: hepatic, renal, or thyroid disease, or hypersensitivity to iodine or contrast medium.

Procedure

• The patient is placed in a supine position on a radiographic table, and the injection site (femoral, carotid, or brachial artery) is shaved.

• The patient is instructed to lie still, with his arms at his sides.

• The skin is cleansed, and a local anesthetic is injected.

• The artery is then punctured with the appropriate needle and catheterized.

• After placement of the needle (or catheter) is verified by radiography or fluoroscopy, the contrast medium is injected.

• A first series of radiographs is taken, developed, and reviewed. Depending on the results of this initial series, more contrast medium may be injected and another series of radiographs taken.

• Arterial catheter patency is maintained by continuous or periodic flushing with normal saline or heparin solution.

• Vital and neurologic signs are monitored throughout the test.

• When an acceptable series of radiographs has been obtained, the needle (or catheter) is withdrawn, and firm pressure is applied to the puncture site for 15 minutes. The patient is observed for bleeding, distal pulses are checked, and a pressure bandage is applied.

• The test takes about 2 hours to perform.

Special precautions

The patient should be assessed for signs of hypersensitivity to the contrast medium.

Patient care checklist

Before the test

☑ Explain or clarify test purpose, preparation, procedure, and post-test care.

☑ Tell the patient that he will be positioned on an X-ray table, with his head immobilized, and will be asked to lie still. Tell him that a local anesthetic will be administered. (Some patients—especially children—may receive a general anesthetic.) Explain that he will probably feel a transient burning sensation as the contrast medium is injected and that he may feel flushed and warm and experience a transient headache or salty taste after injection of the dye.

☑ Evaluate patient understanding.

☑ Restrict food and fluids for 8 to 10 hours before the test.

☑ Make sure that the patient or a responsible family member has signed a consent form.

☑ Check the patient's history for hypersensitivity to iodine, shellfish, anesthetics, or other contrast media. Notify the physician of any hypersensitivity.

☑ If ordered, administer a sedative and anticholinergic 30 to 45 minutes before the test.

☑ Make sure the patient voids before leaving his room.

After the test

☑ Enforce bed rest for 12 to 24 hours.

☑ Provide pain medication, as ordered.

☑ Monitor vital signs and neurologic status, as ordered.

☑ Check the puncture site for signs of extravasation, such as redness and swelling. To ease the patient's discomfort and to minimize swelling, apply an ice bag to the site. If bleeding occurs, apply firm pressure to the puncture site.

CLINICAL ALERT: If the *femoral approach* was used, keep the affected leg straight for at least 12 hours, and routinely check pulses distal to the site (dorsalis pedis and popliteal). Check the temperature, color, and tactile sensations of the affected leg, since thrombosis or hematoma can occlude blood flow. Extravasation can also block blood flow by exerting pressure on the artery.

CLINICAL ALERT: If a *carotid artery* was used as the injection site, watch for dysphagia or respiratory distress, which can result from extravasation. Also watch for disorientation and weakness or numbness in the extremities (signs of thrombosis or hematoma) and for arterial spasms that produce symptoms of transient ischemic attacks. Notify the physician if abnormal signs develop.

CLINICAL ALERT: If the *brachial approach* was used, immobilize the arm for at least 12 hours, and routinely check the radial pulse. Place a sign above the patient's bed warning personnel against taking blood pressure readings from the affected arm. Observe the arm and hand, noting any change in color, temperature, or tactile sensations. If it becomes pale, cool, or numb, notify the physician.

Interfering factors
• Head movement during the test affects the clarity of the radiographs and interferes with accurate interpretation.
• Failure to remove radiopaque objects from the X-ray field interferes with radiologic interpretation.

Chest fluoroscopy

Purpose
• To assess lung expansion and contraction during quiet breathing, deep breathing, and coughing
• To assess movement and paralysis of the diaphragm
• To detect bronchiolar obstructions and pulmonary disease
• To localize poorly defined nodules.

Normal results
Diaphragmatic movement is synchronous and symmetric. Normal diaphragmatic excursion ranges from ¾″ to 1⅝″ (2 to 4 cm).

Abnormal results
Chest fluoroscopy may indicate:
  Pulmonary disease
  Bronchial obstruction
  Diaphragmatic paralysis.

The basics
In chest fluoroscopy, a continuous stream of X-rays passes through the patient, casting shadows of the heart, lungs, and diaphragm on a fluorescent screen. Since fluoroscopy reveals less detail than standard chest radiography, it is indicated when diagnosis requires visualization of physiologic or pathologic motion of thoracic contents, such as to rule out paralysis in patients with diaphragmatic elevation. However, fluoroscopy may not detect such paralysis in patients who compensate for diminished diaphragm function by using forceful contraction of their abdominal muscles to aid expiration. This test may also be used for localizing poorly defined nodules.

Procedure
• If necessary, assist with positioning the patient.
• Move cardiac monitoring cables, I.V. tubing from subclavian lines, and safety pins as far from the X-ray field as possible.
• During the test, the patient's cardiopulmonary motion is observed on a screen.
• Special equipment may be used to intensify the images, or a videotape recording of the fluoroscopy may be made for later study.
• The test takes 5 minutes to perform.

Special precautions
• If the patient is intubated, check that no tubes have been dislodged during positioning.
• To avoid exposure to radiation, leave the room or the immediate area during the test; if you must stay in the area, wear a lead-lined apron.

Patient care checklist
Before the test

☑ Explain or clarify test purpose and procedure.

☑ Tell the patient that he will be asked to follow specific instructions, such as to breathe deeply and to cough, while X-ray images depict his breathing.

☑ Evaluate patient understanding.

Interfering factors
Failure to remove radiopaque objects from the X-ray field interferes with radiologic interpretation.

Chest radiography
[Chest X-ray]

Purpose
• To detect pulmonary disorders, such as pneumonia, atelectasis, pneumothorax, pulmonary bullae, and tumors
• To detect mediastinal abnormalities, such as tumors, and cardiac disease
• To determine the location and size of a lesion
• To help assess pulmonary status.

Normal/abnormal results
For normal and abnormal results, see *Some Clinical Implications of Chest X-ray Films*, pp. 498 to 499.

The basics
In a chest radiograph, X-rays or gamma rays penetrate the chest and react on specially sensitized film. Since normal pulmonary tissue is radiolucent, foreign bodies, infiltrates, fluids, tumors, and other abnormalities appear as densities on the chest film. A chest radiograph is most useful when compared with the patient's previous films, allowing the radiologist to detect changes. For an accurate diagnosis, radiography findings require correlation with additional radiologic and pulmonary tests.

Although chest radiography was once routinely performed as a cancer screening test, the associated expense and exposure to radiation has caused many authorities to question its usefulness. The American Cancer Society now recommends sputum cultures rather than chest radiography—even in patients at high risk—and the Food and Drug Administration has convened a panel for the development of guidelines concerning the use of chest radiography.

Procedure
• If a *stationary X-ray machine* is being used, the patient usually stands in front of the machine so films can be taken, most commonly of the posteroanterior and left lateral views.
• The patient is requested to take a deep breath and hold it when the X-ray is taken.
• If a *portable X-ray machine* is being used at the patient's bedside, assist with the positioning of the patient. Since an upright chest radiograph is preferable, move the patient to the top of the bed, if he can tolerate it. Elevate the head of the bed for maximum upright positioning.
• Move cardiac monitoring cables, I.V. tubing from subclavian lines, pulmonary artery catheter lines, and safety pins as far from the X-ray field as possible.
• Again, the patient is requested to take a deep breath and hold it while the X-ray is taken.

Special precautions
• If the patient is intubated, check that no tubes have been dislodged during positioning.
• To avoid exposure to radiation, leave the room or the immediate area while the films are being taken. If you must stay in the area, wear a lead-lined apron or protective clothing.

Patient care checklist
Before the test

☑ Explain or clarify test purpose and procedure.

☑ Evaluate patient understanding.

Some Clinical Implications of Chest X-ray Films

Normal Anatomic Location and Appearance	Possible Abnormality	Implications
Trachea Visible midline in the anterior mediastinal cavity; translucent tubelike appearance	• Deviation from midline	• Tension pneumothorax, atelectasis, pleural effusion, consolidation, mediastinal nodes, or in children, enlarged thymus
	• Narrowing, with hourglass appearance and deviation to one side	• Substernal thyroid
Heart Visible in the anterior left mediastinal cavity; solid appearance due to blood contents; edges may be clear in contrast with surrounding air density of the lung.	• Shift • Hypertrophy of right heart • Cardiac borders obscured by stringy densities ("shaggy heart")	• Atelectasis • Cor pulmonale, congestive heart failure • Cystic fibrosis
Aortic knob Visible as water density; formed by the arch of the aorta	• Solid densities, possibly indicating calcifications • Tortuous shape	• Atherosclerosis • Atherosclerosis
Mediastinum (mediastinal shadow) Visible as the space between the lungs; shadowy appearance that widens at the hilum of the lungs	• Deviation to nondiseased side; deviation to diseased side by traction • Gross widening	• Pleural effusion or tumor, fibrosis or collapsed lung • Neoplasms of esophagus, bronchi, lungs, thyroid, thymus, peripheral nerves, lymphoid tissue; aortic aneurysm; mediastinitis; cor pulmonale
Ribs Visible as thoracic cavity encasement	• Break or misalignment • Widening of intercostal spaces	• Fractured sternum or ribs • Emphysema
Spine Visible midline in the posterior chest; straight bony structure	• Spinal curvature • Break or misalignment	• Scoliosis, kyphosis • Fractures

(continued)

Some Clinical Implications of Chest X-ray Films *(continued)*

Normal Anatomic Location and Appearance	Possible Abnormality	Implications
Clavicles Visible in upper thorax; intact and equidistant in properly centered X-ray films	• Break or misalignment	• Fractures
Hila (lung roots) Visible above the heart where pulmonary vessels, bronchi, and lymph nodes join the lungs; appear as small, white, bilateral densities	• Shift to one side • Accentuated shadows	• Atelectasis • Emphysema, pulmonary abscess, tumor, enlarged lymph nodes
Mainstem bronchus Visible, part of the hila with translucent tubelike appearance	• Spherical or oval density	• Bronchogenic cyst
Bronchi Usually not visible	• Visible	• Bronchial pneumonia
Lung fields Usually not visible throughout, except for the blood vessels	• Visible • Irregular, patchy densities	• Atelectasis • Resolving pneumonia, silicosis, fibrosis, metastatic neoplasm
Hemidiaphragm Rounded, visible; right side ⅜″ to ¾″ (1 to 2 cm) higher than left	• Elevation of diaphragm (difference in elevation can be measured on inspiration and expiration to detect movement) • Flattening of diaphragm • Unilateral elevation of either side • Unilateral elevation of left side only	• Active tuberculosis, pneumonia, pleurisy, acute bronchitis, active disease of the abdominal viscera, bilateral phrenic nerve involvement, atelectasis • Asthma, emphysema • Possible unilateral phrenic nerve paresis • Perforated ulcer (rare), gas distention of stomach or splenic flexure of colon, free air in abdomen

Interfering factors

• Portable chest radiographs taken in the anteroposterior position may show larger cardiac shadowing than other radiographs, because the distance of the anterior structures from the beam is shorter. Portable chest radiographs—primarily those taken to detect atelectasis, pneumonia, pneumo-thorax, and mediastinal shift, or to evaluate treatment—may be less reliable than stationary radiographs.

• Since chest radiographs vary with the patient's age, sex, and habitus, these factors should be considered when the films are evaluated.

• Failure to remove radiopaque objects from the X-ray field interferes with radiologic interpretation.

Chest tomography
[Laminagraphy, planigraphy, stratigraphy, body-section roentgenography]

Purpose
To demonstrate pulmonary densities (for cavitation, calcification, and presence of fat), tumors (especially those obstructing the bronchial lumen), or lesions (especially those located deep within the mediastinum, such as lymph nodes at the hilum).

Normal results
Structures equivalent to a normal chest X-ray film.

Abnormal results
Chest tomography can:
Suggest whether a lesion is benign, malignant, or granulomatous
Help differentiate blood vessels from nodes at the hilum
Identify bronchial dilation, stenosis, and endobronchial lesions
Detect tumor extension into the hilar lung area
Identify extension of a mediastinal lesion to the ribs or spine.

The basics
Tomography provides clearly focused radiographic images of selected body sections otherwise obscured by shadows of overlying or underlying structures. This procedure produces exposures in which a selected body plane appears sharply defined, and the areas above and below it are blurred.

Tomography is used only for further evaluation of a chest lesion when other tests are inconclusive.

Procedure
• The patient is placed in a supine position or in different degrees of lateral rotation on the X-ray table. The X-ray tube then swings over the patient, taking numerous exposures from different angles.
• The test takes 30 to 60 minutes to perform.

Special precautions
To avoid exposure to radiation, leave the room or the immediate area during the test; if you must stay in the area, wear a lead-lined apron.

Patient care checklist
Before the test
☑ Explain or clarify test purpose and procedure.
☑ Advise the patient to breathe normally during the test, but to remain immobile.
☑ Evaluate patient understanding.

Interfering factors
• The patient's inability to lie still may interfere with test results and necessitate additional X-ray films, with greater exposure to radiation.
• Failure to remove radiopaque objects from the X-ray field interferes with radiologic interpretation.

Cholangiography, percutaneous transhepatic

Purpose
• To distinguish between obstructive and nonobstructive jaundice
• To determine the location, the extent, and often the cause of mechanical obstruction.

Normal results
The biliary ducts are of normal diameter and appear as regular channels homogenously filled with contrast medium.

Abnormal results
Percutaneous transhepatic cholangiography may identify:
Dilated biliary ducts, indicating:
  Obstructive jaundice.
The cause of biliary obstruction:
  Cholelithiasis
  Biliary tract carcinoma
  Carcinoma of the pancreas
  Carcinoma of the papilla of Vater.

The basics
Percutaneous transhepatic cholangiography is the fluoroscopic examination of the biliary ducts after injection of an iodinated contrast medium directly into a biliary radicle. This test opacifies the biliary ducts without depending on the gallbladder's concentrating ability. It is useful for evaluating patients with severe jaundice, since impaired hepatic function often prevents uptake and excretion of the contrast medium during oral cholecystography or intravenous cholangiography.

Although computed tomography scanning or ultrasonography is usually performed first when obstructive jaundice is suspected, percutaneous transhepatic cholangiography may provide the most detailed view of the obstruction; however, this invasive procedure carries a potential risk of complications that include bleeding, septicemia, bile peritonitis, extravasation of the contrast medium into the peritoneal cavity, and subcapsular injection.
Contraindications to this test include: cholangitis, massive ascites, uncorrectable coagulopathy, or hypersensitivity to iodine.

Procedure
• After the patient is placed in a supine position on the radiographic table, the upper right quadrant of his abdomen is cleansed and draped, and a local anesthetic is administered.
• The patient's liver is punctured with a thin, flexible needle (Chiba needle) under fluoroscopic guidance. When bile can be aspirated from the duct, the contrast medium is injected.
• When fluoroscopy reveals placement in a radicle, the needle is held in position and the remaining contrast medium is injected.
• As the contrast medium flows through the biliary ducts, the filling process is visualized by fluoroscopy. Spot films are then taken of any significant findings.
• The test takes about 30 minutes to perform.

Special precautions
The patient should be assessed for signs of hypersensitivity to the contrast medium, although these reactions occur more commonly with I.V. injection.

Patient care checklist
Before the test
☑ Explain or clarify test purpose, preparation, procedure, and post-test care.
☑ Inform the patient that he will be placed on a tilting X-ray table that rotates into vertical and horizontal positions during the procedure. Assure him that he will be adequately secured to the table and assisted to supine and side-lying positions throughout the procedure.
☑ Warn him that injection of the local anesthetic may sting the skin and produce transient pain when it punctures the liver capsule. Also advise him that injection of the contrast medium may produce a sensation of pressure and epigastric fullness and may cause transient upper back pain on his right side.
☑ Tell him that he must rest for at least 6 hours after the procedure.
☑ Evaluate patient understanding.
☑ Make sure that the patient or a re-

sponsible family member has signed a consent form.

☑ Check the patient's history for hypersensitivity to iodine, seafood, contrast media used in other diagnostic tests, and the local anesthetic. Report any hypersensitivity to the physician.

☑ Also check the patient's history for normal bleeding, clotting and prothrombin times, and a normal platelet count. Consult with the physician, as needed.

☑ If ordered, administer 1 g of ampicillin I.V. every 4 to 6 hours for 24 hours before the procedure.

☑ Just before the procedure, administer a sedative, as ordered.

After the test

☑ Check the patient's vital signs until they are stable.

☑ Enforce bed rest for at least 6 hours after the test, preferably with the patient lying on his right side, to help prevent hemorrhage.

CLINICAL ALERT: **Check the injection site for bleeding, swelling, and tenderness. Watch for signs of peritonitis: chills, temperature of 102° to 103° F. (38.9° to 39.4° C.), and abdominal pain, tenderness, and distention. Notify the physician immediately if such complications develop.**

Interfering factors

• Marked obesity or gas overlying the biliary ducts may interfere with the clarity of the X-ray films.

• Failure to remove radiopaque objects from the X-ray field interferes with radiologic interpretation.

Cholangiography, postoperative
[T-tube cholangiography]

Purpose

To detect calculi, strictures, neoplasms, and fistulae in the biliary ducts.

Normal results

Biliary ducts demonstrate homogeneous filling with contrast medium and are normal in diameter. When the sphincter of Oddi is functioning properly and the ducts are patent, the contrast medium flows unimpeded into the duodenum.

Abnormal results

Postoperative cholangiography may indicate:

Biliary duct obstruction due to calculi or neoplasms overlooked during surgery

Fistulae in the biliary ducts.

The basics

Often, immediately after cholecystectomy or common bile duct exploration, a T-shaped rubber tube is inserted into the common bile duct to facilitate drainage. Postoperative cholangiography, performed 7 to 10 days after this surgery, is the radiographic and fluoroscopic examination of the biliary ducts after the injection of contrast medium through the T tube. The contrast flows through the biliary ducts and outlines the size and patency of the ducts, revealing any obstruction overlooked during surgery. (See also *Operative Cholangiography*.)

Procedure

• After the patient is in a supine position on the radiographic table, the injection area of the T tube is cleansed.

• The T tube is held in a vertical position, which allows trapped air to surface, and a needle attached to a long transparent catheter is carefully inserted into the end of the T tube.

• Contrast medium is injected under fluoroscopic guidance. Spot films and plain films are taken.

• The T tube is then clamped, and the patient is assisted to an erect position for additional films; in this position, air bubbles may be distinguished from calculi or other pathology.

• A final film is taken 15 minutes after contrast injection, to record the emp-

Operative Cholangiography

Operative cholangiography is an alternate method of visualizing the biliary ducts and is recommended in patients with suspected cholelithiasis or with jaundice resulting from calculus disease of the biliary tree. The test is performed during surgery by the injection of a contrast medium, such as sodium diatrizoate, directly into the common bile duct, the cystic duct, or the gallbladder through a thin needle or catheter. If the gallbladder has been removed before injection, the contrast medium may be administered through a T tube (shown below)

inserted after cholecystectomy (operative T-tube cholangiography).

As the contrast flows through the biliary ducts, it reveals calculi and small intraluminal neoplasms, permitting the surgeon to remove them before closing the incision. Operative cholangiography can therefore eliminate the need for two surgical procedures, since gallbladder disease requiring cholecystectomy is often associated with biliary tract disease. However, this advantage must be weighed against the risks associated with contrast administration during a simple cholecystectomy.

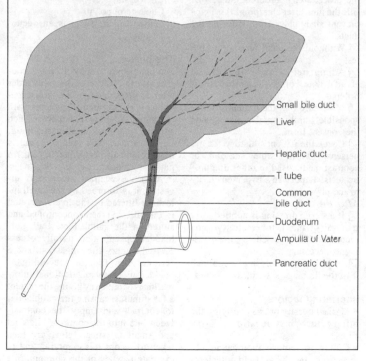

- Small bile duct
- Liver
- Hepatic duct
- T tube
- Common bile duct
- Duodenum
- Ampulla of Vater
- Pancreatic duct

tying of contrast-laden bile into the duodenum.
• If emptying is delayed, additional films may be taken at 15- or 30-minute

intervals until this action is demonstrated.
• The test takes approximately 15 minutes to perform.

Special precautions

The patient should be assessed for signs of hypersensitivity to the contrast medium, although these reactions occur more commonly with I.V. injection.

Patient care checklist

Before the test

☑ Explain or clarify test purpose, preparation, and procedure.

☑ Although this procedure is not painful, warn the patient that he may experience a sensation of bloating in the upper right quadrant as the contrast medium is injected.

☑ Evaluate patient understanding.

☑ Clamp the T tube the day before the procedure, if ordered. Since bile fills the tube after clamping, this helps prevent air bubbles from entering the ducts.

☑ Withhold the meal just before the test.

☑ Administer a cleansing enema about 1 hour before the procedure, if ordered.

☑ Make sure that the patient or a responsible family member has signed the consent form.

☑ Check the patient's history for hypersensitivity to iodine, seafood, or contrast media used in other diagnostic tests. Report any hypersensitivity to the physician.

After the test

☑ If a sterile dressing is applied after removal of the T tube, observe and record any drainage. Change the dressing as necessary.

☑ If the T tube is left in place, attach it to the drainage system, as ordered.

Interfering factors

• Marked obesity or gas overlying the biliary ducts may invalidate X-ray films.

• Failure to remove radiopaque objects from the X-ray field interferes with radiologic interpretation.

Cholecystography
[Gallbladder radiography]

Purpose

• To detect gallstones
• To aid diagnosis of inflammatory disease and tumors of the gallbladder.

Normal results

The gallbladder is visible and normal in size and structure. There is no evidence of inflammation or stones.

Abnormal results

Cholecystography may indicate:
Gallstones (cholelithiasis)
Cholecystitis
Cholesterol polyps
Benign tumor, such as an adenomyoma.

The basics

Oral cholecystography is the radiographic examination of the gallbladder after administration of a contrast medium. It is indicated in patients with symptoms of biliary tract disease, such as upper right quadrant epigastric pain, fat intolerance, and jaundice, and is most commonly performed to confirm gallbladder disease.

After the contrast medium is ingested, it is absorbed by the small intestine, filtered by the liver, excreted in the bile, and then concentrated and stored in the gallbladder. Full gallbladder opacification usually occurs 12 to 14 hours after ingestion, and a series of X-ray films then records gallbladder appearance. Additional information is obtained by giving the patient a fat stimulus, causing the gallbladder to contract and empty the contrast-laden bile into the common bile duct and small intestine. Films are then taken to record this emptying and to evaluate patency of the common bile duct.

When the gallbladder fails to opacify or when only faint opacification occurs, inflammatory disease, such as cholecystitis—with or without gallstone formation— may be present. Gallstones may obstruct the cystic duct and prevent the contrast medium from entering the gallbladder; inflammation may impair the concentrating ability of the gallbladder mucosa and prevent or diminish opacification.

When the gallbladder fails to contract following stimulation by a fatty meal, cholecystitis or common bile duct obstruction may be present. If the X-ray films are inconclusive, oral cholecystography will have to be repeated the following day.

Contraindications to this test include: severe renal or hepatic damage, or hypersensitivity to the contrast medium.

Oral cholecystography should precede barium studies, since retained barium may cloud subsequent X-ray films.

Procedure

• After the patient is in a prone position on the radiographic table, the abdomen is examined fluoroscopically to evaluate gallbladder opacification, and films are taken of significant findings.

• The patient is then examined while in left lateral decubitus and erect positions, to detect possible layering or mobility of any filling defects, and additional films are taken.

• The patient may then be given a fat stimulus, such as a high-fat meal or a synthetic fat-containing agent (for example, Bilevac).

• Fluoroscopy is used to observe the emptying of the gallbladder in response to the fat stimulus, and spot films are taken at 15 and 30 minutes to visualize the common bile duct.

• If the gallbladder empties slowly or not at all, these films are also taken at 60 minutes.

• The test usually takes 30 to 45 minutes to perform but, as mentioned, may take longer.

Patient care checklist
Before the test

☑ Explain or clarify test purpose, preparation, and procedure.

☑ Evaluate patient understanding.

☑ If ordered, provide a meal containing fat at noon the day before the test, and a fat-free meal in the evening. The former stimulates release of bile from the gallbladder, preparing it to receive the contrast-laden bile; the latter inhibits gallbladder contraction, promoting accumulation of bile.

☑ After the evening meal, restrict food and fluids, except water.

☑ Give the patient six tablets (3 g) of iopanoic acid 2 or 3 hours after the evening meal, as ordered. Other commercial contrast agents are available (such as sodium ipodate), but iopanoic acid is most commonly used. Have the patient swallow the tablets one at a time, at 5-minute intervals, with one or two mouthfuls of water, for a total of 8 oz (240 ml) of water. Thereafter, withhold water.

☑ Check the patient's history for hypersensitivity to iodine, seafood, or contrast media used for other diagnostic tests. Report to the physician any such hypersensitivity.

☑ Inform the patient that the possible side effects of dye ingestion include diarrhea (common) and, rarely, nausea, vomiting, abdominal cramps, and dysuria. Tell him to report such symptoms immediately if they develop.

☑ Examine any emesis or diarrhea for undigested tablets. If any tablets were expelled, notify the physician and the X-ray department.

☑ Administer a cleansing enema the morning of the test, if ordered.

After the test

☑ Nonopacification and repeat cholecystography require continuation of a low-fat diet until definitive diagnosis can be made.

☑ If gallstones are discovered during opacification, the doctor will order an appropriate diet—usually one that restricts fat intake, to help prevent acute attacks.

Interfering factors

• Failure to adhere to dietary preparation and restrictions before contrast study can interfere with accurate determination of results.

• Failure to ingest the full dosage of contrast medium, partial loss of the contrast medium through emesis or diarrhea, inadequate absorption of the contrast medium in the small intestine, and barium retained from previous studies of the biliary tract can interfere with accurate determination of test results.

• Impaired hepatic function and moderate jaundice (serum bilirubin levels greater than 3 mg/dl) cause diminished excretion of the contrast medium into the bile, thereby inhibiting adequate visualization of the biliary tract.

Digital subtraction angiography (DSA)

Purpose

• To visualize extracranial and intracranial cerebral blood flow

• To detect and evaluate cerebrovascular abnormalities

• To detect peripheral artery disease

• To identify renal artery stenosis or occlusion

• To identify abnormalities in pulmonary circulation

• To aid postoperative evaluation of vascular surgery, such as arterial grafts and endarterectomies.

Normal results

Normal cerebral vasculature, abdominal aorta and branches, peripheral vasculature, and renal arteries.

Abnormal results

DSA may detect:
  Aneurysms
  Tumors (possibly their vascular supply)
  Arterial stenosis
  Arterial occlusion
  Arteriovenous malformations
  Pulmonary emboli
  Plaques.

The basics

DSA is a sophisticated radiographic technique that uses video equipment and computer-assisted image enhancement to examine the vascular system. As in conventional angiography, X-ray images are obtained after injection of a contrast medium. However, unlike conventional angiography, in which images of bone and soft tissue often obscure vascular detail, DSA provides a better, high-contrast view of blood vessels, without interfering images or shadows.

In addition to superior image quality, DSA has other important advantages over conventional angiography. Because the digital subtraction process allows intravenous, rather than intraarterial, injection of the contrast medium, DSA avoids the risk of arterial puncture and the subsequent complication of emboli, and reduces the pain and discomfort associated with arterial catheterization.

Although DSA has been used to study peripheral and renal vascular disease, it is probably most useful in diagnosing cerebrovascular disorders. It also permits visualization of arterial bypass grafts. DSA can be performed quickly on an outpatient basis.

Contraindications to this test may include: iodine or contrast media hypersensitivity; poor cardiac function; renal, hepatic, or thyroid disease; or multiple myeloma.

Procedure

• The patient is placed in a supine position on an X-ray table and told to lie still with his arms at his sides.

• After an initial series of fluoroscopic pictures (mask images) is taken, the injection site—most commonly the antecubital basilic or cephalic vein—is shaved and cleansed.

• If catheterization is ordered, a local anesthetic is administered, a venipuncture is performed, and a catheter is inserted and advanced to the superior vena cava.

• After placement is verified by X-ray, I.V. lines from a bottle of normal saline solution and from an automatic contrast medium injector are connected. While the saline is administered, the injector delivers the contrast medium at a rate of about 14 ml/second.

• If simple injection of the contrast medium is ordered, a bolus of 40 to 60 ml is administered intravenously by needle.

• The patient's vital signs and neurologic status are monitored.

• After allowing time for the contrast medium to clear the pulmonary circulation, a second series of fluoroscopic images (contrast images) is taken.

• The computer digitizes the information received from both series and compares mask and contrast images, subtracting the common information (images of bone and soft tissue).

• A detailed image of the contrast medium-filled vessels is displayed on a video monitor; the image may be stored on videotape or a videodisc for future reference.

• The test takes approximately 30 to 45 minutes to perform.

Special precautions
The patient should be assessed for signs of a hypersensitivity reaction.

Patient care checklist
Before the test

☑ Explain or clarify test purpose, preparation, procedure, and post-test care.

☑ Stress the importance of lying still for the procedure. (Some patients—especially children—may be given a sedative to prevent movement during the procedure.)

☑ Tell the patient that he will probably feel some transient pain from insertion of the needle or catheter, and that he may experience mild symptoms from injection of the contrast medium, such as a feeling of warmth, a headache, or a metallic taste.

☑ Evaluate patient understanding.

☑ Restrict food for 4 hours before the test. Fluids are permitted.

☑ Make sure that the patient or a responsible family member has signed a consent form.

☑ Check the patient's history for hypersensitivity to local anesthetics, iodine, iodine-containing substances such as shellfish, and radiographic contrast media. Report any hypersensitivities to the physician.

After the test

☑ Because the contrast medium acts as a diuretic, encourage the patient to increase his fluid intake over the 24 hours after this test. Monitor intake and output, as ordered.

☑ Check the venipuncture site for signs of extravasation, such as redness or swelling. If bleeding occurs, apply firm pressure to the puncture site. If a hematoma develops, elevate the arm and apply warm soaks.

Interfering factors
• Patient movement during the procedure may cause blurred images.

• Failure to remove radiopaque objects from the X-ray field interferes with radiologic interpretation.

Hypotonic duodenography

Purpose
• To detect small postbulbar duodenal lesions, tumors of the head of the pancreas, and tumors of the ampulla of Vater

• To aid diagnosis of chronic pancreatitis.

Normal results
Duodenal mucosa appears smooth and even. The regular contour of the head of the pancreas also appears on the duodenal wall.

Abnormal results
Irregular nodules or masses on the duodenal wall may indicate:
Duodenal lesions
Tumors of the ampulla of Vater
Tumors of the head of the pancreas
Chronic pancreatitis.

The basics
Hypotonic duodenography is the radiographic examination of the duodenum after instillation of barium sulfate and air through an intestinal catheter. This test is indicated in patients with symptoms of duodenal or pancreatic pathology, such as persistent upper abdominal pain.

Although these films readily demonstrate small duodenal lesions and tumors of the head of the pancreas that impinge on the duodenal wall, differential diagnosis requires further studies.

Procedure
• While the patient is in a sitting position, a catheter is passed through his nose into his stomach.
• The patient is placed in a supine position on the radiographic table, and the catheter is advanced into the duodenum, under fluoroscopic guidance.
• Glucagon I.V. is administered to the patient, which quickly induces duodenal atony for approximately 20 minutes, or an anticholinergic is injected I.M. Throughout the procedure, the patient is observed for side effects.
• Barium is then instilled through the catheter, and spot films are taken of the duodenum.
• Some of the barium is then withdrawn and air is instilled; then additional spot films are taken.
• When the required films have been obtained, the catheter is removed.
• The test takes about 30 minutes to perform.

Special precautions
CLINICAL ALERT: **Anticholinergics are contraindicated in patients with** severe cardiac disorders or glaucoma.

Patient care checklist
Before the test
☑ Explain or clarify test purpose, preparation, procedure, and post-test care.
☑ Tell the patient that he may experience a cramping pain as air is introduced into the duodenum. Instruct him to breathe deeply and slowly through his mouth if he experiences this pain, to help relax his abdominal muscles.
☑ Evaluate patient understanding.
☑ Restrict food and fluids after midnight before the test.
☑ If an anticholinergic is being administered to an outpatient, advise him to have someone accompany him home.
After the test
☑ Watch for possible side effects after administration of glucagon or an anticholinergic. If an anticholinergic was given, be sure the patient voids within a few hours after the test. Advise the outpatient to rest in a waiting area until his vision clears (about 2 hours), unless someone can accompany him home.
☑ Administer a cathartic, as ordered.
☑ Tell the patient that he may burp instilled air or pass flatus, and that the barium will color his stool chalky white for 24 to 72 hours. Record description of any stool passed by the patient in the hospital, and notify the physician if the patient has not expelled the barium after 2 or 3 days.

Interfering factors
Failure to remove radiopaque objects from the X-ray field interferes with radiologic interpretation.

Hysterosalpingography

Purpose
• To confirm tubal abnormalities, such as adhesions and occlusion

• To confirm uterine abnormalities, such as the presence of foreign bodies, congenital malformations, and traumatic injuries

• To confirm the presence of fistulas or peritubal adhesions.

Normal results

A symmetric uterine cavity with no defects; the contrast medium courses through fallopian tubes of normal caliber, spills freely into the peritoneal cavity, and does not leak from the uterus.

Abnormal results

Hysterosalpingography may help detect:

Intrauterine adhesions
Uterine tumors
Foreign bodies in the uterus
Congenital malformations
Traumatic uterine injuries
Fistulas
Tubal occlusion and adhesions
Peritubal adhesions.

The basics

Hysterosalpingography is the radiologic visualization of the uterine cavity, the fallopian tubes, and the peritubal area. The procedure consists of taking fluoroscopic X-ray films as contrast medium flows through the uterus and the fallopian tubes. Generally performed as part of an infertility study, this test also helps evaluate repeated fetal loss and may be utilized as a follow-up to surgery, especially uterine unification procedures and tubal reanastomosis.

Although ultrasonography has virtually replaced hysterosalpingography in the detection of foreign bodies, such as a dislodged intrauterine device, it cannot evaluate tubal patency, which is the main purpose of hysterosalpingography. Laparoscopy with contrast instillation confirms positive or equivocal findings.

Uterine perforation is a possible complication.

Contraindications to this test include: menses, undiagnosed vaginal bleeding, or pelvic inflammatory disease.

Procedure

• With the patient in lithotomy position, a scout film is taken.

• A speculum is inserted into the patient's vagina, a tenaculum is placed on her cervix, and the cervix is cleansed.

• Next, a cannula is inserted into her cervix and anchored to the tenaculum.

• After the contrast medium is injected through the cannula, the uterus and fallopian tubes are viewed fluoroscopically, and radiographs are taken.

• Films may also be taken later, to evaluate spillage of contrast medium into the peritoneal cavity.

• The test takes about 15 minutes to perform.

Special precautions

The patient should be assessed for signs of a hypersensitivity reaction.

Patient care checklist

Before the test

☑ Explain or clarify test purpose and procedure.

☑ Advise the patient that she may experience moderate cramping from the procedure; however, she may receive a mild sedative, such as diazepam.

☑ Evaluate patient understanding.

☑ Check the patient's history for hypersensitivity to contrast medium, and report any hypersensitivity to the physician.

After the test

☑ Watch for signs of infection, such as fever, pain, increased pulse rate, malaise, and muscle ache.

☑ Assure the patient that cramps and vagal reaction (slow pulse rate, nausea, and dizziness) are transient.

Interfering factors

• Tubal spasm or excessive traction may cause the appearance of a stricture in normal fallopian tubes.

• Excessive traction can displace adhesions, making tubes appear normal.

• Failure to remove radiopaque objects from the X-ray field interferes with radiologic interpretation.

Intracranial computed tomography (CT)

Purpose
• To diagnose intracranial lesions and abnormalities
• To monitor the effects of surgery, radiotherapy, or chemotherapy on intracranial tumors.

Normal results
Intracranial structures are of normal symmetry, density, size, shape, and position.

Abnormal results
Areas of altered density, or displaced structures, may indicate:
    Intracranial tumors
    Cerebral atrophy
    Cerebral infarction
    Brain abscess
    Epidural, subdural, and intracerebral hematomas
    Cerebral edema
    Hydrocephalus
    Arteriovenous malformation.

The basics
Intracranial computed tomography, commonly called CT scanning, is a noninvasive test (if contrast is not used) that provides clear cross-sectional images of various layers (or slices) of the brain. It is based on computer reconstruction of radiation levels absorbed by various tissues. The density of tissue determines the amount of radiation that will pass through it. Tissue densities appear as black, white, or shades of gray on the computerized image obtained by intracranial CT scanning. Bone, the densest tissue, ap-

pears white; brain matter appears in shades of gray; cerebrospinal fluid—the least dense—appears black.

Newer versions of the scanner produce more detailed images than earlier models. The improved images identify intracranial tumors and other brain lesions as areas of altered density. For example, both subdural and epidural hematomas and other acute hemorrhages are normally easy to detect, because the high density of blood contrasts markedly with low-density brain tissue. In fact, in a patient with suspected head injury, intracranial CT may allow diagnosis of subdural hematoma before it causes characteristic symptoms. Displaced structures also signify abnormalities. In children, enlargement of the fourth ventricle generally indicates hydrocephalus.

The increasing availability of CT scanners allows faster and safer diagnosis than in the past. Often, intracranial CT scanning eliminates the need for painful and hazardous invasive procedures, such as pneumoencephalography and cerebral angiography. CT often uses contrast enhancement to help define abnormalities.

Procedure
• The patient is placed in a supine position on a radiographic table, with his head immobilized by straps, and is asked to lie still.
• The head of the table is moved into the scanner, which rotates around the patient's head, taking radiographs at 1-degree intervals in a 180-degree arc.
• When this series of radiographs is complete, contrast enhancement is performed, if ordered. Usually, 50 to 100 ml of contrast medium are injected I.V. or by drip method over 1 to 2 minutes.
• After injection of the contrast medium, another series of scans is taken. Information from the scans is stored on magnetic tapes, fed into a computer, and converted into images on an oscilloscope screen. Photographs of

selected views are taken for further study.
• The test takes about 15 to 30 minutes to perform.

Special precautions
The patient is observed for signs of a hypersensitivity reaction, if contrast enhancement is used. Such reactions usually develop within 30 minutes.

Patient care checklist
Before the test
☑ Explain or clarify test purpose, preparation, and procedure.
☑ Reassure the patient that the test will cause him no discomfort.
☑ Evaluate patient understanding.
☑ Restrict food and fluids for 4 hours before the test, only if contrast enhancement is scheduled. Otherwise, he need not restrict food and fluids.
☑ If the patient is restless or apprehensive, notify the physician, and administer a sedative, if ordered.
☑ Make sure that the patient or a responsible family member has signed the consent form.
☑ Check the patient's history for hypersensitivity to shellfish, iodine, or other contrast media. Inform the physician of any hypersensitivity.
After the test
☑ If a contrast agent was used, watch for residual side effects (headache, nausea, and vomiting).

Interfering factors
• Artifacts caused by the patient moving his head make CT scan images difficult to interpret.
• Failure to remove radiopaque objects from the X-ray field interferes with radiologic interpretation.

Intravenous pyelography
[Excretory urography]

Purpose
• To evaluate the structure and excre-

tory function of the kidneys, ureters, and bladder
• To support a differential diagnosis of renovascular hypertension.

Normal results
Normal size, shape, and position of the kidneys, ureters, and bladder, with no gross evidence of soft- or hard-tissue lesions.

With normal renal functioning, in the first minute after injection the contrast medium should delineate the size and shape of the kidneys. After 3 to 5 minutes, the contrast medium should move into the calyces and pelvises. Finally, the ureters and then bladder are outlined. A postvoiding radiograph should show no mucosal abnormalities and minimal residual urine.

Abnormal results
Intravenous pyelography may demonstrate:
Renal or ureteral calculi
Abnormal size, shape, or position of kidneys, ureters, or bladder
Absent kidney
Supernumerary kidney
Polycystic kidney disease associated with renal hypertrophy
Redundant pelvis or ureter
Pyelonephritis
Renal tuberculosis
Hydronephrosis
Cysts
Tumors
Renovascular hypertension.

The basics
The cornerstone of a urologic workup, this test allows visualization of the renal parenchyma, calyces, and pelvis, as well as the ureters, the bladder, and in some cases the urethra, following I.V. administration of a contrast medium.

Clinical indications for this test include suspected renal or urinary tract disease, space-occupying lesions, congenital anomalies, or trauma to the urinary system.

Procedure

• The patient is placed in supine position on the radiographic table. A plain film of the abdomen is taken.

• If the film confirms the absence of gross abnormalities, contrast medium is injected intravenously.

• The first radiograph, visualizing the renal parenchyma, is obtained about 1 minute after the injection, possibly supplemented by tomography if small space-occupying masses, such as cysts or tumors, are suspected.

• Films are then exposed at regular intervals—usually 5, 10, and 15 or 20 minutes after the injection.

• Sometimes it is necessary to apply painless pressure to the patient's abdomen to facilitate retention of the contrast medium by the upper urinary tract. This is done by inflating two small rubber bladders and securing them tightly on the patient's abdomen, on both sides of the midline.

• At the end of the procedure, the patient voids, and another film may be made immediately to visualize residual bladder content or mucosal abnormalities of the bladder or urethra.

Special precautions

The patient should be observed for signs of a hypersensitivity reaction.

Patient care checklist

Before the test

☑ Explain or clarify test purpose, preparation, and procedure.

☑ Inform the patient that he may experience nausea, a transient burning sensation, and a metallic taste when the contrast medium is injected. Tell him to report any other sensations he may experience.

☑ Evaluate patient understanding.

☑ Be sure that the patient is well hydrated, then restrict food and fluids for 8 hours before the test.

☑ Make sure that the patient or a responsible family member has signed a consent form.

☑ Check the patient's history for hypersensitivity to iodine, iodine-containing foods, or contrast media containing iodine. If the patient has such a history, notify the physician.

☑ Administer a laxative, as ordered, the night before the test.

After the test

☑ If a hematoma develops at the injection site, ease the patient's discomfort by applying warm soaks.

Interfering factors

• Fecal matter or gas in the colon, insufficient injection of contrast medium, or a recent barium enema or gastrointestinal series interferes with accurate testing.

• Failure to remove radiopaque objects from the X-ray field interferes with radiologic interpretation.

Kidney-ureter-bladder (KUB) radiography
[Scout film, flat plate, or plain film of the abdomen]

Purpose

• To evalute the size, structure, and position of the kidneys

• To screen for gross abnormalities in the abdomen.

Normal results

Normal abdominal structures.

Abnormal results

KUB radiography may identify:

Renal enlargement or atrophy

Renal displacement, as from a retroperitoneal tumor

Absence of a kidney

Abnormal renal location or shape, as with congenital anomalies

Urinary calculi

Vascular calcification

Cystic tumors

Fecaliths
Foreign bodies
Ascites.

The basics

Usually the first step in diagnostic testing of the urinary system, KUB radiography surveys the abdomen to determine the position of the kidneys, ureters, and bladder and to detect gross abnormalities. This test does not require intact renal function and may aid differential diagnosis of urologic and gastrointestinal diseases, which often produce similar signs and symptoms. However, a KUB has many limitations and nearly always must be followed by more elaborate tests, such as intravenous pyelography or renal computed tomography. KUB should not follow recent instillation of barium, which obscures the urinary system.

Procedure

• The patient is placed in supine position on a radiographic table.
• His arms are exended overhead, and his iliac crests are checked for symmetrical positioning.
• A single radiograph is taken.

Special precautions

The male patient should have gonadal shielding to prevent irradiation of the testes. The female patient's ovaries cannot be shielded because they are located too close to the kidneys, ureters, and bladder.

Patient care checklist

Before the test
☑ Explain or clarify test purpose and procedure.
☑ Evaluate patient understanding.

Interfering factors

• Gas, feces, contrast medium, or foreign bodies in the intestine may obscure the urinary system.
• Obesity or ascites may result in a radiograph of poor quality.

Lower limb venography
[Ascending contrast phlebography]

Purpose

• To confirm diagnosis of deep vein thrombosis (DVT)
• To distinguish clot formation from venous obstruction (a large tumor of the pelvis impinging on the venous system, for example)
• To evaluate congenital venous abnormalities
• To assess deep vein valvular competence (especially helpful in identifying underlying causes of leg edema)
• To locate a suitable vein for arterial bypass grafting.

Normal results

Normal, patent superficial and deep veins of the lower limb.

Abnormal results

Lower limb venography
Confirms a diagnosis of:
  DVT.
Can also indicate:
  Deep vein valvular incompetence
  Venous obstruction.

The basics

Venography is the radiographic examination of a vein and is often used to assess the condition of the deep leg veins after injection of a contrast medium. It is the definitive test for DVT, an acute condition marked by inflammation and thrombus formation in the deep veins of the legs. Such thrombi usually develop in valve pockets (venous junctions or sinuses of the calf muscle), travel to the deep calf veins, and if untreated may occlude the popliteal, femoral, and iliac vein systems. This condition may lead to pulmonary embolism, a potentially lethal complication.

A venogram that shows consistent filling defects on repeat views, abrupt termination of a column of contrast material, unfilled major deep veins, or diversion of flow (through collaterals, for example) is diagnostic of DVT.

Venography should not be used for routine screening, since it exposes the patient to relatively high doses of radiation and can cause complications such as phlebitis, local tissue damage, and occasionally DVT itself. The ^{125}I fibrinogen scan provides an acceptable, though less accurate, alternative to venography.

Procedure

• The patient lies on a tilting radiographic table, inclined 40 to 60 degrees, so that the leg being tested does not bear any weight.

• The patient is instructed to relax this leg and keep it still; a tourniquet may be tied around the ankle to expedite venous filling.

• Normal saline solution is injected into a superficial vein in the dorsum of the patient's foot.

• Once correct needle placement is achieved, contrast medium is slowly injected and the presence of extravasation is checked. (If a suitable superficial vein cannot be found due to edema, a surgical cutdown of the vein may be performed.)

• Using a fluoroscope, the distribution of the contrast medium is monitored, and spot films may be taken from the anteroposterior and oblique projections and over the thigh and femoro-iliac regions. Then overhead films are taken of the calf, knee, thigh, and femoral area.

• After filming, the patient is repositioned horizontally, the leg being tested is quickly elevated, and normal saline solution is infused to flush the contrast medium from the veins.

• The fluoroscope is checked to confirm complete emptying. Then the needle is removed, and an adhesive bandage is applied to the injection site.

• The test takes 30 to 45 minutes to perform.

Special precautions

The patient should be assessed for signs of a hypersensitivity reaction.

Patient care checklist

Before the test

☑ Explain or clarify test purpose, preparation, procedure, and post-test care.

☑ Warn the patient that he may feel a transient burning sensation in his leg on injection of the contrast medium and some discomfort during the procedure.

☑ Evaluate patient understanding.

☑ Restrict food and permit only clear liquids for 4 hours before the test.

☑ Make sure that the patient or a responsible family member has signed a consent form.

☑ Check the patient's history for hypersensitivity to iodine or iodine-containing foods, such as shellfish, or to contrast media used in previous diagnostic tests. Report any hypersensitivity to the physician.

☑ If ordered, restrict anticoagulant therapy.

☑ Just before the test, instruct the patient to void, to remove all clothing below the waist, and to put on a hospital gown.

☑ If ordered, give the anxious or uncooperative patient a mild sedative.

After the test

☑ Monitor vital signs until stable; check the pulse rate on the dorsalis pedis, popliteal, and femoral arteries.

☑ Administer analgesics, as ordered, to counteract the irritating effects of the contrast medium.

☑ Watch for hematoma, redness, bleeding, or infection (especially if a cutdown of the vein was performed) at the puncture site, and replace the dressing when necessary. Notify the physician if complications develop.

☑ If the venogram indicates DVT, initiate therapy (heparin infusion, bed rest, leg elevation or support, blood chemistry tests), as ordered.

Interfering factors

• If the patient places weight on the leg being tested, the contrast medium may fail to fill the leg veins.

• Movement of the leg being tested, excessive tourniquet constriction, insufficient injection of contrast medium, or delay between injection and radiography interferes with accurate testing.

• Failure to remove radiopaque objects from the X-ray field interferes with radiologic interpretation.

Lymphangiography
[Lymphography]

Purpose

• To detect and stage lymphomas and to identify metastatic involvement of the lymph nodes

• To distinguish primary from secondary lymphedema

• To suggest surgical treatment or to evaluate the effectiveness of chemotherapy and radiation therapy in controlling malignancy.

Normal results

Normal lymph nodes and lymphatic vessels.

Abnormal results

Enlarged, foamy-looking nodes indicate:

Lymphoma, classified as Hodgkin's or non-Hodgkin's.

Filling defects or lack of opacification indicates:

Metastatic involvement of the lymph nodes.

Shortened lymphatic vessels and a deficient number of vessels indicate:

Primary lymphedema.

Abruptly terminating lymphatic vessels indicate:

Secondary lymphedema resulting from retroperitoneal tumors, inflammation, filariasis, surgery, or irradiation.

The basics

Lymphangiography is the radiographic examination of the lymphatic system after the injection of an oil-based contrast medium into a lymphatic vessel in each foot or, less commonly, in each hand. Injection into the foot allows visualization of the lymphatics of the leg, inguinal and iliac regions, and the retroperitoneum up to the thoracic duct. Injection into the hand allows visualization of the axillary and supraclavicular nodes. This procedure may also be used to study the cervical region (retroauricular area), but this is less useful and less common.

X-ray films are taken immediately after injection to demonstrate the filling of the lymphatic system, and then again 24 hours later to visualize the lymph nodes. Since the contrast remains in the nodes for up to 2 years, subsequent X-ray films can assess progression of disease and monitor effectiveness of treatment.

Lymphangiography is usually performed to stage disease in patients with an established diagnosis of lymphoma or cancer. It may also be performed for patients with enlarged lymph nodes, detected by computed tomography or ultrasonography.

Contraindications to this test include: hypersensitivity to iodine, pulmonary insufficiency, cardiac disease, or severe renal or hepatic disease.

Procedure

• A preliminary X-ray of the chest is taken.

• The skin over the dorsum of each foot is cleansed, and blue contrast is injected intradermally into the area between the toes, usually the first and fourth toe webs.

• Within 15 to 30 minutes, the lymphatic vessels appear as small blue lines on the upper surface of the instep of each foot.

• A local anesthetic is then injected into the dorsum of each foot, and a 1″ (2.5 cm) transverse incision is made

to expose the lymphatic vessel.
• Each vessel is cannulated, and contrast medium is injected at a rate of 0.1 to 0.2 ml/minute for about 1½ hours, to avoid injuring delicate lymphatic vessels.
• Fluoroscopy may be used to monitor filling of the lymphatic system. If so, the infusion is stopped when the contrast reaches the level of the third and fourth lumbar vertebrae.
• At this point, or when the injection is completed, the needles are removed, the incisions are sutured, and sterile dressings are applied.
• X-ray films of the legs, pelvis, abdomen, and chest are taken.
• The test takes about 3 hours to perform.
• After the procedure is completed, the patient is taken to his room, but must return 24 hours later for additional films.

Special precautions
The patient should be assessed for signs of a hypersensitivity reaction.

Patient care checklist
Before the test
☑ Explain or clarify test purpose, preparation, procedure, and post-test care.
☑ Inform the patient that the injection of contrast medium causes transient discomfort and that the contrast discolors urine and stool for 48 hours and may give his skin and vision a bluish tinge for 48 hours.
☑ Advise the patient that he must remain as still as possible during injection of the contrast medium.
☑ Warn him that the incision site may be sore for several days afterward.
☑ Evaluate patient understanding.
☑ If this test is performed on an outpatient, advise him to be accompanied by a friend or relative.
☑ Make sure that the patient or a responsible family member has signed a consent form.
☑ Check the patient's history for hypersensitivity to iodine, seafood, or the contrast media used in other diagnostic tests. Report any hypersensitivity to the physician.
☑ Just before the procedure, instruct the patient to void, and check his vital signs for a baseline.
☑ If ordered, administer a sedative.
After the test
☑ Monitor the patient's vital signs, as ordered.
CLINICAL ALERT: **Watch for pulmonary complications, such as shortness of breath, pleuritic pain, hypotension, low-grade fever, and cyanosis, due to embolization of the contrast medium.**
☑ Enforce bed rest for 24 hours, with the patient's feet elevated to help reduce swelling, as ordered.
☑ Apply ice packs to the incision sites to help reduce swelling, and administer an analgesic, as ordered.
☑ Check the incision sites for infection, and leave the dressings in place for 2 days, making sure the wounds remain dry. Tell the patient the sutures will be removed in 7 to 10 days.
☑ Prepare the patient for follow-up X-rays, as ordered.

Interfering factors
Failure to remove radiopaque objects from the X-ray field interferes with radiologic interpretation.

Mammography

Purpose
• To screen for breast malignancy
• To investigate palpable and non-palpable breast masses, breast pain, or nipple discharge
• To help differentiate between benign breast disease and breast malignancy.

Normal results
Normal duct, glandular tissue, and fat architecture. No abnormal masses or calcifications in the breasts.

Abnormal results

Well-outlined, regular, clear spots suggest:

Benign cysts.

Poorly outlined, opaque areas suggest:

Malignancy.

The basics

Mammography is a radiographic technique used to detect breast cysts or tumors, especially those not palpable on physical examination. In xeromammography, an electrostatically charged plate records the X-ray images and transfers them to a special paper. Biopsy of suspicious areas may be required to confirm malignancy. Although 90% to 95% of breast malignancies can be detected by mammography, this test carries a 75% false-positive result rate. The American College of Radiologists and the American Cancer Society have established

Guidelines For Mammography

The American Cancer Society recommends a single baseline mammogram, using low-dose mammography (less than 1 rad for two views), for women between ages 35 and 40. Afterward, women under age 50 should consult their personal physicians about their need for mammography; women over age 50 should have an annual mammogram.

The American College of Radiologists suggests baseline mammograms for all women between ages 35 and 40, repeated every 2 years until age 50, and every year thereafter. Women at high risk (those with fibrocystic breasts; histories of breast, uterine, ovarian, colorectal, or salivary gland cancer; or family histories of breast malignancies) require earlier and more frequent screening than the general population.

Diaphanography

In *diaphanography*, also known as transillumination of the breast, infrared light is directed through the breast with a fiberoptic device, and the transmitted light is photographed with infrared film. The denser the tissues, the darker they appear on the film, allowing a trained examiner to distinguish them. Healthy breast tissue is reddish-yellow and translucent; fluid-filled cysts and fatty tissue appear as bright spots; benign tumors are red; blood vessels are dark red to black, and malignant tumors are dark brown or black. The technique can also be used to guide a needle for biopsy or cyst drainage.

Currently, diaphanography is used by only a few specialists in the United States. Although the method has a detection rate of 98% with modified equipment, it is less reliable than mammography and cannot accurately distinguish cancer from benign mastitis, which causes lumps and inflammation, or from hemorrhage, which resembles malignant tissue in transmitted light. However, this test can be repeated as often as needed without risk to the patient.

guidelines for the use and potential risks of mammography; both agree that despite low radiation levels (0.1 to 0.3 rads), the test is contraindicated during pregnancy. (See *Guidelines for Mammography* and *Diaphanography*.)

Procedure

• The patient is sitting on a chair or is standing and is asked to rest one of her breasts on a table above an X-ray cassette.

• A compressor is placed on the breast, and the patient is asked to hold her breath.

• A radiograph is taken of the craniocaudal view.

• The machine is rotated, the breast is compressed again, and a radiograph of the lateral view is taken.
• The procedure is then repeated on the other breast.
• The test takes about 15 to 30 minutes to perform.

Patient care checklist
Before the test
☑ Explain or clarify test purpose and procedure.
☑ Reassure the patient that the test is painless.
☑ Evaluate patient understanding.

Interfering factors
• Very glandular breasts (common under age 30) and previous breast surgery can impair readability of the films.
• Powders and salves on the breast may cause false-positive results.
• Failure to remove radiopaque objects from the X-ray field interferes with radiologic interpretation.

Myelography

Purpose
• To demonstrate lesions, such as tumors and herniated intervertebral disks, that partially or totally block the flow of cerebrospinal fluid (CSF) in the subarachnoid space
• To aid detection of arachnoiditis, spinal nerve root injury, or tumors in the posterior fossa of the skull.

Normal results
The contrast medium flows freely through the subarachnoid space, showing no obstruction or structural abnormalities.

Abnormal results
Myelography may detect and, if needed, localize:
  Herniated intervertebral disks
  Metastatic (extradural) tumors
  Neurofibromas and meningiomas
  (within the subarachnoid space)
  Ependymomas and astrocytomas
  (within the spinal cord)
  Syringomyelia
  Arachnoiditis
  Spinal nerve root injury
  Posterior fossa tumors.

The basics
Myelography combines fluoroscopy and radiography to evaluate the spinal subarachnoid space after injection of a contrast medium. Because the contrast medium is heavier than CSF, it will flow through the subarachnoid space to the dependent area when the patient, lying prone on a fluoroscopic table, is tilted up or down. The fluoroscope allows visualization of the flow of the contrast medium and the outline of the subarachnoid space. Radiographs are taken for a permanent record. Test results must be correlated with the patient's history and clinical status.

Sometimes, myelography is performed to confirm the need for surgery; in such cases, a neurosurgeon may stand by. If this test confirms a spinal tumor, the patient may be taken directly to the operating room. Immediate surgery may also be necessary when the contrast medium causes the total block of the subarachnoid space. *Contraindications to this test generally include:* increased intracranial pressure, hypersensitivity to iodine or contrast media, or infection at the puncture site.

Procedure
• The procedure is performed in the X-ray department.
• The patient is positioned on his side, and a lumbar puncture is performed. (See "Cerebrospinal Fluid Analysis," p. 287.)
• Fluoroscopy confirms needle position; some CSF may be removed.
• The patient is placed in the prone position and carefully secured.
• With the spinal needle in place, the

contrast medium is injected, and the table is tilted so the contrast flows through the subarachnoid space.

• When the required radiographs have been obtained, if the contrast agent is an oil (i.e., iophendylate) it is withdrawn, since it cannot be excreted. Water-soluble contrast medium (i.e., metrizamide) does not have to be removed.

• The needle is then removed.

• The puncture site is cleansed with povidone-iodine solution, and a small adhesive bandage is applied.

• The test takes 1 hour or more to perform.

Patient care checklist

Before the test

☑ Explain or clarify test purpose, preparation, procedure, and post-test care.

☑ Explain to the patient that he will probably feel a transient burning sensation as the contrast medium is injected, that he may feel flushed and warm, and may experience a headache, a salty taste, or nausea and vomiting after injection of the contrast medium.

☑ Warn him that he may feel some pain during the procedure from the positions he will assume, from insertion of the needle, and in some cases from removal of the contrast medium.

☑ Evaluate patient understanding.

☑ Restrict food and fluids for 8 hours before the test. However, if the test is scheduled for late in the day and if hospital policy permits, the patient may have clear liquids before the test.

☑ Make sure that the patient or a responsible family member has signed the consent form.

☑ Check the patient's history for hypersensitivity to iodine and to iodine-containing substances (such as shellfish), radiographic contrast medium, and other medications associated with the procedure. Report any hypersensitivity to the physician.

☑ If metrizamide is used as the contrast medium, discontinue phenothiazines 48 hours before the test is scheduled to begin. Notify the radiologist if the patient has a history of epilepsy or phenothiazine use.

☑ Administer a cleansing enema, which may be ordered to prevent gas shadows on the film.

☑ Just before the procedure, administer a sedative and anticholinergic (such as atropine sulfate), if ordered.

After the test

☑ Find out which contrast medium was used for the test, and position the patient accordingly. If *iophendylate* was used, the patient must return to his room on a stretcher and lie flat for 24 hours. If *metrizamide* was used, the patient must return to his room in a wheelchair, or on a stretcher with the head elevated at least 60 degrees. He must *not* lie flat for at least 8 hours, because this contrast medium can irritate cervical nerve roots and cranial structures.

☑ Monitor vital signs and neurologic status, as ordered.

☑ Encourage the patient to drink extra fluids. He should void within 8 hours after returning to his room.

☑ If no complications or side effects occur, the patient may resume his usual diet and activities the day after the test. If radicular pain, fever, back pain, or signs of meningeal irritation (headache, irritability, or neck stiffness) develop, keep the room quiet and dark, and provide an analgesic or an antipyretic, as ordered.

Interfering factors

• Incorrect needle placement or patient failure to cooperate may alter results.

• Failure to remove radiopaque objects from the X-ray field interferes with radiologic interpretation.

Nephrotomography

Purpose

• To differentiate between a simple renal cyst and a solid neoplasm

• To assess renal lacerations as well as posttraumatic nonperfused areas of the kidneys
• To localize adrenal tumors when laboratory tests indicate their presence.

Normal results
Normal size, shape, and position of kidneys, with no space-occupying lesions.

Abnormal results
Nephrotomography may detect:
    Cysts
    Solid tumors
    Renal sinus-related lesions
    Ectopic renal lobes
    Adrenal tumors
    Areas of nonperfusion
    Renal lacerations following trauma.

The basics
In nephrotomography, special films are exposed before and after opacification of the renal arterial network and parenchyma with contrast medium. The resulting tomographic slices clearly delineate various linear layers of the kidneys, while blurring structures in front of and behind these selected planes. Nephrotomography can be performed as a separate procedure or as an adjunct to intravenous pyelography.

The test may be performed using either the infusion method or the bolus method. The former is currently the method of choice, because it allows repetition of poorly defined tomograms without additional infusion of contrast.

Complications resulting from either technique are minor and uncommon. Other tests that may resolve nephrotomographic findings include renal angiography and radionuclide renal imaging.

Procedure
Infusion method:
• After test tomograms are reviewed, five vertical slices of renal parenchyma 1 cm apart are selected for filming.

• Contrast medium is then administered through the antecubital vein—the first half in 4 to 5 minutes (rapid phase) and the second half in the following 8 to 10 minutes (slow phase).
• Serial tomograms are made as soon as the slow phase begins.
Bolus method:
• After test tomograms are reviewed, circulation time from arm to tongue is determined by injecting a bolus of a bitter-tasting agent (dehydrocholic acid or sodium dehydrocholate) into the antecubital vein. Arm-to-tongue circulation time is close to arm-to-kidney circulation time (10 to 14 seconds).
• With the needle still in place, a loading dose of a conventional urographic contrast medium is injected, to perform intravenous pyelography.
• Five minutes after this injection, a loading dose of a contrast medium (such as Renografin-76 or Hypaque-M 75%) is quickly injected—within 2 seconds—to ensure a high concentration of the contrast in the kidneys.
• A multifilm tomographic cassette, exposed at the predetermined arm-to-kidney circulation time, visualizes the main renal vessels and possible vessels within tumors.
• A series of individual tomograms measuring 1 cm is then made in rapid succession—less than 2 minutes—through the opacified kidneys.
• The test takes less than 1 hour to perform.

Special precautions
The patient should be assessed for signs of a hypersensitivity reaction.

Patient care checklist
Before the test
☑ Explain or clarify test purpose, preparation, and procedure.
☑ Be sure to tell the patient that he may experience transient side effects from the injection of the contrast medium—usually a burning or stinging sensation at the injection site, flushing, and a metallic taste.

☑ Evaluate patient understanding.

☑ Restrict food and fluids for 8 hours before the test.

☑ Make sure that the patient or a responsible family member has signed the consent form.

☑ Check the patient's history for hypersensitivity to iodine or to iodine-containing foods, such as shellfish, or to contrast media used in other diagnostic tests. Report any hypersensitivity to the physician.

After the test

☑ Monitor vital signs and urinary output, as ordered, usually for 24 hours.

Interfering factors

• Pretest upper or lower gastrointestinal series, or residual barium from a recent barium enema, may obscure sharp delineation of the kidneys.

• Failure to remove radiopaque objects from the X-ray field interferes with radiologic interpretation.

Orbital computed tomography *(CT)*

Purpose

• To evaluate pathologies of the orbit and eye—especially expanding lesions and bone destruction

• To evaluate fractures of the orbit and adjoining structures

• To determine the cause of unilateral exophthalmos.

Normal results

Orbital structures are normal in size, shape, and position.

Abnormal results

Orbital CT scan:

Identify intra- and extraorbital space-occupying lesions:

Infiltrative lesions, such as lymphomas and metastatic carcinomas

Encapsulated tumors, such as benign hemangiomas and meningiomas

Intracranial tumors that invade the orbit.

Determine the cause of unilateral exophthalmos:

Lesions in the ethmoidal cells

Space-occupying lesions in the orbital or paranasal sinuses

Thickening of the medial and lateral rectus muscles resulting from Graves' disease.

The basics

Orbital CT allows visualization of abnormalities not readily seen on standard radiographs, delineating their size, position, and relationship to adjoining structures. The orbital CT scan identifies space-occupying lesions that obscure the normal structures or cause orbital enlargement, indentation of the orbital walls, or bone destruction, earlier and more accurately than other radiographic techniques; it provides three-dimensional images of orbital structures, especially the ocular muscles and the optic nerve.

Contrast enhancement may be used in orbital CT to define ocular tissues and evaluate a patient with such conditions as suspected circulatory disorder, hemangioma, or subdural hematoma. However, use of contrast enhancement is contraindicated in those patients with known hypersensitivity reactions to iodine, shellfish, or radiographic dyes used in other tests. Application of orbital CT to ophthalmology extends beyond the evaluation of the orbital and adjoining structures; it also permits precise diagnosis of many intracranial lesions that affect vision.

Procedure

• The patient is placed in a supine position on the radiographic table, with his head immobilized by straps, and is asked to lie still.

• The head of the table is then moved into the scanner, and radiographs are taken.

• The information is stored on magnetic tapes, and the images are displayed on an oscilloscope screen, which may be photographed if a permanent record is desired.

• When this series of radiographs has been taken, contrast enhancement is performed, if ordered. The contrast agent is injected, and a second series of scans is recorded.

• The test takes 15 to 30 minutes to perform.

Special precautions
If contrast enhancement is performed, the patient should be assessed for signs of a hypersensitivity reaction.

Patient care checklist
Before the test

☑ Explain or clarify test purpose, preparation, and procedure.

☑ Reassure the patient that the test will cause him no discomfort.

☑ Stress the importance of lying still for the procedure.

☑ If a contrast agent will be used, tell the patient that he may feel flushed and warm and may experience a transient headache or a salty taste after the dye is injected.

☑ Evaluate patient understanding.

☑ If contrast enhancement is scheduled, withhold food and fluids from the patient for 4 hours before the test. There are no dietary restrictions if contrast enhancement is not scheduled.

☑ Make sure that the patient or a responsible family member has signed a consent form.

☑ Check the patient's history for hypersensitivity reactions to iodine, shellfish, or radiographic dyes. Report any hypersensitivity to the physician.

Interfering factors
Movement of the patient's head may cause unclear images, interfering with accurate determination of test results.

Orbital radiography

Purpose
• To aid in diagnosis of orbital fractures and pathology
• To help locate intraorbital or intraocular foreign bodies.

Normal results
Size, shape, and position of orbital structures are normal when compared with those on the opposite side.

Abnormal results
Orbital radiography may detect:
  Orbital fracture
  Intraorbital or intraocular foreign bodies.
Enlargement of an orbit generally indicates:
  Growing tumor, such as orbital meningioma, retinoblastoma, or, in children, optic nerve glioma.
Decreased size of an orbit occurs:
  Following childhood enucleation of the eye
  In congenital microphthalmia.
Destruction of the orbital walls may indicate:
  Malignant neoplasm
  Infection.
Clear-cut local indentation of the orbital wall occurs with:
  Benign tumor
  Cyst.
Increased bone density occurs with:
  Osteoblastic metastasis
  Sphenoid ridge meningioma
  Paget's disease.

The basics
The orbit is a deep-set cavity that houses the eye, lacrimal gland, blood vessels, nerves, muscles, and fat. It is enclosed anteriorly by the eyeball and the eyelids. Since portions of the orbit are composed of thin bone that is easily fractured, radiographs of these structures are commonly taken following facial trauma. Radiographs are also

useful in diagnosing ocular and orbital pathology. Special radiographic techniques can visualize foreign bodies in the eye that cannot be seen with an ophthalmoscope. To confirm orbital pathology, however, radiographic findings must be supplemented with results from other appropriate tests and procedures. Tomograms may be taken concurrently with standard radiographs. Computerized tomography and ultrasonography can provide further information.

Procedure

• The patient is placed in a supine position on the radiographic table or is seated in a chair and is instructed to remain still while the radiographs are taken.
• A standard series of orbital radiographs, with various views, is taken.
• The test takes about 15 minutes to perform.

Patient care checklist

☑ Explain or clarify test purpose and procedure.
☑ Reassure the patient that this procedure is usually painless unless he has suffered facial trauma, in which case positioning may cause some discomfort.

Interfering factors

Failure to remove radiopaque objects from the X-ray field interferes with radiologic interpretation.

Pancreatic computed tomography (CT)

Purpose

• To detect pancreatic carcinoma or pseudocysts
• To detect or evaluate pancreatitis
• To distinguish between pancreatic disorders and disorders of the retroperitoneum.

Normal results

Pancreas is normal in size, shape, and position, with no evidence of pathology.

Abnormal results

Pancreatic CT can identify:
  Acute pancreatitis
  Chronic pancreatitis
  Pancreatic carcinoma
  Benign pancreatic tumor
  Pancreatic abscesses
  Pancreatic pseudocysts.

The basics

In pancreatic CT, multiple X-rays penetrate the upper abdomen and are measured, while a detector records the differences in tissue attenuation. A computer then reconstructs this data as a three-dimensional image on a television screen. Since attenuation varies with tissue density, pancreatic CT accurately distinguishes the pancreas, and surrounding organs and vessels if enough fat is present between the structures. Use of an I.V. or P.O. contrast medium can accentuate differences in tissue density.

Pancreatic CT is replacing ultrasonography as the test of choice for pancreatic examination. Ultrasonography costs less and involves less risk for the patient, but is somewhat less accurate.

In retroperitoneal disorders—specifically, when pancreatitis is suspected—CT scanning goes beyond ultrasonography by showing the general swelling that accompanies acute inflammation of the gland. In chronic cases, CT scanning easily detects calcium deposits often missed by simple radiography, particularly in obese patients.

Besides detecting tumors, cysts, and abscesses, CT can also distinguish between benign and malignant tumors, because of its unique sensitivity to variations in tissue density. CT scanning can spot presymptomatic warning signs of pancreatic carcinoma, such as localized swelling in the head, body, or tail of the gland. However, CT cannot detect tumors too small to alter pancreatic size and shape.

Procedure

• The patient is placed in a supine position on a radiographic table, and the table is positioned within the opening in the scanning gantry.

• A series of transverse X-rays is taken and recorded on magnetic tape.

• The varying tissue absorption is calculated by a computer, and the information is reconstructed as images on a television screen.

• These images are studied, and selected ones are photographed. After the first series of films is completed, the images are reviewed.

• Contrast enhancement may then be ordered. After the contrast medium is administered, another series of films is taken.

• The test takes about 1½ hours to perform.

Special precautions

If contrast enhancement is used, the patient should be assessed for signs of a hypersensitivity reaction.

Patient care checklist
Before the test

☑ Explain or clarify test purpose, preparation, and procedure.

☑ Assure the patient that although the test equipment looks formidable, the procedure is painless. Tell him that he will be asked to be still during the test and to hold his breath at certain times. Inform him that he may be given a contrast medium I.V. or P.O. or both to aid visualization of the pancreas.

☑ Evaluate patient understanding.

☑ Restrict food and fluids after midnight before the test.

☑ Make sure that the patient or a responsible family member has signed a consent form.

☑ Check the patient's history for hypersensitivity to iodine, seafood, or the contrast media used in other diagnostic tests. Report any hypersensitivity to the physician.

☑ Give gastrografin, as ordered, to clearly define and demarcate the stomach and intestines.

Interfering factors

• Barium retained in the gastrointestinal tract may obscure visualization.

• Excessive movement by the patient during scanning may produce artifacts.

• Excessive peristaltic movement during scanning may produce artifacts.

• Failure to remove radiopaque objects from the X-ray field interferes with radiologic interpretation.

Paranasal sinus radiography

Purpose

• To detect unilateral or bilateral abnormalities, possibly indicating trauma or disease

• To confirm diagnosis of neoplastic or inflammatory paranasal sinus disease

• To determine the location and size of a malignant neoplasm.

Normal results

Paranasal sinuses are radiolucent and filled with air.

Abnormal results
Paranasal sinus radiography may detect:

Paranasal sinus trauma or fracture
Acute sinusitis
Chronic sinusitis
Wegener's granulomatosis
Malignant neoplasms
Benign tumors of the bone and soft tissue
Cysts
Mucocele
Polyps.

The basics

The paranasal sinuses—air-filled cavities lined with mucous membrane—lie within the maxillary, ethmoid, sphenoid, and frontal bones. Sinus abnormalities, resulting from several conditions, may include distorted bony sinus walls, altered mucous membranes, and fluid or masses within the cavities.

In paranasal sinus radiography, the air that normally fills the paranasal sinuses appears black on film, but fluid in a sinus appears as a clouded to opaque density and may reveal an airfluid level. A bone fracture is visible as a linear, radiolucent defect; cysts, polyps, and tumors are visible as softtissue masses projecting into the sinus.

When surrounding facial structures—superimposed on the paranasal sinuses—interfere with visualization of relevant areas, tomography may be done to provide further information. Tomography is especially useful in evaluating facial trauma and neoplastic disease. (See *Paranasal Sinus Tomography*.)

Procedure

• The patient sits upright (possibly with his head in a foam vise), between the X-ray tube and a film cassette.
• During the test, the X-ray tube is positioned at specific angles and the patient's head is placed in various standard positions, while his paranasal sinuses are filmed from different angles.
• The test takes 10 to 15 minutes to complete.

Patient care checklist

Before the test

☑ Explain or clarify test purpose and procedure.
☑ Evaluate patient understanding.

Interfering factors

Failure to remove radiopaque objects from the X-ray field interferes with radiologic interpretation.

Paranasal Sinus Tomography

Tomography of the paranasal sinuses is performed by moving an X-ray beam and X-ray film simultaneously and in opposite directions around a pivot point during film exposure. The resulting image produces a sharply focused selected section, with blurred areas above and below it. This test supplements radiography when surrounding facial structures obscure relevant areas. Because tomography visualizes the paranasal sinuses in very thin sections, one section at a time, it is especially useful in detecting involvement of bone by tumor and locating fractures of bony sinus walls and foreign bodies.

To prepare a patient for paranasal sinus tomography, describe the procedure to him and advise him to remain motionless while the tomograms are being taken; patient movement during filming interferes with test results. A normal paranasal sinus tomogram shows structures equivalent to a normal X-ray film of this area without superimposition of other structures.

Pulmonary angiography
[Pulmonary arteriography]

Purpose

• To detect pulmonary embolism in a patient who is symptomatic but whose lung scan is indeterminate or normal
• To evaluate pulmonary circulation preoperatively in a patient with congenital heart disease.

Normal results

Normal pulmonary circulatory system.

Abnormal results
Interruption of blood flow may result from:

Pulmonary emboli
Vascular filling defects
Stenosis.

The basics
Pulmonary angiography is the radiographic examination of the pulmonary circulation following injection of a radiopaque iodine contrast agent into the pulmonary artery or one of its branches. Most commonly, it is used to confirm symptomatic pulmonary emboli when scans prove nondiagnostic, especially before anticoagulant therapy or in patients in whom it is contraindicated.

Possible complications include arterial occlusion, myocardial perforation or rupture, ventricular arrhythmias from myocardial irritation, and acute renal failure from hypersensitivity to the contrast agent.

Procedure
• After the patient is placed in a supine position, a local anesthetic is injected, and a cardiac monitor is attached to the patient.
• An incision is made, and a catheter is introduced into the antecubital or femoral vein.
• As the catheter passes through the right atrium, the right ventricle, and the pulmonary artery, pressures are measured and blood samples may be drawn from various regions of the pulmonary circulatory system.
• The contrast agent is then injected and circulates through the pulmonary artery and lung capillaries while X-ray films are taken.
• A pressure dressing is applied over the catheter insertion site.
• The test takes about 1 hour to perform.

Special precautions
CLINICAL ALERT: **The patient should be monitored for ventricular arrhythmias due to myocardial irri-** tation, resulting from passage of the catheter through the heart chambers.
• The patient should be observed for signs of a hypersensitivity reaction.

Patient care checklist
Before the test
☑ Explain or clarify test purpose, preparation, procedure, and post-test care.
☑ Warn the patient that he may experience an urge to cough, a flushed feeling, nausea, or a salty taste for approximately 5 minutes after the injection of the contrast medium. Inform him that his heart rate will be monitored continuously during the procedure.
☑ Evaluate patient understanding.
☑ Restrict food and fluids for 8 hours before the test.
☑ Make sure that the patient or a responsible family member has signed a consent form.
☑ Check the patient's history for hypersensitivity to anesthetics, iodine, seafood, or radiographic contrast agents. Report any hypersensitivity to the physician.
After the test
☑ Check the dressing, and note any bleeding.
CLINICAL ALERT: **Watch for signs of myocardial perforation or rupture by monitoring vital signs, as ordered.**
CLINICAL ALERT: **Be alert for signs of acute renal failure, such as sudden onset of oliguria, nausea, and vomiting.**
☑ Check the catheter insertion site for inflammation or hematoma formation, and report symptoms of a delayed hypersensitivity response to the contrast agent or to the local anesthetic.
☑ Advise the patient about any restriction of activity.

Interfering factors
Failure to remove radiopaque objects from the X-ray field interferes with radiologic interpretation.

Renal angiography

Purpose
• To demonstrate the configuration of total renal vasculature before surgery
• To determine the cause of renovascular hypertension, such as stenosis, thrombotic occlusions, emboli, and aneurysms
• To evaluate chronic renal disease or renal failure
• To investigate renal masses and renal trauma
• To evaluate the volume of residual functioning renal tissue in hydronephrosis
• To evaluate donors and recipients before renal transplantation
• To detect complications following renal transplantation, such as a nonfunctioning shunt or rejection of the donor organ.

Normal results
Normal appearance of the renal vasculature and normal architecture of the renal parenchyma.

Abnormal results
Renal angiography may show:
   Hypervascularity due to renal tumors
   Renal artery stenosis
   Renal artery dysplasia with its alternating aneurysms and stenotic regions
   Renal infarction
   Renal artery aneurysms
   Renal arteriovenous fistula
   Distortion and fibrosis of renal tissue and reduced vascularity, due to severe or chronic pyelonephritis
   Renal abscesses
   Renal cysts
   Intrarenal hematoma, parenchymal laceration, shattered kidney, or areas of infarction from trauma.

The basics
Renal angiography permits radiographic examination of the renal vasculature and parenchyma following arterial injection of a contrast medium. As the contrast pervades the renal vasculature, rapid-sequence radiographs show the vessels during three phases of filling: arterial, nephrographic, and venous. This procedure virtually always follows standard bolus aortography, which shows individual variations in number, size, and condition of the main renal arteries, aberrant vessels, and the relationship of the renal arteries to the aorta.

Clinical indications for renal angiography include renal masses, pseudotumors, unilateral or bilateral kidney enlargement, nonfunctioning kidneys in patients with acute renal failure, positive urograms in patients with renovascular hypertension, vascular malformations, and intrarenal calcifications of unexplained etiology. *Contraindications to this test may include:* pregnancy, bleeding tendencies, allergy to contrast media, and renal failure due to end-stage renal disease.

Procedure
• The patient is placed in a supine position, and a peripheral I.V. infusion is started.
• The skin over the arterial puncture site is cleansed, and a local anesthetic is injected.
• A catheter is inserted into the femoral artery and advanced, under fluoroscopic guidance, up to the aorta. Screening aortograms may be taken before proceeding.
• The renal catheter is then advanced into the renal artery, and contrast medium is injected.
• A series of rapid-sequence X-ray films of the filling of the renal vascular tree is exposed.
• If additional selective studies are required, the catheter remains in place while the films are examined.
• If the films are satisfactory, the catheter is removed, and a sterile sponge is firmly applied to the punc-

ture site for 15 minutes.

• Before the patient is returned to his room, the puncture site is observed for hematoma.

• The test takes about 1 hour to perform.

Special precautions
The patient should be assessed for signs of a hypersensitivity reaction.

Patient care checklist
Before the test

☑ Explain or clarify test purpose, preparation, procedure, and post-test care.

☑ Inform the patient that he may experience transient discomfort (flushing, burning sensation, and nausea) during injection of the contrast medium.

☑ Evaluate patient understanding.

☑ Restrict food and fluids for 8 hours before the test.

☑ Make sure that the patient or a responsible family member has signed the consent form.

☑ Check the patient's history for hypersensitivity to iodine-based contrast media or iodine-containing foods, such as shellfish, or to anesthetics. If the patient has a history of sensitivity, inform the physician.

☑ As ordered, administer medication (usually a sedative and a narcotic analgesic) before the test.

☑ Just before the procedure, instruct the patient to void.

After the test

☑ Keep the patient flat in bed for 8 to 12 hours and nonambulatory for a total of 24 hours.

CLINICAL ALERT: **Check vital signs, as ordered. Monitor popliteal and dorsalis pedis pulses for adequate perfusion at least every hour for 4 hours.**

CLINICAL ALERT: **Watch for bleeding or hematomas at the injection site. Keep the pressure dressing in place. If bleeding occurs, notify the physician, and apply direct pressure to the site.**

Interfering factors
• Recent contrast studies (such as a barium enema or an upper gastrointestinal series) may produce a cloudy radiographic image and interfere with accurate interpretation of test results.

• Patient movement during the test may impair the quality of the radiograms.

• The presence of feces and gas in the gastrointestinal tract may impair the clarity of the radiograms and hinder accurate interpretation of results.

• Failure to remove radiopaque objects from the X-ray field interferes with radiologic interpretation.

Renal computed tomography (CT)

Purpose
• To detect and evaluate renal pathology

• To evaluate the retroperitoneum

• To guide needle placement for percutaneous renal biopsy

• To evaluate for tumor recurrence following nephrectomy

• To determine the kidney's size and location in relation to the bladder, following kidney transplant.

Normal results
Normal size, shape, and position of the kidneys, with no evidence of pathology.

Abnormal results
Renal CT can detect and evaluate:
  Renal cysts
  Renal tumors
  Adrenal tumors
  Renal calculi
  Polycystic kidney disease
  Congenital anomalies of the kidneys
  Perirenal hematomas, lymphoceles,
    or abscesses.

The basics
Renal CT provides a useful image of the kidneys made from a series of to-

mograms or cross-sectional slices, which are then translated by a computer and displayed on an oscilloscope screen. The image density reflects the amount of radiation absorbed by renal tissue and permits identification of masses and other lesions. An I.V. contrast medium may be injected to accentuate the renal parenchyma's density and to help differentiate renal masses.

This highly accurate test is usually performed to investigate diseases found by other diagnostic procedures, such as intravenous pyelography or ultrasound.

Procedure

• The patient is placed in a supine position on the scanning table and is secured with straps.
• The table is moved into the scanner, and the patient is instructed to lie still.
• When the scanner is turned on, it takes multiple images at different angles within each cross-sectional slice.
• When one series of tomograms is complete, contrast enhancement may be performed. Following I.V. injection of contrast medium, another series of tomograms is taken.
• Information from the scan is stored on a disk or on magnetic tape, fed into a computer, and converted into an image for display on an oscilloscope screen. Radiograms are taken of selected views.
• The test takes about 1 hour to perform.

Special precautions

If contrast enhancement is required, the patient should be assessed for signs of a hypersensitivity reaction.

Patient care checklist
Before the test
☑ Explain or clarify test purpose, preparation, and procedure.
☑ Tell the patient that he may experience transient side effects, such as flushing and headache, if contrast enhancement is used.

☑ Evaluate patient understanding.
☑ Restrict food and fluids for 4 hours before the test, if contrast enhancement will be performed. Fasting is not necessary if contrast enhancement is not planned.
☑ Make sure that the patient or a responsible family member has signed the consent form.
☑ Check the patient's history for hypersensitivity to iodine, shellfish, or the contrast media used in other diagnostic tests. Inform the physician of any sensitivities.
☑ Administer a pre-test sedative, if ordered.

Interfering factors

• Patient failure to lie still during the scan results in blurred images.
• Artifacts may be caused by many factors, such as recent contrast studies, foreign bodies, catheters, and surgical clips.
• Failure to remove radiopaque objects from the X-ray field interferes with radiologic interpretation.

Renal venography

Purpose

• To detect renal vein thrombosis
• To evaluate renal vein compression due to extrinsic tumors or retroperitoneal fibrosis
• To assess renal tumors and detect invasion of the renal vein or inferior vena cava
• To detect venous anomalies and defects
• To differentiate renal agenesis from a small kidney
• To collect renal venous blood samples for evaluation of renovascular hypertension.

Normal results

Renal veins and tributaries are normal. Normal renin content of venous blood in a supine adult is 1.5 to 1.6 ng/ml/hr.

Abnormal results

Renal venography detects:
Renal vein thrombosis
Renal tumor that invades the renal vein or inferior vena cava
Venous anomalies
Obstruction or compression of the renal vein due to extrinsic tumor or retroperitoneal fibrosis.

Elevated renin content in renal venous blood from both kidneys usually indicates:
Renovascular hypertension.

Elevated renin levels in one kidney usually indicates:
Unilateral lesion.

The basics

This relatively simple procedure allows radiographic examination of the main renal veins and their tributaries. Contrast medium is injected by percutaneous catheter passed through the femoral vein and inferior vena cava into the renal vein. When catheterization of the femoral vein is contraindicated, the right antecubital vein is punctured, and the catheter is inserted and advanced through the right atrium of the heart into the inferior vena cava.

Indications for renal venography include renal vein thrombosis, tumor, and venous anomalies. This test helps distinguish renal parenchymal disease and aneurysms from pressure exerted by an adjacent mass. When other diagnostic tests yield ambiguous results, renal venography can detect the absence of a renal vein, which definitively differentiates renal agenesis from a small kidney.

Renal venography is also useful in assessing renovascular hypertension. Blood samples can be collected from renal veins during the procedure, and renin assays of the samples can differentiate essential renovascular hypertension from hypertension due to unilateral renal lesions.

Contraindications to this test include:
severe thromboses of the inferior vena cava.

Procedure

• The patient is placed in a supine position on the X-ray table.
• The skin over the right femoral vein is cleansed.
• A local anesthetic is injected, and the femoral vein is cannulated.
• Under fluoroscopic guidance, a guide wire is threaded a short distance through the cannula, which is then removed.
• A catheter is passed over the wire into the inferior vena cava.
• If the inferior vena cava is patent, the catheter is advanced into the right renal vein, and contrast medium is injected.
• When studies of the right renal vasculature are completed, the catheter is withdrawn into the vena cava, rotated, and guided into the left renal vein.
• If visualization of the renal venous tributaries is indicated, epinephrine can be injected into the ipsilateral renal artery by catheter before contrast medium is injected into the renal vein. Epinephrine temporarily blocks arterial flow and allows the filling of distal intrarenal veins. Obstructing the artery briefly with a balloon catheter is an alternate method that produces the same effect.
• After anteroposterior films are made, the patient is placed prone for posteroanterior films. If renin assays are indicated, blood samples are withdrawn under fluoroscopy within 15 minutes after venography is completed.
• The catheter is removed, and a dressing is applied.
• The test takes about 1 hour to perform.

Special precautions

• The guide wire and catheter should be advanced carefully if severe renal vein thrombosis is suspected.
• The patient should be assessed for signs of a hypersensitivity reaction.

Patient care checklist
Before the test

☑ Explain or clarify purpose, preparation, procedure, and post-test care.

☑ Tell the patient that he may feel mild discomfort during injection of the local anesthetic and contrast medium, and that he may feel transient burning and flushing from the contrast medium.

☑ Evaluate patient understanding.

☑ If ordered, restrict food and fluids for 4 hours before the test.

☑ Check the patient's history for hypersensitivity to contrast media, iodine, or iodine-containing foods, such as shellfish, or to local anesthetics. Report any hypersensitivity to the physician.

☑ Check the patient's history and any coagulation studies for indications of bleeding disorders. Consult with the physician, as needed.

☑ If renin assays will be done, check the patient's diet and medications and consult with the physician. As ordered, restrict the patient's salt intake and discontinue antihypertensive drugs, diuretics, estrogen, and oral contraceptives.

☑ Make sure that the patient or a responsible family member has signed a consent form.

☑ Administer a pre-test sedative, as ordered.

After the test

☑ Monitor vital signs and distal pulses, as ordered.

☑ Check the puncture site for bleeding or hematoma; if a hematoma develops, apply warm soaks.

CLINICAL ALERT: **Report signs of vein perforation, embolism, and extravasation of contrast medium. These include chills, fever, rapid pulse and respiration, hypotension, dyspnea, and chest, abdominal, or flank pain. Also report complaints of paresthesias or pain in the catheterized limb—symptoms of nerve irritation or vascular compromise.**

☑ Administer a sedative and antibiotics, as ordered.

Interfering factors

• Recent barium contrast studies of the GI tract or the presence of feces or gas in the bowel impairs visualization of the renal veins.

• Failure to restrict salt, antihypertensive drugs, diuretics, estrogen, and oral contraceptives can interfere with renin assay results.

• Failure to remove radiopaque objects from the X-ray field interferes with radiologic interpretation.

Retrograde cystography

Purpose
To evaluate the structure and integrity of the bladder.

Normal results
Normal bladder contours, capacity, integrity, and urethrovesical angle, with no evidence of displacement, compression, or intrinsic bladder pathology.

Abnormal results
Retrograde cystography can identify:
    Vesical trabeculae
    Vesical diverticula
    Vesicovaginal fistula
    Ruptured bladder
    Bladder tumors
    Bladder calculi
    Blood clots in the bladder
    High- or low-pressure vesicoureteral reflux
    Hypo- or hypertonic bladder.

The basics
Retrograde cystography involves the instillation of contrast medium into the bladder, followed by radiographic examination. This procedure is used to diagnose bladder rupture without urethral involvement, since it can determine the location and extent of the rupture. Other indications for retrograde cystography include neurogenic bladder, recurrent urinary tract infections (especially in children), sus-

pected vesicoureteral reflux, and vesical fistulas, diverticula, and tumors. This test is also performed when cystoscopic examination is impractical, as in male infants, or when intravenous pyelography has not adequately visualized the bladder. Voiding cystourethrography is often performed concomitantly.

Contraindications to this test include: exacerbation of an acute urinary tract infection or an obstruction that prevents passage of a urinary catheter. This test should not be performed in the presence of urethral evulsion or transection, unless catheter passage and flow of contrast medium are monitored fluoroscopically.

Procedure

• The patient is placed in a supine position on the examining table, and a preliminary plain film of the abdomen is taken.

• The bladder is then catheterized, and contrast medium is instilled by gravity or by gentle syringe action. The catheter is then clamped.

• X-ray films are taken with the patient in various positions, to obtain different views.

• The catheter is unclamped, the bladder fluid is allowed to drain, and a radiograph is obtained to detect urethral diverticula, fistulous tracts into the vagina, or intra- or extraperitoneal extravasation of the contrast medium.

• Rarely, to enhance visualization, 100 to 300 ml of air may be insufflated into the bladder by syringe after removal of the contrast medium (double contrast technique).

• The test takes about 30 to 60 minutes to perform.

Patient care checklist

Before the test

☑ Explain or clarify test purpose, preparation, and procedure.

☑ Inform the patient that he may experience some discomfort when the catheter is inserted and when the contrast medium is instilled through the catheter.

☑ Evaluate patient understanding.

☑ Make sure that the patient or a responsible family member has signed a consent form.

☑ Check the patient's history for hypersensitivity to contrast media used in other diagnostic tests. Inform the physician if such sensitivity is present.

After the test

☑ Record the time of the patient's voidings and the color and volume of the urine. Watch for hematuria. If it persists after the third voiding, notify the physician.

CLINICAL ALERT: **Watch for signs of urinary sepsis from urinary tract infection (chills, fever, elevated pulse and respiration rates, hypotension) or similar signs related to extravasation of contrast medium into the general circulation.**

Interfering factors

• Residual barium from recent diagnostic tests or the presence of feces or gas in the bowel may obscure images and interfere with test results.

• Failure to remove radiopaque objects from the X-ray field interferes with radiologic interpretation.

Retrograde pyelography
[Retrograde ureteropyelography]

Purpose

To assess the structure and integrity of the renal collecting system.

Normal results

Normal size and contour of the ureters and kidneys.

Abnormal results

Retrograde pyelography may detect obstruction due to:

Calculus

Tumor (intrinsic or extrinsic)

Stricture
Blood clot.
The test may also detect:
Perinephritic abscess.

The basics

Retrograde pyelography allows radiographic examination of the renal collecting system (calyces, renal pelvis, and ureter) after injection of a contrast medium through a ureteral catheter during cystoscopy. The contrast medium is usually iodine-based, and although some of it may be absorbed through the mucous membranes, this test is preferred for patients with hypersensitivity to iodine (in whom I.V. administration of an iodine-based contrast medium, as in intravenous pyelography, is contraindicated). This test is also indicated when visualization of the renal collecting system by intravenous pyelography is inadequate due to inferior films or marked renal insufficiency, since retrograde pyelography is not influenced by impaired renal function.

Procedure

• A cystoscopic examination is performed. (See "Cystoscopy," p. 420.)
• One or both ureters are catheterized, depending on the condition or abnormality suspected.
• The renal pelvis is emptied by gravity drainage or aspiration.
• Contrast medium is then injected slowly through the catheter.
• When adequate filling and opacification have occurred, X-ray films are taken.
• After the radiograms of the renal pelvis are examined, a few more milliliters of contrast medium are injected to outline the ureters as the catheter is slowly withdrawn.
• Delayed films (10 to 15 minutes after complete catheter removal) are then taken to check for retention of the contrast medium, indicating urinary stasis.
• If ureteral obstruction is present, the ureteral catheter may be kept in place and, together with an indwelling (Foley) catheter, connected to a gravity drainage system until post-test urinary flow is corrected or returns to normal.
• The test takes about 1 hour to perform.

Special precautions

Retrograde pyelography must be done carefully in the presence of urinary stasis caused by ureteral obstruction, to prevent further injury to the ureter.

Patient care checklist
Before the test
☑ Explain or clarify test purpose, preparation, procedure, and post-test care.
☑ Inform the patient that he will be positioned on an examining table, with his feet in stirrups, and that the position may be tiring. If he will be awake throughout the procedure, tell him that he may feel pressure as the instrument is passed and a pressure sensation in the kidney area when the contrast medium is introduced. Also, he may feel an urgency to void.
☑ Evaluate patient understanding.
☑ If a general anesthetic is ordered, restrict food and fluids for 8 hours before the test.
☑ Make sure that the patient is generally well hydrated.
☑ Make sure that the patient or a responsible family member has signed a consent form.
☑ Just before the procedure, administer premedication, as ordered.
After the test
☑ Monitor vital signs, as ordered.
☑ Monitor fluid intake and urinary output for 24 hours. Observe each specimen for hematuria. Gross hematuria or hematuria after the third voiding is abnormal and should be reported. Notify the physician if the patient does not void for 8 hours after the procedure or immediately if the patient feels distress and his bladder is distended. Urethral catheterization may be necessary.

☑ Be especially attentive to catheter output if ureteral catheters have been left in place, since inadequate output may reflect catheter obstruction, requiring irrigation by the physician. Protect ureteral catheters from being dislodged.

☑ Administer analgesics, as ordered, tub baths, and increased fluid intake for dysuria, which commonly occurs after retrograde pyelography.

CLINICAL ALERT: Watch for and report severe pain in the area of the kidneys, as well as any signs of sepsis (such as chills, fever, and hypotension).

Interfering factors

• Previous contrast studies or the presence of feces or gas in the bowel impairs the quality of the radiogram and hinders accurate interpretation.

• Failure to remove radiopaque objects from the X-ray field interferes with radiologic interpretation.

Retrograde urethrography

Purpose

To diagnose urethral strictures, lacerations, and diverticula, and congenital anomalies.

Normal results

The membranous, bulbar, and penile portions of the urethra—and occasionally the prostatic portion—appear normal in size, shape, and course.

Abnormal results

Retrograde urethrography may detect:

  Urethral diverticula
  Urethral fistulas
  Urethral strictures
  False passages
  Calculi
  Urethral lacerations

Congenital anomalies, such as urethral valves and perineal hypospadias
Urethral tumors (very rare).

The basics

Used almost exclusively in males, this radiographic study is performed during instillation or injection of a contrast medium into the urethra, permitting visualization of its membranous, bulbar, and penile portions. Clinical indications for retrograde urethrography include outlet obstructions, congenital anomalies, and urethral lacerations or other trauma. This test may also be performed on patients who require a follow-up examination after surgical repair of the urethra. Although visualization of the anterior portion of the urethra is excellent with this test alone, the posterior portion is more effectively outlined by retrograde urethrography in tandem with voiding cystourethrography.

Procedure

• The male patient is placed in a recumbent position on the examining table.

• After X-rays of the bladder and urethra are taken and studied, the glans and meatus are cleansed.

• The catheter is filled with the contrast medium before insertion, to eliminate air bubbles.

• The catheter is inserted until the balloon portion is inside the meatus; the balloon is then inflated with 1 to 2 ml of water, which prevents the catheter from slipping during the procedure.

• The patient assumes the right posterior oblique position, and contrast medium is injected.

• X-rays are taken. Left lateral oblique views may also be taken.

• Fluoroscopic control may be helpful, especially for evaluating urethral injury.

• In females, this test may be used when urethral diverticula are suspected. A double-balloon catheter is used, which occludes the bladder neck from above and the external meatus from below.

• In children, the procedure is the same as for adults, except that a smaller catheter is used.

• The test takes about 30 minutes to perform.

Special precautions

Retrograde urethrography should be performed cautiously in the presence of urinary tract infection.

Patient care checklist

Before the test

☑ Explain or clarify test purpose, preparation, and procedure.

☑ Inform the patient that he may experience some discomfort when the catheter is inserted and when the contrast medium is instilled through the catheter.

☑ Evaluate patient understanding.

☑ Make sure that the patient or a responsible family member has signed a consent form.

☑ Check the patient's history for hypersensitivity to iodine-based contrast media or iodine-containing foods, such as shellfish. Inform the physician of any such hypersensitivities.

☑ Just before the procedure, administer a sedative, as ordered, and instruct the patient to void before leaving his room.

After the test

CLINICAL ALERT: **Watch for chills and fever related to extravasation of contrast medium into the general circulation for 12 to 24 hours after retrograde urethrography. Also watch for signs of sepsis and allergic manifestations.**

Skull radiography

Purpose

• To detect skull fractures in patients with head trauma

• To help detect and assess increased intracranial pressure (ICP), tumors, bleeding, and infections

• To aid diagnosis of pituitary tumors

• To detect congenital anomalies.

Normal results

The size, shape, thickness, and position of the cranial bones, as well as the vascular markings, sinuses, and sutures, are normal for the patient's age.

Abnormal results

Skull radiography may detect:

Fractures of the vault or base (basilar fractures may not show on an X-ray)

Congenital anomalies

Increased ICP

Calcification from osteomyelitis or chronic subdural hematomas

Bone changes from metabolic disorders, like acromegaly or Paget's disease

Tumors of the skull

Brain tumors containing calcium

Midline shifting of the calcified pineal gland due to a space-occupying lesion.

The basics

Skull radiography is the oldest noninvasive neurologic test. In patients with head injuries, X-ray films of the skull offer limited information about skull fractures. However, this test is extremely valuable for studying increased ICP, abnormalities of the base of the skull and the cranial vault, congenital and perinatal anomalies, and many systemic diseases that produce bone defects of the skull.

Skull radiography evaluates the three groups of bones that make up the skull—the calvaria or vault, the mandible or jawbone, and the facial bones. The calvaria and the facial bones are closely connected by immovable joints with irregular serrated edges, called sutures. The bones of the skull form an anatomic structure so complex that several radiologic views of each area are required for a complete skull examination.

Procedure
• The patient is placed in a supine position on a radiographic table or is seated in a chair and is instructed to remain still while the radiograms are taken.
• Routinely, three, four, or five views of the skull are taken.
• The test takes about 15 minutes to perform.

Patient care checklist
Before the test
☑ Explain or clarify test purpose and procedure.
☑ Evaluate patient understanding.

Interfering factors
• Improper positioning of the patient.
• Excessive head movement by the patient.
• Failure to remove radiopaque objects from the X-ray field.

Spinal computed tomography (CT)

Purpose
• To diagnose spinal lesions and abnormalities
• To monitor the effects of spinal surgery or therapy.

Normal results
Spinal structures are of normal density, size, shape, and position.

Abnormal results
Spinal CT scanning can reveal:
  Spinal tumors
  Herniated intervertebral disks
  Cervical or lumbar spondylosis
  Paraspinal cysts
  Vascular malformations
  Congenital spinal malformations, such as meningocele, myelocele, or spina bifida.

The basics
Much more versatile than conventional radiography, spinal CT provides detailed, clear cross-sectional images of various layers of the spine. It is based on computer reconstruction of radiation levels absorbed by various tissues. Vertebrae, the densest tissues, are white; soft tissues appear in shades of gray; cerebrospinal fluid is black. By highlighting areas of altered density, and depicting structural malformation, spinal CT scanning can reveal all types of spinal lesions and abnormalities. It is particularly useful in detecting and localizing tumors, which appear as masses varying in density. Often, it can identify the type of tumor as well. Spinal CT scanning also reveals degenerative processes and structural changes in detail.

Contrast-enhanced CT further expands the procedure's diagnostic capabilities by accentuating spinal vasculature and highlighting even subtle differences in tissue density.

Air CT, which involves removing a small amount of cerebrospinal fluid and injecting air via lumbar puncture, intensifies the contrast between the subarachnoid space and surrounding tissue.

Procedure
• The patient is placed in a supine position on a table and is told to lie as still as possible.
• The table is then moved into the circular opening of the body CT scanner.
• The scanner takes radiographs at preselected intervals.
• After the first set of radiographs is taken, the patient is removed from the scanner and contrast medium is administered, if ordered.
• After dye injection, the patient is returned to the scanner and another series of radiographs is taken.
• The images obtained from the scan are displayed on a video monitor during the procedure and stored on magnetic tape to create a permanent record for subsequent study.

• The test takes 30 to 60 minutes to perform.

Special precautions
• If contrast enhancement is performed, the patient should be assessed for signs of a hypersensitivity reaction.
• Some patients may experience strong feelings of claustrophobia or anxiety when inside the body CT scanner. For such patients, the physician may order the administration of a mild sedative, to help reduce their anxiety.

Patient care checklist
Before the test
☑ Explain or clarify test purpose, preparation, and procedure.
☑ Reassure the patient that the procedure is painless.
☑ Stress that he should lie as still as possible when asked to do so.
☑ If a contrast medium is used, tell him that he may feel flushed and warm and may experience a transient headache, a salty taste, and nausea or vomiting after injection of the dye.
☑ Evaluate patient understanding.
☑ If contrast enhancement is ordered, restrict food and fluid for 4 hours before the test. Fasting is not necessary if contrast enhancement is not ordered.
☑ Make sure that the patient or a responsible family member has signed a consent form.
☑ Check the patient's history for hypersensitivity reactions to iodine, shellfish, or contrast media. If such reactions have occurred, notify the physician, who may order prophylactic medications or may choose not to use contrast enhancement.
☑ If the patient appears restless or apprehensive about the procedure, notify the physician, who may prescribe a mild sedative.

Interfering factors
• Excessive movement by the patient during the scanning procedure may create artifacts, making the images difficult to interpret.

• Failure to remove radiopaque objects from the X-ray field interferes with radiologic interpretation.

Splenoportography
[Transsplenic portography]

Purpose
• To diagnose or assess portal hypertension
• To stage cirrhosis.

Normal results
Splenic pulp pressure is normally 50 to 180 mmH$_2$O (3.5 to 13.5 mm Hg). Splenic tributary and splenic and portal veins appear normal and patent, with no evidence of collateral veins. Hepatic portal radicles branch in an acute and homogenous fashion throughout the liver and empty normally.

Abnormal results
Splenoportography identifies:
   Portal hypertension
   The stage of cirrhosis.

The basics
Splenoportography is rapid sequence filming of the splenic veins and portal system after injection of a contrast medium into the splenic pulp. It is indicated in patients with confirmed or suspected portal hypertension and in those with cirrhosis, to stage the disease.

In portal hypertension, splenic pulp pressure ranges from 200 to 450 mmH$_2$O (15 to 34 mm Hg). The presence of collateral veins—often associated with esophageal varices, splenomegaly, and in some cases hepatomegaly—can also indicate portal hypertension.

In early-stage cirrhosis, a normal splenogram is characteristic, but emptying of the intrahepatic radicles is delayed. As cirrhosis progresses, collateral veins develop, the intrahepatic radicles become angular and shortened, and emptying is again delayed. In advanced cirrhosis, venous blood flow reverses, preventing visualization of the portal and, usually, the splenic veins. Numerous collateral veins in the hilum of the spleen and the immediate retroperitoneum are also characteristic.

Splenoportography generally provides clearer definition of the venous system than superior mesenteric arteriography; however, superior mesenteric arteriography offers the advantage of outlining the portal and splenic veins even during reversed blood flow and causes fewer complications.

Contraindications to this test include: ascites, uncorrectable coagulopathy, splenomegaly due to infection, markedly impaired liver or kidney function, and hypersensitivity to iodine. This test may cause excessive bleeding that requires transfusion or, occasionally, splenectomy.

Procedure

● The patient is placed in a supine position on the radiographic table, with his left hand under his head.
● The left side of his thorax and abdomen is cleansed.
● A scout film of the spleen is taken.
● A local anesthetic is injected.
● As the patient holds his breath midrespiration, the sheathed needle is rapidly inserted into the spleen, and the inner needle withdrawn.
● The patient is then instructed to maintain shallow respirations with the sheath in place. With flexible plastic tubing, a spinal manometer filled with normal saline solution is connected to the sheath, and the splenic pulp pressure is measured.
● The manometer is then replaced with a syringe containing contrast medium.
● If the sheath is properly positioned, the patient is moved over the angiographic changer, contrast medium is injected, and films are taken.
● When the required films have been obtained, the sheath is withdrawn, and

pressure and a sterile dressing are applied to the puncture site.
● The test takes about 30 to 45 minutes to perform.

Special precautions

The patient should be assessed for signs of a hypersensitivity reaction.

Patient care checklist

Before the test

☑ Explain or clarify test purpose, preparation, procedure, and post-test care.

☑ Inform the patient that he may experience a brief stinging sensation on injection of the local anesthetic and a transient flushed feeling on injection of the contrast medium. Instruct him to report upper left quadrant pain (which indicates subcapsular injection) immediately.

☑ Evaluate patient understanding.

☑ Restrict food and fluids after the evening meal the day before the procedure.

☑ Make sure that the patient or a responsible family member has signed a consent form.

☑ Check the patient's history for hypersensitivity to local anesthetics, iodine, seafood, or contrast media used in other diagnostic tests. Report any such hypersensitivity to the physician.

☑ Check platelet count and bleeding, clotting, and prothrombin times. Consult with the physician if test results are abnormal.

☑ About 30 minutes before the procedure, obtain baseline vital signs and administer a mild sedative and an analgesic, as ordered.

After the test

☑ Monitor vital signs, as ordered.

☑ Observe for bleeding, swelling, and tenderness at the puncture site, and notify the physician if such signs develop.

☑ Instruct the patient to lie on his left side for 24 hours to minimize the risk of bleeding. Advise an additional 24 hours of bed rest.

☑ Encourage fluids to promote excretion of the contrast medium.

☑ Draw a blood sample for hematocrit determination every 8 to 12 hours until hematocrit levels stabilize.

Thoracic computed tomography *(CT)*

Purpose
• To locate suspected neoplasms (such as in Hodgkin's disease), especially with mediastinal involvement
• To differentiate coin-sized calcified lesions (including tuberculosis) from tumors
• To distinguish tumors adjacent to the aorta from aortic aneurysms
• To detect the invasion of a neck mass into the thorax
• To evaluate primary malignancy that may metastasize to the lungs, especially in patients with primary bone tumors, soft-tissue sarcomas, and melanomas
• To evaluate the mediastinal lymph nodes.

Normal results
The lungs, heart, great vessels, and mediastinal lymph nodes are of normal density, size, shape, and position.

Abnormal results
Thoracic CT may detect:
Tumors
Cysts
Aortic aneurysm
Enlarged mediastinal lymph nodes
Pleural effusion
Abscesses
Accumulations of blood, fluid, or fat.

The basics
Thoracic CT provides cross-sectional views of the chest by passing an X-ray beam from a computerized scanner through the body at different angles. Thoracic CT scanning may be done with or without an injected radioiodine contrast agent, which is primarily used to highlight blood vessels and to allow greater visual discrimination.

This test is especially useful in detecting small differences in tissue density. Along with nuclear medicine scanning, thoracic CT is one of the most accurate and informative diagnostic tests and may replace mediastinoscopy in diagnosis of mediastinal masses and Hodgkin's disease; its clinical application in the evaluation of pulmonary pathology is proven.

Procedure
• After the patient is placed in a supine position on the radiographic table and the contrast agent has been injected, the machine scans the patient at different angles while the computer calculates small differences in the densities of various tissues, water, fat, bone, and air.
• This information is displayed as a printout of numerical values and as a projection on an oscilloscope screen. Images may be recorded for future study.
• This test usually takes about 1½ hours to perform.

Special precautions
If contrast enhancement is necessary, the patient should be assessed for signs of a hypersensitivity reaction.

Patient care checklist
Before the test
☑ Explain or clarify test purpose, preparation, and procedure.
☑ Reassure the patient that the procedure will not cause him any discomfort.
☑ Inform him that a radiographic contrast agent may be injected into a vein in his arm. If so, he may experience nausea, warmth, flushing of the face, or a salty taste.
☑ Evaluate patient understanding.
☑ If contrast enhancement is ordered, restrict food and fluids for 4 hours be-

fore the test. Fasting is not necessary if contrast enhancement will not be used.

☑ Make sure that the patient or a responsible family member has signed a consent form.

☑ Check the patient's history for hypersensitivity to iodine, seafood, or contrast media used in other diagnostic studies. Notify the physician of any such hypersensitivity.

Interfering factors

• The patient's inability to lie still during scanning may interfere with accurate diagnosis or may require repetition of the test, which increases his exposure to radiation.

• Failure to remove radiopaque objects from the X-ray field interferes with radiologic interpretation.

Upper gastrointestinal (GI) and small bowel series

Purpose

• To detect hiatal hernia, diverticula, and varices

• To aid diagnosis of strictures, ulcers, tumors, regional enteritis, and malabsorption syndrome

• To help detect motility disorders.

Normal results

Normal size and contour of the esophagus, stomach, and small intestine, and normal peristalsis.

Abnormal results

X-ray studies of the esophagus may reveal:
   Strictures
   Tumors
   Hiatal hernia
   Diverticula
   Varices
   Ulcers
   Achalasia.

X-ray studies of the stomach may reveal:
   Tumors
   Polyps
   Ulcers
   Gastritis
   Pyloric stenosis.

X-ray studies of the small intestine may reveal:
   Regional enteritis
   Malabsorption syndrome
   Tumors.

X-ray studies sometimes suggest:
   Pancreatitis
   Pancreatic cancer.

The basics

The upper GI and small bowel series is the fluoroscopic examination of the esophagus, stomach, and small intestine after the patient ingests barium sulfate, a contrast agent. As the barium passes through the digestive tract, fluoroscopy outlines peristalsis and the mucosal contours of the respective organs, and spot films record significant findings. This test is indicated in patients with upper GI symptoms (difficulty in swallowing, regurgitation, burning or gnawing epigastric pain), signs of small bowel disease (diarrhea, weight loss), and signs of GI bleeding (hematemesis, melena). Although this test can detect various mucosal abnormalities, subsequent biopsy is often necessary to rule out malignancy or to distinguish specific inflammatory diseases. Oral cholecystography, barium enema, and routine radiography should always precede this test, since retained barium clouds anatomic detail on X-ray films.

Contraindications to this test include: colonic obstruction. In patients with this condition, barium may intensify the obstruction or seep into the abdominal cavity. (See *Gastrointestinal Motility Study*.)

Procedure

• With the patient erect, the heart, lungs, and abdomen are examined fluoroscopically.

• The patient is instructed to swallow the barium suspension at appropriate times.

• The passage of barium through the esophagus, stomach, and small intestine is observed fluoroscopically.

• Spot films are then taken, with the patient in various positions.

• When the barium enters the cecum, the examination is ended.

• To perform a double-contrast examination, as barium enters the stomach, the patient is instructed to sip more barium through a perforated straw. As he does so, a small amount of air is also introduced into the stomach; this permits detailed examination of the gastric rugae.

• The test may take up to 6 hours to complete.

Patient care checklist
Before the test

☑ Explain or clarify test purpose, preparation, procedure, and post-test care.

☑ Describe the milkshake consistency and chalky taste of the barium mixture. Although it is flavored, he may find its taste unpleasant, but tell him that he must drink 16 to 20 oz (480 to 600 ml) for a complete examination.

☑ Evaluate patient understanding.

☑ Provide a low-residue diet for the patient for 2 or 3 days before the test, then restrict food and fluids and tell him to avoid smoking after midnight before the test, as well as during it.

☑ As ordered, withhold most oral medications after midnight, and anticholinergics and narcotics for 24 hours, since these drugs affect small intestinal motility. Antacids are also sometimes withheld for several hours if gastric reflux is suspected.

☑ Administer a cathartic and a saline or warm tap-water enema the evening before the test, as ordered.

After the test

☑ Be sure that additional radiographs have not been ordered before allowing

---

Gastrointestinal Motility Study

When intestinal disease is strongly suspected, the gastrointestinal (GI) motility study may follow the upper GI and small bowel series. This study, which evaluates intestinal motility and the integrity of the mucosal lining, records the passage of barium through the lower digestive tract, using spot films taken at specified intervals.

About 6 hours after barium ingestion, the head of the barium column is usually in the hepatic flexure; the tail, in the terminal ileum. The barium completely opacifies the large intestine 24 hours after ingestion. Since the amount of barium passing through the large intestine is insufficient to fully extend the lumen, spot films taken 24, 48, or 72 hours after barium ingestion prove inferior to the barium enema test. However, when spot films suggest intestinal abnormalities, the barium enema test and colonoscopy can provide more specific, confirming diagnostic information.

---

the patient food, fluids, and oral medications (if applicable).

☑ Administer a cathartic or enema to the patient, as ordered. Tell him that his stool will be lightly colored for 24 to 72 hours. Record and describe any stool passed by the patient in the hospital. Since retention of barium in the intestine may cause obstruction or fecal impaction, notify the physician if the patient does not pass barium within 2 or 3 days.

☑ Encourage bed rest, since this test exhausts most patients.

Interfering factors

• Failure to observe restrictions of diet, smoking, and medications may interfere with accurate determination of test results.

• Failure to remove radiopaque objects from the X-ray field interferes with radiologic interpretation.

Vertebral radiography

Purpose
• To detect vertebral fractures, dislocations, subluxations, and deformities
• To detect vertebral degeneration, infection, and congenital disorders
• To detect disorders of the intervertebral disks
• To determine the vertebral effects of arthritic and metabolic disorders.

Normal results
Normal vertebral structure and alignment.

Abnormal results
Vertebral radiography readily shows:
  Spondylolisthesis
  Fractures
  Subluxations
  Dislocations
  Wedging
  Kyphosis
  Scoliosis
  Lordosis.
Vertebral radiography may help to detect or to evaluate:
  Torticollis
  Absence of sacral or lumbar vertebrae
  Congenital abnormalities
  Degenerative processes, such as osteoarthritis
  Tuberculosis (Pott's disease)
  Intraspinal tumors
  Ruptured disk
  Cervical disk syndrome
  Systemic disorders, such as rheumatoid arthritis, Charcot's disease, and Paget's disease.

The basics
Vertebral radiography, a commonly performed test, visualizes all or part of the vertebral column. All vertebrae are similar in structure, but vary in size, shape, and articular surface, according to their location in the vertebral column. Fibrocartilaginous intervertebral disks allow some movement between the individual vertebrae.

The type and extent of vertebral radiography depends on the patient's clinical condition. For example, a patient with suspected scoliosis usually requires radiographic study of the entire vertebral column; one with lower back pain requires only study of the lumbar and sacral segments.

Procedure
• Initially, the patient is placed in a supine position on the radiographic table for an anteroposterior view.
• He may then be repositioned, depending on the vertebral segment or adjacent structure of interest, and X-rays are taken.
• The test takes 15 to 30 minutes to perform.

Special precautions
CLINICAL ALERT: **Exercise extreme caution when handling trauma patients with suspected spinal injuries, particularly of the cervical area. Such patients should be filmed while on the stretcher to avoid further injury during transfer to the radiographic table.**

Patient care checklist
Before the test
☑ Explain or clarify test purpose and procedure.
☑ Evaluate patient understanding.

Interfering factors
• Improper positioning of the patient or movement during radiography may produce inaccurate films.
• Failure to remove radiopaque objects from the X-ray field interferes with radiologic interpretation.

Voiding cystourethrography

Purpose
To detect abnormalities of the bladder and urethra.

Normal results
Normal structure and function of the bladder and urethra.

Abnormal results
Voiding cystourethrography may detect or evaluate:
   Urethral stricture
   Urethral valves
   Vesical or urethral diverticula
   Ureteroceles
   Prostatic enlargement
   Vesicoureteral reflux
   Neurogenic bladder.

The basics
Voiding cystourethrography, radiographic examination of the bladder and urethra after instillation of contrast medium into the bladder, may be performed to investigate possible causes of chronic urinary tract infection. Other indications for voiding cystourethrography include a suspected congenital anomaly of the lower urinary tract, abnormal bladder emptying, and incontinence. In males, this test can assess hypertrophy of the lobes of the prostate, urethral stricture, and the degree of compromise of a stenotic prostatic urethra.

Contraindications to this test include: acute or exacerbated urethral or bladder infection, or acute urethral injury. Hypersensitivity to contrast medium may also contraindicate this test.

Procedure
• The patient is placed in a supine position, and an indwelling (Foley) catheter is inserted into the bladder.
• The contrast medium is instilled through the catheter until the patient's bladder is full.

• The catheter is clamped, and X-ray films are exposed with the patient in various positions.
• The catheter is then removed, and the patient is repositioned and instructed to void.
• Four high-speed exposures of the bladder and urethra, coned down to reduce radiation exposure, are usually made on one film during voiding. (Male patients should wear a lead shield over their testes to prevent irradiation of the gonads; female patients cannot be shielded without blocking the urinary bladder.)
• The most reliable voiding cystourethrograms are obtained with the patient recumbent. Patients who cannot void recumbent may do so standing (not sitting).
• Expression cystourethrography may have to be performed under general anesthesia for young children who cannot void on command.
• The test takes about 30 to 45 minutes to perform.

Special precautions
The patient should be assessed for signs of a hypersensitivity reaction, although reactions are more common with intravenous administration of contrast medium.

Patient care checklist
Before the test
☑ Explain or clarify test purpose, preparation, and procedure.
☑ Evaluate patient understanding.
☑ Make sure that the patient or a responsible family member has signed a consent form.
☑ Check the patient's history for hypersensitivity to iodine-based contrast media or iodine-containing foods, such as shellfish; notify the physician of any sensitivities.
☑ Just before the procedure, administer a sedative, as ordered.
After the test
☑ Observe and record the time, color, and volume of the patient's voidings.

If hematuria is present after the third voiding, notify the physician.

☑ Encourage the patient to drink large quantities of fluids to reduce burning on urination and to flush out any residual contrast medium.

CLINICAL ALERT: Monitor the patient for chills and fever related to extravasation of contrast material or urinary sepsis.

Interfering factors
• Embarrassment may inhibit the patient's ability to void on command.

• Pain on voiding resulting from urethral trauma during catheterization may cause an interrupted or less vigorous stream, muscle spasm, or incomplete sphincter relaxation.

• Previous radiographic testing using contrast media or the presence of feces or gas in the bowel may obscure visualization of the urinary tract.

• Failure to remove radiopaque objects from the X-ray field interferes with radiologic interpretation.

Selected References

Arnell, Iris, and Nassberg, Barbara R. "A Clean, Quick Way to Administer a Barium Enema Through a Colostomy," *Nursing81* 11:81-82, February 1981.

Berkow, Robert, ed. *The Merck Manual of Diagnosis and Therapy,* 14th ed. Rahway, N.J.: Merck Sharp & Dohme, 1982.

Brunner, Lillian S., and Suddarth, Doris S. *Textbook of Medical-Surgical Nursing,* 5th ed. Philadelphia: J.B. Lippincott Co., 1984.

"CT Technology: Scanning Advances in Tomography Today," *Patient Care* 15:147-48, February 28, 1981.

Diagnostics, 2nd ed. Nurse's Reference Library. Springhouse, Pa.: Springhouse Corp., 1986.

Farrell, Jane. *Illustrated Guide to Orthopedic Nursing,* 2nd ed. Philadelphia: J.B. Lippincott Co., 1982.

Feldman, Frieda. *Radiology, Pathology, and Immunology of Bones and Joints.* East Norwalk, Conn.: Appleton-Century-Crofts, 1979.

Fischbach, Frances. *A Manual of Laboratory Diagnostic Tests,* 2nd ed. Philadelphia: J.B. Lippincott Co., 1984.

Griffiths, Harry J., and Sarno, Robert C. *Contemporary Radiology: An Introduction to Imaging.* Philadelphia: W.B. Saunders Co., 1979.

Grossman, Zachary D., et al. *The Clinician's Guide to Diagnostic Imaging.* New York: Raven Press Pubs., 1983.

Michaels, Davida, ed. *Diagnostic Procedures.* New York: John Wiley & Sons, 1983.

Pagana, Kathleen D., and Pagana, Timothy James. *Diagnostic Testing and Nursing Implications,* 2nd ed. St. Louis: C.V. Mosby Co., 1986.

Proto, A.V., et al. "The Chest Radiologic Workup—Special Studies," *Basics of RD* 9:1-6, September 1980.

Randall, Brendal Joy. "Reacting to Anaphylaxis," *Nursing86* 16:34-39, March 1986.

Respiratory Disorders. Nurse's Clinical Library. Springhouse, Pa.: Springhouse Corp., 1984.

Swett, Henry A. "Thoracic CT: When X-rays Are Not Enough," *Journal of Respiratory Diseases* 1(8):48-64, July/August 1980.

11 NUCLEAR MEDICINE TESTING

Introduction

Nuclear medicine tests allow us to study the distributive characteristics of a radioactive tracer that has been introduced into the body. The basis of these diagnostic tests is that specific pathologic conditions will alter normal distribution of the tracer. Nuclear medicine includes in vitro tests, such as T_3 resin uptake and T_4 radioimmunoassay, in vivo imaging or scanning, and therapeutic uses of unsealed sources of the isotopes.

Radiopharmaceuticals, the chemical compounds used in nuclear medicine, are composed of radionuclides labeled for human use. The term *nuclide* refers to any specific nucleus, stable or unstable, plus its orbiting electrons. The term *radionuclide* refers specifically to an unstable nucleus plus its orbiting or radioactive electrons. Radionuclides become stable following emission of alpha (α), beta (β), or gamma (γ) rays. The emitted gamma rays are used in these diagnostic tests. In nuclear medicine, radionuclides are rarely used in their simplest chemical form. Instead, they are labeled to a variety of chemical compounds that have favorable biochemical, physiologic, and metabolic properties. Radiopharmaceuticals are chosen for tests based on their tissue affinity for the organ or system being studied. The importance of radiopharmaceuticals cannot be overemphasized, since the growth of nuclear medicine depends heavily upon their continuing development.

Nuclear scanning, often referred to as scintiscan, scintigraphy, or radionuclide imaging, constitutes about 90% of all nuclear medicine testing in most hospitals. The scanning is aimed at diagnosing pathologic conditions. Some nuclear scanning procedures require patient preparation. For example, a patient needs to be in a fasting state before the stress thallium myocardial scan or the hepatobiliary scan. Different radiopharmaceuticals are used for different nuclear scanning tests. For example, a technetium-labeled phosphate compound such as Tc-99m-methylene diphosphonate (MDP) is used for bone scans, since the tracer localizes in the bone. Following administration of the radiopharmaceutical, through oral or (more frequently) intravenous routes, the patient undergoes nuclear scanning. The time between administration of the radiopharmaceutical and the scanning procedure varies, depending on how long it takes for the radioactive agent to reach and concentrate in the desired tissue.

The gamma camera has essentially replaced the rectilinear scanner in nuclear scanning. The gamma camera maps the distribution of emitted radioactivity and produces an image of a certain organ on a scan. On the scan, pathologic findings are shown by either "cold" or "hot" spots. A cold spot refers to an area of decreased radiotracer distribution, as in a liver scan, while a hot spot shows an area of increased uptake, as in a bone scan. In general, nuclear physicians can identify a hot spot more easily than a cold spot. Nuclear imaging depicts anatomic information as well as physiologic information, such as blood flow and excretion. However, anatomic resolution is usually inferior to ultrasound, computed tomography (CT), and magnetic resonance imaging (MRI); functional assessment is usually superior.

Nuclear scanning always includes a radiation risk for the patient. However, this risk is usually less significant than that of a comparable X-ray study. Still, pregnancy and breast-feeding are contraindications to most of the studies. New mothers are often told to stop nursing for a specific time period if a nuclear scan is planned.

Advances in nuclear medicine include the development of new and promising techniques. Unlike the plain (planar) imaging of standard nuclear images, **single-photon emission computed tomography** (SPECT) can generate tomographic slices of the organs, using computer algorithms similar to those used in CT and MRI. This means lesions that may not be detected by standard imaging may be found using SPECT. This procedure is also being used investigationally for noninvasive analysis of cerebral blood flow.

Positron emission tomography (PET), also known as positron computed tomography (PCT), is a form of nuclear computed tomography that generates cross-sectional images based on the biochemical and physiologic characteristics of the tissue of interest, such as brain, heart, and various tumors. PET scanning requires positron-emitting isotopes, a positron scanner, and a computer for reconstruction of the cross-sectional images. Unlike ultrasound, CT, and MRI, PET provides *functional* images of biochemical changes and metabolism in the brain,

heart, and tumors of various types. PET uses radioisotopes of biologically important elements —oxygen (O-15), nitrogen (N-13), carbon (C-11), and fluorine (F-18)—that emit particles called positrons. These positron emitters are produced by a cyclotron; several hundred positron radiopharmaceuticals have been evaluated so far.

During positron emission, pairs of gamma rays are emitted. The PET scanner detects these rays and relays the information to a computer for reconstruction as an image. About 50 PET centers currently exist in the world, with about 25 in the United States. PET's clinical uses include detection of neuropsychiatric problems (such as Alzheimer's disease, Parkinson's disease, multiple sclerosis, amyotrophic lateral sclerosis, Huntington's chorea, partial complex seizures, schizophrenia, bipolar affective disorder, and stroke) and cardiac problems (such as ischemic heart disease), as well as the grading and detection of malignant tumors. Various neurotransmitters and neuroreceptors can also be studied using PET. Despite the PET scanner and cyclotron's high cost (about $2 million), PET is expected to be used as a clinical tool rather than strictly as a research tool within a few years.

Patient-teaching guidelines
Patient-learner objectives:
• Define the test.
• State the specific purpose of the test.
• Explain the procedure.
• Discuss test preparation, procedure, and post-test care.
• Identify possible risks or adverse effects.
Teaching content:
• Define the test in terms the patient can understand.
• Explain the specific purpose of the test.
• Describe the procedure. Explain that a radionuclide will be administered

before scanning takes place. Tell the patient that a radionuclide is a substance that contains a very small amount of radioactive material that will concentrate in the part of his body being tested. Explain whether the radionuclide will be administered orally, parenterally, or by inhalation. Tell the patient how long it will be before scanning takes place and where the procedure will be performed. Describe the scanning procedure. Tell the patient that, although the equipment may look large and foreboding, the procedure (except for a cisternogram) is painless. The scanner detects radiation emitted from the radionuclide in the patient's body and creates an image of the organ, allowing the physician to check for abnormalities.

• Inform the patient that the radiation risk from the radionuclide is small, usually no more than an X-ray. Tell the patient that no special precautions are generally needed and that the substance will be eliminated from the body within hours to days.

• If the patient is pregnant or breast-feeding, explain that the nuclear scan may not be performed at this time, because of the increased radiation risk for the fetus or child, who is especially sensitive.

• Inform the patient about special preparations (if any) for the test. Be sure to specify if there are dietary restrictions, and indicate the applicable time period.

• Caution the patient to follow directions carefully. He may be told not to move during the scanning procedure; this is to prevent image distortion. Failure to follow directions may necessitate a repeat test.

Evaluation:
After the patient-teaching session is completed, evaluate whether the patient has satisfactorily met each patient-learner objective, by obtaining necessary patient feedback. Refocus teaching as needed.

Bone scan
[Radionuclide scan of the bone; radionuclide bone imaging]

Purpose
• To detect and stage osseous metastatic disease
• To detect osteomyelitis and differentiate it from cellulitis
• To detect subtle fractures
• To aid in work-up of possible battered child
• To detect aseptic necrosis, bone infarction
• To evaluate viability of bone grafts
• To detect if a joint prosthesis is loose or infected
• To aid in choosing a biopsy site in an abnormal bone
• To evaluate the skeleton in patients with bone pain but who have normal radiographs
• To evaluate the extent and progression of certain arthritides
• To monitor degenerative bone disorders.

Normal results
In adults, the radioisotope is distributed evenly throughout the skeletal tissue. In children, the epiphyses of growing bone are normal sites of high concentration, or "hot spots." Activity is normally seen in the urinary tract and in breast tissue.

Abnormal results
The bone scan may identify:
   Most types of primary or metastatic
     bone malignancy
   Osteomyelitis
   Fracture
   Degenerative bone disease
   Loosening of orthopedic prostheses
   Nonviability of bone graft
   Reflex sympathetic dystrophy
   Areas of abnormal soft tissue uptake.

The basics

A bone scan permits imaging of the skeleton by a scanning camera after I.V. injection of a radioactive tracer compound, usually radioactive technetium diphosphonate. This compound collects in bone tissue in increased concentrations at sites of abnormal metabolism. When scanned, these sites appear as "hot spots" that are often detectable months before a radiograph can reveal any lesion. Alternatively, areas of bone ischemia or total replacement by tumor may actually appear as "cold spots." However, this test must be interpreted in light of the patient's medical and surgical history, radiographs, and other laboratory tests.

Contraindications to this test include: pregnancy and lactation.

Procedure

• The patient receives an I.V. injection of ^{99m}Tc diphosphonate.

• For the next 1 to 3 hours, the patient drinks several glasses of fluid.

• The patient is asked to void immediately before the scan.

• The patient is positioned on the scanner table, and the scanner takes as many views as are needed to cover the specified area. The scan takes about 1 hour to perform.

Patient care checklist

Before the test

☑ Explain or clarify test purpose and procedure.

☑ Stress the importance of the patient's drinking at least 32 ounces of any fluid for 2 to 3 hours following injection (unless the patient is fluid restricted).

☑ Tell the patient that he can eat during the waiting period.

☑ Evaluate patient understanding.

Interfering factors

• A distended bladder may obscure pelvic detail, and may mask lesions.

• Improper preparation of the bone scan agent will result in breakdown of the components, causing overall poor skeletal uptake, as well as excretion of the unbound radionuclide by the salivary glands and the stomach.

• Improper injection technique will allow the tracer to seep into subcutaneous tissue at the injection site and possibly permit regional lymphatic uptake, producing erroneous hot spots.

• Ingestion of an inadequate amount of fluid during the waiting period will result in poor soft tissue clearance of activity and will make the skeleton unclear in the images.

Brain scan
[Radionuclide scan of the brain; radionuclide brain imaging]

Purpose

• To detect an intracranial mass or vascular lesion

• To locate areas of ischemia, cerebral infarction, and intracerebral hemorrhage

• To evaluate the course of certain lesions postoperatively and during chemotherapy.

Normal results

A barrier between the bloodstream and brain substance is revealed. Minimal background uptake occurs in each cerebral hemisphere. (The amount signifying abnormality must be carefully interpreted by an experienced examiner.)

Abnormal results

The brain scan can detect:

Lesions, such as malignant gliomas, meningiomas, metastases, and abscesses (quite readily)

Cerebral infarctions and arteriovenous malformations (with variable accuracy, depending on the extent of the lesion and the interim after onset)

Cerebritis and subdural hematomas (early).

The brain scan is less accurate in determining:

Certain benign or low-grade malignant tumors.

The basics

The brain scan permits imaging of the brain after I.V. injection of a radionuclide, usually technetium-99m glucoheptonate. Normally, the radionuclide cannot permeate the blood-brain barrier. If pathologic changes have destroyed the barrier, however, the radionuclide may concentrate in the abnormal area. This test is nonspecific, however, and results must be correlated with the patient's clinical condition. A negative scan, in the presence of clinical features indicating an abnormality, necessitates further testing.

This test has largely been replaced by the more versatile and precise computed tomography.

Contraindications to this test include: pregnancy and lactation.

Procedure

• A bolus of ^{99m}Tc glucoheptonate is injected I.V. while the patient lies supine on a radiographic table.

• If a cerebral blood-flow study has been ordered, rapid-sequence images are taken immediately to follow passage of the radionuclide through the carotid and vertebral arteries and cerebral hemispheres.

• The radionuclide should circulate for at least 1 hour; then static imaging is performed.

• For a clearer picture of radionuclide accumulation, additional imaging is performed 3 or 4 hours after injection.

Patient care checklist

Before the test

☑ Explain or clarify test purpose and procedure.

☑ Evaluate patient understanding.

Interfering factors

Significant head movement by the patient distorts the image.

Cardiac blood pool scanning

[Cardiac blood pool imaging; nuclear ventriculogram; multigated nuclear ventriculogram (MUGA)]

Purpose

• To evaluate left ventricular function

• To detect aneurysms of the left ventricle and other myocardial wall motion abnormalities (areas of akinesia or dyskinesia)

• To detect intracardiac shunting.

Normal results

The left ventricle contracts symmetrically and the isotope appears evenly distributed in the scans. The normal ejection fraction is approximately 50% to 65%.

Abnormal results

Left ventricular abnormalities may be associated with:

Coronary artery disease

Aneurysms of the left ventricle

Cardiomyopathies

Congestive heart failure

Intracardiac shunting.

The basics

In cardiac blood pool scanning, the blood within the heart's chambers is imaged, not the myocardium itself. The test evaluates regional and global ventricular performance after I.V. injection of serum albumin or red blood cells tagged with the isotope technetium-99m (^{99m}Tc) pertechnetate. In first-pass imaging, a scintillation camera records the radioactivity emitted by the isotope in its initial pass through the left ventricle. Higher counts of radioactivity occur during diastole when there is more blood in the ventricle; lower counts occur during systole as the blood is ejected. The portion of isotope ejected during each heartbeat can be calculated to determine the ejection fraction.

Gated cardiac blood pool imaging, performed after first-pass imaging or as a separate test, has several forms; most use electrocardiogram (EKG) signals to trigger the scintillation camera. In two-frame gated imaging, the camera records left ventricular end-systole and end-diastole for 500 to 1,000 cardiac cycles; superimposition of these gated images allows assessment of left ventricular contraction to find areas of dyskinesia or akinesia. In multiple-gated acquisition (MUGA) scanning, the camera records 14 to 64 points of a single cardiac cycle, yielding sequential images that can be studied like motion-picture films to evaluate regional wall motion and determine the ejection fraction and other indices of cardiac function. In the stress MUGA test, the same test is performed at rest and after exercise to detect changes in ejection fraction and cardiac output. In the nitro MUGA test, the scintillation camera records points in the cardiac cycle after the sublingual administration of nitroglycerin, to assess its effect on ventricular function.

Blood pool imaging is more accurate and involves less risk to the patient than left ventriculography in assessing cardiac function.
Contraindications of this test include: pregnancy and lactation.

Procedure
• The patient is placed in supine position beneath the detector of a scintillation camera.
• 15 to 20 mCi of albumin or red blood cells tagged with technetium-99m pertechnetate are injected I.V.

• For the next minute, the scintillation camera records the first pass of the isotope through the heart.
• Using an EKG, the camera is gated.
• The patient may be asked to assume various positions so that nearly all ventricular segments can be imaged.
• Additional gated images may be obtained following administration of 0.4 mg nitroglycerin sublingually, or as the patient exercises.

Patient care checklist
Before the test
☑ Explain or clarify test purpose and procedure.
☑ Stress that the patient must remain silent and motionless during imaging.
☑ Evaluate patient understanding.

Cisternogram *[RISA scan; radionuclide scan of the cisterns and ventricles of the brain; CSF flow scan]*

Purpose
• To detect or rule out normal pressure hydrocephalus
• To detect or rule out other communicating hydrocephalus or external obstructive hydrocephalus
• To detect or rule out cerebrospinal fluid (CSF) leak.

Normal results
Rapid flow into the cisterna magna and other cisterns, such as the Sylvian cistern. No abnormal entry of the radionuclide into the ventricles; activity over the parasagittal convexity.

Abnormal results
The scan may identify:
Normal pressure hydrocephalus
Other communicating hydrocephalus and external obstructive hydrocephalus
CSF leak.

The basics

A cisternogram permits the imaging of the ventricles of the brain after an injection of a radioactive tracer, [111]indium, into the lumbar subarachnoid space. This radioactive tracer travels with the CSF and outlines the cisterns. When scanned, the flow over the cerebral convexity and parasagittal activities is outlined within 24 hours if the flow is normal. Any other findings confirm an abnormality, such as ventricular entry due to hydrocephalus. This test is usually done to confirm a diagnosis suspected by changes in the patient's clinical behavior and history.

Contraindications to this test include: infection or deformity at the lumbar puncture site and, in most cases, increased intracranial pressure.

Procedure

• A lumbar puncture is performed, and the radionuclide is injected into the lumbar subarachnoid space.

• The patient is sent back to his room with instructions to lie flat for 4 to 6 hours, per physician's orders.

• Scans are taken at 4-, 24-, and possibly 48- and 72-hour intervals (anterior and lateral skull images).

• The scans take approximately 3 to 5 minutes each.

Patient care checklist

Before the test:

☑ Have a lumbar puncture tray ready.

☑ Obtain written consent for the lumbar puncture procedure from the patient or his family.

☑ Explain or clarify test purpose and procedure.

☑ Evaluate patient understanding.

After the test:

☑ Instruct the patient to lie flat, as ordered.

Interfering factors

Improper injection, or leakage from the subarachnoidal space, will result in suboptimal flow pattern, necessitating a repeat study (not within a week).

Gallbladder scan

[Cholescintigraphy; radionuclide imaging of hepatobiliary excretion]

Purpose

• To assist in the diagnosis of cholecystitis, cholelithiasis, biliary obstruction, biliary tract leaks, biliary anomalies, liver disease, and tumors or cancer of the hepatobiliary system

• To determine bile-enteric patency after diversionary procedures

• To identify cystic duct remnant after cholecystectomy

• To determine liver rejection after transplantation.

Normal results

Within 60 minutes, the gallbladder (as well as the liver, bile ducts, and part of the small bowel) is visualized, revealing size, shape, and function. Normal results are classified as negative.

Abnormal results

The scan may identify:

Acute, chronic, or acalculous cholecystitis

Cholelithiasis

Cholestasis as a result of hepatocellular disease or bile duct obstruction

Bile leak or fistula

Biliary atresia

Liver metastasis

Liver rejection after transplantation.

The basics

After the inexpensive and readily available radionuclide tracer ^{99m}Tc IDA (technetium-labeled iminodiacetic acid) is injected I.V., it is rapidly excreted by the hepatobiliary system. A gallbladder scan allows serial imaging by a scintillation camera, thus demonstrating the radioactivity not only in the gallbladder, but in the liver, bile ducts, and duodenum as well. Full visualization requires a healthy liver, gallbladder, and hepatobiliary tract.

Radionuclide imaging of the gallbladder is impaired in cholecystitis, cholelithiasis, hepatocellular disease, and biliary obstruction, which block release of IDA into the gallbladder.

The gallbladder scan has been referred to as the HIDA scan. However, since there are now four other IDA compounds that can be used for this scan, the term HIDA is not really accurate.

This scan is quicker and more accurate than the oral cholecystogram, and is replacing it as a more up-to-date test.

Contraindications to this test include: pregnancy and lactation.

Procedure

• The patient is placed on the scanner table, and the camera is placed as close as possible without actually touching the right upper abdominal quadrant.

• The patient is injected with I.V. ^{99m}Tc IDA. The adult dosage is relatively standardized, whereas the amount injected in a child is calculated based on body weight.

• After injection with the radionuclide, scanning begins immediately, and a series of images is taken every 5 minutes for up to 1 hour.

• With severe hepatocellular disease, delayed images may be taken 6 to 48 hours after injection, in an attempt to visualize the gallbladder.

Patient care checklist

Before the test:

☑ Explain or clarify test purpose, preparation, and procedure.

☑ Evaluate patient understanding.

☑ Ask the patient if he has had previous gallbladder or liver disease, or gallbladder surgery. If so, be sure the patient's physician and the radiologist are aware of this.

☑ Restrict food and fluid for 2 hours, if needed, but preferably for 4 hours before the test.

Interfering factors

• Recent food ingestion may cause contraction of the gallbladder, and may result in nonvisualization.

• The presence of barium in the intestines may obscure visualization of the gallbladder.

• Hepatocellular and alcoholic liver disease may delay excretion of the radionuclide into the gallbladder.

• Total parenteral nutrition may cause the same results as if the patient had ingested food.

• Improper injection of IDA into subcutaneous tissues will not allow the radionuclide to be excreted into the hepatobiliary system.

Gallium scan

Purpose

• To detect primary or metastatic neoplasms and inflammatory lesions

• To evaluate malignant lymphoma and identify recurrent tumors following chemotherapy or irradiation therapy

• To clarify focal defects in the liver and evaluate bronchogenic carcinoma.

Normal results

Gallium activity is normally demonstrated in the liver, spleen, bones, and large bowel.

Abnormal results

Gallium scanning may reveal:

Inflammatory lesions—discrete abscesses or diffuse infiltration, such as bacterial peritonitis; inflammatory disease such as sarcoidosis Malignancy, including various sarcomas, Wilms' tumor, and neuroblastomas; carcinoma of the kidney, uterus, vagina, and stomach; and testicular tumors

The extent of Hodgkin's disease and non-Hodgkin's lymphoma.

The basics

This test, a total body scan, is usually performed 24 to 48 hours after the I.V. injection of radioactive gallium (^{67}Ga) citrate; occasionally, it is performed 72 hours after the injection.

Although the liver, spleen, bones, and large bowel normally take up gallium, certain neoplasms and inflammatory lesions also attract it. However, many neoplasms and a few inflammatory lesions may fail to demonstrate abnormal gallium activity. Because gallium has an affinity for both benign and malignant neoplasms and inflammatory lesions, exact diagnosis requires additional confirming tests, such as ultrasonography and computed tomography.

Gallium scanning is usually indicated when the site of the disease (usually malignancy) has not been clearly defined, and when the patient's condition will not be jeopardized by the time required for the procedure. It is also used to detect inflammatory lesions. It can clarify focal hepatic defects when liver-spleen scanning and ultrasonography prove inconclusive, and can evaluate suspected bronchogenic carcinoma when a sputum culture proves positive for malignancy, but other tests are normal.

After chemotherapy or radiation therapy, gallium scanning may be used to detect new or recurrent tumors. These forms of therapy tend to diminish tumor affinity for gallium, however, without necessarily eliminating the tumor.

Contraindications to this test include: pregnancy and lactation.

Procedure

• The patient receives a ^{67}Ga citrate injection I.V.
• Scans are taken 24 to 48 hours after injection from anterior and posterior views and, occasionally, lateral views. The scan takes 30 to 60 minutes.

Patient care checklist

Before the test:

☑ Explain or clarify test purpose, preparation, and procedure.
☑ Evaluate patient understanding.
☑ Administer a high-fiber diet, if ordered.
☑ Administer a laxative and/or cleansing enema, as ordered.

After the test:

☑ If the initial gallium scan suggests bowel disease and additional scans are necessary, administer a cleansing enema, as ordered, before continuing the test.

Interfering factors

• Hepatic and splenic uptake may obscure the detection of abnormal para-aortic nodes in Hodgkin's disease, causing false-negative scans.
• Fecal accumulation can hinder visualization of the retroperitoneal space.
• Barium studies within 1 week before this scan can interfere with visualization of gallium activity in the bowel.

Indium-III leukocyte total body scan
[Indium-III abscess scan]

Purpose

To detect or rule out an inflammatory process.

Normal results

Normal uptake in organs such as liver, spleen, and bone marrow.

Abnormal results

The scan may identify:

The site or source of infection, especially a soft-tissue abscess.

The basics

An ^{111}indium leukocyte scan permits imaging by a camera after an I.V. injection of ^{111}indium–labeled autologous leukocytes. These labeled leukocytes collect at the site of infection. When imaged, this site will appear as a hot spot. This test must be interpreted with knowledge of the patient's medical and surgical history, radiographs, and other laboratory findings.

Contraindications to this test include: pregnancy and lactation.

Procedure
• Approximately 30 ml of blood are drawn from the patient; the leukocytes are separated and labeled with a radioactive [111]indium oxine. This process takes about 2 hours.
• The [111]indium–labeled leukocytes are then injected back into the patient.
• The following day, the patient is positioned under the camera and imaged. As many views as necessary are taken to cover the area suspected of infection. The scan takes about 1 hour.

Patient care checklist
Before the test:
☑ Explain or clarify test purpose and procedure.
☑ Evaluate patient understanding.

Interfering factors
• Improper injection technique will allow the tracer to seep into subcutaneous tissue, producing poor images.
• Results will not be good on leukopenic patients and on patients with chronic infection.

Liver-spleen scan

Purpose
• To screen for hepatic metastases and hepatocellular disease, such as cirrhosis and hepatitis
• To detect focal disease, such as tumors, cysts, and abscesses, in the liver and spleen
• To demonstrate hepatomegaly, splenomegaly, and splenic infarcts
• To assess the condition of the liver and spleen after abdominal trauma.

Normal results
The liver and spleen are normal in size, shape, and position. Since the liver and spleen contain equal numbers of reticuloendothelial cells per area, both organs normally appear equally bright on the image. Distribution of radioactive colloid, however, is generally more uniform and homogeneous in the spleen than in the liver. The liver has various normal indentations and impressions, such as the gallbladder fossa and falciform ligament, that may mimic focal disease.

Abnormal results
Focal defects that fail to take up the radioactive colloid may be due to:
Hepatic or splenic disorders, such as cysts, abscesses, primary tumors, metastasis, and hematoma.
A shift in radioactive colloid from the liver to the spleen and bone marrow occurs with:
Hepatocellular disease, such as hepatitis and cirrhosis, and also accompanies portal hypertension from extrahepatic uptake.
Increased uptake of the radioactive colloid in certain lobes of the liver occurs with:
Obstruction of the superior vena cava and with Budd-Chiari syndrome.
A peripheral defect is seen with:
Splenic infarct.

The basics
This test permits imaging of the liver and spleen after I.V. injection of a radioactive colloid. The agent most commonly used, technetium-99m (^{99m}Tc) sulfur colloid, concentrates in the reticuloendothelial cells through phagocytosis. About 80% to 90% of the injected colloid is taken up by Kupffer's cells in the liver, 5% to 10% by the spleen, and 3% to 5% by bone marrow.

Liver-spleen scanning is indicated in patients with palpable abdominal masses, to demonstrate hepatomegaly or splenomegaly. It is also indicated in those with suspected hepatic or splenic injury after abdominal trauma. It is generally one of the most reliable screening tests for detecting hepatocellular disease, hepatic metastases, and focal disease, such as tumors, cysts, and abscesses. However, such scanning demonstrates focal disease nonspecifically as a cold spot (a defect that fails to take up the colloid) and may fail to detect focal lesions smaller than ¾" (2 cm) in diameter. Also, this test may fail to detect early hepatocellular disease.

Although clinical signs and symptoms may aid diagnosis, liver-spleen scanning frequently requires confirmation by ultrasonography, computed tomography, gallium scanning, or biopsy. After metastasis is confirmed, serial liver-spleen studies are useful to evaluate the effectiveness of therapy. *Contraindications to this test include:* pregnancy and lactation.

Procedure

• ⁹⁹ᵐTc sulfur colloid is injected I.V.
• After 10 to 15 minutes, the patient's abdomen is scanned with the patient placed in various positions.
• With the patient supine, liver mobility and pliability may be evaluated by marking the costal margin and scanning as the patient breathes deeply. (Since the liver normally moves and changes shape with deep breathing, fixation suggests pathology.)
• Additional views are taken, if needed. The test takes about 1 hour.

Patient care checklist

Before the test:
☑ Explain or clarify test purpose and procedure.
☑ Evaluate patient understanding.
After the test:
☑ Assess the patient for anaphylactoid or pyrogenic reactions that may result from a stabilizer, such as dextran or gelatin, added to the ⁹⁹ᵐTc.
(Also see *Liver Flow Studies.*)

Liver Flow Studies

In contrast to static liver-spleen scanning, which provides static nuclear images, flow studies (dynamic scintigraphy) record in rapid sequence the stages of perfusion after I.V. injection of a radionuclide, such as technetium 99m sulfur colloid. Since flow studies demonstrate the vascularity of a nonspecific focal defect, they sometimes help distinguish among metastases, tumors, cysts, and abscesses.

In flow studies, a hot defect demonstrates an early, increased uptake of the radionuclide when compared to the surrounding parenchyma, and then appears as a filling defect, or cold spot, on later routine images. Cysts and abscesses, which are avascular, fail to take up the radionuclide; hemangiomas appear characteristically hot because of their enlarged vessels. Tumors and metastases are generally more difficult to evaluate, since their vascularity is more variable. Although vascular metastases may appear hot, most metastases demonstrate poor uptake of the radionuclide. Hepatomas can also appear hot or can show perfusion similar to normal parenchyma.

Lung perfusion scan
[Lung scintiscan]

Purpose

• To assess arterial perfusion of the lungs
• To detect pulmonary emboli
• To evaluate, preoperatively, the pulmonary function of a patient with marginal lung reserves.

Normal results

Hot spots—areas with normal blood perfusion—show a high uptake of the radioactive substance; a normal lung shows a uniform uptake pattern.

Abnormal results
Cold spots—areas of low radioactive uptake—indicate:
Poor perfusion, such as from an embolism.
Decreased regional blood flow that occurs without vessel obstruction may indicate:
Pneumonitis.

The basics
The lung perfusion scan, performed with a lung ventilation scan, assesses ventilation-perfusion patterns. This lung scan produces a visual image of pulmonary blood flow after I.V. injection of a radiopharmaceutical—human serum albumin microspheres (particles) or macroaggregated albumin, both of which are bonded to technetium. This test is useful in confirming pulmonary vascular obstruction, such as pulmonary emboli; however, a ventilation scan is necessary to confirm the diagnosis.
Contraindications to this test include: pregnancy and lactation.

Procedure
• The radiopharmaceutical is injected I.V. while the patient is in a supine position.
• After the uptake of the radiopharmaceutical, the gamma camera takes a series of single stationary images in the anterior, posterior, oblique, and both lateral chest views.
• Images projected on an oscilloscope screen and film show the distribution of radioactive particles. The test takes 30 to 45 minutes.

Patient care checklist
Before the test:
☑ Explain or clarify test purpose and procedure.
☑ Evaluate patient understanding.

Interfering factors
• I.V. injection of the radiopharmaceutical while the patient is sitting can produce abnormal images, since a large proportion of the particles settle in the lung bases.
• Preexisting conditions, such as chronic obstructive pulmonary disease, vasculitis, pulmonary edema, tumor, sickle-cell disease, or parasitic disease, may cause abnormal perfusion, interfering with accurate determination of the presence of pulmonary emboli.

Monoclonal antibody imaging

Purpose
To detect primary and metastatic sites of active tumor.

Normal results
No accumulation of the radioactive-labeled antibody within the body.

Abnormal results
Accumulation of the radioactive-labeled antibody in areas of the body indicates the presence of a certain type of tumor.

The basics
Monoclonal antibody imaging is currently in the experimental development stage. Each type of tumor cell expresses specific antigens on its surface. When B lymphocytes encounter an antigenic substance, they produce a variety of antibodies (immunoglobulins) that are specifically directed against certain surface antigens of the offending agent. These aid in the body's recognition and destruction of this foreign material. In order to increase specificity in detecting and treating a certain malignancy, it is desirable to isolate and administer antibodies of a single species (mono-

Production of Monoclonal Antibodies

Monoclonal antibodies are produced in the laboratory based upon the immune response. They may detect a tumor's location and extent earlier and more accurately than traditional methods. Typically, a selected antigen is injected into a mouse, stimulating B lymphocyte antibody production. After a few days, the mouse's spleen cells—rich in B lymphocytes—are removed and fused with rapidly dividing mouse myeloma cells that secrete no antibodies. These fused cells, or hybridomas, are grown in culture, tested for the desired antibody, and cloned. Hybridomas with the desired antibody are either grown in a culture or injected into a mouse's peritoneum, so the monoclonal antibodies can proliferate for later retrieval and purification. A new synthetic in vitro method is also available to produce monoclonal antibodies in bulk.

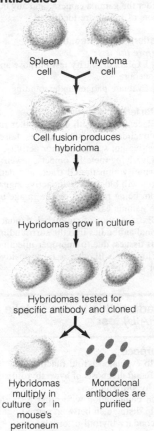

Spleen cell   Myeloma cell

Cell fusion produces hybridoma

Hybridomas grow in culture

Hybridomas tested for specific antibody and cloned

Hybridomas multiply in culture or in mouse's peritoneum

Monoclonal antibodies are purified

clonal antibodies). (See *Production of Monoclonal Antibodies.*)

For imaging purposes, radiolabels (usually [131]iodine, [111]indium, and [67]copper) are attached to the monoclonal antibodies. The radioactive-labeled monoclonal antibodies are injected intravenously into a patient who is suspected or known to have a specific kind of tumor. After an appropriate waiting period, the patient is scanned under the gamma camera, and areas of accumulation (hot spots) are detected, indicating sites of active tumor, possibly earlier and more accurately than traditional methods.

Contraindications to this test include: pregnancy and lactation.

Procedure

• The radioactive-labeled monoclonal antibodies specific for a certain tumor type are injected intravenously into the patient.

• After a required waiting period, regions of the patient's body are scanned under the gamma camera, and any hot spots of tumor are identified.

Patient care checklist
Before the test:
☑ Explain or clarify test purpose and procedure.
☑ Evaluate patient understanding.

Interfering factors
• Recent scans with certain other radionuclides may show up as false-positive hot spots of tumor activity.
• Overlying metallic objects, jewelry, barium within the GI tract, and dentures will block the radioactive signal from being recorded on the image by the gamma camera.
• Extravasation of radiolabeled monoclonal antibodies into the surrounding soft tissues, due to improper injection technique, will give a false-positive hot spot there.

Radioactive iodine uptake (RAIU) test

Purpose
• To evaluate thyroid function
• To aid diagnosis of hyperthyroidism or hypothyroidism
• In combination with other tests, to help distinguish between primary and secondary thyroid disorders.

Normal results
After 6 hours, 3% to 16% radioactive iodine should have accumulated in the thyroid; after 24 hours, 8% to 29%. The remaining radioactive iodine is excreted in the urine. (Local variations in the normal range of iodine uptake may occur due to regional differences in dietary iodine intake, and procedural differences among individual laboratories.)

Abnormal results
Below-normal percentages of iodine uptake may indicate:
  Hypothyroidism
  Subacute thyroiditis
  Iodine overload.
Above-normal percentages may indicate:
  Hyperthyroidism (however, the rate of turnover may be so rapid that the 24-hour measurement appears falsely normal)
  Early Hashimoto's thyroiditis
  Hypoalbuminemia
  Lithium ingestion
  Iodine-deficient goiter.

The basics
The RAIU test evaluates thyroid function by measuring the amount of orally ingested ^{123}I or ^{131}I that accumulates in the thyroid gland after 6 and after 24 hours. An external single counting probe measures the radioactivity in the thyroid as a percentage of the original dose, thus indicating the ability of the gland to trap and retain iodine. The test accurately diagnoses hyperthyroidism (about 90%) but is less accurate for hypothyroidism. When performed concurrently with radionuclide thyroid imaging and the T_3 resin uptake test, the RAIU test helps differentiate Graves' disease from hyperfunctioning toxic adenoma. Indications for this test include abnormal results of chemical tests used to evaluate thyroid function.
Contraindications to this test include: pregnancy and lactation.

Procedure
• The patient receives an oral dose of radioactive iodine.
• At 6 and 24 hours following the administration, the patient's thyroid is scanned by placing the anterior portion of his neck in front of an external single counting probe.
• The amount of radioactivity that the probe detects is compared to the amount in the original dose, in order

to determine the percentage of radio-active iodine retained by the thyroid.

Patient care checklist
Before the test:
☑ Explain or clarify test purpose, preparation, and procedure.
☑ Evaluate patient understanding.
☑ Restrict food and fluids after midnight.
After the test:
☑ As ordered, instruct the patient to resume a light diet 2 hours after taking the oral dose of ^{123}I or ^{131}I.
☑ After the study is complete, the patient may resume a normal diet.

Interfering factors
• Renal failure, diuresis, severe diarrhea, X-ray contrast media studies, ingestion of iodine preparations (including iodized salt, cough syrups, and some multivitamins) or of other drugs (thyroid hormones, salicylates, penicillin, antihistamines, anticoagulants, corticosteroids, and phenylbutazone) can decrease iodine uptake.
• Iodine-deficient diet or ingestion of phenothiazines can increase iodine uptake.

Red blood cell *(RBC)* survival time

Purpose
• To help evaluate unexplained anemia, particularly hemolytic anemia
• To identify sites of abnormal RBC sequestration and destruction.

Normal results
Normal half-life for RBCs labeled with radioactive chromium-51 sodium chromate (^{51}Cr) is 25 to 35 days. Normal gamma camera scans reveal slight radioactivity in the spleen, liver, and sometimes the bone marrow.

Abnormal results
Decreased RBC survival time indicates a hemolytic disease, such as:

Chronic lymphocytic leukemia
Congenital nonspherocytic hemolytic anemia
Hemoglobin C disease
Hereditary spherocytosis
Idiopathic acquired hemolytic anemia
Paroxysmal nocturnal hemoglobinuria
Elliptocytosis
Pernicious anemia
Sickle-cell anemia
Sickle-cell hemoglobin C disease
Hemolytic-uremic syndrome.

The basics
This test aids evaluation of unexplained anemia. Normally, RBCs are destroyed only when they reach senility. However, in hemolytic diseases, RBCs of all ages are randomly destroyed, resulting in anemia.

Survival time is measured by labeling a random sample of RBCs with ^{51}Cr. The ^{51}Cr quickly crosses RBC membranes, reduces to chromium ion, and binds to hemoglobin. This labeled group of RBCs is injected back into the patient. Serial blood samples measure the percent of labeled cells per unit volume over 3 to 4 weeks, until 50% of the cells disappear (disappearance rate corresponds to destruction of a random cell population). A normal RBC survives about 120 days (half-life of 60 days); the ^{51}Cr-labeled RBCs have a shorter half-life (25 to 30 days) because about 1% of senescent RBCs are removed from the circulation each day and about 1% of ^{51}Cr is spontaneously eluted from the labeled RBCs each day.

During the test period, a gamma camera scans the body for sites of abnormally high radioactivity, which indicate sites of excessive RBC sequestration and destruction. This provides direction for treatment. For example, abnormally high RBC sequestration in the spleen may require a splenectomy.

Other tests performed with the RBC survival time test may include spot-checks of the stool to detect gastro-intestinal (GI) blood loss; hematocrit; blood volume studies; and radionuclide iron uptake and clearance tests to aid differential diagnosis of anemia. If hemolytic anemia is diagnosed, additional tests using cross-transfusion of labeled RBCs can determine if anemia results from an intrinsic RBC defect or an extrinsic factor.

Contraindications to this test include: pregnancy or lactation, active bleeding, or poor clotting function.

Procedure
• A 30-ml blood sample is drawn and mixed with 100 microcuries of ^{51}Cr for an adult (less for a child).
• After an incubation period, the mixture is injected intravenously into the patient. A blood sample is drawn 30 minutes after injection to determine blood and RBC volumes.
• A 6-ml sample is collected in a green-top tube after 24 hours; follow-up samples are collected at 3-day intervals for 3 to 4 weeks. (The intervals between samples may vary, depending on the laboratory.)
• To avoid error from physical decay of the ^{51}Cr, each sample is measured with a scintillation well counter on the day it is drawn.
• Radioactivity per ml of RBCs is calculated; these values are plotted to determine mean RBC survival time.
• Simultaneous gamma camera scans of the precordium, sacrum, liver, and spleen detect radioactivity at sites of excessive RBC sequestration.
• A hematocrit is done on a small portion of each blood sample, to check for blood loss.
• At the end of the study, a sample is drawn to compare ending blood and RBC volumes with beginning volumes.
• The patient should not receive blood transfusions during the test period, and should not have blood samples drawn for other tests, as a precaution.

Patient care checklist
Before the test:
☑ Explain or clarify test purpose and procedure.
☑ Evaluate patient understanding.
After the test:
☑ If the test was necessary for a patient with poor clotting function, observe venipuncture sites carefully for signs of hemorrhage.

Interfering factors
• Dehydration, overhydration, or blood loss (from hemorrhage or blood samples drawn for other tests) can change the circulating RBC volume and invalidate test results.
• Blood transfusions during the test period alter the proportion of labeled RBCs to total RBCs, thus altering results.

Renal scan

Purpose
• To detect or rule out masses
• To check patency of the urinary system
• To check kidney function
• To check blood flow to help rule out a renovascular cause for hypertension.

Normal results
Uniform dispersion of the radionuclide bilaterally throughout the kidneys; kidneys are normal in size, shape, position, and function.

Abnormal results
The scan may identify:
—Decreased kidney function
—Masses within the kidneys
—Obstruction
—Organ rejection posttransplant.

The basics
The scan permits imaging of the kidneys by a scanning camera after I.V.

Radionuclide Renography

ISOTOPE RENOGRAM CURVES

Commonly performed with the kidney function study following the administration of ^{131}I-orthoiodohippurate I.V., this test provides a curve illustrating renal activity. Known as a renogram, this curve represents uptake, transit, and excretion time of the radionuclide by each kidney.

Detectors placed posteriorly at each kidney record radiation counts, which, when plotted, form a curve over minute integrals. The amount of radiation detected over certain periods of time and the shape of the curve have diagnostic significance. The illustration below, however, shows a normal absorption and excretion curve for one normal kidney (string of x markers) compared with examples of possible curves associated with renal pathology (solid lines). For example, an obstructed kidney absorbs but fails to excrete the radionuclide; a kidney with a constricted renal artery takes up the radionuclide more slowly and to a lesser degree than normal, and excretes it more slowly; a nonfunctioning kidney fails to absorb the

radionuclide, so the radiation counter detects only background radiation.

Renal uptake is represented by an initial sharp rise in the curve. Known as the vascular phase, this filling of the renal and perirenal space usually occurs within 30 to 45 seconds following radionuclide administration. Renal transit time, the tubular phase, occurs next and is seen as a slower rise in the curve that lasts for 2 to 5 minutes. Finally, the excretory phase represents drainage of the radionuclide from the kidneys.

Although certain curves are characteristic of specific disorders, the curve represents activity of the entire kidney and does not distinguish between its different areas. Consequently, renographic findings must be correlated with the patient's clinical status and results from other urologic tests. When analyzed and correlated with images from the kidney function study, however, the renogram can provide valuable diagnostic information. It is also invaluable for comparing the transit time of both kidneys pre- and posttreatment.

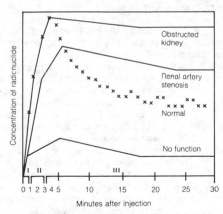

Key:
I = Vascular phase
II = Tubular phase
III = Excretory phase

Normal renogram supplied by Marc S. Lapayowker, M.D., Temple University, Philadelphia; abnormal curve reprinted with permission from J. Stewart Cameron, et al, *Nephrology for Nurses: A Modern Approach to the Kidney* (2nd ed.; Garden City, N.Y.: Medical Examination Publishing Co., 1976).

injection of a radioactive tracer, usually technetium 99m. It is used to evaluate the functioning of one or both kidneys. There should be equal distribution bilaterally in the kidneys. Abnormalities may appear as space-occupying lesions, decreased uptake in one or both kidneys, or dilatation of the collecting system of a kidney, indicating an obstruction. The test should be interpreted with knowledge of the patient's medical history. Renal scanning may be substituted for intravenous pyelography in patients with a hypersensitivity to contrast agents. It may be performed in conjunction with a renogram to give additional information on renal perfusion. (See *Radionuclide Renography*, p. 561.)
Contraindications to this test include: pregnancy and lactation.

Procedure
• The patient is usually placed in a supine position while the camera takes posterior views (except for renal transplants: then the scanning is done anteriorly).
• The patient receives an I.V. injection of the radionuclide.
• Images are taken of the blood flow to the kidneys.
• Static images are taken after blood flow imaging and then at intervals designated by the physician.
• The scan takes approximately 30 minutes to 1 hour. Delayed images may be obtained, as needed, possibly following furosemide (Lasix) injection.

Patient care checklist
Before the test:
☑ Explain or clarify test purpose and procedure.
☑ Evaluate patient understanding.

Interfering factors
Improper injection techniques will result in poor blood flow and picture quality.

Schilling test

Purpose
To differentiate pernicious anemia from other causes of vitamin B_{12} deficiency.

Normal results
Normally, values greater than 7% to 10% of the original doses of radioactive (^{58}Co) vitamin B_{12} and radioactive (^{57}Co) vitamin B_{12} coupled with the intrinsic factor will be excreted.

Abnormal results
Normal excretion of (^{57}Co) vitamin B_{12} coupled with the intrinsic factor and decreased excretion of (^{58}Co) vitamin B_{12}:
    Pernicious anemia
    Patients with total gastrectomy (lack of intrinsic factor production).
Decreased excretion of both (^{57}Co) vitamin B_{12} coupled with the intrinsic factor and (^{58}Co) vitamin B_{12}:
    Malabsorption syndromes, such as:
        Sprue
        Extensive resection of the ileum
        Celiac disease.

The basics
The Schilling test is used in the differential diagnosis of megaloblastic anemia. The intrinsic factor is essential for vitamin B_{12} absorption. When the intrinsic factor is missing, pernicious anemia develops. Patients with pernicious anemia can absorb vitamin B_{12} and eventually excrete it only when the intrinsic factor is administered.

In patients with malabsorption syndromes, however, administration of the intrinsic factor does not help absorption. Absorption and eventual excretion of vitamin B_{12} remains decreased.

Two isotopes are utilized in this test. One isotope is vitamin B_{12} tagged with radioactive cobalt (^{58}Co). The second and different isotope is vitamin B_{12} bound to a purified extract of an intrinsic factor and tagged with a different type of radioactive cobalt (^{57}Co). Following an overnight fast, the patient receives the isotopes orally. The patient is then administered nonradioactive vitamin B$_{12}$ by parenteral injection to saturate the binding capacity of the plasma and ultimately the liver. The parenteral dose of vitamin B$_{12}$ is referred to as the "flushing dose" and is used to ensure maximum excretion of the radioactive vitamin B$_{12}$.

Prior to conducting the Schilling test, it is imperative that all other diagnostic procedures be completed, since the test replenishes the vitamin B$_{12}$ level in the patient.

Contraindications to this test include: pregnancy and lactation.

Procedure
• Have the patient empty his bladder. Note the time.
• The two isotopes (^{58}Co vitamin B$_{12}$ and ^{57}Co vitamin B$_{12}$ bound to intrinsic factor) are orally administered.
• The nonradioactive "flushing dose" of vitamin B$_{12}$ is parenterally administered.
• Following parenteral administration, begin collection of all urine samples for 24 hours. (See "Timed collection," p. xviii.)
• Send the 24-hour urine sample to the clinical laboratory or radiology department for testing.

Patient care checklist
Before the test:
☑ Explain or clarify test purpose and procedure.
☑ Stress that ALL urine samples for the 24-hour period must be saved.
☑ Evaluate patient understanding.
☑ Restrict food and fluids after midnight prior to the test.

Interfering factors
• Improper collection of all urine samples for the 24-hour period will alter test results.
• Urinary excretion of vitamin B$_{12}$ is depressed in enteritis, diabetes, hypothyroidism, and renal disease.

Scrotal scan
[Testicular scan; radionuclide scan of the scrotum or testes]

Purpose
• To detect or rule out torsion of the testes
• To detect or rule out malignancy
• To detect or rule out epididymitis or abscess.

Normal results
Uniform flow and distribution bilaterally throughout the scrotal sac.

Abnormal results
The scan may identify:
   Torsion of the testes
   Hydrocele
   Testicular malignancy
   Epididymitis or abscess.

The basics
A scrotal scan permits imaging of the testes and scrotal sac by a scanning camera after I.V. injection of a radioactive tracer, usually radioactive technetium pertechnetate. Abnormalities may appear as cold or hot spots. Cold spots may indicate hydrocele; hot spots may indicate malignancy or abscess. With torsion of the testes, there is no uniform flow or distribution of the radionuclide. The test should be read with knowledge of the patient's medical history.

Procedure
• The patient first receives potassium perchlorate by mouth. (This is a nonradioactive blocking agent used to prevent the thyroid from concentrating the radioactive agent.)
• The patient is positioned under the camera.
• An I.V. injection of ^{99m}Tc pertechnetate is given to the patient.
• Immediately a flow study is done, watching the blood supply to the scrotum.

• Blood pool images are taken, as are other images, at the physician's discretion.
• The scan takes about 20 to 30 minutes.

Patient care checklist
Before the test:
☑ Explain or clarify test purpose and procedure.
☑ Evaluate patient understanding.

Interfering factors
Improper injection technique or positioning will result in poor images.

Tagged RBC scan
[G.I. bleed scan]

Purpose
To detect the site or origin of GI bleeding.

Normal results
Even distribution of radioisotope throughout the blood pool.

Abnormal results
The scan may identify:
Site of active bleeding in the bowel.

The basics
The tagged RBC scan permits imaging of the blood pool, such as heart, liver, spleen and major blood vessels, after an I.V. injection of radioactive technetium-labeled autologous RBCs. The radioactive compound collects in increasing concentration at the site of active GI bleeding. When imaged, these sites appear "hotter" than normal, identifying the origin of bleeding.
Contraindications to this test include: pregnancy and lactation.

Procedure
• The patient receives an I.V. injection of cold (nonradioactive) pyrophosphate, followed in 15 minutes by another I.V. injection of radioactive technetium. (The pyrophosphate tags

to red blood cells, then the technetium tags to the pyrophosphate.)
• The patient is positioned on the scanning table, and images are taken every 5 minutes, or at the physician's discretion. (Active bleeding may be seen within 30 to 45 minutes.)
• If bleeding does not occur, delayed pictures are taken, as ordered; this might be a 15-minute, 30-minute, 2-hour, or longer interval.

Special precautions
The patient should be monitored for signs and symptoms of shock during the scanning procedure.

Patient care checklist
Before the test:
☑ Explain or clarify test purpose and procedure.
☑ Evaluate patient understanding.

Interfering factors
Improper tagging technique will result in poor picture quality.

Technetium pyrophosphate scanning
[Hot spot myocardial imaging; infarct avid imaging]

Purpose
• To confirm recent myocardial infarction (MI)
• To define the size and location of a recent MI
• To assess prognosis after acute MI.

Normal results
No accumulation of the isotope in the myocardium.

Abnormal results
Hot spots indicate:
Acute MI (typically seen 48 to 72 hours after onset; possibly apparent 12 hours after onset. Typically disappears after 1 week.)

The basics

This test is used to detect recent MI and to determine its location and extent. An I.V. tracer isotope (technetium-99m pyrophosphate) accumulates in damaged myocardial tissue (possibly by combining with calcium in the damaged myocardial cells), where it forms a hot spot on a scan made with a scintillation camera.

This test is most useful for confirming recent MI in patients suffering from obscure cardiac pain (postoperative cardiac patients), when electrocardiograms (EKGs) are equivocal (as with left bundle-branch block or old myocardial scars, for example), or when serum enzyme tests are unreliable. It may also be used to assess prognosis after acute MI. Since hot spots usually disappear after 1 week, those that persist longer than 1 week usually suggest ongoing myocardial damage and a poorer prognosis.

Procedure

• Usually, 20 microcuries of technetium-99m pyrophosphate are injected I.V.
• After 2 or 3 hours, the patient is placed in a supine position.
• Electrocardiography electrodes are attached for continuous monitoring during the test.
• Generally, scans are taken with the patient in several positions, including anterior, left anterior oblique, right anterior oblique, and left lateral.
• The scanning procedure takes 30 to 60 minutes.

Patient care checklist
Before the test
☑ Explain or clarify test purpose and procedure.
☑ Caution the patient to remain quiet and motionless during the scanning.
☑ Evaluate patient understanding.

Interfering factors

In about 10% of patients, isotope accumulations may result from ventricular aneurysm associated with dystrophic calcification, pulmonary neoplasm, recent cardioversion, and from valvular heart disease associated with severe calcification.

Thallium myocardial imaging
[Cold spot myocardial imaging; thallium scintigraphy]

Purpose

• To assess myocardial scarring and perfusion
• To demonstrate the location and extent of acute or chronic myocardial infarction (MI), including transmural and postoperative infarction (resting imaging)
• To diagnose coronary artery disease, or CAD (stress imaging)
• To evaluate the patency of grafts after coronary artery bypass surgery
• To evaluate the effectiveness of antianginal therapy or balloon angioplasty (stress imaging).

Normal results

Characteristic distribution of the isotope throughout the ventricles and no visible defects (cold spots).

Abnormal results

Persistent defects generally indicate:
MI.
Transient defects (present during peak exercise but not after 3- to 6-hour rests) usually indicate:
Ischemia from CAD.

The basics

This test evaluates myocardial blood flow after I.V. injection of the radioisotope thallium-201 (thallous chloride Tl201, or ^{201}TlCl). Thallium, the physiologic analogue of potassium, concentrates in healthy myocardial tissue but not in necrotic or ischemic tissue. Hence, areas of the heart with normal blood supply and intact cells rapidly take up the isotope; areas with poor blood flow and ischemic cells fail to take up the isotope, and appear as cold spots on a scan.

This test is performed in a resting state or after stress (treadmill exercise). Resting imaging can detect acute MI (including transmural and postoperative) within the first few hours of symptoms, but does not distinguish an old from a new infarct. Stress imaging, performed after the patient exercises on a treadmill until he experiences angina or rate-limiting fatigue, can assess known or suspected coronary artery disease. Complications of stress testing include arrhythmias, angina pectoris, and MI.

Contraindications to this test include: impaired neuromuscular function, pregnancy, lactation, locomotor disturbances, acute MI and myocarditis, aortic stenosis, acute infection, unstable metabolic conditions (such as poorly controlled diabetes), digitalis toxicity, and recent pulmonary infarction.

After coronary artery bypass surgery, this test may show improved regional perfusion, which suggests patency of the graft. Increased perfusion noted on imaging after ingestion of antianginal drugs can demonstrate their effectiveness in relieving ischemia. Improved perfusion after balloon angioplasty suggests increased coronary artery flow.

Procedure
Stress imaging
• The patient, wired with electrodes, walks on a treadmill at a regulated pace that is gradually increased, while his EKG, blood pressure, and heart rate are monitored.
• When the patient reaches peak stress, the examiner injects 1.5 to 3 mCi of thallium into the antecubital vein and flushes it with 10 to 15 ml of normal saline solution.
• The patient exercises an additional 45 to 60 seconds to permit circulation and uptake of the isotope, then lies on his back under the scintillation camera.

• If the patient is asymptomatic, the precordial leads are removed.
• Scanning begins after 3 to 5 minutes, with the patient in various positions.
• Additional scans may be taken after the patient rests for 3 to 6 hours.
Resting imaging
• Within the first few hours of symptoms of MI, or if stress testing is contraindicated, the patient receives an injection of thallium I.V.
• Scanning begins after 3 to 5 minutes, with the patient in various positions.

Special precautions
CLINICAL ALERT: **Stress imaging is stopped at once if the patient develops chest pain, dyspnea, fatigue, syncope, hypotension, ischemic EKG changes, significant arrhythmias, or critical signs and symptoms (pallor, clammy skin, confusion, or staggering gait).**

Patient care checklist
Before the test
☑ Explain or clarify test purpose, preparation, and procedure.
☑ For stress imaging, instruct the patient to wear walking shoes during the treadmill exercise and to report fatigue, pain, or shortness of breath immediately.
☑ Also, for stress imaging, instruct the patient to restrict use of alcohol, tobacco, and unprescribed medications for 24 hours before the test and to have nothing by mouth for 6 hours before the test.
☑ Evaluate patient understanding.
☑ For stress imaging, make sure the patient has signed a consent form.
After the test
☑ If the patient must return for future scanning, instruct him to rest in the interim and to restrict his diet to clear liquids before redistribution studies.

Interfering factors
• Cold spots—although usually due to coronary artery disease—may result from sarcoidosis, myocardial fibrosis, cardiac contusion, attenuation due to

soft tissue and artifacts (for example, diaphragm, breast implants, electrodes), apical thinning, and coronary spasm.

• Absence of cold spots in the presence of coronary artery disease may result from insignificant obstruction, inadequate stress, delayed imaging, single-vessel disease (particularly the right or left circumflex coronary arteries), and collateral circulation.

Thyroid scan
[Radionuclide thyroid imaging]

Purpose
• To assess the size, structure, and position of the thyroid gland
• To evaluate thyroid function in conjunction with specific thyroid uptake studies.

Normal results
Normal size, shape, position, and function of the thyroid, with uniform uptake of the radioisotope.

Abnormal results
Hot spots indicate:
  Hyperfunctioning nodules.
Cold spots indicate:
  Hypofunctioning nodules.
(See *Thyroid Scanning and Thyroid Disorders,* p. 568, for specific implications.)

The basics
In this test, thyroid imaging occurs after administration of a radioisotope—usually ^{123}I, ^{99m}Tc pertechnetate, or, less commonly, ^{131}I. Thyroid imaging is usually recommended after discovery of a palpable mass, enlarged gland, or asymmetric goiter. Generally, this test is performed concurrently with measurement of serum triiodothyronine (T_3) and serum thyroxine (T_4) levels, and thyroid uptake tests.

The presence of hot spots requires a follow-up T_3 (Cytomel) thyroid suppression test to determine if the hyperfunctioning areas are autonomous. (See *T_3 Thyroid Suppression Test,* p. 569.)

If a cold spot appears, subsequent thyroid ultrasonography may be performed to rule out cysts; in addition, fine-needle aspiration and biopsy of such nodules may be performed to rule out malignancy.

Contraindications to this test include: pregnancy or lactation.

Procedure
• Scanning follows oral administration of ^{123}I or ^{131}I by 24 hours, I.V. injection of ^{99m}Tc pertechnetate by 20 to 30 minutes.
• The patient's thyroid gland is palpated.
• With the patient in a supine position with his neck extended, his thyroid gland is scanned. Three views are obtained.
• Scanning takes about 30 minutes.

Patient care checklist
Before the test
☑ Explain or clarify test purpose, preparation, and procedure.
☑ As ordered, inform the patient to discontinue administration of thyroid hormones, thyroid hormone antagonists, and iodine preparations (Lugol's solution, some multivitamins, and cough syrups) for 2 to 3 weeks before the test. One week before the test, he should discontinue phenothiazines, as ordered. Also, as ordered, instruct the patient to avoid ingesting iodized salt, iodinated salt substitutes, and seafood during this period.
☑ Evaluate patient understanding.
☑ Restrict food and fluid from midnight the night before the test, if he is scheduled to receive an oral dose of ^{123}I or ^{131}I. (No fasting is necessary if he is to receive I.V. ^{99m}Tc pertechnetate.) Fasting continues for another 2 hours after oral administration of the radioisotope.

Thyroid Scanning and Thyroid Disorders

Condition	Findings	Causes
Hypothyroidism	• Glandular damage or absent gland	• Surgical removal of gland • Inflammation • Radiation • Neoplasm (rare)
Hypothyroid goiter	• Enlarged gland • Decreased uptake if glandular destruction is present • Increased uptake possible from congenital error in thyroxine synthesis	• Insufficient iodine intake • Hypersecretion of TSH caused by thyroid hormone deficiency
Myxedema (cretinism in children)	• Normal or slightly reduced gland size • Uniform pattern • Decreased uptake	• Defective embryonic development, resulting in congenital absence or underdevelopment of thyroid gland • Maternal iodine deficiency
Hyperthyroidism (Graves' disease)	• Enlarged gland • Uniform pattern • Increased uptake	• Unknown, but may be hereditary • Production of thyroid-stimulating immunoglobulins
Toxic nodular goiter	• Multiple hot spots	• Long-standing simple goiter
Hyperfunctioning adenomas	• Solitary hot spot	• Adenomatous production of T_3 and T_4, suppressing TSH secretion and producing atrophy of other thyroid tissue
Hypofunctioning adenomas	• Solitary cold spot	• Cyst or nonfunctioning nodule
Benign multinodular goiter	• Multiple nodules with variable or no function	• Local inflammation • Degeneration
Thyroid carcinoma	• Usually a solitary cold spot with occasional or no function	• Neoplasm

☑ Check patient history for diet and medication. Ask the patient if he has undergone tests that used radiographic contrast media within the past 60 days. Note on the X-ray request slip any drugs or previous radiographic contrast media exposure that may interfere with iodine uptake.

☑ Instruct the patient to remove dentures and jewelry that may interfere with visualization of the thyroid, just prior to scanning.

T₃ Thyroid Suppression Test

The T₃ (Cytomel) thyroid suppression test helps determine whether areas of excessive iodine uptake in the thyroid (hot spots) are autonomous (as in some cases of Graves' disease) or reflect pituitary overcompensation (as in iodine-deficient goiter). Autonomous hot spots function independently of pituitary control. However, hot spots caused by iodine deficiency stem from reduced T₄ production, which decreases T₃ production and increases thyroid-stimulating hormone (TSH) production. Increased TSH production, in turn, overstimulates the thyroid and causes excessive iodine uptake.

After a baseline reading of thyroid function is obtained by a radioactive iodine uptake (RAIU)

test, a dosage of 100 mcg of synthetic T₃ (Cytomel) is administered for 7 days. (Normally, T₃ acts through a negative feedback mechanism to suppress pituitary release of TSH; TSH then suppresses thyroid function and iodine uptake.) During the last 2 days of Cytomel administration, RAIU tests are repeated to assess thyroid response. Suppression of RAIU to at least 50% of baseline indicates that the hot spot is under pituitary control and suggests iodine deficiency as the cause of increased iodine uptake. Failure to suppress RAIU by 50% suggests autonomous thyroid hyperfunction, resulting perhaps from Graves' disease or a toxic thyroid nodule.

Interfering factors

• Iodine-deficient diet and phenothiazines increase uptake of radioactive iodine.

• Uptake of radioactive iodine is decreased by renal disease and by ingestion of iodized salt, iodine preparations, iodinated salt substitutes, seafood, thyroid hormones, thyroid hormone antagonists, aminosalicylic acid, corticosteroids, multivitamins, and cough syrups containing inorganic iodides. Severe diarrhea and vomiting can also decrease uptake by impairing gastrointestinal absorption of radioiodine.

Ventilation scan

Purpose

• To help diagnose pulmonary emboli
• To identify areas of the lung capable of ventilation
• To help evaluate regional respiratory function
• To locate regional hypoventilation

that usually results from excessive smoking or chronic obstructive pulmonary disease.

Normal results

There is an equal distribution of gas in both lungs, and normal wash-in and wash-out phases.

Abnormal results

Unequal gas distribution in both lungs indicates:

Poor ventilation or airway obstruction in areas with low radioactivity.

Abnormal ventilation within areas of consolidation occurs with:

Parenchymal disease, such as pneumonia.

Regional hypoventilation usually results from:

Excessive smoking or chronic obstructive pulmonary disease.

The basics

Ventilation scan—a nuclear scan performed after inhalation of air mixed with radioactive gas—delineates areas of the lung ventilated during respiration. The scan consists of recording the distribution of the gas during three phases: during the buildup of radioactive gas (wash-in phase), after the patient rebreathes from a bag and the radioactivity reaches a steady level (equilibrium phase), and after removal of the radioactive gas from the lungs (wash-out phase). Performed with a perfusion scan (see "Lung perfusion scan," p. 555), a ventilation scan helps distinguish between parenchymal disease, such as bronchogenic carcinoma, and conditions due to vascular abnormalities, such as pulmonary emboli. With pulmonary embolism, perfusion to the embolized area is decreased, but ventilation to this area is maintained.

In a patient on mechanical ventilation, krypton gas must be substituted for xenon gas during the test.

Contraindications to this test include: pregnancy and lactation.

Procedure
• The patient inhales (through a mask) air mixed with a small amount of radioactive gas.
• The patient is asked to hold his breath for a short time after inhaling the gas.
• The distribution of the gas in the lungs is monitored on a nuclear scanner. The patient's chest is scanned as he exhales. The test takes 30 to 45 minutes.

Special precautions
CLINICAL ALERT: **It is important to watch for leaks in the closed system of radioactive gas, such as through the mask, which can contaminate the surrounding atmosphere.**

Radionuclide Venography

Although venography accurately detects deep vein thrombosis (DVT), it is an expensive and sometimes hazardous invasive test, since the injection can cause localized clots. Currently, radionuclide tests, such as the ^{125}I fibrinogen scan, screen for DVT or attempt to detect the disorder in a patient who is too ill for venography or is hypersensitive to the contrast medium. In the ^{125}I fibrinogen scan, labeled fibrinogen injected I.V. collects at sites of active thrombus formation. A scintillation counter records radioactivity at several sites on the calf and thigh after 6, 24, 48, and 72 hours (the time required for the isotope to concentrate in possible thrombi).

An increase of more than 20% in radioactivity between any adjacent sites on the same leg, from results of previous scans or from a corresponding scan on the opposite leg, suggests DVT; an abnormality that persists for more than 24 hours confirms DVT.

The ^{125}I fibrinogen scan is highly sensitive to calf vein thrombi in a patient at high risk, but proves insensitive to groin and pelvic thrombi because of high background radiation from large veins and arteries, and unfavorable anatomic relationships; this is a major limitation since large thrombi can originate in the groin and pelvis, especially after local trauma, such as hip surgery.

Lugol's solution is administered for a week before and a week after this test, to keep the radioactive iodine out of the thyroid gland. The sodium pertechnetate ^{99m}Tc scan, another radionuclide test, can detect peripheral vascular disease—usually in the veins, less often in the arteries. When tagged to albumin, the isotope can image both the lower leg and pulmonary veins. Xenon-133 washout and radioactive centrosome tests, used in research, evaluate peripheral arterial blood flow in the lower legs.

Gastroesophageal Reflux Scanning

When results of a barium swallow are inconclusive, gastroesophageal reflux scanning may be done to evaluate esophageal function and detect reflux. This test delivers less radiation than a conventional barium swallow and is a much more sensitive indicator of reflux. It also allows reflux to be measured without insertion of an esophageal tube—an important consideration in testing infants, small children, and other patients for whom intubation is contraindicated.

The patient is instructed to fast after midnight before the test, to clear stomach contents that impede passage of the imaging agent. As the test begins, the patient is placed in a supine or upright position and is asked to swallow a solution containing a radiopharmaceutical, such as technetium-99m (^{99m}Tc) sulfur colloid. A gamma counter placed over the patient's chest records passage of the ^{99m}Tc sulfur colloid through the esophagus into the stomach, to determine transit time and to evaluate esophageal function. If gastroesophageal reflux is suspected, the patient is repositioned as his stomach distends, and continuous recordings visualize reflux and estimate its quantity. (Depending on hospital policy, manual pressure may be applied to the patient's upper abdomen, and recordings may be taken at specific intervals.)

Normally, ^{99m}Tc sulfur colloid descends through the esophagus in about 6 seconds; radioactivity is then detected only in the stomach and small bowel. However, diffuse spasm of the esophagus, achalasia, or other esophageal motility disorders may prolong transit time; in gastroesophageal reflux, radioactivity may be detected in the esophagus.

Like other radionuclide studies, this scan is usually contraindicated during pregnancy and lactation. It can be modified for use in infants and children.

Patient care checklist
Before the test
☑ Explain or clarify test purpose and procedure.

☑ Evaluate patient understanding.
(Also see *Radionuclide Venography* and *Gastroesophageal Reflux Scanning*.)

Selected References

Bernier, Donald, et al., eds. *Nuclear Medicine Technology and Techniques.* St. Louis: C.V. Mosby Co., 1981.

Conn, Rex B., ed. *Current Diagnosis,* 7th ed. Philadelphia: W.B. Saunders Co., 1985.

Diagnostics, 2nd ed. Nurse's Reference Library. Springhouse, Pa.: Springhouse Corp., 1986.

Diseases, 2nd ed. Nurse's Reference Library. Springhouse, Pa.: Springhouse Corp., 1987.

Early, Paul J., and Soder, D. Bruce. *Principles and Practice of Nuclear Medicine.* St. Louis: C.V. Mosby Co., 1984.

Fischbach, Frances. *A Manual of Laboratory Diagnostic Tests,* 2nd ed. Philadelphia: J.B. Lippincott Co., 1984.

Grossman, Zachary D., et al. *The Clinician's Guide to Diagnostic Imaging.* New York: Raven Press Pubs., 1983.

Harvey, A. McGehee, ed. *The Principles and Practice of Medicine,* 21st ed. East Norwalk, Conn.: Appleton-Century-Crofts, 1984.

Mettler, Fred A., and Guiberteau, Milton J. *Essentials of Nuclear Medicine Imaging,* 2nd ed. Orlando, Fla.: Grune

& Stratton, 1986.

Michaels, Davida, ed. *Diagnostic Procedures*. New York: John Wiley & Sons, 1983.

Neoplastic Disorders. Nurse's Clinical Library. Springhouse, Pa.: Springhouse Corp., 1985.

Pagana, Kathleen D., and Pagana, Timothy James. *Diagnostic Testing and Nursing Implications*, 2nd ed. St. Louis: C.V. Mosby Co., 1986.

Pantaleo, Nancy, et al. "Thallium Myocardial Scintigraphy and Its Use in the Assessment of Coronary Artery Disease," *Heart and Lung* 10(1):61-70, January/February 1981.

Petersdorf, Robert G., and Adams, Raymond D., eds. *Harrison's Principles of Internal Medicine*, 10th ed. New York: McGraw-Hill Book Co., 1983.

Soin, Jacneet S., and Brooks, Harold L. *Nuclear Cardiology for Clinicians*. Mount Kisco, N.Y.: Futura Publishing Co., 1980.

Zeluff, G.W., et al. "Evaluation of Coronary Arteries and Myocardium by Radionuclide Imaging," *Heart and Lung* 9(2):344-47, March/April 1980.

12 ULTRA-SONOGRAPHIC TESTING

Introduction

Ultrasonography is a noninvasive procedure using high-frequency sound waves (beyond the range of human hearing) to examine internal structures of the body. During the procedure, a transducer is moved over the structure being examined, and an ultrasound beam is directed into the body. The beam travels through the tissue and reflects back to the transducer. There, the sound waves are converted into electrical impulses and amplified to show a series of cross-sectional images on a display screen. A coupling agent, such as mineral oil, is used to eliminate air trapped between the transducer and the skin, promoting good acoustic contact.

How ultrasonography works

Although the procedure itself is relatively simple, the principles behind ultrasonography are complex. Sound waves travel at different speeds, depending on the density and elasticity of the structures they pass through. They travel fastest through structures with the most compact molecules (bone) and slowest through structures with the least compact molecules (air-filled organs such as the lungs, bowel, and stomach).

Each time the sound waves hit an interface (the border between two adjacent structures), some of the waves reflect back to the transducer and cause an image to appear on the display screen, while the rest continue moving until they hit the next interface.

The screen image actually shows the different densities of adjacent tissues. (Abnormal tissue often has a density and elasticity different from the surrounding normal tissue.) A small difference in tissue densities causes the sound waves to reflect at different speeds, producing a good image on the screen. But a large difference in tissue densities causes most of the sound waves to reflect right back to the transducer, producing a meaningless image (called an *artifact*). This usually happens when sound waves hit the interface between bone and soft tissue and between air-filled organs and soft tissue; therefore, ultrasound cannot be used to evaluate bones or air-filled organs. To get a good image, sound waves must pass through medium-density soft tissue.

Uses of ultrasonography

Most internal structures can be examined with ultrasound (see *What Can Be Examined by Ultrasonography?*, p. 574). For example, ultrasound can show the size, consistency, and shape of internal structures and can detect abnormalities such as masses, edema, inflammation, stones, and free fluid. It can also be used to differentiate between cystic and solid masses (for example, to examine the breast—see *Breast Ultrasonography*, p. 575), to outline the boundaries of lesions and show displacement of adjacent tissues, to scan a body area to examine several structures at once, and to show motion and allow continuous viewing of a

What Can be Examined by Ultrasonography?

Head and neck
brain
eyes
thyroid
any palpable mass

Chest
pleura
mediastinum
breasts
any palpable mass
heart:
    all four chambers
    pericardium
    mitral valve
    aortic valve
    pulmonic valve
    tricuspid valve

Abdomen
pancreas
liver
spleen
kidney
adrenal glands
gallbladder and biliary system
retroperitoneum
free fluid
masses
peritoneal cavity

Pelvis
uterus
ovaries and adnexa
bladder
prostate
testicles

Blood vessels
carotid artery
abdominal aorta
thoracic aorta
aortic arch
right pulmonary artery
left atrium
popliteal artery
arteriovenous shunt grafts

Extremities
any lump on surface
blood supply

Ultrasonography can be used on a pregnant patient to examine the placenta or fetal anatomy and to determine the biparietal diameter. It can also be used to calculate the age of a fetus and the fetal heart rate.

structure (for example, to examine a fetus).

Advantages and disadvantages

Ultrasonography is quick, relatively inexpensive, comfortable, and safe for both patient and examiner. It requires little or no patient preparation and can be repeated without harmful effects. Since the procedure requires no contrast medium, structural changes in organs that are not functioning properly can be visualized. For instance, ultrasonography can be used to visualize the gallbladder when the common bile duct is blocked with gallstones—while an oral cholecystogram *cannot* be used because the bile duct must be patent so that the contrast medium can circulate to the gallbladder.

The disadvantages are minimal. As mentioned before, ultrasonography cannot be used to examine bones or air-filled organs. It is also difficult to perform on certain patients. For instance, the transducer must be moved very carefully over a new surgical incision, and if a patient has abdominal scars, scar tissue can attenuate the ultrasound beam. Ultrasonography is also difficult to perform on obese patients (sound waves cannot pass through fat layers easily).

Patient-teaching guidelines
Patient-learner objectives:
• Define the test.
• State the specific purpose of the test.
• Explain the procedure.
• Discuss test preparation and procedure.

Teaching content:
• Define the test in terms the patient can understand.
• Explain the specific purpose of the test.
• Describe the procedure. Be sure to describe the equipment, which may be large, unfamiliar, and anxiety-producing. Also explain the use of the coupling agent.
• Reassure the patient that the procedure is safe and painless. Explain that all the patient will feel is the transducer moving over the skin.
• If the patient is pregnant, reassure her that the test will not harm the fetus.
• Tell the patient what position is required for the test; when appropriate, explain that he will have to change positions so that his organs can be visualized at different angles.
• Caution the patient to follow other directions carefully. The patient may be required to hold his breath briefly during the procedure and to remain still, since movement distorts results.
• Inform the patient of any special preparation necessary to help ensure a good image on the screen.
Evaluation:
After the patient-teaching session is completed, evaluate whether or not the patient has satisfactorily met each patient-learner objective by obtaining necessary patient feedback. Refocus teaching as needed.

Abdominal aorta ultrasonography
[abdominal aorta sonogram]

Purpose
• To detect and measure suspected abdominal aortic aneurysm
• To measure expansion of known abdominal aortic aneurysm.

Normal results
In adults, the abdominal aorta tapers from about 1″ to ½″ (2.5 to 1.5 cm) in diameter along its length from the diaphragm to the bifurcation. It descends through the retroperitoneal space, anterior to the vertebral column and slightly left of the midline. Four of its major branches are usually well visualized: the celiac trunk, the renal arteries, the superior mesenteric artery, and the common iliac arteries.

Abnormal results
Luminal diameter of the abdominal aorta greater than 1½″ (4 cm) is aneurysmal; greater than 2¾″ (7 cm), aneurysmal with high risk of rupture.

The basics
In this safe, noninvasive test, a transducer directs high-frequency sound waves into the abdomen over a wide area from the xiphoid process to the

Breast Ultrasonography

Ultrasonography is a test that helps distinguish cysts from solid tumors in dense breast tissue. As in other diagnostic ultrasound techniques, a transducer is used to focus a beam of high-frequency sound waves through the patient's skin and into the breast. The sound waves bounce back to the transducer as an echo that varies in strength with the density of the underlying tissues. A computer processes these echoes and displays them on a screen for interpretation.

Ultrasound can show all areas of a breast, including the area close to the chest wall, which is hard to study with radiographs. When used as an adjunct to mammography, the technique increases diagnostic accuracy. When used alone, it is more accurate than mammography in examining the denser breast tissue of young patients. While still largely experimental, ultrasonography is being studied as a possible replacement for mammography in breast cancer screening programs.

umbilical region. The sound waves, echoing to the transducer from interfaces between tissues of different densities, are transmitted as electrical impulses and displayed on an oscilloscope or television screen. Internal organs, the vertebral column, and, most importantly, the size and course of the abdominal aorta and other major vessels are revealed.

Ultrasonography helps confirm a suspected aortic aneurysm and is the method of choice for determining its diameter. However, angiography is indicated preoperatively to visualize the extent of atherosclerotic changes and to reveal anatomic anomalies, such as three renal arteries. Once an aneurysm is detected, ultrasonography is used every 6 months to monitor changes in patient status.

Procedure
• The patient is assisted to a supine position, and a conductive gel is applied to his abdomen.
• Longitudinal and transverse scans are made.
• Appropriate views are photographed or videotaped.
• The procedure takes 30 to 45 minutes to perform.

Patient care checklist
Before the test
☑ Explain or clarify test purpose and procedure.
☑ Tell the patient that the test is safe and painless, although mild pressure may be experienced as the transducer is moved over the skin. If he has a known aneurysm, reassure him that the sound waves will not cause it to rupture.
☑ Tell the patient that a conductive gel will be applied to the midline of his abdomen, and a transducer will be passed over the area, directing sound waves into his abdomen.
☑ Evaluate patient understanding.
☑ Restrict food and fluids for 12 hours before the test to minimize bowel gas and motility.

☑ If ordered, give simethicone to reduce bowel gas.
After the test
☑ Remove any remaining conductive gel from the patient's skin.

Interfering factors
• Bowel gas and motility, excessive body movement, surgical wounds, and severe dyspnea may prevent adequate imaging.
• Residual barium from gastrointestinal contrast studies within the previous 24 hours, and air introduced during endoscopy within the previous 12 to 24 hours hinder ultrasound transmission.
• In obese patients, mesenteric fat may impair transmission of ultrasound waves during testing.

Doppler ultrasonography

Purpose
• To aid in diagnosis of chronic venous insufficiency and of superficial and deep vein thromboses (popliteal, femoral, iliac)
• To aid in diagnosis of peripheral artery disease and arterial occlusion
• To monitor patients who have had arterial reconstruction and bypass grafts
• To detect abnormalities of carotid artery blood flow associated with such conditions as aortic stenosis
• To evaluate possible arterial trauma.

Normal results
The ankle-arm pressure index (API)—the ratio between ankle systolic pressure and brachial systolic pressure—is normally equal to or greater than 1. (The API is also known as the arterial ischemia index, the ankle/brachial index, or the pedal/brachial index.) Proximal thigh pressure is normally 20 to 30 mm Hg higher than arm pressure, but pressure measurements at adjacent sites are similar. In the arms, pressure readings should remain un-

changed despite postural changes. Segmental pressures in the limbs are equal. Audible signals indicate unobstructed venous and arterial blood flow bilaterally.

Abnormal results

An abnormal API is directly proportional to the degree of circulatory impairment: mild ischemia, 1 to 0.75; claudication, 0.75 to 0.50; pain at rest, 0.50 to 0.25; and pregangrene, 0.25 to 0. Diminished blood flow velocity signals indicate venous or arterial stenosis or occlusion. An absent venous flow velocity signal indicates venous thrombosis.

The basics

This noninvasive test evaluates blood flow in the major veins and arteries of the arms and legs and in the extracranial cerebrovascular system. (See *Carotid Imaging Tests*.) Developed as an alternative to arteriography and venography, Doppler ultrasonography is safer, less costly, and requires a shorter test period than invasive tests. Although this test has a 95% accuracy rate in detecting arteriovenous disease that significantly impairs blood flow (by at least 50%), it may fail to detect mild arteriosclerotic plaques and smaller thrombi and generally fails to detect major calf vein thrombosis.

In Doppler ultrasonography, a hand-held transducer directs high-frequency sound waves to the artery or vein being tested. The sound waves strike moving red blood cells and are reflected back to the transducer at frequencies that correspond to the velocity of blood flow through the vessel. The transducer then amplifies the sound waves to permit direct listening and graphic recording of blood flow.

Measurement of systolic pressure during this test helps detect the presence, location, and extent of peripheral arterial occlusive disease. Observation of changes in sound wave frequency during respiration helps detect

Carotid Imaging Tests

What is it? Carotid imaging is a diagnostic test that assesses the carotid arteries for occlusive disease. In this test, a pulsed Doppler ultrasonic flow transducer or a real-time imager permits imaging and recording of the carotid artery.

• Real-time imaging uses the echo technique, which also permits visualization of the carotid artery. In this technique, a Doppler signal can be directed to specific points along the vessel. The audio signal is then evaluated.

• Pulsed Doppler technique uses a transducer with a range-gating system that allows alternate transmission and reception of ultrasonic signals. The sound reflected from moving red blood cells within the lumen is then collected and stored in a computer for subsequent intraluminal image reconstruction.

How is it done? The patient is placed in a supine position, and the probe is placed on his neck and is moved slowly from the vicinity of the common carotid artery to that of the bifurcation, then to the site of the internal and external carotids.

What are its advantages? Carotid imaging detects ulcerating plaques that cannot be detected by other methods; it can also differentiate between total and near-total arterial occlusion.

What are its disadvantages? Intramural calcification prevents sound penetration and may lead to false-positive results.

venous occlusive disease, since venous blood flow normally fluctuates with respiration. Use of compression maneuvers also helps detect occlusion of the veins as well as occlusion or stenosis of carotid arteries.

Pulse volume recorder testing may be performed along with Doppler ultrasonography to yield a quantitative recording of changes in blood volume or flow in an extremity or organ.

Procedure
A conductive gel is applied to the tip of the transducer.

Peripheral arterial evaluation:
• The patient is instructed to remove all clothing above or below the waist, depending on the test site.
• After he is assisted to a supine position, brachial blood pressure is measured, and the transducer is placed at various points along the test arteries.
• The signals are monitored and the waveforms recorded for later analysis.
• Segmental limb blood pressure is obtained to localize arterial occlusive disease.
• For lower extremity tests, a blood pressure cuff is wrapped around the calf, pressure readings are obtained, and waveforms are recorded from the dorsalis pedis and posterior tibial arteries. Then, the cuff is wrapped around the thigh, and waveforms are recorded at the popliteal artery.
• For upper extremity tests, a blood pressure cuff is wrapped around the forearm, pressure readings are taken and waveforms recorded over both the radial and the ulnar arteries. Then, the cuff is wrapped around the upper arm, pressure readings are taken, and waveforms are recorded with the transducer over the brachial artery.
• Blood pressure readings and waveform recordings are repeated with the arm in extreme hyperextension and hyperabduction to check for possible compression factors that may interfere with arterial blood flow.
• The patient is assisted to a sitting position, and the upper extremity examination is performed again on the same arm.
• The examination is then repeated on the other arm.

Peripheral venous evaluation:
• The patient is instructed to remove all clothing above or below the waist, depending on the test site.
• He is assisted to a supine position and instructed to breathe normally.
• The transducer is placed over the appropriate vein, waveforms are recorded, and respiratory modulations are noted.
• Proximal limb compression maneuvers are performed and augmentation noted after release of compression, to evaluate venous valve competency. Changes in respiration are monitored.
• For lower extremity tests, the patient is asked to perform Valsalva's maneuver, and venous blood flow is recorded.
• The procedure is repeated on the other arm or leg.

Patient care checklist
Before the test
☑ Explain or clarify test purpose and procedure.
☑ Tell the patient that the test is safe and painless, although mild pressure may be experienced as the transducer is moved over the skin.
☑ Tell him that blood pressure will be taken at several sites along the limb being examined.
☑ Evaluate patient understanding.
After the test
☑ Remove any remaining conductive gel from the patient's skin.

Interfering factors
If the patient is uncooperative, test results may be invalid.

Echocardiography
[heart sonogram, sonocardiogram]

Purpose
• To diagnose and evaluate valvular abnormalities
• To measure the size of the heart's chambers

• To evaluate chambers and valves in congenital heart disorders
• To aid in diagnosis of hypertrophic and related cardiomyopathies
• To detect atrial tumors
• To evaluate cardiac function or wall motion after myocardial infarction
• To detect pericardial effusion.

Normal results
Normal heart size and position. Normal motion pattern and structure of the four valves and chamber walls.

Abnormal results
Echocardiography aids in the diagnosis of:
    Mitral stenosis
    Mitral valve prolapse
    Aortic insufficiency
    Aortic stenosis
    Subaortic stenosis
    Tricuspid valve disease
    Left atrial tumor
    Pericardial effusion
    Congenital heart disease
    Enlarged heart chamber.

The basics
This widely used, noninvasive test examines the size, shape, and motion of cardiac structures and is useful for evaluating patients with chest pain, enlarged cardiac silhouettes on X-ray films, electrocardiographic changes unrelated to coronary artery disease, and abnormal heart sounds on auscultation. In echocardiography, a special transducer placed at an acoustic window (an area where bones and lung tissue are absent) on the patient's chest directs ultra–high-frequency sound waves toward cardiac structures, which reflect these waves. The transducer picks up the echoes, converts them to electrical impulses, and relays them to an echocardiography machine for display on an oscilloscope screen and for recording on a strip chart or videotape. Electrocardiography and phonocardiography may be performed simultaneously to time events in the cardiac cycle.

The techniques most commonly used in echocardiography are M-mode (motion-mode) and two-dimensional (cross-sectional). In M-mode echocardiography, a single pencil-like ultrasound beam strikes the heart, producing a vertical view of cardiac structures; this method is especially useful for precisely recording the motion and dimensions of intracardiac structures. In two-dimensional echocardiography, the ultrasound beam rapidly sweeps through an arc, producing a cross-sectional or fan-shaped view of cardiac structures; this technique is useful for recording lateral motion and providing the correct spatial relationship between cardiac structures. Often, these techniques complement each other. Test results should be correlated with clinical history, physical examination, and results of additional tests.

Procedure
• The patient is assisted to a supine position.
• Conductive gel is applied to the third or fourth intercostal space to the left of the sternum, and the transducer is placed directly over it.
• The transducer is systematically angled to direct ultrasonic waves at specific parts of the patient's heart.
• During the test, the oscilloscope screen, which displays the returning echoes, is observed; significant or oscilloscopic findings are recorded on a strip chart recorder (M-mode echocardiography) or on a videotape recorder (two-dimensional echocardiography).
• For a different view of the heart, the transducer is placed beneath the xiphoid process or directly above the sternum.
• For a left lateral view, the patient may be positioned on his left side.
• To record heart function under various conditions, the patient is asked to inhale and exhale slowly, to hold his breath, or to inhale amyl nitrite.

• The procedure takes 15 to 30 minutes to perform.

Patient care checklist
Before the test

☑ Explain or clarify test purpose and procedure.

☑ Tell the patient that the test is safe and painless, although mild pressure may be experienced as the transducer is passed over his skin.

☑ Tell the patient that a conductive gel will be applied to the skin under his left breast, and that a transducer will be passed over the area, directing sound waves to the heart.

☑ Inform the patient that he may be asked to breathe in and out slowly, to hold his breath, or to inhale a gas with a slightly sweet odor (amyl nitrite) while changes in heart function are recorded. Describe the possible adverse effects of amyl nitrite (dizziness, flushing, and tachycardia), but assure the patient that such symptoms quickly subside.

☑ Tell the patient that he must remain still during the test, since movement distorts results.

☑ Evaluate patient understanding.
After the test

☑ Remove any remaining conductive gel from the patient's skin.

Interfering factors
• Incorrect transducer placement and excess movement interfere with results.
• Patients with thick chests, chronic obstructive lung disease, or chest wall abnormalities may be difficult to test.

Echoencephalography
[brain sonogram]

Purpose
To determine the position and size of midline cerebral structures.

Normal results
In a healthy person, an echoence-phalogram shows the third ventricle centered in the skull, no more than 2 to 3 mm from the midline. Other midline structures, such as the right and the left lateral ventricles, also appear in their normal anatomic positions.

Abnormal results
A shift in midline structures of more than 3 mm indicates an abnormality. If the third ventricle is enlarged by 10 mm or more (7 mm or more in children), further investigation for a possible space-occupying lesion is necessary. However, two sets of identical impulses are required to confirm abnormal results. Echoencephalography may also reveal structural shifts caused by cerebral edema or by subdural and extradural hemorrhage.

The basics
In echoencephalography, an ultrasonic beam is transmitted through the skull by a transducer. The time required for midline cerebral structures to reflect the beam back to the transducer is converted to an electrical impulse. This impulse is then displayed on an oscilloscope screen and measured to determine the position of the brain's midline structures, particularly the third ventricle. Echoencephalography has largely been replaced by computerized tomography.

Procedure
• The patient is assisted to a supine position on a radiographic table.
• A conductive gel is applied to the tip of the transducer, which is then placed on the temporoparietal region of the patient's head.
• The transducer transmits an ultrasonic beam to the underlying structures.
• The time required for cerebral structures to reflect the beam to the transducer is converted to an electrical impulse, and is visualized on an oscilloscope screen. This image is photographed for later study and a permanent record.

- The procedure takes approximately 1 hour to perform.

Patient care checklist
Before the test
☑ Explain or clarify test purpose and procedure.
☑ Tell the patient that the test is safe and painless, although mild pressure may be experienced as the transducer is moved on his scalp, directing sound waves to the brain.
☑ Tell the patient that he may hear an echo that sounds like repetitious humming or a musical note.
☑ Evaluate patient understanding.
☑ Just before the test, ask the patient to remove jewelry or other metal objects from his head and neck.
After the test
☑ Remove any remaining conductive gel from the patient's scalp.

Interfering factors
Failure to remove jewelry or metal objects from the patient's head and neck interferes with test results.

Gallbladder and biliary system ultrasonography
[gallbladder and biliary system sonogram]

Purpose
- To confirm diagnosis of cholelithiasis
- To diagnose acute cholecystitis
- To distinguish between obstructive and nonobstructive jaundice.

Normal results
Normal size, contour, and position of gallbladder, cystic duct, and common bile duct.

Abnormal results
Gallbladder and biliary system ultrasonography may reveal:
  Cholelithiasis
  Cholecystitis

Polyps within the gallbladder
Carcinoma of the gallbladder.

The basics
In ultrasonography of the gallbladder and the biliary system, a focused beam of high-frequency sound waves passes into the upper right quadrant of the abdomen, creating echoes that vary with changes in tissue density. When these echoes are converted to electrical energy and amplified by a transducer, they appear on an oscilloscope screen as a pattern of spikes or dots. This pattern reveals the size, shape, and position of the gallbladder, and may outline a portion of the biliary system.

Ultrasonography can also evaluate the gallbladder after injection of sincalide, a hormonal analogue that causes the organ to contract and expel bile. Although oral cholecystography is frequently performed first in diagnosing cholelithiasis or cholecystitis, ultrasonography is used if cholecystography is inconclusive or does not adequately visualize the gallbladder. Since the accuracy of ultrasonography does not depend on hepatic and gallbladder function, it is especially useful for evaluating patients with elevated serum bilirubin levels when contrast radiography may prove ineffective. It is the procedure of choice for evaluation of jaundice, since it readily distinguishes between obstructive and nonobstructive types, and for emergency diagnosis of patients with signs of acute cholecystitis, such as upper right quadrant pain, with or without local tenderness.

Procedure
- The patient is assisted to a supine position.
- A conductive gel is applied to the face of the transducer, and the transducer is passed over the right upper quadrant.

• Scans are taken; during each scan, the patient is asked to exhale deeply and hold his breath. The patient will also be asked to change positions.
• When gallbladder contractility is to be evaluated, an I.V. injection of sincalide is administered.
• Within 5 to 30 minutes after injection, the gallbladder normally contracts, and the scans are repeated.
• The procedure takes 15 to 30 minutes to perform.

Patient care checklist
Before the test
☑ Explain or clarify test purpose, preparation, and procedure.
☑ Tell the patient that the test is safe and painless, although mild pressure may be experienced as the transducer is moved over his skin, directing sound waves to his gallbladder.
☑ If sincalide will be injected to stimulate gallbladder contraction, tell the patient that he may experience abdominal cramping, tenesmus, nausea, dizziness, sweating, and flushing.
☑ Evaluate patient understanding.
☑ Provide a fat-free meal the evening before the test, and restrict food and fluids for 8 to 12 hours before the test. This promotes accumulation of bile in the gallbladder and enhances ultrasonic visualization.
After the test
☑ Remove any remaining conductive gel from the patient's skin.

Interfering factors
• Patient failure to observe pretest dietary restrictions interferes with accurate testing.
• Overlying bowel gas or retention of barium from a preceding test hinders ultrasound transmission.
• In a patient who is dehydrated, ultrasonography can fail to demonstrate the boundaries between organs and tissue structures because of deficiency of body fluids.

Liver ultrasonography
[liver sonogram]

Purpose
• To distinguish between obstructive and nonobstructive jaundice
• To screen for hepatocellular disease
• To detect hepatic metastases and hematoma
• To define cold spots as tumors, abscesses, or cysts.

Normal results
Normal size, shape, and position of the liver.

Abnormal results
Liver ultrasonography may reveal:
  Biliary duct obstruction
  Metastasis to liver
  Primary hepatic tumors
  Intrahepatic abscesses, cysts, or hematomas.

The basics
This ultrasonographic examination produces cross-sectional images of the liver by channeling high-frequency sound waves into the upper right quadrant of the abdomen. The resultant echoes are converted to electrical energy that appears as a pattern of spikes or dots on an oscilloscope screen. Since this pattern varies with tissue density, it can depict intrahepatic structures as well as organ size, shape, and position. Liver ultrasonography is indicated in patients with jaundice of unknown etiology, with unexplained hepatomegaly and abnormal biochemical test results, with suspected metastatic tumors and elevated serum alkaline phosphatase levels, and with recent abdominal trauma.

When used to complement liver-spleen scanning, ultrasonography can define cold spots—focal defects that fail to pick up the radionuclide—as tumors, abscesses, or cysts; it also provides better views of the periportal and perihepatic spaces than liver-spleen scanning. If ultrasonography fails to provide definitive diagnosis, computerized tomography, gallium scanning, or liver biopsy may provide more specific information.

Procedure
• The patient is assisted to a supine position.
• A conductive gel is applied to the face of the transducer, and transverse, longitudinal, and parallel scans are taken.
• During each scan, the patient is asked to hold his breath briefly in deep inspiration.
• The procedure takes 15 to 30 minutes to perform.

Patient care checklist
Before the test
☑ Explain or clarify test purpose and procedure.
☑ Tell the patient that the test is safe and painless, although mild pressure may be experienced as the transducer is moved over the skin, directing sound waves to the liver.
☑ Evaluate patient understanding.
☑ Restrict food and fluids for 8 to 12 hours before the test to reduce bowel gas, which hinders transmission of ultrasound.
After the test
☑ Remove any remaining conductive gel from the skin.

Interfering factors
• Overlying ribs, and gas or residual barium in the stomach or colon hinder transmission of ultrasound.
• In a patient who is dehydrated, ultrasonography may fail to demonstrate the boundaries between organs and tissue structures because of a lack of body fluids.

Ocular ultrasonography
[eye and orbit sonogram]

Purpose
• To aid in evaluating the fundus in an eye with an opaque medium, such as a cataract
• To aid in diagnosis of vitreous disorders and retinal detachment
• To diagnose and differentiate between intraocular and orbital lesions, and to follow their progression through serial examinations
• To help locate intraocular foreign bodies.

Normal results
The optic nerve and posterior lens capsule produce echoes that take on characteristic forms on A- and B-scan images. The posterior wall of the eye appears as a smooth, concave curve; retrobulbar fat can also be identified. The lens and vitreous, which do not produce echoes, can also be identified.

Abnormal results
Ocular ultrasonography may reveal:
  Vitreous hemorrhage
  Vitreous abnormalities
  Retinal or choroidal detachment
  Intraocular tumors
  Retinoblastomas
  Orbital lesions
  Cystic lesions
  Intraocular foreign bodies
  Inflammatory conditions.

The basics
Ocular ultrasonography involves the transmission of high-frequency sound waves through the eye and the measurement of their reflection from ocular structures. An A-scan converts the resulting echoes into waveforms whose crests represent the positions of different structures, giving a linear dimensional picture. The B-scan converts the echoes into patterns of dots that form a two-dimensional,

cross-sectional image of the ocular structure.

Because the B-scan is easier to interpret than the A-scan, it is used more often to evaluate the structures of the eye and to diagnose abnormalities. However, the A-scan is of much greater value in measuring the axial length of the eye and characterizing the tissue texture of abnormal lesions. Thus, the combination of A- and B-scans produces the most useful test results.

Illustrating the eyes' structures through ultrasound is especially helpful in evaluating a fundus clouded by an opaque medium, such as a cataract. In such a condition, this test can identify pathologies that are normally undetectable through ophthalmoscopy.

Ophthalmologists may also perform this test before surgery—for example, cataract removal—to ensure the integrity of the retina. If an intraocular lens is to be implanted, ultrasound may be used preoperatively to measure the length of the eye and the curvature of the cornea, as a guide for the surgeon. Unlike computed tomography, ocular ultrasonography is readily available and has the advantage of providing information immediately. The test takes approximately 5 minutes to perform.

Procedure
• The patient is assisted to a supine position on a radiographic table.
• For the A-scan, the patient's eye is numbed with anesthetizing drops, and a clear plastic eye cup is placed directly on the eyeball. Water-soluble jelly is then applied to the eye cup, and the transducer is positioned on this medium.
• For the B-scan, the patient is asked to close his eyes, and water-soluble jelly (such as Goniosol) is applied to his eyelid. The transducer is then placed on the eyelid.
• The transducer then transmits high-frequency sound waves into the patient's eye, and the resulting echoes are transformed into images or waveforms

on the oscilloscope screen, which may be photographed.

Patient care checklist
Before the test
☑ Explain or clarify test purpose and procedure.
☑ Reassure the patient that the procedure is safe and painless.
☑ For the A-scan, tell the patient that his eye will be numbed with anesthetizing drops and an eye cup will be placed directly on the eyeball. The transducer will then be placed on the eye cup.
☑ For the B-scan, tell the patient that a conductive gel will be put on his eyelid and a small transducer will be placed on the closed eyelid.
☑ Inform the patient that he may be asked to move his eyes or change his gaze during the procedure.
☑ Evaluate patient understanding.

After the test
☑ Remove any remaining conductive gel from the patient's eyelid(s).

Pancreas ultrasonography
[pancreas sonogram]

Purpose
To aid in diagnosis of pancreatitis, pseudocysts, and pancreatic carcinoma.

Normal results
Normal size and position of the pancreas.

Abnormal results
Pancreas ultrasonography may reveal:
    Pancreatitis
    Pancreatic carcinoma
    Pseudocyst.

The basics
In this noninvasive test, cross-sectional images of the pancreas are produced by channeling high-frequency sound

waves into the epigastric region, converting the resultant echoes to electrical impulses, and then displaying these impulses as a pattern of spikes or dots on an oscilloscope screen. The pattern varies with tissue density and so represents the size, shape, and position of the pancreas and surrounding viscera. Although ultrasonography cannot provide a sensitive measurement of pancreatic function, it can help detect anatomic abnormalities, such as pancreatic carcinoma and pseudocysts, and can guide the insertion of biopsy needles.

Since ultrasonography does not expose the patient to radiation, it has largely replaced hypotonic duodenography, endoscopic retrograde cholangiopancreatography, radioisotope studies, and arteriography. However, computed tomography and biopsy of the pancreas may be necessary to confirm diagnosis suggested by ultrasonography.

Procedure

• The patient is assisted to a supine position.
• A conductive gel is applied to the epigastric area.
• The transducer is passed over this area, and scans are taken; during the scanning, the patient may be asked to hold his breath.
• The procedure takes 30 to 40 minutes to perform.

Patient care checklist
Before the test

☑ Explain or clarify test purpose and procedure.

☑ Tell the patient that the test is safe and painless, although mild pressure may be experienced as the transducer is passed over the skin.

☑ Tell the patient that a conductive gel will be applied to his upper abdomen, and that a transducer will be passed over the area, directing sound waves to the pancreas.

☑ Tell the patient that he will be asked to inhale deeply during scanning, and instruct him to remain as still as possible during the procedure to ensure accurate testing.

☑ Evaluate patient understanding.

☑ Restrict food and fluids for 8 to 12 hours before the test to reduce bowel gas, which hinders transmission of ultrasound.

☑ If the patient is a smoker, ask him to abstain before the test; this eliminates the risk of swallowing air while inhaling, which interferes with test results.

After the test

☑ Remove any remaining conductive gel from the skin.

Interfering factors

• Gas, air, or residual barium in the stomach and intestine hinders ultrasound transmission.
• If the patient is dehydrated, ultrasonography may fail to demonstrate the boundaries between organs and tissue structures because of a lack of body fluids.
• Obesity interferes with ultrasound transmission, and fatty infiltration of the gland makes it difficult to delineate the pancreas from surrounding tissue.

Pelvic ultrasonography
[pelvic sonogram]

Purpose

• To detect foreign bodies, such as intrauterine devices
• To distinguish between cystic and solid masses (tumors)
• To measure organ size
• To evaluate fetal viability, position, gestational age, and growth rate
• To detect multiple pregnancy
• To confirm fetal abnormalities (such as molar pregnancy, and abnormalities of the arms and legs, spine, heart, head, kidneys, and abdomen) and maternal abnormalities (such as posterior placenta and placenta previa)
• To guide amniocentesis by deter-

mining placental location and fetal position.

Normal results
The uterus is normal in size and shape. The ovaries are normal in size, shape, and sonographic density. No other masses are visible. If the patient is pregnant, the gestational sac and fetus are of normal size for date. Multiple pregnancy can be revealed after 13 to 14 weeks' gestation.

Abnormal results
Pelvic ultrasonography may reveal:
Cystic mass
Solid mass
Foreign body
Placenta previa
Abruptio placentae
Fetal abnormalities
Fetal malpresentation
Cephalopelvic disproportion
Inappropriate fetal size for date
Dead fetus.

The basics
In pelvic ultrasonography, a piezoelectric crystal generates high-frequency sound waves that are reflected to a transducer, which in turn converts sound energy into electrical energy and forms images of the interior pelvic area on an oscilloscope screen. Techniques of sound imaging include A-mode, a one-dimensional image; B-mode, a two-dimensional or cross-sectional image; gray scale, a representation of organ texture in shades of gray; and realtime imaging, instantaneous images of the tissues in motion, similar to fluoroscopic examination.

The most common uses of pelvic ultrasonography include evaluation of pelvic disease, determination of fetal growth during pregnancy, and determination of fetal position before amniocentesis.

Procedure
• The patient is assisted to a supine position.

• A conductive gel is applied to the pelvic area.
• The transducer crystal is guided over the area, images are observed on the oscilloscope screen, and a good image is photographed.
• The procedure takes from 5 minutes to several hours to perform, depending on the indication for the test.

Patient care checklist
Before the test
☑ Explain or clarify test purpose and procedure.
☑ Tell the patient that the procedure is safe, noninvasive, and painless. If the patient is pregnant, reassure her that the test will not harm the fetus.
☑ Tell the patient that a conductive gel will be applied to the pelvic area, and a transducer will be passed over the area, directing sound waves into the pelvis.
☑ Evaluate patient understanding.
☑ Give the patient 4 cups of water or other liquid to drink before the test, and tell her not to void until the test is over, since a full bladder is a landmark to define pelvic organs.
After the test
☑ Remove any remaining conductive gel from the skin.

Interfering factors
Obesity, failure to fill the bladder, the presence of barium, or fetal head positioned deep in the pelvis can render the image uninterpretable.

Renal ultrasonography
[kidney sonogram]

Purpose
• To determine the size, shape, and position of the kidneys, their internal structures, and perirenal tissues
• To evaluate and localize urinary obstruction and abnormal accumulation of fluid
• To assess and diagnose complications following kidney transplantation.

Normal results
Normal size, shape, and position of kidneys.

Abnormal results
Renal ultrasonography may reveal:

Cysts, tumors, or abscesses involving the kidneys

Cysts or tumors involving the adrenal glands

Advanced pyelonephritis or glomerulonephritis

Hydronephrosis

Obstruction of ureters

Congenital anomalies

Renal hypertrophy

Rejection of renal transplant.

The basics
In this test, high-frequency sound waves are transmitted from a transducer through the kidneys and perirenal structures. The resulting echoes, amplified and converted into electrical impulses, are displayed on an oscilloscope screen as anatomic images. Usually performed with other urologic tests, renal ultrasonography can detect abnormalities or clarify those detected by other tests. A safe, painless procedure, it is especially valuable when excretory urography is ruled out—for example, by hypersensitivity to the contrast medium or the need for serial examinations. Unlike excretory urography, this test is not dependent on renal function, and therefore can be useful in patients with renal failure. Evaluation of urologic disorders may also include ultrasonography of the ureter, bladder, and scrotum.

Procedure
• The patient is assisted to a prone position.

• Conductive gel is applied to the lower back.

• The longitudinal axis of the kidneys is located, and these points are marked on the skin and connected with straight lines.

• Sectional images are obtained by moving the transducer longitudinally and transversely or at any other angle required.

• During the test, the patient may be asked to breathe deeply to assess the kidneys' movement during respiration.

• The procedure takes appoximately 30 minutes to complete.

Patient care checklist
Before the test

☑ Explain or clarify test purpose and procedure.

☑ Tell the patient that the test is safe and painless, although mild pressure may be experienced as the transducer is moved over the skin.

☑ Tell the patient that a conductive gel will be applied to the lower back, and a transducer will be passed over the area, directing sound waves to the kidneys.

☑ Evaluate patient understanding.

After the test

☑ Remove any remaining conductive gel and markings from the skin.

Interfering factors
The presence of barium from recent abdominal X-rays hinders ultrasound transmission.

Spleen ultrasonography
[spleen sonogram]

Purpose
• To demonstrate splenomegaly

• To monitor progression of primary and secondary splenic disease, and to evaluate the effectiveness of therapy

• To evaluate the spleen after abdominal trauma

• To help detect splenic cysts and subphrenic abscesses.

Normal results
Normal size, shape, and position of spleen.

Abnormal results
Spleen ultrasonography may reveal:
Splenomegaly
Rupture
Hematoma
Abscess
Cysts
Tumors.

The basics
In ultrasonography of the spleen, a focused beam of high-frequency sound waves passes into the upper left quadrant of the abdomen, creating echoes that vary with changes in tissue density. These echoes, when converted to electrical energy and amplified by a transducer, appear on an oscilloscope screen as a pattern of spikes or dots. This pattern represents the size, shape, and position of the spleen and surrounding viscera.

Ultrasonography is indicated in patients with an upper left quadrant mass of unknown origin; with known splenomegaly, to evaluate changes in splenic size; with upper left quadrant pain and local tenderness; and with recent abdominal trauma. Although ultrasonography can show splenomegaly, it usually does not identify the cause; computerized tomography can provide more specific information. However, as a supplementary diagnostic procedure after liver-spleen scanning, ultrasonography can clarify the nature of cold spots or detect focal defects not infiltrated by tracer radioisotopes.

Procedure
• The patient is assisted to a supine position.
• Conductive gel is applied to the left upper quadrant of the abdomen.
• A transducer is moved over the area to obtain images of the spleen.
• During scanning, the patient may be repositioned several times and asked to hold his breath briefly at varying stages of inspiration.
• The procedure takes 15 to 30 minutes to perform.

Patient care checklist
Before the test
☑ Explain or clarify test purpose and procedure.
☑ Tell the patient that the test is safe and painless, although mild pressure may be experienced as the transducer is passed over the skin.
☑ Tell the patient that a conductive gel will be applied under the left breast, and a transducer will be passed over the area, directing sound waves to the spleen.
☑ Evaluate patient understanding.
☑ Restrict food and fluids for 8 to 12 hours before the test to reduce bowel gas, which hinders transmission of ultrasound.
After the test
☑ Remove any remaining conductive gel from the skin.

Interfering factors
• Overlying ribs, an aerated left lung, or gas or residual barium in the colon or stomach may prevent visualization of the spleen.
• If the patient is dehydrated, ultrasonography may fail to demonstrate the boundaries between organs and tissue structures because of a lack of body fluids.
• Body physique affecting splenic shape, or adjacent masses displacing the spleen, may be confused with splenomegaly.
• The patient with splenic trauma may be unable to tolerate the procedure because of pain caused by the transducer moving across his abdomen.

Thyroid ultrasonography
[thyroid sonogram]

Purpose
• To evaluate thyroid structure
• To differentiate between a cyst and a tumor
• To determine the depth and dimension of thyroid nodules

• To monitor the size of the thyroid gland during suppressive therapy.

Normal results
Normal size and shape of the thyroid gland.

Abnormal results
Thyroid ultrasonography may reveal:
  Cysts
  Tumors
  Thyroid nodules.

The basics
In this safe, noninvasive procedure, ultrasonic pulses emitted from a transducer and directed at the thyroid gland are reflected back to the transducer. These pulses are then converted electronically to produce structural visualization on an oscilloscope screen.

When a mass is located by palpation or by thyroid imaging, thyroid ultrasonography can differentiate between a cyst and a tumor larger than ⅜″ (1 cm) with about 85% accuracy.

Thyroid ultrasonography is particularly useful in the evaluation of thyroid nodules during pregnancy, since it does not expose the fetus to the radioactive iodine used in other diagnostic procedures.

See *Parathyroid Ultrasonography* for information on examination of the parathyroid gland by this technique.

Procedure
• The patient is assisted to a supine position, with a pillow under his shoulder blades to hyperextend his neck.
• Conductive gel is applied to the middle of the neck.
• A transducer is passed over the area of the thyroid gland, and scans are taken.
• The test takes approximately 30 minutes.

Patient care checklist
Before the test
☑ Explain or clarify test purpose and procedure.

Parathyroid Ultrasonography

On ultrasonography, the parathyroid glands appear as solid masses, 5 mm or smaller in size, with an echo pattern of less amplitude than thyroid tissue. Glandular enlargement is usually characteristic of tumor growth or of hyperplasia. Normally, on a scan, the parathyroid glands are indistinguishable from the nearby neurovascular bundle.

☑ Tell the patient that the test is safe and painless, although mild pressure may be experienced as the transducer is passed over the skin.
☑ Tell the patient that a conductive gel will be applied to his neck and that a transducer will be passed over the area, directing sound waves to the thyroid gland.
☑ Evaluate patient understanding.
After the test
☑ Remove any remaining conductive gel from the skin.

Urinary bladder ultrasonography
[urinary bladder sonogram]

Purpose
• To determine the presence of residual urine
• To detect bladder tumors or cystitis
• To detect an overdistended bladder
• To determine the extent of a known bladder tumor.

Normal results
The bladder is normal in contour and volume. There is no significant residual urine. No masses are identified within the bladder or external to it.

Abnormal results

The ultrasound may identify:
Abnormally distended bladder
Residual urine
Bladder tumors
Masses or collections external to bladder
Extent of malignant tumors of bladder
Bladder calculi
Cystitis
Bladder diverticula
Ureteroceles.

The basics

In urinary bladder ultrasonography, the bladder is examined by placing the ultrasound transducer on the abdominal wall over the full bladder, thereby imaging the bladder and its adjacent structures. The patient is then asked to void completely; the bladder is examined again, and the volume of residual urine, if any, is calculated.

Procedure

• The patient is assisted to a supine position, and a conductive gel is then placed on the skin over the bladder.
• The ultrasound probe is placed on the skin and pictures are obtained.
• The patient then voids and is re-scanned.
• The films are processed and shown to the radiologist, who may or may not order more scanning.
• The examination takes about 20 minutes.

Patient care checklist

Before the test
☑ Explain or clarify test purpose and procedure.
☑ Tell the patient the procedure is safe and painless.
☑ Evaluate patient understanding.
☑ Ask the patient to drink several glasses of fluid since a full bladder is necessary when performing the test.
After the test
☑ Remove any remaining conductive gel from the skin.

Interfering factors

Obesity or scar tissue may interfere with accurate test results.

Selected References

Diagnostics, 2nd ed. Nurse's Reference Library. Springhouse, Pa.: Springhouse Corp., 1986.

Fischbach, Frances. *A Manual of Laboratory Diagnostic Tests,* 2nd ed. Philadelphia: J.B. Lippincott Co., 1984.

Grossman, Zachary D., et al. *The Clinician's Guide to Diagnostic Imaging.* New York: Raven Press Pubs., 1983.

Haughey, Cynthia. "Preparing Your Patient for Echocardiography," *Nursing84* 14:68-71, May 1984.

Haughey, Cynthia. "Understanding Ultrasonography," *Nursing81* 11:100-04, April 1981.

Hudson, Barbara. "Sharpen Your Assessment Skills with the Doppler Ultrasound Stethoscope," *Nursing83* 13:55-57, May 1983.

Kee, Joyce LeFever. *Laboratory and Diagnostic Tests with Nursing Implications.* East Norwalk, Conn.: Appleton-Century-Crofts, 1983.

Michaels, Davida, ed. *Diagnostic Procedures.* New York: John Wiley & Sons, 1983.

Pagana, Kathleen D., and Pagana, Timothy James. *Diagnostic Testing and Nursing Implications,* 2nd ed. St. Louis: C.V. Mosby Co., 1986.

Sanders, R., and James, A.E., Jr., eds. *Principles and Practice of Ultrasonography in Obstetrics and Gynecology,* 2nd ed. East Norwalk, Conn.: Appleton-Century-Crofts, 1980.

SPECIAL ORGAN AND BODY SYSTEM TESTS

Introduction

Special organ and body system tests are necessary for a variety of reasons. Some confirm a diagnosis; many identify the cause and/or severity of signs or symptoms; others monitor the effectiveness of therapy; still others are used as screening tests and may indicate the need for more refined tests such as computerized tomography scans and ultrasonography.

Many of the noninvasive tests discussed in this chapter require minimal patient preparation and cause little or no discomfort. Tests that involve invasive procedures, such as cardiac catheterization, involve serious risks to the patient. Informed consent is required. Patient care during and after these tests involves careful assessment for complications.

Patient-teaching guidelines
Patient-learner objectives:
• Define the test.
• State the specific purpose of the test.
• Explain the procedure.
• Discuss test preparation, procedure, and post-test care.
• Identify possible risks or adverse effects.

Teaching content:
• Define the test in terms the patient can understand.
• Explain the specific purpose of the test.
• Describe the procedure. Explain where the test will be performed and who will be performing it. Describe the equipment, what discomfort or other sensations (if any) to expect, and what positions the patient will be placed in, since unfamiliarity with the test may provoke extreme anxiety.
• If a local anesthetic will be administered, explain that this will alleviate much discomfort, but that the patient will remain alert.
• If any other medication will be administered prior to, during, or following the test, explain the purpose, route, and possible adverse effects of the drug.
• Inform the patient of any special preparations for the test. Be sure to specify dietary restrictions and indicate the applicable time period.
• Explain whether discomfort or any other problem is a normal consequence of the test. Reassure the patient that it is only temporary and, when possible, explain what will be done to alleviate the problem.
• Describe any other special care, positioning, or restrictions following the test. Be sure to explain why these are necessary. If assessment measures will be implemented frequently, alleviate undue patient anxiety by explaining them as a routine precaution.
• If there are risks associated with the test, answer any questions the patient may still have after the physician's explanation.

Evaluation:
After the patient-teaching session is completed, evaluate whether or not the patient has satisfactorily met each patient-learner objective by obtaining necessary patient feedback. Refocus teaching as needed.

Ambulatory electrocardiography
[ambulatory monitoring, EKG, Holter monitoring]

Purpose
• To detect cardiac dysrhythmias
• To evaluate chest pain
• To evaluate cardiac status after acute myocardial infarction (MI) or pacemaker implantation
• To evaluate effectiveness of antiarrhythmic drug therapy
• To assess and correlate dyspnea, central nervous system symptoms—such as syncope and light-headedness—and palpitations with actual cardiac events and the patient's activities.

Normal results
When compared with the patient's diary of daily activities, emotional reaction, and physical symptoms, if any, the normal EKG pattern shows no significant dysrhythmias or ST segment changes. Changes in heart rate normally occur during various activities.

Abnormal results
Abnormalities of the heart detected by ambulatory EKG include:
   Premature ventricular contractions
   Conduction defects
   Tachyarrhythmias
   Bradyarrhythmias
   Brady-tachyarrhythmia syndrome.

The basics
Ambulatory electrocardiography, commonly called *Holter monitoring* after the scientist who developed the technique, is the continuous recording of heart activity as the patient follows his normal routine. In this test, which is usually performed for 24 hours or about 100,000 cardiac cycles, the patient wears a small reel-to-reel or cassette tape recorder connected to electrodes placed on his chest, and keeps a diary of his activities and any associated symptoms. At the end of the recording period, the tape is analyzed by a microcomputer and a report is printed, permitting correlation of cardiac irregularities, such as dysrhythmias and ST segment changes, with the activities in the patient's diary. For example, ST-T wave changes associated with ischemia may coincide with chest pain or increased patient activity. ST segment changes associated with an acute MI require careful study, since smoking, eating, postural changes, certain drugs, Wolff-Parkinson-White syndrome, bundle branch block, myocarditis, myocardial hypertrophy, anemia, hypoxemia, and abnormal hemoglobin binding can produce a similar tracing on the EKG. Monitoring the MI patient 1 to 3 days before discharge and again 4 to 6 weeks after discharge may detect ST-T wave changes associated with ischemia or dysrhythmias; such information aids patient therapy and rehabilitation and refines prognosis.

Although ambulatory electrocardiography correlates patient symptoms and EKG changes, it does not always identify their causes. If initial monitoring proves inconclusive, the test may be repeated.

Ambulatory electrocardiography is not a substitute for coronary care unit surveillance, but it can detect sporadic dysrhythmias missed by an exercise or resting EKG. In a patient with an artificial pacemaker, it can also detect a dysrhythmia, such as bradycardia, that the pacemaker fails to override.

Patient-activated monitors can be worn for 5 to 7 days. With these devices, the patient manually initiates recording of heart activity only when he experiences symptoms. Intermittent monitoring, triggered only by an unusual heart rhythm, is used in cardiac research.

Procedure
• Shave electrode sites, if necessary; cleanse them with an alcohol sponge,

and gently abrade them until they redden.

• Peel off the electrode backings, check that all pads have a sufficient amount of conductive gel, and apply them to the correct sites (see "Electrocardiography," p. 607).

• Press the sides and bottom of each electrode firmly to ensure that the adhesive portion of each electrode is securely fastened to the skin.

• Press the center of each electrode lightly to make good contact between the gel and the patient's skin.

• Check to ensure that the electrode cable is securely attached to the monitor.

• Position the monitor and case as the patient will wear them. Then attach the lead wires to the electrodes.

• Install a new or fully charged battery in the recorder, insert the tape, and turn the recorder on.

• Test the electrode attachment circuit by connecting the recorder to a standard EKG machine. Watch for artifacts while the patient moves normally (sits, stands).

• Show the patient how to position the recorder when he lies down.

• Show the patient how to check the recorder to make sure it is working properly. Explain that, if the monitor light flashes, one of the electrodes may be loose, and he should depress the center of each one. Tell him to notify you if one comes off.

• If the patient will not be returning to the office or hospital immediately after the monitoring period, show him how to remove and store the equipment. Remind him to bring the diary when he returns.

• If applicable to the monitor, demonstrate how to mark the tape at the onset of symptoms. (If a patient-activated monitor is being used, show the patient how to press the event button to activate the monitor if he experiences any unusual sensations.)

• Instruct the patient to begin his diary.

Patient care checklist
Before the test
☑ Explain or clarify test purpose, preparation, and procedure. Be sure to explain preparation of electrode sites.

☑ Tell the patient that he must wear a small tape recorder for 24 hours (for 5 to 7 days if a patient-activated monitor is being used). Mention that a shoulder strap or a special belt will be provided to carry the recorder, which weighs about 2 lb (0.9 kg).

☑ Encourage the patient to continue his routine activities during the monitoring period.

☑ Show the patient a sample diary. Stress the importance of logging his usual activities (walking, stair climbing, urinating, sleeping, sexual activity, for example), emotional upsets, physical symptoms (dizziness, palpitations, fatigue, chest pain, and syncope), and ingestion of medication.

☑ Advise the patient to wear loose-fitting clothing with front-buttoning tops during monitoring.

☑ Instruct him not to tamper with the monitor or to disconnect the lead wires or electrodes.

☑ If he must bathe, advise a sponge bath, since the equipment must not get wet. Tell him to avoid magnets, metal detectors, high-voltage areas, and electric blankets.

☑ Evaluate patient understanding.
After the test
☑ Remove all chest electrodes, and clean the electrode sites.

Interfering factors
• Failure to apply the electrodes correctly can cause muscle or movement artifact.

• Patient failure to carefully record daily activities and symptoms or to maintain his normal routine interferes with accurate testing.

• If a patient-activated monitor is used, patient failure to turn on the monitor during symptoms interferes with accurate testing.

• Physiologic variation in frequency and severity of dysrhythmias may cause a dysrhythmia to be missed on the 24-hour ambulatory EKG.

Apexcardiography (ACG)

Purpose
• To aid in evaluation of left ventricular function
• To help identify effects of ventricular enlargement, infarction, and/or ischemia; ventricular aneurysm; and pericarditis
• To aid in identification of heart sounds.

Normal results
Reading an Apexcardiogram shows a normal ACG waveform and describes what each component represents in the cardiac cycle.

Abnormal results
Absence of the a wave characterizes:
  Atrial fibrillation
  Mitral stenosis.

Series of small a waves characterizes:
  Atrial flutter.
Abnormally large a waves may occur in:
  Systemic hypertension
  Aortic valve stenosis
  Idiopathic hypertrophic subaortic stenosis.
Abnormal a wave configuration during isometric exercises may indicate:
  Latent left ventricular abnormality.
Late systolic apical impulse or systolic bulge:
  characteristically occurs in:
    Left ventricular aneurysm
    Ischemia
    Infarction.
  may occur in:
    Systemic hypertension
    Aortic stenosis
    Primary myocardial disease
    Coronary artery disease.
Decrease in the slope of the normally steep rf wave (because of rapid ventricular filling) indicates:
  Mitral stenosis.

Reading An Apexcardiogram

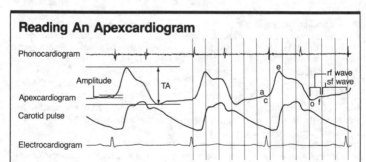

This illustration shows a normal apexcardiogram (ACG) accompanied by a simultaneous phonocardiogram, carotid pulse wave tracing, and electrocardiogram. The ACG waveform provides the following information about the cardiac cycle:
a wave: atrial systole (normally less than 15% of total apical amplitude); ventricular filling
c point: isovolumetric ventricular systole
e point: ventricular systole; aortic valve opens
o point: mitral valve opens (approximate time)
rf wave: rapid ventricular filling
f point: marks change from rapid to slow ventricular filling
sf wave: slow, passive ventricular filling.

Increase in the slope of the rf wave indicates:
  Myocardial failure
  Mitral regurgitation
  Constrictive pericarditis.

The basics
Apexcardiography is the graphic recording of chest movement caused by low-frequency precordial cardiac pulsations. A transducer placed on the patient's chest at the cardiac apex picks up these pulsations and converts them from kinetic to electrical energy. A recorder then converts this electrical energy into waveforms, or apexcardiograms, that depict cardiac events during systole and diastole. The components of the ACG waveform include the a wave, c point, e point, o point, rf wave, f point, sf wave, and stasis.

Apexcardiography alone usually does not provide sufficient information to make an accurate diagnosis; however, when it is performed simultaneously with electrocardiography, phonocardiography, or carotid and/or jugular pulse tracings, it aids in diagnosis of cardiac abnormalities, especially left ventricular dysfunction, and helps identify heart sounds. Additional tests, such as echocardiography and cardiac catheterization, may be needed to clarify or confirm results.

Procedure
• Place the patient in left oblique position.
• Attach electrocardiography electrodes to the patient's arms and legs for continuous recording throughout the procedure.
• Palpate the patient's chest wall to locate the point of maximum impulse (PMI).
• Place the transducer (to which conductive gel has been applied) on the PMI, making sure that it does not interfere with chest wall motion.
• Begin the recording.
• Ask the patient to breathe in and out slowly, to hold his breath, and to do isometric hand-grip exercises during the recording. (These exercises increase systemic resistance; the resultant recordings demonstrate their effect on ventricular function.)
• Remove the transducer and the electrodes when the recordings are complete.
• The test takes approximately 15 minutes.

Patient care checklist
Before the test
☑ Explain or clarify test purpose, preparation, and procedure.
☑ Reassure the patient that the test, performed simultaneously with electrocardiography, is safe and painless. When appropriate, tell him that phonocardiography and pulse wave tracings will also be performed.
☑ Advise the patient not to talk or move during the procedure unless asked to do so; this helps ensure a clear recording.
☑ Evaluate patient understanding.
☑ Just before the procedure, instruct the patient to remove any metallic objects above the sites where the electrodes are to be placed.

Interfering factors
• Respiratory excursions can distort recordings.
• Incorrect patient positioning, transducer placement, or transducer tension can distort recordings.

Breast thermography

Purpose
• To screen for breast cancer
• To predict the risk of breast cancer
• To detect breast cancer, fibrocystic disease of the breast (Schimmelbusch's disease), and breast abscesses
• To evaluate the prognosis of breast cancer.

Normal results
Breasts appear symmetric on the thermogram.

Abnormal results
Breast thermography may reveal:
Malignancy
Fibrocystic disease
Abscesses.

The basics
Breast thermography is an infrared photographic procedure that measures and records heat patterns within breast tissue. Since body changes that increase the breast's metabolic rate raise the breast's surface temperature, thermography can aid in detection of breast cancer. However, because of a high rate of false-positive results with this test (possibly 25%), thermography is being replaced by ultrasonography and low-dose mammography.

Asymmetric appearance of the breasts or the appearance of white areas, or "hot spots," on the thermogram may indicate abnormalities. "Hot spots" may mean inflammatory or malignant lesions; these have a greater vascularity than normal tissue, which increases venous drainage and raises the surface temperature of the skin. Additional tests, such as mammography and biopsy, are necessary to confirm breast cancer.

Procedure
• After the patient has been in the room where the test is to be performed for about 10 minutes (to lower the skin temperature of the breasts), photographs of the breasts are taken from three different angles, usually with the patient's hands above her head or on her hips.
• After the procedure, the patient may be asked to wait while the films are checked for readability.
• The test takes about 15 minutes.

Patient care checklist
Before the test
☑ Explain or clarify test purpose and procedure.
☑ Tell the patient that the test is painless.

☑ Instruct her to avoid excessive exposure to sunlight before the test, since a recent sunburn invalidates results, and not to put ointment or powder on her breasts the day of the test.
☑ Tell the patient that the temperature in the room where the test will be performed may be a little cool.
☑ Inform her that test results are usually available in 1 or 2 days.
☑ Evaluate patient understanding.
☑ Just before the test, provide a gown for her to wear that opens in the front, and ask her to remove all clothing and jewelry above the waist.

Interfering factors
Insufficient cooling of the breasts, recent sunburn, skin lesions, or ointment on the breasts can cause false-positive results by altering skin temperature.

Cardiac catheterization

Purpose
To evaluate valvular insufficiency or stenosis, septal defects, congenital anomalies, myocardial function and blood supply, and cardiac wall motion.

Normal results
Cardiac catheterization reveals normal heart chamber size and configuration, wall motion and thickness, direction of blood flow, and valve motion; the coronary arteries should have a smooth and regular outline. The graph on page 597 shows normal pressure events during a single cardiac cycle. The chart on page 598 shows upper limits of normal chamber and vessel pressures in a recumbent adult: higher pressures than these are significant; lower pressures, except in shock, usually are not. (See *Normal Pressure Curves,* and *Upper Limits of Normal Pressures in Cardiac Chambers and Great Vessels in Recumbent Adults,* p. 598.)

A normal ejection fraction (60% to 70%) is a good indicator for successful cardiac surgery.

Abnormal results

Cardiac catheterization can detect, evaluate, and document nearly all types of congenital or acquired anatomic intracardiac conditions or defects, including:

Coronary artery disease
Valvular heart disease
Septal defect (atrial and ventricular)
Ventricular aneurysm
Left ventricular enlargement.

The basics

Simply stated, cardiac catheterization is the passing of a catheter into the right or the left side of the heart. Catheterization can determine blood pressure and blood flow in the chambers of the heart, permit collection of blood samples, or record films of the heart's ventricles (contrast ventriculography) or arteries (coronary arteriography or angiography). During the procedure, percutaneous transluminal coronary angioplasty can be performed, intracoronary streptokinase can be injected, or the patient's left ventricular function can be evaluated prior to coronary artery bypass graft surgery.

In left heart catheterization, a catheter is inserted into an artery in the antecubital fossa or into the femoral artery through a puncture or cutdown procedure and, guided by fluoroscopy, the catheter is advanced retrograde through the aortic valve into the coronary artery orifices and/or left ventricle. Then, injection of a contrast medium into the ventricle permits radiographic visualization of the ventricle and the coronary arteries, and filming (cineangiography) of heart activity. Left heart catheterization assesses coronary artery patency, mitral and aortic valve function, and left ventricular function. With the use of angiography, it is possible to observe the heart's pumping performance, detect coronary artery disease (CAD), and

Normal Pressure Curves

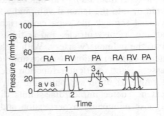

Right Heart Chambers

Two pressure complexes are represented for each chamber. Complexes at far right in this diagram represent simultaneous recordings of pressures from the RA, RV, and PA. The numbered tracings are: 1, RV peak systolic pressure; 2, RV end-diastolic pressure; 3, PA peak systolic pressure; 4, PA dicrotic notch; 5, PA diastolic pressure.

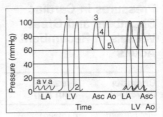

Left Heart Chambers

Overall pressure configurations are similar to those of the right heart, but left heart pressures are significantly higher because systemic flow resistance is much greater than pulmonary resistance.

Key:	
PA =	Pulmonary artery
RV =	Right ventricle
RA =	Right atrium
a wave =	Contraction
v wave =	Passive filling
LV =	Left ventricle
LA =	Left atrium
Asc Ao =	Ascending aorta

From H. Kasparian et al., "Interpreting Cardiac Catheterization Data," *Postgraduate Medicine*, 57:4:66 (April 1975).

identify vessels in need of bypass grafting.

In right heart catheterization, the catheter is inserted into an antecubital vein or into the femoral vein and advanced through the vena cava, right atrium, right ventricle, and at times, into the pulmonary artery. With right heart catheterization, it is possible to assess right ventricular function, determine tricuspid and pulmonic valve patency, detect intracardiac shunts, diagnose pulmonary hypertension and, if thermodilution catheters are used, calculate cardiac output.

In *CAD*, catheterization shows constriction of the lumen of the coronary arteries. Constriction greater than 70% is especially significant, particularly in proximal lesions. Narrowing of the left main coronary artery and occlu-

---

Upper Limits of Normal Pressures in Cardiac Chambers and Great Vessels in Recumbent Adults

Chamber or vessel	Pressure (mm Hg)
Right atrium	6 (mean)
Right ventricle	30/6*
Pulmonary artery	30/12* (mean, 18)
Left atrium	12 (mean)
Left ventricle	140/12*
Ascending aorta	140/90* (mean, 105)
Pulmonary artery wedge	Almost identical (± 1 to 2 mm Hg) to left atrial mean pressure

*Peak systolic and end-diastolic

Adapted with permission from H. Kasparian, et al., "Interpreting Cardiac Catheterization Data," *Postgraduate Medicine*, 57:4:67, April 1975.

---

sion or narrowing high in the left anterior descending artery are often indications for revascularization surgery. (This lesion responds best to coronary bypass grafting.)

Impaired wall motion can indicate *myocardial incompetency* from coronary artery disease, aneurysm, cardiomyopathy, or congenital anomalies. Comparing the size of the left ventricle in systole and diastole helps assess the efficiency of cardiac muscular contraction, segmental wall motion, chamber size, and ejection fraction (comparison of the amount of blood pumped out of the left ventricle during systole with the amount of blood remaining at end diastole). An ejection fraction under 35% generally increases the risk of complications and decreases the probability of successful surgery.

Valvular heart disease is indicated by a gradient, or difference in pressures above and below a heart valve. For example, systolic pressure measurements on both sides of a stenotic aortic valve show a gradient across the valve. The higher the gradient, the greater the degree of stenosis. If left ventricular systolic pressure measures 200 mm Hg and aortic systolic pressure is 120 mm Hg, the gradient across the valve is 80 mm Hg. Since these pressures should normally be equal during systole when the aortic valve is open, a gradient of this magnitude indicates the need for corrective surgery. Incompetent valves can be visualized in ventriculography by watching retrograde flow of the contrast medium across the valve during systole.

Septal defects (both atrial and ventricular) can be confirmed by measuring blood oxygen content in both sides of the heart. Elevated blood oxygen on the right side indicates a left-to-right atrial or ventricular shunt; decreased oxygen on the left side indicates a right-to-left shunt.

Cardiac output can be measured by analyzing blood oxygen levels in the cardiac chambers; by injecting contrast medium into the venous circulation and measuring its concentration as it moves past a thermodilution catheter; or by drawing blood from cardiac chambers.

Contraindications to both left and right heart catheterization include: coagulopathy, poor renal function, or debilitation. Unless a temporary pacemaker is inserted to counteract induced ventricular asystole, left bundle branch block contraindicates right heart catheterization. Acute myocardial infarction (MI) once contraindicated left heart catheterization; now, many physicians perform catheterization and surgically bypass blocked vessels during acute ischemic episodes to prevent myocardial necrosis.

Procedure

• The patient is placed in supine position on a tilt-top table and secured by restraints.

• Electrocardiogram (EKG) leads are applied for continuous monitoring and an I.V. line, if not already in place, is started with 5% dextrose in water or normal saline solution at keep-vein-open rate.

• After the local anesthetic is injected at the catheterization site, a small incision or percutaneous puncture is made into the artery or vein, depending on whether left-side or right-side studies are to be performed, and the catheter is passed through the needle into the vessel; the catheter is guided to the cardiac chambers or coronary arteries using fluoroscopy.

• When the catheter is in place, the contrast medium is injected through it to visualize the cardiac vessels and structures.

• The patient may be asked to cough or breathe deeply. Coughing helps counteract nausea or light-headedness caused by the contrast medium and can correct dysrhythmias produced by its depressant effect on the myocardium; deep breathing can ease catheter placement into the pulmonary artery

or the wedge position and moves the diaphragm downward, making the heart easier to visualize.

• During the procedure, the patient may be given nitroglycerin to eliminate catheter-induced spasm or measure its effect on the coronary arteries. Ergonovine maleate, a vasoconstrictor, may be administered to provoke coronary artery spasm (a risky but valuable test in Prinzmetal's angina).

• The heart rate and rhythm, respiration, pulse rate, and blood pressure are monitored frequently during the procedure.

• After completing the procedure, the catheter is removed and a pressure dressing is applied to the incision site.

• The test takes 2 to 3 hours. See *Complications of Cardiac Catheterization*, p. 600.

Special precautions

If the patient has valvular heart disease, prophylactic antibiotic therapy may be indicated to guard against subacute bacterial endocarditis.

Patient care checklist

Before the test

☑ Explain or clarify test purpose and procedure.

☑ Restrict food and fluids for at least 6 hours before the test.

☑ Inform the patient that he may receive a mild sedative but will remain conscious during the procedure.

☑ Inform the patient that he will be strapped to a padded table, and the table may be tilted so his heart can be examined from different angles.

☑ Warn the patient that the catheterization team wears gloves, masks, and gowns to protect him from infection, and that the changing X-ray plates and advancing film make clacking noises.

☑ Inform him that he will have an I.V. needle inserted in his arm to allow administration of medication.

☑ Assure him that the electrocardiography electrodes attached to his chest during the procedure cause no pain.

Complications of Cardiac Catheterization

Because cardiac catheterization is an invasive test usually done on high-risk patients, it imposes more patient risk than most other diagnostic tests. Although the incidence of such complications is low, they are potentially life-threatening and require careful observation during the procedure.

Keep in mind that some complications are common to *both* left heart and right heart catheterization; others result only from catheterization of one side. In either case, complications require that you notify the physician and carefully document the complication and its treatment.

Complication	Signs and Symptoms	Nursing Considerations
LEFT- OR RIGHT-SIDE CATHETERIZATION		
Myocardial infarction *Possible causes:* • Emotional stress induced by procedure • Blood clot dislodged by catheter tip travels to a coronary artery (left-side catheterization only) • Air embolism	• Chest pain, possibly radiating to left arm, back, and/or jaw • Cardiac dysrhythmias • Diaphoresis, restlessness, and/or anxiety • Thready pulse • Fever • Peripheral cyanosis, causing cool skin	• Keep resuscitation equipment available. • Give oxygen or other drugs, as ordered. • Monitor patient continuously, as ordered.
Dysrhythmias *Possible cause:* • Cardiac tissue irritated by catheter	• Irregular heartbeat • Irregular apical pulse • Palpitations	• Monitor patient continuously, as ordered. • Administer antiarrhythmic drugs, if ordered.
Cardiac tamponade *Possible cause:* • Perforation of heart wall by catheter	• Sudden shock • Dysrhythmias • Increased heart rate • Decreased blood pressure • Chest pain • Diaphoresis and cyanosis • Distant heart sounds	• Give oxygen, if ordered. • Prepare patient for emergency surgery, if ordered. • Monitor patient continuously, as ordered. • Keep emergency equipment available.
Infection (systemic) *Possible causes:* • Poor aseptic technique • Catheter contaminated during manufacture, storage, or use	• Fever • Increased pulse rate • Chills and tremors • Unstable blood pressure	• Collect urine, sputum, and blood samples for culture, as ordered. • Monitor vital signs.

(continued)

Complications of Cardiac Catheterization (continued)

Complication	Signs and Symptoms	Nursing Considerations
LEFT- OR RIGHT-SIDE CATHETERIZATION (continued)		
Hypovolemia *Possible cause:* • Diuresis from angiography contrast medium	• Increased urinary output • Hypotension	• Replace fluids by giving patient one or two glasses of water every hour, or maintain I.V. at a rate of 150 to 200 ml/hr, as ordered. • Monitor fluid intake and output closely. • Monitor vital signs.
Pulmonary edema *Possible cause:* • Excessive fluid administration	• Early stage: tachycardia, tachypnea, dependent rales, diastolic (S_3) gallop • Acute stage: dyspnea; rapid, noisy respirations; cough with frothy, blood-tinged sputum; cyanosis with cold, clammy skin; tachycardia; hypertension	• Administer oxygen, as ordered. • Give medication (digitalis, diuretics, morphine), as ordered. • Restrict fluids. Insert indwelling (Foley) catheter. • Monitor the patient continuously, as ordered. • Maintain the patient's airway, and keep him in semi-Fowler position. • Apply rotating tourniquets, as ordered. • Keep resuscitation equipment available.
Hematoma or blood loss at insertion site *Possible cause:* • Bleeding at insertion site from vein or artery damage	• Bloody dressing • Limb swelling • Decreased blood pressure • Increased heart rate	• Elevate limb, and apply direct manual pressure. • When the bleeding has stopped, apply a pressure bandage. • If bleeding continues, or if vital signs are unstable, notify the physician.
Reaction to contrast medium *Possible cause:* • Allergy to iodine	• Fever • Agitation	• Administer antihistamines to relieve itching, (continued)

Complications of Cardiac Catheterization *(continued)*

Complication	Signs and Symptoms	Nursing Considerations
LEFT- OR RIGHT-SIDE CATHETERIZATION *(continued)*		
Reaction to contrast medium *(continued)*	• Hives • Itching • Decreased urinary output, indicating kidney failure	as ordered. • Administer diuretics toi treat kidney failure, as ordered. • Monitoir fluid intake and output closely
Infection at insertion site *Possible cause:* • Poor aseptic technique	• Swelling, warmth, redness, and soreness at site • Purulent discharge at site	• Obtain drainage sample for culture. • Clean site, and apply antimicrobial ointment, if ordered. Cover site with sterile gauze pad. • Review and improve aseptic technique.
LEFT-SIDE CATHETERIZATION		
Arterial embolus or thrombus in limb *Possible causes:* • Injury to artery during catheter insertion, causing blood clot • Plaque dislodged from artery wall by catheter	• Slow or faint pulse distal to insertion site • Loss of warmth, sensation, and color in arm or leg distal to insertion site	• Notify physician. He may perform an arteriotomy and Fogarty catheterization to remove embolus or thrombus. • Protect affected arm or leg from pressure. Keep it at room temperature, and maintain it at a level or slightly dependent position. • Administer a vasodilator, such as papaverine, to relieve painful vasospasm, if ordered.
Cerebrovascular accident *Possible cause:* • Blood clot or plaque dislodged by catheter tip travels to brain	• Hemiplegia • Aphasia • Lethargy • Confusion, or decreased level of consciousness	• Monitor vital signs closely. • Keep suctioning equipment nearby. • Administer oxygen, as ordered. *(continued)*

Complications of Cardiac Catheterization (continued)

Complication	Signs and Symptoms	Nursing Considerations
RIGHT-SIDE CATHETERIZATION		
Thrombophlebitis *Possible cause:* • Vein damaged during catheter insertion	• Vein is hard, sore, cordlike, and warm. Vein may look like a red line above catheter insertion site. • Swelling at site	• Elevate arm or leg, and apply warm, wet compresses. • Administer anticoagulant or fibrinolytic drugs, if ordered.
Pulmonary embolism *Possible cause:* • Blood clot or plaque dislodged by catheter tip travels to lungs	• Shortness of breath • Tachypnea • Increased heart rate • Chest pain	• Place patient in high Fowler position. • Administer oxygen, if ordered. • Monitor vital signs.
Vagal response *Possible causes:* • Vagus nerve endings irritated in sinoatrial node, atrial muscle tissue, or atrioventricular junction • Complete heart block	• Hypotension • Decreased heart rate • Nausea	• Monitor heart rate closely. • Administer atropine, if ordered. • Keep patient supine and quiet. • Give liquids.

☑ Tell the patient that the catheter will be inserted into an artery or vein in his arm or leg. If the skin above the vessel is hairy, it will be shaved and cleansed with an antiseptic.

☑ Tell him that he will experience a transient stinging sensation when the local anesthetic is injected to numb the incision site for catheter insertion, and that he may feel pressure as the catheter moves along the blood vessel; assure him that these sensations are normal.

☑ Inform him that injection of a contrast medium through the catheter may produce a hot, flushing sensation or nausea that quickly passes; instruct him to follow directions to cough or breathe deeply.

☑ Tell him that he will be given medication if he experiences chest pain during the procedure and may also receive nitroglycerin periodically to dilate coronary vessels and aid visualization.

☑ Assure him that complications, such as MI or thromboemboli, are rare.

☑ Make sure that the patient or a responsible family member has signed a consent form.

☑ Check patient hypersensitivity to shellfish, iodine, or the contrast media used in other diagnostic tests; notify the physician if such hypersensitivities exist.

☑ If the patient is scheduled for right heart catheterization, discontinue any anticoagulant therapy, as ordered, to reduce the risk of complications from venous bleeding. If he is scheduled for left heart catheterization, begin or continue anticoagulant therapy, as ordered.

☑ Evaluate patient understanding.

☑ Just before the procedure, tell the patient to void and put on a hospital gown.

After the test

CLINICAL ALERT: **Monitor vital signs every 15 minutes for the first hour after the procedure, then every hour until stable. If unstable, check every 5 minutes and notify the physician.**

☑ Observe the insertion site for a hematoma or blood loss, and replace the pressure dressing, as needed.

☑ Check the patient's color, skin temperature, and peripheral pulse below the puncture site.

☑ Enforce bed rest for 8 hours. If the femoral route was used for catheter insertion, keep the patient's leg extended for 6 to 8 hours; if the antecubital fossa was used, keep the patient's arm extended for at least 3 hours.

☑ Review with the physician the resuming of medications withheld before the test. Administer analgesics, as ordered.

☑ Unless the patient is scheduled for surgery, encourage intake of fluids high in potassium, such as orange juice, to counteract the diuretic effect of the contrast medium.

CLINICAL ALERT: **Make sure that a post-test EKG is scheduled to check for possible myocardial damage.**

Interfering factors

• Improperly functioning equipment or poor technique interferes with accurate testing.

• Patient anxiety increases the heart rate and cardiac chamber pressure.

Cold stimulation test for Raynaud's syndrome

Purpose
To detect Raynaud's syndrome.

Normal results
Digital temperature returns to the prebath level within 15 minutes.

Abnormal results
If digital temperature takes longer than 20 minutes to return to the prebath level, Raynaud's syndrome is indicated.

The basics
The cold stimulation test demonstrates Raynaud's syndrome by recording temperature changes in the patient's fingers before and after their submersion in an ice-water bath. However, digital blood pressure recording or examination of the arteries in the arm and palmar arch should precede this test to rule out arterial occlusive disease.

Raynaud's syndrome is an arteriospastic disorder characterized by intense episodic constriction (vasospasm) of the small cutaneous arteries and arterioles of the hands or, less often, the feet, after exposure to cold or stress. In this syndrome, the skin on the fingers characteristically blanches and becomes cyanotic and hyperemic after such exposure; in some patients, color changes are variable. If the syndrome is primary, it is called *Raynaud's disease;* if it is secondary to connective tissue disorders, such as scleroderma, systemic lupus erythematosus, or rheumatoid arthritis, it is called *Raynaud's phenomenon*. Although the cause of Raynaud's disease is unknown, several theories attempt to explain the reduced digital blood flow: intrinsic vascular wall hypersensitivity to cold, increased vasomotor tone caused by sympathetic stimulation, and antigen-antibody immune response. Raynaud's disease requires no

specific treatment and has no serious sequelae. Its more serious form, Raynaud's phenomenon, may not be clinically apparent for several years. Distinguishing between Raynaud's phenomenon and Raynaud's disease is difficult.
Contraindications to this test include: gangrenous fingers or open, infected wounds.

Procedure
• To minimize extraneous environmental stimuli, the test room should be neither too warm nor too cold.
• A thermistor is taped to each of the patient's fingers (but not so tightly as to restrict circulation), and the temperature is recorded.
• The patient's hands are submerged in an ice-water bath for 20 seconds.
• Then, he is instructed to remove his hands from the water, and the temperature of his fingers is recorded immediately and every 5 minutes thereafter until it returns to the prebath level.
• The test takes 20 to 40 minutes.

Patient care checklist
Before the test
☑ Explain or clarify test purpose and procedure.
☑ Tell the patient that he may experience discomfort when his hands are briefly immersed in ice water.
☑ Evaluate patient understanding.
☑ Suggest to the patient that he remove his watch or other jewelry.

Interfering factors
An excessively warm or cold test environment may cause inaccurate results.

Cystometry

Purpose
• To evaluate detrusor muscle function and tonicity

• To help determine the cause of bladder dysfunction.

Normal results
Normal bladder filling pattern; first desire to void at about 150 ml of infused fluid; strong desire to void at 250 to 300 ml; maximum capacity at 300 to 500 ml, with contraction occurring at capacity.

Abnormal results
Urinary problems:
   Lower urinary tract obstruction, such as bladder tumors.
Neurologic problems, such as:
   Multiple sclerosis
   Stroke
   Spinal cord pathology (cord injury, myelomeningocele, spinal cord tumor).

The basics
Cystometry assesses the bladder's neuromuscular function by measuring the efficiency of the detrusor muscle reflex, intravesical pressure and capacity, and the bladder's reaction to thermal stimulation.

Cystometry alone can provide ambiguous results. Consequently, cystometry results should always be supported by the results of other tests of the urinary system, such as cystourethrography, excretory urography, and voiding cystourethrography.

Cystometry can be performed by the instillation of physiologic saline solution or sterile water, or by the insufflation of a gas. In either method, characteristics of the urinary stream and bladder reaction to thermal stimulation may furnish accurate pathophysiologic information.

In chronic urinary tract infection, adjustments can be made to allow accurate interpretation of results, and the procedure is less likely to cause complications.
Contraindications to this test include: acute urinary tract infections, because uninhibited contractions may cause erroneous readings and the test may lead

Supplemental Cystometric Tests

Test	Purpose	Description
Ice-water test	Tests integrity of vesical reflex arc	After deflation of balloon catheter, 60 to 100 ml of sterile ice water is instilled into bladder
Bulbocavernosus reflex test	Determines integrity of sacral portion of spinal cord	Insertion of gloved finger into rectum, followed by squeezing of glans penis or clitoris
Saddle sensation test	Tests reflex activity of conus medullaris	Anocutaneous line of perineum is pricked or stroked with pin
Bethanechol sensitivity test	Defines patient with uninhibited or reflex-type neurogenic bladder	Bethanechol chloride (2.5 mg/68 kg body weight) administered subcutaneously, followed by cystometric measurement at 10, 20, and 30 minutes
Stress incontinence	Tests loss of voluntary control of vesicourethral sphincters	After filling of bladder, catheter is withdrawn and patient asked to cough, bend over, or lift heavy object

to pyelonephritis and septic shock. (See *Supplemental Cystometric Tests*.)

Procedure
• First, the patient voids into a device that gauges amount, flow, and time of voiding.
• Time and effort required to initiate the stream, its strength and continuity, and terminal dribbling are also noted.
• Next, as the patient lies supine on an examination table, a catheter is passed into his bladder to measure residual urine, if any. Difficult catheter insertion may indicate an obstructed meatus or urethra.
• The patient's response to thermal sensation is then tested by instilling sterile water or saline solution into the bladder, followed by an equal volume of warm fluid.
• The patient is asked to describe what he feels (discomfort, the need to void, nausea, or flushing).

• After the fluid is drained from the bladder, the catheter is attached to the cystometer, and fluid is dripped into the bladder. The patient is asked to tell when he feels the first urge to void, then when he feels he must void.
• The related pressure and volume are automatically plotted on a graph.
• When his bladder is full, he is asked to void, and maximal intravesical pressure is noted.
• If no more tests are needed, the catheter is removed; otherwise, the catheter is left in place to measure the urethral pressure profile or to provide supplemental findings.
• The procedure takes about 40 minutes.

Special precautions
CLINICAL ALERT: **If the patient has a spinal cord injury that has caused motor impairment, transport him on a stretcher so the test can be performed without transferring him to the examining table.**

Normal Response

Rapid expulsion of catheter and water through urethra

Constriction of anal sphincter

Visible constriction of anal sphincter

Manometric pressure > 15 cm H_2O

No dribbling of urine from urethra (dribbling indicates stress incontinence)

Patient care checklist
Before the test
☑ Explain or clarify test purpose and procedure.
☑ Tell the patient not to strain at voiding; it can cause ambiguous cystometric readings.
☑ Evaluate patient understanding.
☑ Have the patient or a responsible family member sign a consent form.
After the test
☑ Administer a sitz bath or warm tub bath if the patient experiences discomfort after the test.
CLINICAL ALERT: **Measure fluid intake and urinary output for 24 hours. Notify the physician if hematuria persists after the third voiding, or if the patient develops signs of sepsis (such as fever or chills).**

Interfering factors
• Poor patient response because of a misunderstanding of instructions or

embarrassment may interfere with test results.
• Inability to urinate in the supine position may interfere with test results.
• Concurrent use of drugs that may interfere with bladder function (such as antihistamines) affects test results.
• Inconclusive results are likely if cystometry is performed within 6 to 8 weeks after surgery for spinal cord injury.

Electrocardiography
(EKG, ECG)

Purpose
• To help identify primary conduction abnormalities, cardiac dysrhythmias, cardiac hypertrophy, pericarditis, electrolyte imbalances, myocardial ischemia, and the site and extent of myocardial infarction (MI)
• To monitor recovery from MI
• To evaluate the effectiveness of cardiac medication (cardiac glycosides, antiarrhythmics, antihypertensives, and vasodilators)
• To observe pacemaker performance. (See *Testing Pacemaker Function*, p. 608.)

Normal results
The lead II waveform, known as the rhythm strip, is described because it depicts the heart's rhythm more clearly than any other waveform.
In lead II:
   The P wave normally does not exceed 2.5 mm (0.25 mV) in height or last longer than 0.11 second.
   The PR interval (includes the P wave plus the PR segment) persists for 0.12 to 0.20 second for cardiac rates over 60 beats/minute.
   The QT interval varies with cardiac rate.
In V_1 through V_6 leads:
   R wave voltage does not exceed 27 mm.
   The QRS interval lasts 0.06 to 0.10 second.

Testing Pacemaker Function

Using the EKG machine and a magnet, you can easily test your patient's pacemaker. Set up a 12-lead EKG, and run and mark strips for leads I and II. Then, set the selector to lead II, and hold the magnet about 1″ (2.5 cm) above the pacemaker site (some magnets may be placed on the skin). If the pacemaker is functioning properly, the magnet causes it to fire regularly. In some pacemakers, the magnet rate is normally faster than the set rate. Check the patient's pacemaker identification card to identify the normal rate.

Run a strip for about 1 minute indicating that a magnet was used. Then, set aside the magnet, and run the other 10 leads. Determine the pacemaker rate by calculating the distance between each spike instead of between each QRS complex. If the pacemaker does not maintain a regular rate, notify the physician.

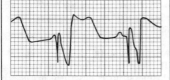

The lead II waveform illustrated above shows a regular 75 beat/minute rate. Notice the spike preceding the QRS complex; this indicates that the pacemaker has fired.

Abnormal results

An abnormal EKG may show:

MI

Right or left ventricular hypertrophy

Dysrhythmias

Right or left bundle branch block

Ischemia

Conduction defects

Pericarditis

Electrolyte abnormalities, such as hyperkalemia

Effects of cardioactive drugs.

The basics

The most commonly used procedure for evaluating cardiac status, electrocardiography records the conduction, magnitude, and duration of the electrical activity of the heart. It detects the presence and location of MI, ischemia, conduction delay, chamber enlargement, or dysrhythmias, and helps to assess the effects of electrolyte disturbances and cardiac drugs. In the 12-lead EKG, five electrodes attached to the patient's arms, legs, and chest measure the electrical potential generated by the heart. This potential is analyzed from twelve different views, or leads: three standard bipolar limb leads (I, II, III), three unipolar augmented limb leads (aV_R, aV_L, aV_F), and six unipolar chest leads (V_1 to V_6). Lead I measures the electrical potential between the left and right arms; lead II, the electrical potential between the left leg and right arm; and lead III, the electrical potential between the left leg and left arm. Using the same electrode placement, leads aV_R, aV_L, and aV_F measure electrical potential between one augmented limb lead and the electrical midpoint of the remaining two leads (determined electronically by the EKG machine). Both standard and augmented leads view the heart from the front, in the vertical plane. The six unipolar chest leads view it from the horizontal plane, helping to locate pathology in the lateral and posterior walls. The EKG machine averages the electrical potentials of the three limb electrodes (I, II, and III) and compares this with the electrical potential of the chest electrode. Recordings made with the V connection show variations in electrical potential that occur under the chest electrode as its position is changed.

After electrical potentials are transmitted to the EKG machine, these forces are amplified and graphically displayed on a strip chart recorder. The graphic display, or tracing, usually consists of the P wave, the QRS complex, and the T wave. The P wave shows atrial depolarization; the QRS complex, ventricular depolarization; and the T wave, ventricular repolarization. (See *EKG Strip: What It Shows.*)

Sometimes an EKG may reveal abnormal waveforms only during episodes of symptoms such as angina or during exercise (see "Exercise electrocardiography," p. 620, and "Ambulatory electrocardiography," p. 592).

Procedure

• Instruct the patient to disrobe to the waist and expose both legs for electrode placement. Drape the female patient's chest until chest leads are applied.
• Place the patient in the supine position. (However, if he is orthopneic, place him in semi-Fowler position.)
• Instruct him to avoid touching the metal handrail of the bed or allowing his feet to touch the footboard, to prevent current leakage that distorts the EKG tracing.
• Turn on the EKG machine and set the lead selector to the standby mode to warm up the stylus machine.
• Check the paper supply and center the stylus on the paper.
• Cleanse the electrode placement sites with alcohol and shave them, if necessary.
• Apply electrode gel to the inner aspect of the forearms and the medial aspect of the lower legs.
• Rub the skin vigorously when applying the electrodes to create an erythema that will enhance skin contact with the electrode.
• Secure the limb electrodes with rubber straps, but avoid overtightening the straps to prevent circulatory impairment and the onset of muscle spasms, which may distort the recording.
• Position the leg electrodes with their connector ends pointing upward to avoid bending or straining the lead wires.
• Connect each lead wire to an electrode by inserting the wire prong into the terminal post and tightening the screw. Be sure to match each color-

EKG Strip: What It Shows

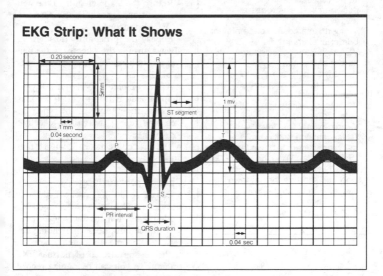

Chest Lead Positions and Marks

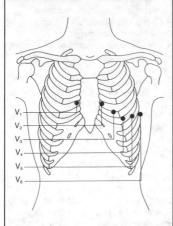

Limb leads

I: -
II: --
III: ---
aV_R: - ---
aV_L: -- ---
aV_F: --- ---

Chest leads

V_1: --- -
V_2: --- --
V_3: --- ---
V_4: --- ----
V_5: --- -----
V_6: --- ------

To prevent spurious test results, position chest electrodes as follows:
V_1: fourth intercostal space at right border of sternum
V_2: fourth intercostal space at left border of sternum
V_3: halfway between V_2 and V_4
V_4: fifth intercostal space at midclavicular line
V_5: anterior axillary line (halfway between V_4 and V_6)
V_6: midaxillary line, level with V_4.

Use marking button on EKG machine to identify chest leads (shown above) and limb leads. Depress button to print a code of long and short dashes (shown above) directly on the EKG strip. (*Note:* Since code varies, check manufacturer's instructions.)

coded lead wire to the corresponding electrode. (If necessary, replace metal electrodes and straps with suction cups for limb leads to enhance baseline stability. Position the cups on the outer aspect of the upper arms instead of the forearms, and on the upper thighs instead of the lower legs.)

• Turn the lead selector to lead I. Then write the lead number on the paper strip, or push the marking button on the machine, to identify the lead with a series of dots and dashes (see *Chest Lead Positions and Marks*). Record for 3 to 6 seconds, then return the machine to the standby mode.

• Repeat the procedure for leads II to aV_F.

• After completing the aV_F run, turn the lead selector to a neutral position before running chest leads V_1 to V_6. This prevents the stylus from swinging wildly and possibly damaging the paper.

• Connect the chest lead wire to the suction cup electrode, apply electrode gel to the chest lead sites, and press the cup firmly to the V_1 position. Apply enough gel to produce efficient suction and low skin resistance.

• Return the lead selector to the neutral position, reposition the electrode to V_2, and record.

• Repeat the procedure through V_6, always turning the selector to the neutral position before moving the suction cup.

• After completing V_6, run a rhythm strip on lead II for at least 6 seconds.

• Assess the quality of the whole series, and repeat individual lead tracings as needed.

• The procedure takes about 15 minutes.

Special precautions

• Before recording, recheck the lead positions and the lead wire and electrode connections to avoid lead reversal, which produces misleading test results. Become thoroughly familiar with the appearance of normal EKG tracings so you can recognize recording errors. For example, the leads for right and left arms, when reversed, may falsely indicate MI. A normal lead I has a positive deflection; similarly, the P waves in lead II normally have a positive deflection. The R waves in the chest leads should appear increasingly positive as they progress from V_2 to V_6. Avoid positioning V_3 at the same level as V_4 to V_6 to prevent a spurious Q wave tracing.

• If the patient with left ventricular hypertrophy exhibits large R wave tracings that run off the paper, change the sensitivity setting to half-standard, but be sure to mark the run as such. If the patient experiences chest pains during a lead run, note it on the appropriate strip.

• If he has a pacemaker in place, you can perform electrocardiography with or without a magnet, but be sure to indicate the presence of a pacemaker and the use of the magnet on the strip. (Many pacemakers function only when the heartbeat falls below a preset rate; a magnet makes the pacemaker fire regularly, permitting evaluation of its performance.)

• The recording equipment and other nearby electrical equipment should be properly grounded to prevent electrical interference that distorts EKG recording.

Patient care checklist
Before the test
☑ Explain or clarify test purpose, preparation, and procedure.

☑ Instruct the patient to relax, lie still, and breathe normally.

☑ Advise the patient not to talk during the procedure, because the sound of his voice may distort the EKG tracing.

☑ Check the patient's history for cardiac drugs, and note any current therapy on the test request form.

☑ Evaluate patient understanding.
After the test
☑ Disconnect the equipment, and wash the conductive gel from the patient's skin with a damp cloth.

Interfering factors
• Mechanical difficulties, such as EKG machine malfunction, inadequate or ineffective conductive gel, or electromagnetic interference, can produce artifacts.

• Improper placement of electrodes, patient movement or muscle tremor, strenuous exercise before the test, or medication reactions can produce inaccurate test results.

• Exceptionally oily, scaly, or diaphoretic skin can cause baseline wander and interference in the tracings. Rub the electrode site with alcohol and dry it with a cotton ball before applying the electrode, to prevent this problem.

Electroencephalography
(EEG)

Purpose
• To determine the presence and type of epilepsy

• To aid in diagnosis of intracranial lesions, such as abscesses and tumors

• To evaluate the brain's electrical activity in metabolic disease, head injury, meningitis, encephalitis, mental retardation, and psychological disorders

• To confirm brain death.

Normal results
Characteristics, amplitude, and frequency of brain waves are normal.

Abnormal results
EEGs are helpful in diagnosing:
Seizure disorders, such as epilepsy

Intracranial lesions, such as tumors or abscesses

Vascular lesions, such as cerebral infarcts and intracranial hemorrhages

Any condition that causes a diminishing level of consciousness, including metabolic disorders (such as meningitis or encephalitis), increased intracranial pressure, and brain death.

The basics

In electroencephalography, electrodes attached to standard areas of the patient's scalp record a portion of the brain's electrical activity. These electrical impulses are transmitted to an electroencephalograph, which magnifies them one million times and records them as brain waves on moving strips of paper.

Usually, 100′ to 200′ (30 to 60 m) of the recording are evaluated, with particular attention paid to basic waveforms, symmetry of cerebral activity, transient discharges, and responses to stimulation. Some waves are irregular, while others demonstrate frequent patterns. (See *EEGs: Recording the Brain's Electrical Activity.*) A specific diagnosis depends on the patient's clinical status. In patients with epilepsy, EEG patterns may identify the specific disorder, such as petit mal epilepsy, grand mal epilepsy, or temporal lobe epilepsy.

The procedure is usually performed in a room designed to eliminate electrical interference and minimize distractions. Portable units are available, however, to perform electroencephalography at bedside, which is commonly done to confirm brain death.

Procedure

• The patient is positioned comfortably on a bed or a reclining chair, and electrodes are attached to his scalp.
• Before the recording procedure begins, the patient is instructed to close his eyes, relax, and remain still.
• During the recording, the patient is carefully observed through a window in an adjacent room, and blinking, swallowing, talking, or other movements that may cause artifacts on the tracing are noted.
• The recording may be stopped periodically to allow the patient to reposition himself and get comfortable. This is important, since restlessness and fatigue can alter brain wave patterns.
• After an initial baseline recording, the patient may be tested in various stress situations to elicit abnormal patterns not obvious in the resting state. For example, the patient may be asked to breathe deeply and rapidly for 3 minutes (hyperventilate), which may elicit brain wave patterns typical of seizure disorders or other abnormalities. This technique is commonly used to detect petit mal epilepsy. Photic stimulation—another technique—tests central cerebral activity in response to bright light, accentuating abnormal activity in petit mal or myoclonic seizures. A strobe light placed in front of the patient is flashed 1 to 20 times/second. Recordings are made with the patient's eyes opened and closed.

EEGs: Recording the Brain's Electrical Activity

In electroencephalography (EEG), electrodes attached to the patient's scalp detect electrical impulses generated by the brain's nerve cells. Lead wires then transmit these impulses to an EEG machine, which translates them into waveforms. Among the basic waveforms are the alpha, beta, theta, and delta rhythms. Alpha waves occur at frequencies of 8 to 12 cycles/second in a regular rhythm and are most prominent in the occipital region of the brain. They are present only in the waking state, when the patient's eyes are closed but he is mentally alert; usually, they disappear with visual activity or mental concentration. Beta waves (13 to 30 cycles/second)—generally associated with anxiety, depression, or sedative drugs—are seen most readily in the frontal and central regions of the brain. Theta waves (4 to 7 cycles/second) are most common in children and young adults and appear in the frontal and temporal regions. Delta waves (0.5 to 3.5 cycles/second) normally occur only in young children and during sleep.

Special precautions

<u>CLINICAL ALERT:</u> **Observe the patient carefully for seizure activity. Record seizure patterns, and be prepared to provide assistance in the rare event of a severe seizure. Have suction equipment and diazepam for I.V. injection readily available.**

Patient care checklist

Before the test

☑ Explain or clarify test purpose, preparation, and procedure.

☑ Tell the patient that he must refrain from drinking fluids that contain caffeine, such as coffee and colas, before the test.

☑ Tell the patient that he should not skip a meal before the test, since this can cause relative hypoglycemia and alter brain wave patterns.

☑ Tell the patient that his hair must be thoroughly washed and dried. All hair sprays, creams, and oils must be removed.

☑ Tell the patient that electrodes will be attached to his scalp. Assure him that the electrodes will not shock him. (If needle electrodes are used, he will feel pricking sensations when they are inserted; however, flat electrodes are more commonly used.) Do your best to allay the patient's fears, since mental tension can affect brain wave patterns.

☑ Evaluate patient understanding.

☑ As ordered, withhold anticonvulsants, tranquilizers, barbiturates, and other sedatives for 24 to 48 hours before the test.

☑ If ordered, sedate infants and very young children to prevent crying and restlessness during the test.

☑ If a "sleep EEG" is ordered, keep the patient awake the night before the test and, as ordered, administer a sedative (such as chloral hydrate) to help him sleep during the test.

After the test

☑ Review with the physician the reinstatement of anticonvulsant medication or other drugs that were withheld before the test.

☑ Carefully observe the patient for seizure activity.

☑ Help the patient remove electrode paste from his hair with acetone.

☑ If the patient received a sedative before the test, take safety precautions, such as raising the side rails.

Interfering factors

• Excessive artifacts may be caused by extraneous electrical activity; head, body, eye, or tongue movement; and muscular contractions.

• Anticonvulsants, tranquilizers, barbiturates, and other sedatives interfere with the accurate determination of test results.

• Acute drug intoxication or severe hypothermia resulting in loss of consciousness causes a flat EEG.

Electromyography *(EMG)*

Purpose

• To aid in differentiation between primary muscle disorders, such as the muscular dystrophies, and those that are secondary

• To help diagnose diseases characterized by central neuronal degeneration, such as amyotrophic lateral sclerosis

• To aid in diagnosis of neuromuscular disorders, such as myasthenia gravis.

Normal results

At rest, a normal muscle exhibits minimal electrical activity. During voluntary contraction, however, electrical activity increases markedly. A sustained contraction or one of increasing strength causes a rapid "train" of motor unit potentials that can be heard as a crescendo of sounds.

Abnormal results

EMG aids in the diagnosis of:

Muscular dystrophies
Amyotrophic lateral sclerosis
Peripheral nerve disorders
Myasthenia gravis.

Nerve Conduction Studies

Nerve conduction studies aid in diagnosis of peripheral nerve injuries and diseases affecting the peripheral nervous system, such as peripheral neuropathies. To measure nerve conduction time, a nerve is stimulated electrically through the skin and underlying tissues. The patient experiences mild electrical shock discomfort with each stimulation. At a known distance from the point of stimulation, a recording electrode detects the response from the stimulated nerve. The time between stimulation of the nerve and the detected response is measured on an oscilloscope. The speed of conduction along the nerve is then calculated by dividing the distance between the point of stimulation and the recording electrode by the time between stimulus and response. In peripheral nerve injuries and diseases such as peripheral neuropathies, nerve conduction time is abnormal.

The basics

EMG is the recording of the electrical activity of selected skeletal muscle groups at rest and during voluntary contraction. In this test, a needle electrode is inserted percutaneously into a muscle. The electrical discharge (or motor unit potential) of the muscle is then displayed and measured on an oscilloscope screen. Nerve conduction time (see *Nerve Conduction Studies*) is often measured simultaneously.

EMG is a useful diagnostic technique for evaluating muscle disorders. The interpreter makes a distinction between waveforms that indicate a muscle disorder and those that indicate denervation. Findings must be correlated with the patient's history, clinical features, and other neurodiagnostic test results.

Contraindications to this test include: bleeding disorders.

Procedure

• The patient lies on a stretcher or bed or sits in a chair, depending on the muscles to be tested.
• The arm or leg is positioned so the muscle to be tested is at rest.
• The needle electrodes are then quickly inserted into the selected muscle.
• The muscle's resulting electrical signal is recorded during rest and contraction, amplified one million times, and displayed on an oscilloscope screen.
• Photographs are taken of the display for a permanent record.
• Usually, the lead wires of the recorder are attached to an audioamplifier, so the fluctuation of voltage within the muscle can be heard.
• The procedure takes 1 to 2 hours to perform.

Patient care checklist

Before the test

☑ Explain or clarify test purpose and procedure.
☑ Tell the patient that a needle will be inserted into selected muscles and that he may experience some pain.
☑ Evaluate patient understanding.
☑ Restrict cigarettes, coffee, tea, or cola for 2 to 3 hours before the test, as ordered.
☑ Make sure that the patient or a responsible family member has signed a consent form.

After the test

☑ If the patient experiences residual pain, apply warm compresses and administer analgesics, as ordered.

Interfering factors

• The patient's inability to comply with instructions during the test may invalidate results.
• Drugs that affect myoneural junctions, such as cholinergics, anticholinergics, and skeletal muscle relaxants, interfere with test results.

Esophageal acidity test

Purpose
To evaluate competency of the lower esophageal sphincter.

Normal results
The pH of the esophagus is more than 5.0.

Abnormal results
An intraesophageal pH of 1.5 to 2.0 indicates gastric acid reflux resulting from incompetency of the lower esophageal sphincter.

The basics
In contrast with the high acidity of the stomach (pH 1.1 to 2.4), the esophagus normally maintains a pH greater than 5.0. Although some reflux of gastric juices into the lower esophagus is common, a sharp increase in such backflow may acidify the intraesophageal pH to as low as 1.5. When repeated reflux occurs, the esophageal mucosa becomes inflamed by the acidic gastric juices, resulting in pyrosis (heartburn).

The esophageal acidity test evaluates the competency of the lower esophageal sphincter—the major barrier to reflux—by measuring intraesophageal pH with an electrode attached to a manometric catheter. This test, the most sensitive indicator of gastric reflux, is indicated in patients who complain of persistent heartburn, with or without regurgitation. The esophageal manometry test may be performed to measure esophageal sphincter pressure (see *Esophageal Manometry,* p. 616).

Procedure
• The patient is assisted to a high Fowler's position.
• A catheter with a pH electrode is introduced into the patient's mouth, and he is instructed to swallow.
• The lower esophageal sphincter is located manometrically, and the patient is asked to perform Valsalva's maneuver or to lift his legs, to stimulate reflux.
• After he does so, the intraesophageal pH is determined.
• If the pH remains normal, the catheter is passed into the patient's stomach and 300 ml of 0.1% N HCl is instilled over 3 minutes.
• The catheter is passed to ¾" (2 cm) above the sphincter. The patient is again asked to perform Valsalva's maneuver or lift his legs.
• After he does so, the intraesophageal pH is again determined.
• The procedure takes approximately 45 minutes to perform.

Special precautions
• During insertion, the electrode may enter the trachea instead of the esophagus. If the patient develops cyanosis or paroxysms of coughing, remove the electrode immediately.
• Observe the patient closely during intubation, since dysrhythmias may develop.
• The catheter must be clamped before removal to prevent aspiration of fluid into the lungs.

Patient care checklist
Before the test
☑ Explain or clarify test purpose and procedure.
☑ Inform the patient that he may experience slight discomfort or may cough or gag as the catheter is passed through his mouth to his esophagus.
☑ Evaluate patient understanding.
☑ Restrict food, fluids, and smoking after midnight before the test.
☑ Withhold medications that may interfere with test results, as ordered.
☑ Just before the test, take vital signs and ask the patient to void.

Interfering factors
• Failure to adhere to pretest dietary

Esophageal Manometry

Esophageal manometry measures esophageal sphincter pressure and records the duration and sequence of peristaltic contractions to detect motility disorders, such as achalasia, diffuse esophageal spasm, and scleroderma. In this test, the patient is asked to swallow a manometric catheter that contains a small pressure transducer along its length. With the catheter placed at various levels in the esophagus, baseline measurements of pressures are made, followed by measurement of pressures in the lower esophageal sphincter immediately before and after swallowing, and then peristaltic contractions are recorded. It may be necessary to ask the patient to take wet swallows, as well as swallows with ice water, to obtain more specific information. Cholinergic and anticholinergic drugs are withheld and the patient is told to avoid tobacco and alcohol for 24 hours before the test; he is instructed to fast for 4 hours. These restrictions help prevent esophageal sphincter pressures from increasing or decreasing, which would interfere with test results. Normally, baseline sphincter pressure is about 20 mm Hg; relaxation pressure (the pressure immediately before swallowing) is at least 18 mm Hg. Peristalsis usually appears as a series of high-pressure peaks, representing sequential contractions of the esophagus.

In **achalasia,** baseline sphincter pressure commonly reaches 50 mm Hg; relaxation pressure, less than 25 mm Hg. Peristalsis is usually weak and nonpropulsive. Food and fluids accumulate in the esophagus until their weight can overcome sphincter resistance.

In **diffuse spasm of the esophagus,** sphincter pressure is generally normal, but peristalsis is disordered. Instead of sequential, orderly contractions, different segments of the esophagus contract simultaneously—and often with abnormal force—after swallowing. Contractions may also occur without the stimulus of swallowing, or more than one contraction may follow a single swallow.

In **esophageal scleroderma,** impaired sphincter function and peristalsis result from replacement of smooth muscle by fibrous tissue in the lower two thirds of the esophagus. Both baseline and relaxation pressures are depressed. Peristalsis is normal in the upper third of the esophagus, where striated muscle predominates, but it is weak or absent in the lower two thirds.

and smoking restrictions interferes with accurate testing.

• Antacids, anticholinergics, and cimetidine may depress intraesophageal pH by decreasing gastric secretion or reducing its acidity; cholinergics, reserpine, alcohol, adrenergic blockers, and corticosteroids may elevate intraesophageal pH by increasing gastric secretion or by promoting reflux by relaxing the lower esophageal sphincter.

Evoked potential studies

Purpose
• To aid in diagnosis of nervous system lesions and abnormalities
• To assess neurologic function
• To differentiate between cochlear and retrocochlear lesions.

Normal results
Visual evoked potentials:
Because many physical and technical

factors affect P100 latency, normal results vary greatly between laboratories and patients.

Auditory brain stem evoked potential:
Values vary among patients and may also be influenced by the specific instrument and laboratory used.

Somatosensory evoked potential:
The waveforms obtained vary, depending on locations of the stimulating and recording electrodes.

See *Normal Findings in Evoked Potential Studies,* p. 618, for typical responses.

Abnormal results

Visual evoked potentials:
  Abnormal unilateral P100 latencies indicate:
    Lesion anterior to optic chiasm.
  Abnormal bilateral P100 latencies are associated with:
    Multiple sclerosis
    Optic neuritis
    Retinopathies
    Amblyopias
    Spinocerebellar degeneration
    Adrenoleukodystrophy
    Sarcoidosis
    Parkinson's disease
    Huntington's chorea.

Auditory brain stem evoked potentials:
  Abnormal responses are associated with:
    Cochlear hearing loss
    Retrocochlear lesions
    Multiple sclerosis
    Cerebrovascular accident.

Somatosensory evoked potentials:
  Abnormal upper limb responses may indicate:
    Cervical spondylosis
    Intracerebral lesions
    Sensorimotor neuropathies.
  Abnormal lower limb responses are associated with:
    Guillain-Barré syndrome
    Compressive myelopathies
    Multiple sclerosis
    Transverse myelitis
    Traumatic spinal cord injury.

The basics

These tests evaluate the integrity of visual, somatosensory, and auditory nerve pathways by measuring *evoked potentials*—the brain's electrical response to stimulation of the sense organs or peripheral nerves. Evoked potentials are recorded as electronic impulses by surface electrodes attached to the scalp and to the skin over various peripheral sensory nerves. A computer extracts these low-amplitude impulses from background brain wave activity and averages the signals from repeated stimuli.

Three types of responses are measured. *Visual evoked potentials,* produced by exposing the eye to a rapidly reversing checkerboard pattern, help evaluate demyelinating disease, traumatic injury, and puzzling visual complaints. *Auditory brain stem evoked potentials,* produced by delivering clicks to the ear, help locate auditory lesions and evaluate brain stem integrity. *Somatosensory evoked potentials,* produced by electrically stimulating a peripheral sensory nerve, help diagnose peripheral nerve disease and locate brain and spinal cord lesions.

Evoked potential studies are also useful for monitoring comatose patients and patients under anesthesia, monitoring spinal cord function during spinal cord surgery, and evaluating neurologic function in infants whose sensory systems normally cannot be adequately assessed. Information from evoked potential studies is useful but insufficient to confirm a specific diagnosis. Test data must be interpreted in light of clinical information.

Procedure

• The patient is assisted to a reclining chair or a bed and is instructed to relax and remain still.

To measure visual evoked potentials:
• Electrodes are attached to the patient's scalp at occipital, parietal, and vertex locations; a reference electrode is placed on the midfrontal area or on the ear.

Normal Findings in Evoked Potential Studies

Visual evoked potential: In this test, visual neural impulses are recorded as they travel along the pathway from the eye to the occipital cortex. Wave P100 is the most significant component of the resultant waveform—normal P100 latency is approximately 100 msec after the application of visual stimulus.

Normal tracing

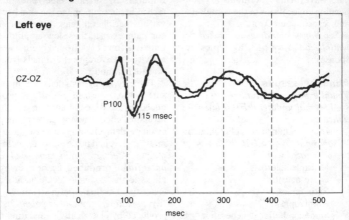

Auditory brain stem evoked potential: In this test, auditory neural activity is recorded as it passes from the peripheral or cochlear end organ through the brain stem to the cortex. Wave I is associated with the acoustic nerve response, while Wave V is associated with an upper brain stem response. Waves I and V are considered to be the most clinically useful. The test is repeated for accuracy; thus each graph shows two sets of waveforms.

Normal tracing

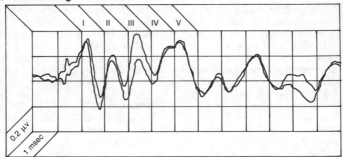

(continued)

Normal Findings in Evoked Potential Studies *(continued)*

Somatosensory evoked potentials: These tests measure the conduction time of an electrical impulse traveling along a somatosensory pathway to the cortex. Interwave latency is the most significant component of the resultant waveform.

Upper limb

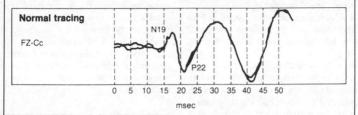

FZ = midfrontal   Cc = sensoparietal cortex contralateral to stimulated limb

Lower limb

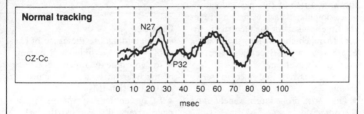

CZ = vertex   Cc = sensoparietal cortex contralateral to stimulated limb

• The patient is positioned 1 m from the pattern shift stimulator.
• One eye is occluded, and the patient is instructed to fix his gaze on a dot in the center of the screen.
• A checkerboard pattern is projected and then rapidly reversed or shifted 100 times, once or twice per second.
• A computer amplifies and averages the brain's response to each stimulus, and the results are plotted as a waveform.
• The procedure is repeated for the other eye.

To measure auditory brain stem evoked potentials:
• Electrodes are placed at the vertex of the patient's scalp (active), the mastoid process, or earlobe of the stimulated ear (reference) and the mastoid process or earlobe of the opposite ear (ground).
• Stimuli, in the form of clicks or rapid rise time (1 msec) tone pips, are presented at 10 per second until 2,000 time-locked responses are collected and averaged.
• To estimate thresholds, responses to stimuli are collected at decreasing intensities until wave V disappears from the trace.
• Cochlear and retrocochlear lesions are differentiated by presenting click stimuli at high intensities and comparing the absolute latencies of waves I, III, and V to the interwave latency

differences between ears and to normal data.

To measure somatosensory evoked potentials:

• Electrodes are attached to the patient's skin over somatosensory pathways to stimulate peripheral nerves. Electrode sites usually include the wrist, knee, and ankle.

• Recording electrodes are placed on the scalp over the sensory cortex of the hemisphere opposite the limb to be stimulated.

• A painless electric shock is delivered to the peripheral nerve through the stimulating electrode. The intensity of the shock is adjusted to produce a minor muscle response, such as a thumb twitch upon median nerve stimulation at the wrist.

• The shock is delivered at least 500 times, at a rate of five per second.

• A computer measures and averages the time it takes for the electrical current to reach the cortex; the results, expressed in milliseconds, are recorded as waveforms.

• The test is repeated once to verify results.

• The entire procedure is repeated on the other side.

Patient care checklist

Before the test

☑ Explain or clarify test purpose and procedure.

☑ Tell the patient that he will be positioned in a reclining chair or on a bed. If visual evoked potentials will be measured, tell him that electrodes will be attached to his scalp. If auditory brain stem evoked potentials will be measured, tell him that the electrodes will be placed on his scalp and on both earlobes. If somatosensory evoked potentials will be measured, explain that electrodes will be placed on his scalp, neck, lower back, wrist, knee, and ankle. Assure the patient that the electrodes will not hurt him.

☑ Encourage him to relax during testing, since tension can affect neurologic function and interfere with test results.

☑ Evaluate patient understanding.

☑ Just before the test, ask the patient to remove all jewelry.

Interfering factors

• Incorrect placement of electrodes or equipment failure can alter test results.

• Patient tension or failure to cooperate can impair the accuracy of test results.

• Extremely poor visual acuity can hinder accurate determination of visual evoked potentials; severe hearing loss can interfere with accurate determination of auditory brain stem evoked potentials.

Exercise electrocardiography
[stress test]

Purpose

• To help diagnose the cause of chest pain or other possible cardiac pain

• To determine the functional capacity of the heart after surgery or myocardial infarction (MI)

• To screen for asymptomatic coronary artery disease (particularly in men over age 35)

• To help set limitations for an exercise program

• To identify cardiac dysrhythmias that develop during physical exercise

• To evaluate the effectiveness of antiarrhythmic or antianginal therapy.

Normal results

In a normal exercise EKG, the P wave, QRS complex, T wave and the ST segment change slightly; slight ST segment depression occurs in some patients, especially women. Heart rate rises in direct proportion to the work load and metabolic oxygen demand; systolic blood pressure also rises as work load increases. The normal patient attains the endurance levels predicted by his age and the appropriate exercise protocol.

Abnormal results

Although criteria for judging test results vary, two findings strongly suggest an abnormality: a flat or down-sloping ST segment depression of 1 mm or more for at least 0.08 second after the junction of the QRS complex and ST segments (J point); and a markedly depressed J point, with an up-sloping but depressed ST segment of 1.5 mm below the baseline 0.08 second after the J point. Initial ST segment depression on the resting EKG must be further depressed by 1 mm during exercise to be considered abnormal.

Hypotension resulting from exercise, ST segment depression of 3 mm or more, down-sloping ST segments, and ischemic ST segments appearing within the first 3 minutes of exercise and lasting 8 minutes into the post-test recovery period may indicate multivessel or left coronary artery disease. ST segment elevation may indicate dyskinetic left ventricular wall motion or severe transmural ischemia.

The basics

Exercise electrocardiography evaluates heart action during physical stress—to test cardiac reaction to increased demand for oxygen—and so provides important diagnostic information that cannot be obtained from resting electrocardiography alone. An EKG and blood pressure readings are taken while the patient walks on a treadmill or pedals a stationary bicycle, and his response to a constant or an increasing work load is observed.

Unless complications develop, the test continues until the patient reaches the target heart rate (determined by an established protocol) or experiences chest pain or fatigue. The patient with a recent MI or coronary artery surgery may walk the treadmill at a slow pace to determine his activity tolerance before discharge from the hospital.

The risk of MI during exercise electrocardiography is less than 1 in 500; the risk of death, less than 1 in 10,000.

The predictive value of this test for coronary artery disease varies with the patient's history and sex; however, false-negative and false-positive test results are common. To detect coronary artery disease accurately, thallium imaging and stress testing, cardiac blood pool scanning, or coronary angiography may be necessary. *Contraindications to this test may include:* ventricular or dissecting aortic aneurysm, uncontrolled dysrhythmias, pericarditis, myocarditis, severe anemia, uncontrolled hypertension, unstable angina, and congestive heart failure, since exercise electrocardiography places considerable stress on the heart.

Procedure

• The electrode sites are shaved, if necessary, and the skin is thoroughly cleansed with an alcohol sponge.
• The superficial epidermal cell layer and excess skin oils are removed with a gauze pad, fine sandpaper, or dental burr; adequately prepared sites appear slightly red.
• Chest electrodes are placed according to the lead system selected and are secured with adhesive tape or a rubber belt.
• The lead wire cable is placed over the patient's shoulder, and the lead wire box is placed on his chest.
• The cable is secured by pinning it to the patient's clothing or taping it to his shoulder or back.
• Then, the lead wires are connected to the chest electrodes.
• The monitor is started, and a stable baseline tracing is obtained. A baseline rhythm strip is checked for dysrhythmias.
• A blood pressure reading is taken, and the patient is auscultated for presence of S_3 or S_4 gallops or rales.
Treadmill test:
• The treadmill is turned on to a slow speed, and the patient is shown how to step onto it and how to use the support railings to maintain balance, but not to support weight.

• Then, the treadmill is turned off.
• The patient is instructed to step onto the treadmill, and it is turned on to slow speed until the patient gets used to walking on it.

Bicycle ergometer test:
• The patient is instructed to sit on the bicycle, and the seat and handlebars are adjusted, if necessary, so that he can pedal the bike comfortably.
• The patient is instructed not to grip the handlebars tightly, but to use them only for maintaining balance, and to pedal until he reaches the desired speed, as shown on the speedometer.

In both tests:
• A monitor is observed continuously for changes in the heart's electrical activity. The rhythm strip is checked at preset intervals for dysrhythmias, premature ventricular contractions (PVCs), or ST segment changes. The test level and the elapsed time into the test level are marked on each strip.
• Blood pressure is monitored at predetermined intervals—usually at the end of each test level—and changes in systolic readings are noted.
• Testing stops when the patient reaches the target heart rate or if he experiences severe dizziness, lightheadedness, leg fatigue, dyspnea, diaphoresis, or an ataxic gait.
• As the treadmill speed slows, the patient may be instructed to continue walking for several minutes to prevent nausea or dizziness. The treadmill is then turned off, the patient is helped to a chair, and his blood pressure and EKG are monitored for 10 to 15 minutes.

Special precautions
CLINICAL ALERT: **Stop the test immediately if the EKG shows three consecutive PVCs, if systolic blood pressure falls below resting level, if heart rate falls to 10 beats/minute below resting level, or if the patient becomes exhausted. Depending on the patient's condition, the test may be stopped if the EKG shows bundle branch block, ST segment depression that exceeds 3 mm, or frequent or complicated PVCs; if blood pressure fails to rise above resting level; if systolic pressure exceeds 220 mm Hg; or if the patient experiences angina. Rarely, persistent ST segment elevation may indicate transmural myocardial ischemia and should end the test.**

Patient care checklist
Before the test
☑ Explain or clarify test purpose, preparation, and procedure.
☑ Inform the patient that the test will cause him to feel fatigued, slightly breathless, and sweaty, but assure him that it has few risks; he may, in fact, stop the test if he experiences extreme fatigue or chest pain.
☑ Advise the patient to wear comfortable socks and shoes and loose, lightweight shorts or slacks during the procedure; men usually do not wear a shirt during the test, and women generally wear a bra and a lightweight short-sleeved blouse or a patient gown with a front closure.
☑ Inform the patient that several areas on his chest and, possibly, on his back will be cleansed, shaved (if necessary), and abraded to prepare the skin for the electrodes. Reassure him that he will not feel any current from the electrodes, but the electrode sites may itch slightly.
☑ Tell the patient that his blood pressure and heart rate will be checked periodically throughout the procedure, and for 10 to 15 minutes after the test.
☑ If the patient is scheduled for a multistage *treadmill test,* explain that the speed and incline of the treadmill will increase at predetermined intervals, and tell him that he will be informed of each adjustment. If he is scheduled for a *bicycle ergometer test,* explain that the resistance he experiences in pedaling will increase gradually as he tries to maintain a specific speed.

☑ Encourage him to report his feelings during the test.
☑ Evaluate patient understanding.
☑ Instruct the patient not to eat, smoke, or drink alcoholic or caffeinic beverages for 3 hours before the test, but to continue any drug regimen unless the physician directs otherwise.
☑ Make sure that the patient or a responsible family member has signed a consent form.

After the test
☑ Tell the patient to wait at least 1 hour before showering. Caution him to use warm water; hot water may cause him to faint or feel dizzy.

Interfering factors
• Patient failure to observe pretest restrictions hinders the heart's ability to respond to stress.
• Use of beta blockers may make test results difficult to interpret.
• Inability to exercise to the target heart rate because of fatigue or uncooperativeness interferes with accurate testing.
• Wolff-Parkinson-White syndrome (anomalous atrioventricular excitation), electrolyte imbalance, and digitalis may cause false-positive results.
• Conditions that cause left ventricular hypertrophy (congenital abnormalities, hypertension) may interfere with testing for ischemia.

External sphincter electromyography

Purpose
• To assess neuromuscular function of the external urinary sphincter
• To assess the functional balance between bladder and sphincter muscle activity.

Normal results
The International Continence Society does not specify normal findings for sphincter electromyography.

The electromyogram shows increased muscle activity when the patient tightens the external urinary sphincter and decreased muscle activity when he relaxes it. If electromyography and cystometrography are done together, a comparison of results shows that muscle activity of the normal sphincter increases as the bladder fills. During voiding and with bladder contraction, muscle activity decreases as the sphincter relaxes. This comparison is important in assessing external sphincter efficiency and the functional balance between bladder and sphincter muscle activity.

Abnormal results
Failure of the sphincter to relax or an increase in muscle activity during voiding demonstrates detrusor–external sphincter dyssynergia. Confirmation of such muscle activity by electromyography may indicate neurogenic bladder, spinal cord injury, multiple sclerosis, Parkinson's disease, or stress incontinence.

The basics
This procedure measures electrical activity of the external urinary sphincter. The electrical activity can be measured in three ways: by needle electrodes inserted in perineal or periurethral tissues, by electrodes in an anal plug, or by skin electrodes. Skin electrodes are commonly used.

The primary indication for external sphincter electromyography is incontinence. Often, this test is done with cystometry and voiding urethrography as part of a full urodynamic study, to provide a thorough evaluation of detrusor and sphincter coordination.

Procedure
• The patient is placed in lithotomy position for electrode placement, then may lie supine.
• Patient position, type of electrode used, measuring equipment used, and any other tests done at the same time are recorded. (To obtain comparable

results, subsequent studies must be done the same way.)

• Electrode paste is applied to the ground plate, which is taped to the thigh and grounded.

• The electrodes are then placed, as described below, and connected to electrode adapters.

Placing skin electrodes:

• The skin is cleansed with antiseptic solution and dried.

• A small area may be shaved for optimum electrode contact.

• Electrode paste is applied and the electrodes taped in place: for females, in the periurethral area; for males, in the perineal area beneath the scrotum.

Placing needle electrodes:

• With the male patient, a gloved finger is inserted into the rectum. The needles and wires are inserted 1½″ through the perineal skin toward the apex of the prostate. While the needles are withdrawn, the wires are held in place and then taped to the thigh.

• With the female patient, the labia are spread, and the needles and wires inserted periurethrally. The needles are withdrawn and the wires taped to the thigh.

Placing anal plug electrodes:

• The plug is lubricated, and the patient is informed again that only the tip will be inserted into the rectum.

• The patient is asked to relax by breathing slowly and deeply.

• He is asked to relax the anal sphincter to accommodate the plug by bearing down as if for a bowel movement.

After placing the appropriate electrodes and connecting them to adapters:

• The adapters are inserted into the preamplifier and recording is begun.

• The patient is asked to alternately relax and tighten the sphincter.

• When sufficient data have been recorded, he is asked to bear down and exhale while the anal plug and needle electrodes are removed.

• Remove skin electrodes gently to avoid pulling hair and tender skin.

• Cleanse and dry the area before the patient dresses.

• The test takes 30 to 60 minutes.

Special precautions

• Insert needles quickly to minimize discomfort.

• The ground plate should be properly applied and anchored; wires should be taped securely to prevent artifact.

Patient care checklist

Before the test

☑ Explain or clarify test purpose and procedure.

☑ If needle electrodes will be used, tell the patient where they will be placed, and explain that the discomfort will be equivalent to that of an intramuscular injection. Assure him that he will feel discomfort only during insertion.

☑ Advise the patient that the needles are connected to wires leading to the recorder, but that there is no danger of electrical shock.

☑ Explain to the female patient that she may notice slight bleeding at the first voiding.

☑ If an anal plug will be used, inform the patient that only the tip of the plug will be inserted into the rectum, that he may feel fullness but no discomfort, and that bowel movements during testing are rare but easily managed.

☑ Evaluate patient understanding.

☑ Withhold medications that may interfere with test results, as ordered.

After the test

☑ Watch for and report hematuria after the first voiding in the female patient tested with needle electrodes.

☑ Watch for and report symptoms of mild urethral irritation, such as dysuria, hematuria, and urinary frequency.

☑ Advise the patient to take a warm sitz bath, and encourage fluids (2 to 3 liters/day) unless contraindicated.

Interfering factors

• Patient movement during electromyography may distort recordings.

• Anticholinergic or cholinergic drugs affect detrusor and sphincter activity.
• Improperly placed and anchored electrodes will cause inaccurate recordings.

Fetal monitoring, external

Purpose
• To measure fetal heart rate (FHR) and the frequency of uterine contractions
• To evaluate antepartum and intrapartum fetal health during stress and nonstress situations
• To detect fetal distress
• To determine the necessity for internal fetal monitoring.

Normal results
Baseline FHR ranges from 120 to 160 beats/minute, with 5 to 25 beats/minute variability.
Antepartum nonstress test:
If two fetal movements associated with more than a 15 beats/minute heart rate acceleration from baseline FHR occur within 20 minutes, the fetus is considered healthy and should remain so for another week.
Contraction stress test (CST):
If three contractions occur during a 10-minute period, with no late decelerations, the fetus is considered healthy and should remain so for another week.

Abnormal results
Bradycardia (FHR of less than 120 beats/minute) may indicate:
    Fetal heart block
    Malposition
    Hypoxia
    Drug use by mother.
Tachycardia (FHR of more than 160 beats/minute) may result from:
    Vagolytic drugs
    Maternal fever, tachycardia, or hyperthyroidism
    Early fetal hypoxia
    Fetal infection or dysrhythmia.

Decreased variability (a fluctuation of less than 5 beats/minute in the FHR) may be caused by:
    Fetal cardiac dysrhythmia or heart block
    Fetal hypoxia
    Central nervous system malformation
    Infections
    Vagolytic drugs.
Positive antepartum nonstress test (less than two accelerations of FHR that last longer than 15 seconds each, with a heart rate acceleration over 15 beats/minute) indicates:
    Exaggerated risk of perinatal morbidity and mortality
    A need to perform the CST.
Positive CST test (persistent late decelerations during two or more contractions) indicates:
    Increased risk of fetal morbidity or mortality.

The basics
In external fetal monitoring, a noninvasive test, an electronic transducer and cardiotachometer amplify and record FHR, while a pressure-sensitive transducer, the tokodynamometer, simultaneously records uterine contractions. This procedure records the baseline FHR (average FHR over two contraction cycles or 10 minutes), periodic fluctuations in the baseline FHR, and beat-to-beat heart rate variability. Fluctuations in FHR can occur as baseline changes (unrelated to uterine contractions) or as periodic changes (in response to uterine contractions). Such fluctuations are described in terms of amplitude (difference in beats per minute between baseline readings and maximum or minimum fluctuation), lag time (difference between the peak of the contraction and the lowest point of deceleration), and recovery time (difference between the end of the contraction and the return to the baseline FHR). (See *Comparison of Decelerated Fetal Heart Rates and Uterine Contractions,* p. 626.)

Comparison of Decelerated Fetal Heart Rates and Uterine Contractions

Unlike variable decelerations, early and late decelerations in the FHA correspond to uterine contractions.

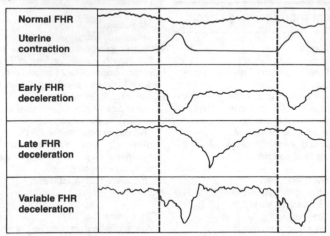

Decelerations in fetal heart rate (FHR) may be affected by uterine contractions. The three types of FHR decelerations—early, late, and variable—occur at different points in the contraction phase.

Early FHR decelerations occur at onset of uterine contraction and reach their lowest point at the peak of the contraction. In early deceleration, FHR returns to the average baseline by the end of the contraction. FHR produces a smooth wave pattern that mirrors the uterine contraction. There is a consistent relationship between the fall in FHR and the uterine contractions. Early deceleration is usually benign and is most commonly caused by compression of the fetal head.

Late decelerations begin about 20 seconds after onset of a contraction and reach their lowest point well after the contraction has peaked. In late deceleration, FHR recovery occurs later than 15 seconds following the contraction. Although the FHR tracing in late deceleration resembles the smooth wave of early deceleration, its implications are far more serious. Late decelerations usually result from uteroplacental insufficiency and may lead to fetal death. When associated with increased variability or with tachycardia and no variability, late decelerations indicate fetal central nervous system depression and myocardial hypoxia.

Variable decelerations—sudden drops in FHR—may occur at any time during a contraction. Following the decline, baseline FHR recovery may be rapid or prolonged. Since the fall in FHR is unrelated to uterine contractions, wave patterns also vary. Variable decelerations are common, occurring in about 50% of all labors, and are usually associated with transitory umbilical cord compression. However, a severe drop (to less than 70 beats per minute for more than 60 seconds) may indicate fetal acidosis, hypoxia, and low Apgar scores.

When FHR patterns indicate fetal distress, fetal oxygenation can often be improved by turning the mother on her side (preferably the left) to alleviate supine hypoxia; by giving oxygen to the mother; or by loading maternal fluids to increase placental perfusion. If the FHR returns to normal, labor may continue. If abnormal FHR patterns persist, cesarean birth may be required.

Accelerations in FHR may result from early hypoxia. They may precede or follow variable decelerations and may indicate a breech position. External fetal monitoring is also used for other tests of fetal health—the nonstress test and the CST. (See *Contraction Stress Test*.) The relationship between FHR and the uterine contraction pattern is described by acceleration (transient rise in FHR lasting longer than 15 seconds and associated with a uterine contraction) and deceleration (transient fall in FHR related to a uterine contraction).

The CST produces a high rate of false-positive results; therefore, further testing is essential. If hyperstimulation (long or frequent uterine contractions) or suspicious results occur, repetition of the test on the following day is necessary. If results are still positive, internal fetal monitoring or cesarean birth may be necessary.

External fetal monitoring can be performed before (antepartum) or during (intrapartum) labor. Antepartum monitoring may be repeated weekly as long as indications, such as pregnancy over 42 weeks' gestation or fetal growth retardation, persist. (Also see *Using the Doppler Stethoscope*, p. 628.)

Procedure

• Place the patient in semi-Fowler or left lateral position, with her abdomen exposed.
• Cover the ultrasonic transducer receiver crystal with ultrasound transmission gel.
• After palpating the abdomen to identify the fetal chest area, locate the most

distinct fetal heart sounds, and secure the ultrasound transducer over this area with the elastic band, stockinette, or abdominal strap.
• Check the recordings to ensure an adequate printout, and verify the fetal monitor's alarm boundaries.
• During monitoring, periodically check the elastic band, stockinette, or abdominal strap securing the transducer to ensure that the fit is tight enough to produce a good tracing but loose enough to be comfortable.
• As labor progresses, reposition the pressure transducer, as necessary, so that it remains on the fundal portion of the uterus. You may have to reposition the ultrasonic transducer as fetal position changes.

Antepartum monitoring with non-stress tests:
• Tell the patient to hold the pressure transducer in her hand and to push it each time she feels the fetus move.
• Within a 20-minute period, monitor the baseline FHR until you record two fetal movements that last longer than

---

Contraction Stress Test

The contraction stress test (CST) measures fetal ability to withstand the stress of contractions induced before actual labor begins. Late decelerations in the fetal heart rate in response to uterine contractions during this test may indicate that the placenta cannot deliver enough oxygen to the fetus. Placental insufficiency may result from maternal vascular disease, associated with diabetes mellitus, preeclampsia, or chronic hypertension. Intrauterine growth retardation, postmaturity syndrome, and Rh isoimmunization may also cause fetal compromise.

Since the CST mimics labor, it is contraindicated in patients with placenta previa or when premature labor is likely, as in premature rupture of the membranes, multiple pregnancy, or incompetent cervix.

Using the Doppler Stethoscope

The Doppler stethoscope is used antepartum and intrapartum to confirm fetal life by monitoring the fetal heart rate (FHR) through continuous ultrasonic vibration electronically converted to audible sound. Testing for fetal life takes only a few seconds; evaluating fetal health may take several hours. No risks or adverse effects are associated with this procedure.

To perform this test, mineral oil or water-soluble jelly is rubbed on the patient's abdomen, and the transducer attached to the Doppler stethoscope is moved over the abdomen until fetal heart tones are heard. For continuous FHR monitoring, the transducer is strapped to the mother's abdomen.

Obesity or hydramnios may absorb sound waves and make it difficult to obtain results.

15 seconds each and cause heart rate accelerations of more than 15 beats/minute from the baseline.

• If you cannot obtain two FHR accelerations, wait 30 minutes, shake the patient's abdomen to stimulate the fetus, and repeat the test.

Antepartum monitoring with CST:

• Induce contractions by oxytocin infusion or nipple stimulation (endogenous oxytocin).

• If you administer oxytocin, infuse a dilute solution at a rate of 1 μU/minute, and increase the oxytocin rate until the patient experiences three contractions within 10 minutes, each lasting longer than 45 seconds.

• If nipple stimulation is used, tell the patient to stimulate one nipple by hand until contractions begin. If a second contraction does not occur in 2 minutes, have her restimulate the nipple. Stimulate both nipples if contractions do not occur in 15 minutes. Continue the test until three contractions occur in 10 minutes.

• If no decelerations occur during three contractions, the patient may be discharged. Late decelerations during any of the contractions require notification of the physician and additional testing.

Intrapartum monitoring:

• Secure the pressure transducer with an elastic band, stockinette, or abdominal strap over the area of greatest uterine electrical activity during contractions (usually the fundus).

• Adjust the machine to record 0 to 10 mm Hg of pressure between palpable contractions. (Readings during contractions vary, depending on the tightness of the bands, the amount of adipose tissue, and the placement of the pressure transducer.)

• Reposition the ultrasound and pressure transducers, as necessary, to ensure continuous accurate readings.

• Review the tracings frequently for baseline abnormalities, periodic changes, variability changes, and uterine contraction abnormalities.

• Record maternal movement, administration of drugs, and procedures performed directly on the tracing so changes in the tracing can be evaluated in view of these activities.

• Report any abnormalities immediately.

Patient care checklist
Before the test

☑ Explain or clarify test purpose and procedure.

☑ If monitoring is to be performed antepartum, instruct the patient to eat a meal just before the test to increase fetal activity, which decreases the test time.

☑ Assure the patient that external fetal monitoring is painless and noninvasive, and that it will not hurt the fetus or interfere with the normal progress of labor.

☑ Tell the patient that she may have to restrict movement during baseline readings, but that she may change position between the readings.

☑ Evaluate patient understanding.
☑ Have the patient sign a consent form.

Interfering factors
• Drugs that affect the sympathetic and the parasympathetic nervous systems may depress FHR.
• Maternal position, particularly if the patient is lying supine, may cause artifactual fetal distress.
• Maternal obesity or excessive maternal or fetal activity may inhibit recording of uterine contractions or of FHR.
• Loose or dirty leads or transducer connections may cause artifacts.

Fetal monitoring, internal

Purpose
• To monitor fetal heart rate (FHR), especially beat-to-beat variability
• To measure the frequency and pressure of uterine contractions
• To evaluate intrapartum fetal health
• To supplement or replace external fetal monitoring.

Normal results
FHR ranges from 120 to 160 beats/minute, with a variability of 5 to 25 beats/minute from FHR baseline. (Also see *Normal Intrauterine Pressure Readings During Labor*, p. 630.)

Abnormal results
Bradycardia—FHR of less than 120 beats/minute—may indicate:
 Fetal heart block
 Fetal malposition
 Fetal hypoxia
 Effect on fetus from maternal ingestion of drugs such as propranolol or narcotic analgesics.
Tachycardia—FHR greater than 160 beats/minute—may result from:
 Vagolytic drugs
 Maternal fever, tachycardia, or hyperthyroidism

 Early fetal hypoxia
 Fetal infection or dysrhythmia
 Prematurity.
Decreased variability—fluctuation of less than 5 beats/minute from FHR baseline—may result from:
 Vagolytic drugs
 Fetal cardiac dysrhythmia
 Fetal heart block
 Fetal hypoxia
 Central nervous system malformation
 Infections.
Early decelerations (slowing of FHR at onset of contraction, with recovery to baseline no longer than 15 seconds after completion of uterine contraction) are related to:
 Fetal head compression (and usually ensure fetal health).
Late decelerations (slowing of FHR, with onset after the start of the contraction, a lag time longer than 20 seconds, and a recovery time longer than 15 seconds) may be related to:
 Uteroplacental insufficiency
 Fetal hypoxia, or acidosis.
Recurrent and persistent late decelerations with decreased variability usually indicate:
 Serious fetal distress that may result from conduction (spinal, caudal, or epidural) anesthesia or fetal depression.
Variable decelerations (sudden, precipitous drops in FHR unrelated to uterine contractions) are commonly related to:
 Cord compression.
A severe drop in FHR (to less than 70 beats/minute for longer than 60 seconds) with decreased variability indicates:
 Fetal distress, and may result in a depressed neonate.
Decreased intrauterine pressure during labor that is not progressing normally may require:
 Oxytocin stimulation.
Elevated intrauterine pressure readings may indicate:
 Abruptio placentae
 Overstimulation from oxytocin.

Normal Intrauterine Pressure Readings During Labor

Stage of Labor	Frequency (Number of contractions per 10 minutes)	Baseline Pressure (mm Hg)	Pressure During Contraction (mm Hg)
Prelabor	1 to 2	—	25 to 40
First stage	3 to 5	8 to 12	30 to 40 (or more)
Second stage	5	10 to 20	50 to 80

The basics

In internal fetal monitoring, an invasive procedure, an electrode attached directly to the fetal scalp measures the FHR—especially its beat-to-beat variability—and a fluid-filled catheter that has been introduced into the uterine cavity measures the frequency and pressure of uterine contractions. This procedure is performed exclusively during labor, after the membranes have ruptured and the cervix has dilated 1¼" (3 cm), with the fetal head lower than the -2 station. Internal monitoring is indicated when external monitoring provides inadequate or suspicious data. Since internal monitoring records FHR directly, it supplies more accurate information about fetal health than external monitoring; measuring the pressure of uterine contractions allows better assessment of the progress of labor. Consequently, internal monitoring is especially useful in determining if cesarean birth is necessary.

When FHR patterns indicate fetal distress, fetal oxygenation can often be improved by loading maternal fluids to increase placental perfusion, turning the mother on her side (preferably the left) to alleviate supine hypotension, and administering oxygen to the mother. If these measures return heart rate patterns to normal, labor may continue. If abnormal patterns persist, cesarean birth may be necessary. Poor beat-to-beat variability without periodic patterns may indicate fetal stress, requiring further evaluation such as analysis of fetal blood gases.

Risks to the mother (perforated uterus or intrauterine infection) or to the fetus (scalp abscess or hematoma) from internal fetal monitoring are small, and the benefit is more accurate information about fetal health.

Contraindications to this test include: uncertainty as to the fetal presenting part, technical inability to attach the lead, or cervical or vaginal herpes lesions.

Procedure

Measuring FHR:

• Place the patient in dorsal lithotomy position, and prepare her perineal area for a vaginal examination, explaining each step of the procedure as it is performed.

• As the procedure begins, ask the patient to breathe through her mouth and to concentrate on relaxing her abdominal muscles.

• After the vaginal examination, the fetal scalp is palpated, and an area not over a fontanelle is identified.

• The plastic guide tube surrounding the small corkscrew-type electrode is introduced into the cervix, pressed firmly against the fetal scalp, and rotated 180° clockwise to insert the electrode into the scalp.

• After the electrode wire is tugged slightly to make sure it is attached properly, the tube is withdrawn, leaving the electrode in place.

• After a conduction medium is applied to a leg plate, the leg plate is strapped to the mother's thigh. The electrode wires are attached to the leg plate, and a cable from the leg plate is plugged into the fetal monitor.

• To check proper placement of the scalp electrode, the monitor is turned on and the EKG button is pressed; an FHR signal indicates proper electrode attachment.

Measuring uterine contractions:

• Before inserting the uterine catheter, fill it with sterile normal saline solution to prevent air emboli. Explain each step of the procedure to the patient, and ask her to breathe deeply through her mouth and to concentrate on relaxing her abdominal muscles.

• After the vagina has been examined and the presenting part of the fetus has been palpated, the fluid-filled catheter and catheter guide are inserted ⅜″ to ¾″ (1 to 2 cm) into the cervix, usually between the fetal head and the posterior cervix.

• The catheter is then gently inserted into the uterus until the black mark on the catheter is flush with the vulva (the catheter guide should *never* be passed deeply into the uterus).

• The guide is removed and the catheter is connected to a transducer that converts the intrauterine pressure, as measured by the fluid in the catheter, into an electrical signal.

• To standardize pressure readings, the transducer is exposed to air (it should measure zero pressure).

• The system is then closed to the air, and intrauterine pressure readings are checked.

Special precautions

• Prevent artifactual pressure readings by flushing the pressure transducer with normal saline solution; to relieve catheter obstruction (by vernix caseosa, for example), inject a small amount of sterile normal saline solution into the catheter while the transducer is isolated from the system.

• Be sure that a low heart rate is actually the FHR (the fetal tachometer may be recording a maternal heart rate).

• Check that the fetal scalp electrode and the uterine catheter are removed before cesarean birth.

Patient care checklist

Before the test

☑ Explain or clarify test purpose and procedure.

☑ Warn the patient that she may feel mild discomfort when the uterine catheter and scalp electrode are inserted, but reassure her that this part of the procedure takes only a few minutes.

☑ Evaluate patient understanding.

☑ Make sure the patient has signed a consent form.

After the test

☑ After removal of the fetal scalp electrode, apply antiseptic or antibiotic solution to the site of attachment.

☑ Watch for signs of fetal scalp abscess or maternal intrauterine infection.

Interfering factors

Drugs that affect the parasympathetic and the sympathetic nervous systems may influence FHR.

Fluorescein angiography

Purpose

To document retinal circulation as an aid in evaluating intraocular abnormalities such as retinopathy, tumors, and circulatory or inflammatory disorders.

Normal results

Normal retinal vessels with no leakage; normal retina and choroidal circulation.

Abnormal results
Fluorescein angiography may reveal:
Microaneurysms
Arteriovenous shunts
Neovascularization
Arterial occlusion
Stenosis
Prolonged venous drainage
Venous occlusion
Increased vascular tortuosity
Capillary hemangiomas
Tumors
Retinal edema or inflammation
Fibrous tissue
Papilledema.

The basics
In this test, rapid-sequence photographs of the fundus are taken with a special camera following I.V. injection of sodium fluorescein, a contrast medium. The fluorescein dye and the use of sophisticated photographic equipment enhance the visibility of microvascular structures of the retina and choroid, allowing evaluation of the entire retinal vascular bed, including retinal circulation. Thus, fluorescein angiography records the appearance of blood vessels inside the eye.

Procedure
• Mydriatic eye drops are administered.
• The patient is seated comfortably in the examining chair, facing the camera.
• The patient is asked to loosen or remove any restrictive clothing around his neck, and to place his chin in the chin rest and his forehead against the bar.
• The antecubital vein is prepared and punctured.
• Preinjection photographs are taken, and then the dye is injected into the vein.
• As the dye is injected, 25 to 30 photographs are taken in rapid sequence.
• The needle and syringe are removed, and pressure and a dressing are applied to the injection site.

• If late-phase photographs have been requested, the patient may relax for 20 minutes.
• After 20 minutes, the patient is positioned for 5 to 10 late-phase photographs.
• If ordered, photographs may be taken up to 1 hour after the injection.

Special precautions
• Be sure to check for proper placement of the needle in the patient's vein, since extravasation of the dye around the injection site is very painful.
• The patient may briefly experience nausea and a feeling of warmth. Reassure him, as necessary, and observe for hypersensitivity reactions, such as vomiting, dry mouth, metallic taste, sudden increased salivation, sneezing, light-headedness, fainting, and hives. Rarely, anaphylactic shock may result.

Patient care checklist
Before the test
☑ Explain or clarify test purpose and procedure.
☑ Explain to the patient that eye drops will be instilled to dilate his pupils, and that a dye will be injected into his arm. Tell him that his eyes will be photographed with a special camera before and after the injection.
☑ Warn him that his skin and urine may appear yellow after the test, but these effects will disappear within 24 to 48 hours.
☑ Tell the patient that his near vision will be blurred for up to 12 hours.
☑ Evaluate patient understanding.
☑ Check the patient's history for glaucoma and hypersensitivity to contrast media and dilating eye drops.
☑ Withhold medications that may interfere with test results, as ordered.
☑ Make sure that the patient or a responsible family member has signed a consent form.

Interfering factors
• The use of miotic eye drops will prevent an adequate view of the fundus.

• Cataracts, media opacity, or inability of the patient to keep his eyes open and to maintain fixation will interfere with accuracy of test results.

His bundle electrography

Purpose
• To diagnose dysrhythmias and conduction anomalies
• To determine the need for implanted pacemakers and cardioactive drugs, and to evaluate their effects on the conduction system and ectopic rhythms
• To locate the site of a bundle branch block, especially in asymptomatic patients with conduction disturbances.

Normal results
Normal conduction intervals in adults:
H-V interval, 35 to 55 msec
A-H interval, 45 to 150 msec
P-A interval, 20 to 40 msec.
(Also see *Normal His Bundle Electrogram*.)

Abnormal results
A prolonged H-V interval can result from:
    Acute or chronic disease.
Atrioventricular nodal (A-H interval) delays can stem from:
    Atrial pacing
    Chronic conduction system disease
    Carotid sinus pressure
    Recent myocardial infarction
    Drugs.
Intraatrial (P-A interval) delays can result from:
    Atrial disease (acquired, surgically induced, or congenital)
    Atrial pacing.

The basics
His bundle electrography permits measurement of discrete conduction intervals by recording electrical conduction during the slow withdrawal of a bipolar or tripolar electrode catheter

from the right ventricle through the His bundle to the sinoatrial node. The catheter is introduced into the femoral vein and passed through the right atrium and across the septal leaflet of the tricuspid valve.

The His bundle electrogram can lo-

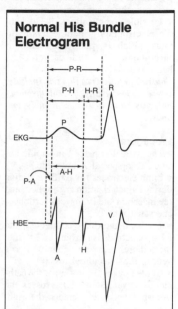

Normal His Bundle Electrogram

In a normal His bundle electrogram, atrial activation appears as a sharp diphasic or triphasic wave (A) during the P wave, followed by His bundle deflection (H) and ventricular activation (V). By measuring the interval between the beginning of the P wave and His bundle activation (P-H interval) or the interval between the beginning of the atrial wave and His bundle activation (A-H interval), abnormally prolonged A-V nodal conduction can be detected.

Adapted with permission from H.H. Hecht and C.E. Kossmann, "Atrioventricular and Intraventricular Conduction," *American Journal of Cardiology,* 31:232-244.

calize disturbances within the atrioventricular conduction system. When an ectopic site takes over as pacemaker of the heart, the electrogram can help pinpoint its origin. The test also aids in diagnosis of syncope, evaluates a candidate for permanent artificial pacemaker implantation, and helps select or evaluate antiarrhythmic drugs.

Possible complications of His bundle electrography include dysrhythmias, phlebitis, pulmonary emboli, thromboemboli, and catheter-site hemorrhage.

Contraindications to this test include: severe coagulopathy, recent thrombophlebitis, and acute pulmonary embolism.

Procedure

• The patient is placed in supine position on a special X-ray table.
• Limb electrodes for EKG recording during catheterization are applied, and the insertion site is shaved, scrubbed, and sterilized.
• The local anesthetic is injected, and a J-tip electrode is introduced I.V. into the femoral vein (occasionally, into a vein in the antecubital fossa).
• Guided by the fluoroscope, the catheter is advanced until it crosses the tricuspid valve and enters the right ventricle.
• The catheter is slowly withdrawn from the tricuspid area, and recordings of conduction intervals are made from each pole of the catheter, either simultaneously or sequentially.
• After recordings and measurements are completed, the catheter is removed and a pressure dressing is applied to the site.
• The procedure takes 1 to 3 hours to perform.

Special precautions

CLINICAL ALERT: **Be sure emergency medication is available in case the patient develops dysrhythmias during the test.**

Patient care checklist
Before the test
☑ Explain or clarify test purpose, preparation, procedure, and post-test care.
☑ Evaluate patient understanding.
☑ Restrict food and fluids for at least 6 hours before the test.
☑ Make sure that the patient or a responsible member of the family has signed a consent form.
☑ Just before the test, advise the patient to void.
After the test
☑ Monitor the patient's vital signs, as ordered. Observe for shortness of breath, chest pain, pallor, or changes in pulse rate or blood pressure.
☑ Enforce bed rest for 4 to 6 hours.
☑ Check catheter insertion site for bleeding, as ordered—usually every 30 minutes for 8 hours; apply a pressure bandage until the bleeding stops.
☑ Be sure a 12-lead resting EKG is scheduled to assess for changes.

Interfering factors
Malfunctioning recording equipment or improper catheter positioning interferes with accurate testing.

Impedance plethysmography
[occlusive impedance phlebography]

Purpose
• To detect deep-vein thrombosis (DVT) in the proximal deep veins of the leg
• To screen patients at high risk for thrombophlebitis
• To evaluate patients with a suspected pulmonary embolism (since most pulmonary emboli are complications of DVT in the leg).

Normal results
Temporary venous occlusion normally produces a sharp rise in venous volume; release of the occlusion produces

rapid venous outflow, as recorded on a strip chart tracing.

Abnormal results

With DVT, the strip chart tracing indicates impeded venous volume and venous outflow.

The basics

Impedance plethysmography—a reliable, widely used, noninvasive test for measuring venous flow in the limbs—aims principally to detect DVT in the leg. Electrodes from a plethysmograph are applied to the patient's leg to record changes in electrical resistance (impedance) caused by blood volume variations—the result of respiration or venous occlusion. If a pressure cuff applied to the thigh is inflated to temporarily occlude venous return without interfering with arterial blood flow, blood volume in the calf distal to the cuff normally increases. However, in DVT, blood volume increases less than expected because the veins are already at capacity, and cuff release causes an abnormally slow return of blood volume to physiologic levels.

This test is especially sensitive for DVT in the popliteal and iliofemoral venous systems. It is less sensitive for calf vein clots or partially occlusive thrombi, since these are less likely to cause detectable obstruction in veins below the knee.

Procedure

• The patient is placed in supine position, with the leg being tested elevated 30 to 35 degrees to promote venous drainage (the calf should be above heart level).
• He is asked to flex his knee slightly and to rotate his hips by shifting his weight to the same side as the leg being tested.
• After the electrodes (connected to the plethysmograph) have been loosely attached to the calf, about 3″ to 4″ (7.5 to 10 cm) apart, the pressure cuff (connected to an air pressure system) is wrapped snugly around the thigh—about 2″ (5 cm) above the knee.
• The pressure cuff is inflated with 45 to 60 cm of water, allowing full venous distention without interfering with arterial blood flow.
• Pressure is maintained for 45 seconds or until the tracing stabilizes. (In a patient with reduced arterial blood flow, pressure is maintained for 2 minutes or longer to permit complete venous filling, then the pressure cuff is rapidly deflated.)
• The strip chart tracing, which records the increase in the venous volume following cuff inflation and the decrease in venous volume 3 seconds after deflation, is checked.
• The test is repeated for the other leg.
• If necessary, three to five tracings for each leg are obtained to confirm full venous filling and outflow; the tracing showing the greatest rise and fall in venous volume is used as the test result. If the result is ambiguous, the position of the patient's leg and placement of the cuff and electrode are checked.
• The test takes 30 to 45 minutes to perform.

Patient care checklist

Before the test

☑ Explain or clarify test purpose and procedure.

☑ Emphasize that accurate testing requires that the leg muscles be relaxed and breathing be normal. Reassure the patient that, if he experiences pain that may interfere with leg relaxation, a mild analgesic will be administered, as ordered.

☑ Evaluate patient understanding.

☑ Just before the test, instruct the patient to void and to put on a hospital gown.

After the test

☑ Be sure the conductive gel is removed from the patient's skin.

Interfering factors

• Decreased peripheral arterial blood flow resulting from shock, increased vasoconstriction, low cardiac output, or arterial tree occlusive disease may interfere with test results.

• Extrinsic venous compression, such as from pelvic tumors, large hematomas, or constricting clothing or bandages, may alter test results.

• Patient failure to relax leg muscles completely or to breathe normally may interfere with accurate determination of test results.

• Coldness of extremities because of environmental factors can interfere with accurate readings.

Lumbar, thoracic, and cervical thermography

Purpose
To evaluate sensory nerve irritation or significant soft-tissue injury.

Normal results
Thermograms show diffused heat patterns with relative left-right symmetry.

Abnormal results
A difference of 1° C. between 25% of the surface area on one side of the spine and the other side is abnormal. If the abnormality follows the course of a specific dermatome, sensory nerve irritation may exist at this level. Soft-tissue injuries appear as local abnormalities.

The basics
Using infrared sensors, thermography measures and compares the heat emitted from two adjacent areas of skin surface. Irritation of a nerve root may produce an abnormal heat pattern along the course of its dermatome, the area of skin supplied with afferent fibers by the nerve root; thermography can often graphically demonstrate such changes. Lumbar, thoracic, and cervical thermography, specifically, can thus be helpful in evaluating sensory nerve irritation or significant soft-tissue injury. The usual clinical indication for this test is back pain—often severe and possibly chronic—such as chronic lumbar pain.

The patient should not undergo physical therapy or electromyography on the same day that thermography is to be performed.

To verify test results, thermography is repeated three times at 20-minute intervals. An abnormality caused by organic disease should be reproducible on the thermogram at any given time. Thermography complements tests such as electromyography, myelography, and computerized tomography scans.

Procedure
• After the patient undresses, his back is cooled with room-temperature water (68° F. [20° C.]) and is blown dry with cool air from a hair dryer.

• The patient may then relax for 10 to 15 minutes before the procedure begins.

• A lumbar examination includes scans of the low back, the buttocks, and both legs.

• For a thoracic examination, only the posterior chest is scanned.

• For a cervical examination, thermograms of the back of the neck, the back of the shoulders, and both arms are taken.

• The procedure takes about 1½ hours.

Patient care checklist
Before the test

☑ Explain or clarify test purpose, preparation, and procedure.

☑ Reassure the patient that thermography is painless and does not expose him to radiation.

☑ Instruct him not to smoke for several hours before the test.

☑ Evaluate patient understanding.

Interfering factors

• Smoking affects vascular distribution, producing abnormalities that reflect impaired circulation and do not follow the course of sensory dermatomes.

• A patient history of fractures, surgery, or grossly asymmetrical varicose veins may cause abnormal test results.

• Direct or indirect drafts on the patient during testing will interfere with test results.

Magnetic resonance imaging
(MRI) [Nuclear magnetic resonance (NMR)]

Purpose
To aid in diagnosis of intracranial and spinal lesions and of cardiovascular and soft-tissue abnormalities.

Normal results
The image shows normal anatomic and biochemical tissue details in any plane, without bone interference. Tissue color and shading will vary, depending on the radio frequency (RF) energy, magnetic strength, and degree of computer enhancement.

Abnormal results
MRI can detect:
  Cerebral edema
  Demyelinating disease, such as multiple sclerosis
  Plaque formations
  Infarctions
  Tumors
  Blood clots
  Hemorrhage
  Abscesses.

The basics
Although its full range of clinical applications has yet to be established, MRI is already recognized as a safe, valuable tool for neurologic diagnosis. MRI's greatest advantages are its ability to "see through" bone and to de-

lineate fluid-filled soft tissue in great detail. It provides greater tissue discrimination than computerized tomography scanning without the risk of ionizing radiation or injected contrast solutions, and may permit safe serial studies of children and pregnant women.

MRI, a noninvasive imaging technique, relies on the magnetic properties of the atom. (Hydrogen, the most abundant and magnetically sensitive of the body's atoms, is most commonly selected for MRI studies.) The scanner uses a powerful magnetic field and RF energy to produce images based on the hydrogen (primarily water) content of body tissues. Exposed to an external magnetic field, positively charged atomic nuclei and their negatively charged electrons align uniformly in the field. RF energy is then directed at the atoms, knocking them out of this magnetic alignment and causing them to *precess,* or spin. When the RF pulse is discontinued, the atoms realign themselves with the magnetic field, emitting RF energy as a tissue-specific signal based on the relative density of nuclei and the realignment time. These signals are monitored by the MRI computer, which processes them and displays the information on a video monitor as a high-resolution image.

The magnetic fields and RF energy used for MRI are imperceptible by the patient; no harmful effects have been documented. Research is continuing on the optimal magnetic fields and RF waves for each type of tissue.

In cardiovascular testing, MRI may allow visualization of blood flow, cardiac chambers, the intraventricular septum, and valvular areas. Phosphorous MRI may aid in diagnosis of peripheral vascular disease. Uses of MRI are still evolving. Soon, in fact, it may be able to provide *in vivo* information about cellular processes.

Contraindications to MRI include: ferrous metal implants, such as pacemakers, intracranial aneurysm clips, or orthopedic screws, because MRI works through a powerful magnetic field.

Procedure

• The patient is placed in a supine position on a narrow bed and asked to lie still.

• The bed then slides him to the desired position inside the scanner, where RF energy is directed at his head, spine, or other area of interest.

• The resulting images are displayed on a monitor and recorded on film or magnetic tape for permanent storage.

• The radiologist may vary RF waves and use the computer to manipulate and enhance the images.

• The procedure may take up to 90 minutes to perform.

Patient care checklist

Before the test

☑ Explain or clarify test purpose, preparation, and procedure.

☑ Stress that the test is painless and involves no exposure to radiation.

☑ Evaluate patient understanding.

☑ Ask the patient to wear a loose-fitting hospital gown. (Outpatients may wear any comfortable clothing.)

☑ Since watches and jewelry can be damaged by the strong magnetic field, ask the patient to remove all metal objects before the test begins.

Interfering factors

Excessive movement can blur images.

Oculoplethysmography
(OPG)

Purpose

To aid in detection and evaluation of carotid occlusive disease.

Normal results

OPG:

All pulses should occur simultaneously.

Ocular pneumoplethysmography (OPG-Gee):

The difference between ophthalmic artery pressures should be less than 5 mm Hg. Ophthalmic artery pressure divided by the higher brachial systolic pressure should be more than 0.67.

Abnormal results

For OPG, a delay in pulse arrival in the ipsilateral eye or ear indicates:

Carotid occlusive disease.

For OPG-Gee, a difference between ophthalmic artery pressures of more than 5 mm Hg suggests:

Carotid occlusive disease on the side with the lower pressure.

For OPG-Gee, a ratio between the ophthalmic artery pressure and the higher brachial systolic pressure of less than 0.67 reinforces:

Diagnosis of carotid occlusive disease. (The lower the ratio, the more severe the stenosis.)

The basics

An important cerebrovascular test, OPG is a noninvasive procedure that indirectly measures blood flow in the ophthalmic artery. Since the ophthalmic artery is the first major branch of the internal carotid artery, its blood flow accurately reflects carotid blood flow and ultimately that of cerebral circulation. Two techniques are used for this test. In OPG, pulse arrival times in the eyes and ears are measured and compared to detect carotid occlusive disease. Although the length of the delay is related to the degree of carotid artery stenosis, this test only estimates the extent of stenosis and cannot give an exact percentage.

In OPG-Gee, ophthalmic artery pressures are indirectly measured and compared with the higher brachial pressure and with each other. As in OPG, OPG-Gee only estimates the degree of stenosis present, and angiography may be necessary for precise evaluation.

Indications for both oculoplethysmographic techniques include symp-

Carotid Phonoangiography

An often valuable complement to oculoplethysmography, carotid phonoangiography graphically records the intensity of carotid bruits during systolic and diastolic phases. It thus helps identify the presence, site, and severity of carotid artery occlusive disease.

For this test, the patient assumes a supine position and holds his breath while a transducer is placed at several sites along the carotid artery. Soundings are made directly over the clavicle (common carotid artery), midway up the neck (carotid bifurcation), and directly below the mandible (internal carotid artery). Oscillographic recordings are obtained and stored on both Polaroid film and magnetic tape for later study.

Absence of bruits generally indicates an absence of significant carotid artery disease. However, bruits may also be absent when stenosis approaches total occlusion. Bruits heard at all three sites, but loudest over the clavicle, usually originate in the aortic arch or within the heart. Blood flow in the carotid artery itself is unobstructed. Bruits heard over the carotid bifurcation and internal carotid sites, but louder over the latter, indicate turbulent blood flow within the internal carotid artery and the likely presence of a lesion of greater than 40% occlusion.

Carotid phonoangiography is a quick test and relatively simple to perform, but it is less sensitive and less specific than other noninvasive techniques, such as carotid imaging with Doppler ultrasound. Nevertheless, this test is approximately 85% accurate in detecting stenosis of the carotid artery of more than 40%.

toms of transient ischemic attacks, asymptomatic carotid bruits, and non-hemispheric neurologic symptoms such as dizziness, ataxia, or syncope. This test may also be performed as a follow-up procedure after carotid endarterectomy or with carotid phonoangiography or carotid imaging.

Contraindications for oculoplethysmography include recent eye surgery (within 2 to 6 months), previous enucleation, a history of retinal detachment or lens implantation, or hypersensitivity to the local anesthetic. Contraindications for OPG-Gee include current anticoagulant therapy because of the risk of scleral hematoma or erythema.

(Also see *Carotid Phonoangiography*.)

Procedure

For OPG:

• Anesthetic eye drops are instilled to minimize patient discomfort during the test.

• Small photoelectric cells are attached to the earlobes; these cells can detect blood flow to the ear through the external carotid artery.

• Tracings for both ears are taken and compared, but only right-ear tracings are compared with tracings of the eyes. (Tracings for the ears should be the same; if they are not, this is considered during interpretation of test results.)

• Eyecups resembling contact lenses are applied to the corneas and are held in place with light suction (40 to 50 mm Hg).

• Tracings of the pulsations within each eye are compared with each other and with tracings for the right ear.

For OPG-Gee:

• Anesthetic eye drops are instilled, as for OPG, and eyecups like those used in OPG are attached to the scleras of the eyes.

• A vacuum of 300 mm Hg is applied to each eye, corresponding to a mean pressure of 100 mm Hg in the ophthalmic artery, and gradually released.

• With the application of suction, the pulse in both eyes disappears; with the gradual release of suction, both pulses should return simultaneously.
• Pulse arrival times are converted to ophthalmic artery pressures, and then compared.
• Both brachial pressures are taken. The higher systolic pressure is then compared with the ophthalmic artery pressures.

Special precautions
To limit the risk of corneal abrasion, both techniques must be performed only by specially trained personnel.

Patient care checklist
Before the test
☑ Explain or clarify test purpose, preparation, procedure, and post-test care.
☑ Warn the patient that his eyes may burn slightly after the eye drops are instilled.
☑ If OPG-Gee is scheduled, warn him that he may experience transient loss of vision when suction is applied to the eyes.
☑ Instruct him not to blink or move during the procedure.
☑ If he wears contact lenses, tell him to remove them before the test.
☑ Inform patients with glaucoma that they may take their usual medications and eye drops.
☑ Evaluate patient understanding.
After the test
☑ To prevent corneal abrasions, instruct the patient not to rub his eyes for 2 hours after the test. Observe for symptoms of corneal abrasion, such as pain or photophobia, and report them to the physician.
☑ Mild burning as the eye drops wear off is normal. Report severe burning.
☑ If the patient wears contact lenses, instruct him not to reinsert them for about 2 hours after OPG to allow the effect of the anesthetic drops to wear off.

Interfering factors
• In patients with hypertension, OPG-Gee test results may be more difficult to interpret due to elevated ophthalmic artery pressures.
• Constant blinking or nystagmus may cause an artifact, making the tracings difficult to interpret.
• Severe cardiac dysrhythmias may alter test results.

Phonocardiography *(PCG)*

Purpose
• To aid in the precise timing of cardiac events
• To aid in calculation of systolic time intervals
• To help diagnose valvular abnormalities and other cardiac disorders.

Normal results
A normal PCG has a smooth baseline interrupted by vibrations from the major heart sounds. The first and second heart sounds, S_1 and S_2, generate the strongest vibrations, which appear as spikes above and below the baseline. The third and fourth heart sounds, S_3 and S_4, generate weaker vibrations than the S_1 and S_2. S_3, or ventricular gallop, may be normal in children and in adults with high cardiac output. S_4, or atrial gallop, may sometimes occur under normal conditions. (See *Understanding Heart Sounds*.)

Abnormal results
Phonocardiography can help reveal:
  Valvular disorders
  Hypertrophic cardiomyopathies
  Left ventricular failure.

The basics
Phonocardiography graphically records audible vibrations produced as blood courses through the heart and great vessels. This test is valuable for locating and timing abnormal heart sounds detected on auscultation, and for diagnosing valvular abnormalities.

Understanding Heart Sounds

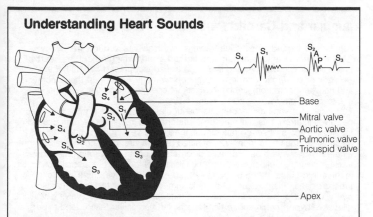

Base
Mitral valve
Aortic valve
Pulmonic valve
Tricuspid valve

Apex

Although the physiologic cause of heart sounds has not been clearly defined, S_1 probably results from closure of the mitral and tricuspid valves; S_2, closure of the aortic and pulmonic valves; S_3, early rapid filling of the ventricles with limited distensibility; and S_4, atrial contraction against increasing ventricular resistance, as shown above. The accompanying phonocardiogram shows the S_3 and S_4 sounds in relation to the S_1 and S_2 sounds.

During phonocardiography, microphones are placed on the patient's chest, usually at the apex and the base of the heart. A transducer in each microphone picks up heart sounds, amplifies them, converts them to electrical impulses, and relays these impulses to a recorder, which produces a graph of heart sounds in waveform—a PCG.

Phonocardiography is usually performed simultaneously with electrocardiography, carotid and/or jugular pulse wave tracings, and apexcardiography. Together, these tests permit precise timing of heart sounds and cardiac events.

(Also see *Jugular and Carotid Pulse Wave Tracings*, p. 642, and *Measuring Systolic Time Intervals*, p. 643.)

Procedure
• The patient is placed in supine position and is prepared for electrocardiography, apexcardiography, and carotid and/or jugular pulse wave tracing.

• The apex and base of the heart are located with a stethoscope, and microphones are strapped to the patient's chest.

• Both sites may be recorded simultaneously, or the base site may be recorded first; 4 complete cardiac cycles are recorded in patients with sinus rhythm, and 7 to 10 cycles in those with cardiac dysrhythmias.

• To record changes in heart sounds under different conditions, the patient may be asked to assume various positions (supine, upright, and left lateral oblique), to breathe in and out slowly or to hold his breath, to perform isometric exercises, or to inhale amyl nitrite.

• The procedure takes 15 to 30 minutes.

Jugular and Carotid Pulse Wave Tracings

Jugular and carotid pulse wave tracings graphically record low-frequency vibrations from the jugular vein and carotid artery, which reflect the heart's pulsations during diastole and systole. A transducer placed over either the jugular vein or carotid artery, 1 to 2 cm below the jaw, picks up these vibrations and converts them from kinetic to electrical energy. A recorder then shapes this electrical energy into pulse wave tracings.

The superior vena cava connects the jugular vein and the right atrium. Since no valves interrupt this pathway, pressure changes in the right atrium caused by diastole and systole are reflected in the jugular vein. Jugular pulse wave tracings can thus help identify right sided heart failure, causing increased right atrial pressure, and tricuspid valve disorders. In contrast, carotid pulse wave tracings primarily reflect events on the left side of the heart, especially changes in the aortic pulse. When blood is ejected from the left ventricle, aortic pressure rises; this pressure change is immediately reflected in the carotid artery. Carotid pulse wave tracings can thus help identify aortic valve disease, idiopathic hypertrophic subaortic stenosis, left ventricular failure, and hypertension.

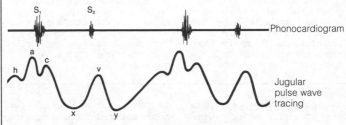

The jugular pulse wave tracing normally has three positive waves (a, c, and v) and two negative waves (x and y). The a wave shows right atrial contraction, usually as a dominant positive wave; the c wave, right ventricular contraction causing bulging of the tricuspid valve into the atrium; the x wave, right atrial relaxation; the v wave, passive filling of the right atrium; the y wave, opening of the tricuspid valve and emptying of the right atrium; and the h wave, conclusion of right ventricular filling.

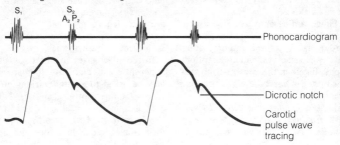

The carotid pulse wave tracing normally has a prominent positive wave coinciding with systole and a smaller positive wave coinciding with diastole. The characteristic dicrotic notch marks the closure of the aortic (A_2) and pulmonic (P_2) valves.

Patient care checklist
Before the test
☑ Explain or clarify test purpose and procedure.
☑ Reassure the patient that the procedure is safe and painless. Mention that additional tests (electrocardiography, carotid and/or jugular pulse wave tracings, and apexcardiography) are usually performed simultaneously with phonocardiography.
☑ Evaluate patient understanding.

Interfering factors
• Incorrect placement of or pressure on the microphone, background noise, or patient movement (muscle tremors, shivering) interferes with accurate determination of test results.
• Obesity makes heart sounds difficult to detect.

Measuring Systolic Time Intervals

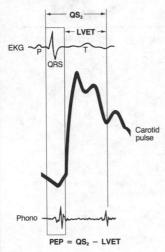

$$PEP = QS_2 - LVET$$

Systolic time intervals are made up of the pre-ejection period (PEP), left ventricular ejection time (LVET), and total electromechanical systole (QS_2). As shown above, they can be measured by correlating the results from three simultaneously performed tests: phonocardiography, electrocardiography, and carotid pulse wave tracing. The PEP:LVET ratio reflects the efficiency of left ventricular contraction and thus helps identify cardiac abnormalities. For example, in left ventricular dysfunction, PEP increases and LVET decreases; conversely, in hypertension, PEP decreases and LVET increases.

Pulmonary artery catheterization
[Swan-Ganz catheterization, balloon flotation catheterization of the pulmonary artery, right heart catheterization]

Purpose
• To help assess right and left ventricular failure.
• To monitor therapy for complications of acute myocardial infarction, such as cardiogenic shock, pulmonary edema, fluid-related hypovolemia and hypotension, systolic murmur, unexplained sinus tachycardia, and various cardiac dysrhythmias
• To monitor fluid status in patients with serious burns, renal disease, or shock lung (noncardiogenic pulmonary edema) after open-heart surgery
• To monitor the effects of cardiovascular drugs, such as nitroglycerin and nitroprusside.

Normal results
Normal pressures are as follows:
Right atrial: 1 to 6 mm Hg
Systolic right ventricular: 20 to 30 mm Hg
End diastolic right ventricular: < 5 mm Hg
Systolic pulmonary artery pressure (PAP): 20 to 30 mm Hg (same as right ventricular pressure)
Diastolic PAP: about 10 mm Hg (same as left atrial pressure)

Pulmonary Artery Catheter Insertion

As the catheter is directed through the right heart chambers to its wedge position, it produces distinctive waveforms on the oscilloscope screen that are important indicators of the catheter's position in the heart.

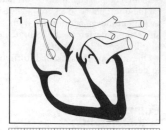

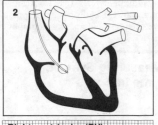

Right atrial (RA) pressure

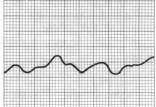

Right ventricular (RV) pressure

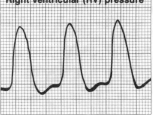

1. When the catheter tip reaches the right atrium from the superior vena cava, the waveform on the oscilloscope screen or readout strip looks like this. When it does, the physician inflates the catheter's balloon, which floats the tip through the tricuspid valve into the right ventricle.

2. When the catheter tip reaches the right ventricle, the waveform looks like this.

Mean PAP: < 20 mm Hg
Pulmonary artery wedge pressure (PAWP): 6 to 12 mm Hg
Left atrial: about 10 mm Hg.

Abnormal results

Increased right atrial pressure can indicate:
    Pulmonary disease
    Right ventricular failure
    Fluid overload
    Cardiac tamponade

    Tricuspid stenosis and regurgitation
    Pulmonary hypertension.
Increased right ventricular pressure can result from:
    Pulmonary hypertension
    Pulmonary valvular stenosis
    Right ventricular failure
    Pericardial effusion
    Constrictive pericarditis
    Chronic congestive heart failure
    Ventricular septal defects.

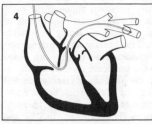

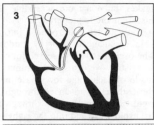

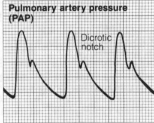

Pulmonary artery pressure (PAP)

Dicrotic notch

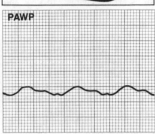

PAWP

3. A waveform like this one indicates that the balloon has floated the catheter tip through the pulmonic valve into the pulmonary artery. A dicrotic notch should be visible in the waveform, indicating the closing of the pulmonic valve.

4. Blood flow in the pulmonary artery then carries the catheter balloon into one of the pulmonary artery's many smaller branches. When the vessel becomes too narrow for the balloon to pass through, the balloon wedges in the vessel, occluding it. The monitor then displays a pulmonary artery wedge pressure (PAWP) waveform like this one.

Increased PAP is characteristic in:
  Increased pulmonary blood flow, such as in left-to-right shunt secondary to atrial or ventricular septal defect
  Increased pulmonary arteriolar resistance, such as in pulmonary hypertension or mitral stenosis
  Chronic obstructive pulmonary disease
  Pulmonary edema or embolus
  Left ventricular failure.

Increased PAWP can result from:
  Left ventricular failure
  Mitral stenosis and regurgitation
  Cardiac tamponade
  Cardiac insufficiency.
Decreased PAWP results from:
  Hypovolemia.

The basics
Pulmonary artery catheterization uses a balloon-tipped, flow-directed catheter to provide intermittent occlusion

of the pulmonary artery. Once the catheter is in place, this procedure permits measurement of both PAP and PAWP—the latter also known as pulmonary capillary wedge pressure. The PAWP reading accurately reflects left atrial pressure and left ventricular end-diastolic pressure, although the catheter itself never enters the left side of the heart. Such a reading is possible because the heart momentarily relaxes during diastole as it fills with blood from the pulmonary veins; at this instant, the pulmonary vasculature, left atrium, and left ventricle act as a single chamber, and all have identical pressures. Thus, changes in PAP and PAWP reflect changes in left ventricular filling pressure, permitting detection of left ventricular impairment.

Pulmonary artery systolic pressure is the same as right ventricular systolic pressure. Pulmonary artery diastolic pressure is the same as left atrial pressure, except in patients with severe pulmonary disease causing pulmonary hypertension; in such patients, catheterization still provides important diagnostic information.

Pulmonary artery catheterization is usually performed at bedside in an intensive care unit. The catheter is inserted through the cephalic vein in the antecubital fossa or the subclavian (sometimes, femoral) vein. It is threaded into the right atrium, the balloon is inflated, and the catheter follows the blood flow through the tricuspid valve into the right ventricle and out into the pulmonary artery.

In addition to measuring atrial and pulmonary aterial pressures, this procedure evaluates pulmonary vascular resistance and tissue oxygenation, as indicated by mixed venous oxygen content. It should be performed cautiously in patients with left bundle branch block or implanted pacemakers.

Procedure

• A two-, three-, or four-lumen (thermodilution) catheter is chosen, depending on the purpose of catheterization. The equipment is set up and checked according to the manufacturer's directions and hospital procedure.

• The patient is placed in a supine position, with his head and shoulders slightly lower than his trunk; this makes the vein more accessible. The insertion site is prepared.

• The catheter is introduced into the vein percutaneously or by cutdown. The oscilloscope is observed for characteristic waveforms, and printouts are made of each stage for a baseline as the catheter is advanced through the right atrium and passes through the tricuspid valve and into the right ventricle and pulmonary artery. (See *Pulmonary Artery Catheter Insertion*, pp. 644 and 645.)

• PAWP is recorded by inflating the balloon with air or carbon dioxide, using the smallest syringe possible. The catheter tip floats into the wedge position, indicated by the waveform; the pressure is recorded; the air is allowed to return to the syringe; and the catheter tip returns to the pulmonary artery. The system is then flushed and recalibrated.

• When the catheter's correct positioning and function are established, the catheter is sutured to the skin, and antibiotic ointment and an airtight dressing are applied to the insertion site.

• A chest X-ray film is obtained, as ordered, to verify catheter placement. (The radiology department should be notified before the procedure that a catheter is to be inserted.)

• Alarms are set on the EKG and pressure monitors.

• Vital signs, PAP waveforms, PAWP, and cardiac output are monitored routinely and as ordered. (See *Measuring Cardiac Output*.)

• When the catheter is no longer needed, the patient's blood pressure and radial pulse are taken. Then, the balloon is deflated, the dressing is removed, and the catheter is slowly withdrawn. The EKG is monitored for

Measuring Cardiac Output

Cardiac output—the amount of blood ejected from the right and left ventricles every 60 seconds—can be measured by a 4-lumen thermodilution catheter. One catheter lumen houses a thermistor, a pair of wires that terminate in a small bead located about 4 cm behind the catheter tip. The thermistor detects changes in blood temperature and transmits this information to a monitoring computer that calculates and displays cardiac output.

To measure cardiac output, 5 to 10 ml of cooled normal saline solution or 5% dextrose in water is injected into the proximal lumen over a period of 2 to 3 seconds. The fluid travels quickly through the right atrium and ventricle and into the pulmonary artery, where the thermistor bead records the temperature change.

Normal cardiac output is 4 to 8 liters/minute, the mean being 5 liters/minute. Cardiac output relates to body surface area, which is determined from the patient's height and weight using a nomogram. The cardiac output is divided by the figure obtained from the nomogram to get the *cardiac index*, which is a less size-dependent figure. A normal cardiac index is 2.5 to 5.0 liters/minute/m².

Decreased cardiac output and cardiac index may indicate impaired myocardial contractility caused by myocardial infarction or drugs (negative inotropics, such as procainamide, quinidine, or propranolol); acidosis or hypoxia; decreased left ventricular filling pressure caused by fluid depletion; increased systemic vascular resistance from arteriosclerosis or hypertension, or valvular heart disease causing decreased blood flow from the ventricles.

dysrhythmias. If any difficulty is encountered in removing the catheter, the procedure is stopped at once, and the physician is notified immediately.
• After the catheter is withdrawn, pressure, an antibiotic ointment, and a sterile dressing are applied to the insertion site. Blood pressure and radial pulse are checked.
• Insertion takes about 30 minutes. The catheter remains in place for 48 to 72 hours.

Special precautions
CLINICAL ALERT: As the catheter is passed into the right ventricular chamber, the oscilloscope screen is observed for frequent premature ventricular contractions and tachycardia—the results of catheter irritation of the right ventricle. If irritation occurs, the catheter may be partially withdrawn or medication administered to suppress the

dysrhythmia or right bundle branch block.
CLINICAL ALERT: The balloon catheter should not be overinflated. Overinflation could distend the pulmonary artery, causing vessel rupture.
• All connections are checked for air leaks that may have prevented balloon inflation, particularly if the patient is confused or uncooperative.
• After each PAWP reading, flush and recalibrate the monitoring system and make sure the balloon is completely deflated.
CLINICAL ALERT: If you encounter difficulty in flushing the system, notify the physician. Balloon rupture may cause a life-threatening air embolism.
• Maintain 300 mm Hg of pressure in the pressure bag to permit fluid flow of 3 to 6 ml/hour. Instruct the patient to extend the appropriate arm (or leg,

if the catheter is in the femoral vein). If the patient develops fever while the catheter is in place, remove the catheter and send the catheter tip to the laboratory for culture.

CLINICAL ALERT: **Make sure all stopcocks are properly positioned and all connections are secure. Loose connections during the test can allow rapid, massive arterial blood loss.**

• Be sure the lumen hubs are properly identified to serve the appropriate catheter ports. Do not add or remove fluids from the distal pulmonary artery port; this may cause pulmonary extravasation or damage the artery.

• If the catheter has not been sutured to the skin, tape it securely to prevent dislodgement.

Patient care checklist
Before the test

☑ Explain or clarify test purpose and procedure.

☑ Tell the patient that he will be conscious for the procedure, and that he may feel transient local discomfort from the administration of the local anesthetic.

☑ Instruct the patient to report any discomfort immediately.

☑ Have the patient or a responsible family member sign a consent form.

After the test

☑ Observe the catheter insertion site for signs of infection—redness, swelling, and discharge.

CLINICAL ALERT: **For 24 hours, watch for complications such as pulmonary emboli, pulmonary artery perforation, heart murmurs, thrombi, and dysrhythmias.**

Interfering factors

• Malfunctioning monitoring and recording devices, loose connections, clot formation at the catheter tip, air in the fluid column, or a ruptured balloon interfere with accurate testing.

• Incorrect catheter placement causes catheter fling—excessive catheter movement that produces a dampened pressure tracing.

• Migration of the catheter against a vessel wall may cause constant occlusion (permanent wedging) of the pulmonary artery.

• Mechanical ventilators with positive pressure cause increased intrathoracic pressure, which raises catheter pressure.

Pulmonary function tests

Purpose

• To determine the cause of dyspnea
• To assess the effectiveness of a specific therapeutic regimen
• To determine whether a functional abnormality is restrictive (inspiration impaired) or obstructive (expiration impaired)
• To estimate the degree of pulmonary dysfunction.

Normal results

Normal values are predicted for each patient based on age, height, weight, and sex and are expressed as a percentage. Usually, results are considered abnormal if they are less than 80% of these values. (See *Interpreting Pulmonary Function Tests*, p. 650.)

Abnormal results

The following pulmonary function test results indicate restrictive lung impairment: decreased total lung capacity, inspirational capacity, and vital capacity; decreased or normal functional residual capacity, inspiratory reserve volume, expiratory reserve, residual volume, and tidal volume; normal flow rates; and decreased lung compliance.

The following pulmonary function test results indicate obstructive lung impairment: decreased expiratory flow rates (including forced expiratory volume in 1 second, maximal breathing capacity, forced expiratory flow rate, and maximal midexpiratory flow rate);

and increased residual volume, functional residual capacity, and residual volume/total lung capacity ratio.

Also, see specific tests in *Interpreting Pulmonary Function Tests,* p. 650.

The basics

Pulmonary function tests (volume and capacity tests) are a series of measurements that evaluate ventilatory function through spirometric measurements and are performed on patients with suspected pulmonary dysfunction. Of the seven tests to determine volume, tidal volume (V_T) and expiratory reserve volume (ERV) are direct spirographic measurements; minute volume (V_E), carbon dioxide response, inspiratory reserve volume (IRV), and residual volume (RV) are calculated from the results of other pulmonary function tests; and thoracic gas volume (TGV) is calculated from body plethysmography.

Of the pulmonary capacity tests, vital capacity (VC), inspiratory capacity (IC), functional residual capacity (FRC), total lung capacity (TLC), and maximal midexpiratory flow (MMEF) may be measured directly or calculated from the results of other tests. Forced vital capacity (FVC), flow-volume curve, forced expiratory volume (FEV), peak expiratory flow rate (PEFR), and maximal voluntary ventilation (MVV) are direct spirographic measurements. The diffusing capacity for carbon monoxide (DL_{CO}) is calculated from the amount of carbon monoxide exhaled.

Contraindications to these tests include: acute coronary insufficiency, angina, or recent myocardial infarction.

Procedure

V_T:
• Tell the patient to breathe normally into the mouthpiece 10 times.

ERV:
• The patient is told to breathe into the mouthpiece 10 times and to exhale as completely as possible after each breath.

VC:
• The patient is told to inhale as deeply as possible and to exhale into the mouthpiece as completely as possible.
• This procedure is repeated three times, and the test result showing the largest volume is used.

IC:
• The patient is instructed to inhale fully, to exhale normally into the mouthpiece, and then to breathe normally 10 times, inhaling as deeply as possible after the 10th breath.

FRC:
• The patient is told to breathe normally into a spirometer that contains a known concentration of an insoluble gas (usually helium or nitrogen) in a known volume of air.
• After a few breaths, the concentrations of gas in the spirometer and in the lungs reach equilibrium.
• The point of equilibrium and the concentration of gas in the spirometer are recorded.
• Alternatively, the patient is placed in an airtight box called a *body plethysmograph,* and told to breathe air through a tube connected to a transducer.
• At end-expiration, the tube is occluded, the patient is told to pant, and changes in intrathoracic and plethysmographic pressures are measured.
• The results are used to calculate total TGV and FRC.

FVC and FEV:
• The patient is instructed to inhale as slowly and deeply as possible, and then asked to exhale into the mouthpiece as quickly and completely as possible.
• This procedure is repeated three times, and the largest volume is recorded.
• The volume of air expired at 1 second (FEV_1), at 2 seconds (FEV_2), and at 3 seconds (FEV_3) during all three repetitions is also recorded.

Interpreting Pulmonary Function Tests

Measurement of pulmonary function	Method of calculation	Abnormal results
Tidal volume (V_T): amount of air inhaled or exhaled during normal breathing	Determine the spirographic measurement for 10 breaths, and then divide by 10.	Decreased V_T may indicate restrictive disease and requires further testing, such as full pulmonary function studies or chest radiography.
Minute volume (V_E): total amount of air breathed per minute	Multiply V_T by the respiration rate.	Normal V_E can occur in emphysema; decreased V_E may indicate other diseases, such as pulmonary edema. Increased V_E can occur with acidosis, increased carbon dioxide (CO_2), decreased Po_2, exercise, and low compliance states.
CO_2 response: increase or decrease in V_E after breathing various CO_2 concentrations	Calculated by plotting changes in V_E against increasing inspired CO_2 concentrations	Reduced CO_2 response may indicate chronic bronchitis or other obstructive disease.
Inspiratory reserve volume (IRV): amount of air inspired over above-normal inspiration	Subtract V_T from inspiratory capacity.	Abnormal IRV alone does not indicate respiratory dysfunction; IRV decreases during normal exercise.
Expiratory reserve volume (ERV): amount of air exhaled after normal expiration	Direct spirographic measurement	ERV varies, even in healthy persons, but usually decreases in the obese.
Residual volume (RV): amount of air remaining in the lungs after forced expiration	Subtract ERV from functional residual capacity.	RV greater than 35% of total lung capacity (TLC) after maximal expiratory effort may indicate obstructive disease.
Vital capacity (VC): total volume of air that can be exhaled after maximum inspiration	Direct spirographic measurement, or add V_T, IRV, and ERV.	Normal or increased VC with decreased flow rates may indicate any condition that causes a reduction in functional pulmonary tissue. Decreased VC with normal or increased flow rates may indicate decreased respiratory effort, decreased thoracic expansion, or limited movement of the diaphragm.

(continued)

Interpreting Pulmonary Function Tests (continued)

Measurement of pulmonary function	Method of calculation	Abnormal results
Inspiratory capacity (IC): amount of air that can be inhaled after normal expiration	Direct spirographic measurement, or add IRV and V_T.	Decreased IC indicates restrictive disease.
Thoracic gas volume (TGV): total volume of gas in lungs from both ventilated and nonventilated airways	Body plethysmography	Increased TGV indicates air trapping, which may result from obstructive disease.
Functional residual capacity (FRC): amount of air remaining in lungs after normal expiration	Body plethysmography, helium dilution technique, or add ERV and RV	Increased FRC indicates overdistention of lungs, which may result from obstructive pulmonary disease.
Total lung capacity (TLC): total volume of the lungs when maximally inflated	Add V_T, IRV, ERV, and RV; or FRC and IC; or VC and RV.	Low TLC indicates restrictive disease; high TLC indicates overdistended lungs caused by obstructive disease.
Forced vital capacity (FVC): measurement of the amount of air exhaled forcefully and quickly after maximum inspiration	Direct spirographic measurement; expressed as a percentage of the total volume of gas exhaled	Decreased FVC indicates flow resistance in respiratory system from obstructive disease, such as chronic bronchitis, or from restrictive disease, such as pulmonary fibrosis.
Flow-volume curve (also called flow-volume loop): greatest rate of flow (Vmax) during FVC maneuvers versus lung volume change	Direct spirographic measurement at 1-second intervals; calculated from flow rates (expressed in liters/second) and lung volume changes (expressed in liters) during maximal inspiratory and expiratory maneuvers	Decreased flow rates at all volumes during expiration indicate obstructive disease of the small airways, such as emphysema. A plateau of expiratory flow near TLC, a plateau of inspiratory flow at mid-VC, and a square wave pattern through most of VC indicate obstructive disease of large airways. Normal or increased peak expiratory flow (PEF), decreased flow with decreasing lung volumes, and markedly decreased VC indicate restrictive disease.
Forced expiratory volume (FEV): volume of air expired in the 1st, 2nd, or 3rd second of FVC maneuver	Direct spirographic measurement; expressed as percentage of FVC	Decreased FEV; increased FEV_2 and FEV_3 may indicate obstructive disease; decreased or normal FEV_1 may indicate restrictive disease. (continued)

Interpreting Pulmonary Function Tests (continued)

Measurement of pulmonary function	Method of calculation	Abnormal results
Maximal midexpiratory flow (MMEF)—also called forced expiratory flow (FEF) or FEF 25%-75%: average rate of flow during middle half of FVC	Calculated from the flow rate and the time needed for expiration of middle 50% of FVC	Low MMEF indicates obstructive disease of the small airways.
Peak expiratory flow (PEF): Vmax during forced expiration	Calculated from flow-volume curve, or by direct spirographic measurement, using a pneumotachometer or electronic tachometer with a transducer to convert flow to electrical output display	Decreased PEF may indicate a mechanical problem, such as upper airway obstruction or obstructive disease. PEF is usually normal in restrictive disease but decreases in severe cases. Because PEF is effort-dependent, it is also low in a person who has poor expiratory effort or does not understand the procedure.
Maximal voluntary ventilation (MVV)—also called maximum breathing capacity (MBC): greatest volume of air breathed per unit of time	Direct spirographic measurement	Decreased MVV may indicate obstructive disease; normal or decreased MVV may indicate restrictive disease, such as myasthenia gravis.
Diffusing capacity for carbon monoxide (DL$_{CO}$): milliliters of carbon monoxide diffused per minute across the alveolar-capillary membrane	Calculated from analysis of amount of carbon monoxide exhaled compared with amount inhaled	Decreased DL$_{CO}$ in the presence of thickened alveolar-capillary membrane indicates interstitial pulmonary disease, such as pulmonary fibrosis and emphysema.

MVV:
• The patient is told to breathe into the mouthpiece as quickly and deeply as possible for 15 seconds.

DL$_{CO}$:
• The patient is told to inhale a gas mixture with a low concentration of carbon monoxide and then to hold his breath for 10 seconds before exhaling.

Special precautions
CLINICAL ALERT: **During pulmonary function testing, watch for respira-** tory distress, changes in pulse rate and blood pressure, coughing, or bronchospasm.

Patient care checklist
Before the test
☑ Explain or clarify test purpose, preparation, and procedure.
☑ Assure the patient that the procedure is painless and that he will be able to rest between tests.
☑ Tell the patient that he will be instructed to put on a nose clip before

the tests, and advise him that the accuracy of the tests depends on his cooperation.

☑ Evaluate patient understanding.

☑ Instruct him not to eat a heavy meal before the tests and not to smoke for 4 to 6 hours before the tests.

☑ Withhold medications that may interfere with test results and intermittent positive-pressure breathing therapy, as ordered. If they must be continued, note them on the request slip.

☑ Just before the test, tell the patient to void and to loosen tight clothing. If he wears dentures, tell him to wear them during the test to help form a seal around the mouthpiece.

Interfering factors

• Hypoxia, metabolic disturbances, or lack of patient cooperation can make testing difficult or impossible.

• Pregnancy or gastric distention may displace lung volume.

• A poor seal around the mouthpiece or the tube can decrease volumes.

• A narcotic analgesic or sedative administered before the test can decrease inspiratory and expiratory forces.

• Bronchodilators may temporarily improve pulmonary function, thereby producing misleading results.

Skin tests

Purpose

• To help diagnose and differentiate infectious diseases

• To evaluate primary and secondary immune responses

• To detect sensitivity to microorganisms that can cause disease, such as tuberculosis

• To help evaluate a patient's response to immunotherapy

• To detect sensitivity to various allergens, such as certain types of foods and pollens.

Normal results

Tests of immune response:

Positive reaction (5 mm or more of induration at the test site) to each antigen tested in the recall antigen test.

Tests to detect exposure to specific disease-causing microorganisms:

Negative reaction (no inflammation at test site, or inflammation less than 5 mm in diameter).

Tests to detect specific allergens:

Negative reaction (no inflammation at test site, or inflammation less than 5 mm in diameter).

Abnormal results

Tests of immune response:

Recall antigen test:

A positive response to less than two of the six test antigens, a persistent unresponsiveness to intradermal injection of higher-strength antigens, or a generalized diminished reaction (causing less than 10 mm combined induration) indicates diminished delayed hypersensitivity, and thus an immune system problem.

Tests to detect exposure to specific disease-causing microorganisms:

Coccidioidomycosis test:

Positive reaction (induration of 5 mm or more. Erythema is not considered indicative of a delayed hypersensitivity reaction. The test is read at 24 hours and at 48 hours, with reaction peaking at 36 hours.)

Histoplasmosis test:

Positive reaction (induration of 5 mm or more. The test is read at 24 to 48 hours. Occasionally, maximum reactions may not be present until the 4th day.)

Mumps skin test:

Positive reaction (induration of 5 mm or more. Erythema is not considered indicative of a delayed hypersensitivity reaction. The test is read at 24-, 48-, and 72-hour intervals.)

Tuberculosis tests:

Mantoux (tuberculin purified protein derivative [TPPD]): Significant reaction, formerly called positive reaction (induration of 10 mm or greater; read in 48 to 72 hours after injection). The significance of a reaction is determined not only by the size of the reaction, but by circumstances. For example, a reaction of 5 mm or more may be considered significant in a close relative of a person with known tuberculosis. A reaction of 2 mm may be considered significant in infants and children. The amount of induration—not erythema—at the site determines the significance of the reaction.

Multiple puncture tests (tine test, Mono-Vacc test, Aplitest, Sclarotest, Sterneedle): Currently, the only significant reaction is vesiculation (blistering). Other measurable induration reactions are considered doubtful and the patient should be retested with a Mantoux test. These tests are read in 48 to 72 hours.

Tests to detect specific allergens:
Intradermal tests:

Positive reaction (induration of 5 mm or more within a given period of time).

Patch and scratch tests:

See *Patch and Scratch Allergy Tests.*

The basics

In general, skin tests determine immunity or hypersensitivity. Immunity is the body's resistance to the effects of harmful agents. Hypersensitivity indicates a change in the strength with which the body can react to an antigen. Skin testing is one of the most important methods for evaluating the cellular immune response of a patient with severe recurrent infection, infection caused by unusual organisms, or suspected disorders associated with delayed hypersensitivity. Since diminished delayed hypersensitivity may be associated with a poor prognosis in patients with certain malignancies, this test may also be useful in determining the prognosis in such patients.

Skin tests employ new and recall antigens. New antigens—those not previously encountered by the patient, such as dinitrochlorobenzene (DNCB)—evaluate the patient's primary immune response when a sensitizing dose is given, followed by a challenge dose. (For more information, see *Testing for DNCB Sensitization,* p. 656.)

Recall antigens—those to which a patient has had, or may have had, previous exposure or sensitization—evaluate the secondary immune response; these antigens include candidin, trichophytin, streptokinase-streptodornase (SK-SD), purified protein derivative (PPD), staphage lysate, mumps, and mixed respiratory vaccine, among others. The specific antigens chosen for this intradermal testing are those to which exposure is common and will usually provoke an immune response. If there is no inflammatory reaction to these antigens at the test site, the patient's immune system is probably impaired.

When skin tests are used to detect the presence of microorganisms that can cause disease, hypersensitivity is evidenced by a positive delayed inflammatory response at the test site. In this case, the positive reaction indicates that the patient has an intact cell-mediated immune function, and that the patient has had recent or past exposure to the specific antigen. A negative response (no inflammation at the test site) indicates that the patient has had no exposure to the antigen, or it may mean that the patient has an active infection with a loss of cell-mediated immune function. This is known as anergy. Anergy can occur in advanced stages of many infectious diseases, as well as in some chronic diseases such as Hodgkin's disease, in people receiving immunosuppressant drugs, and in the elderly. In general,

Patch and Scratch Allergy Tests

Patch and scratch skin tests are used to evaluate the immune system's ability to respond to known allergens, which are applied to hairless areas of the patient's body, such as the scapula, the volar surface of the forearm, or the anterior surface of the thigh. In patch testing, each allergen (a dilute solution, an ointment, or a dry preparation) is applied directly to the skin and covered with gauze secured by tape, or prepared gauze patches impregnated with the antigens are applied to the skin. Test results are read 48 to 72 hours later; erythema, papules, vesicles, or edema indicates a positive reaction.

Results are read as follows:

? + = doubtful reaction
 + = weak (nonvesicular) reaction—
    erythema and papules
 + + + = extreme reaction—all of
    the above, plus large
    vesicles, bullae, and at
    times ulceration
IR = irritant reaction

Scratch tests involve scarifying the patient's skin with a special tool or needle and introducing the allergens into the scratched area. Test sites are examined 30 to 40 minutes later and compared with a control site; erythema or edema indicates a positive reaction.

Both kinds of tests provoke delayed hypersensitivity reactions mediated by T cells in the patient's immune system. Although minute amounts of test allergens can usually demonstrate an intact immune response, the test may also indicate an anergic (diminished or absent) reaction in patients with acute leukemia, Hodgkin's disease, congenital immunodeficiencies, or overwhelming infections, and in elderly patients.

If a patient is thought to be anergic, he may be exposed to a new antigen, such as dinitrochlorobenzene, to confirm anergy.

Patch and scratch tests are contraindicated in patients with inflammation, skin diseases, or significantly impaired immune response. These tests have limited value in infants because of their immature, poorly sensitized immune system.

negative reactions mean active infection is highly unlikely. False-positive and false-negative reactions may occur, so skin tests alone are not diagnostic.

Tuberculin tests (such as the tine, Aplitest, Mono-Vacc, or Mantoux) and the recall antigen tests for coccidioidomycosis and histoplasmosis are examples of this type of testing for hypersensitivity. The recall antigen and the Mantoux tests are intradermal injection tests. The tine, Aplitest, Mono-Vacc, Sclavo, and Sterneedle tests are multiple puncture tests.

Tests to detect allergies, another form of hypersensitivity, are intradermal tests, scratch tests, or patch tests.

Patch and scratch testing is discussed in *Patch and Scratch Allergy Tests*. Intradermal testing for allergies is performed in much the same manner as described for recall antigen tests, but the antigens introduced are usually environmental material, such as dust, pollen, and foods.

Contraindications for tuberculin tests include current reactions to smallpox vaccinations or any rash or other skin disorder, and known tuberculin-positive reactions. Contraindications for recall antigen tests include known hypersensitivity to the test antigen. Intradermal tests have limited value in infants, because their immune systems are immature and inadequately sensitized. (See also *Schick Test*, p. 657.)

Testing For DNCB Sensitization

The patient who shows little or no reaction (anergy) to the panel of test antigens during skin testing may not have been previously exposed to them or may be immunodeficient. In such a patient, the dinitrochlorobenzene (DNCB) sensitization test can verify the presence of cell-mediated immune function.

In the DNCB test, this chemical, when applied to the patient's skin, acts like a "new" antigen, combining with skin proteins to form a substance that stimulates T cell sensitization to DNCB. Ten to fourteen days after this sensitizing dose, a challenge dose should produce a positive reaction, indicating intact cell-mediated immunity. A negative reaction confirms anergy.

To perform this test, wear gloves and a mask to prevent self-sensitization to the chemical. You will need a sterile gauze pad, an adhesive bandage, alcohol sponges, acetone, and cotton-tipped applicators. Follow these steps:
• Explain the procedure to the patient, and tell him the DNCB will be reapplied after 2 weeks. Check your hospital's policy on DNCB. This test usually requires a record of informed consent and possibly Food & Drug Administration approval.

• Dissolve the DNCB in acetone, as ordered. Position the patient's arm as for a patch test. Using an alcohol sponge, cleanse a small, hairless area midway between the wrist and elbow and allow it to dry. Then, using a cotton-tipped applicator, apply the prescribed amount of DNCB (sensitizing dose) and allow the DNCB to dry. Cover the area with a sterile gauze pad or adhesive bandage for 24 to 48 hours.
• Tell the patient to watch for a spontaneous flare reaction 10 to 14 days after the first DNCB application. If a reaction occurs, use a smaller dose of test solution for the DNCB challenge dose.
• After 14 days, apply the challenge dose to the same site, using the same procedures; inspect the site 48 to 96 hours later for reactivity. If test results are negative, the challenge dose can be repeated 2 weeks later (1 month after the sensitizing dose).
• Score the patient's response to the test as follows:

0 = No reaction

1+ = Erythema only

2+ = Erythema with induration

3+ = Vesicles, erythema, and induration

4+ = Bullae and/or ulceration.

Procedure
To prepare the test site:
Cleanse the test site (usually the volar surface of the forearm, about 2 or 3 fingerbreadths distal to the antecubital space) with alcohol to protect the wheal from infection. Also, if necessary, cleanse the area with acetone to remove skin oils that may interfere with test results. (Be sure the test site you have chosen has adequate subcutaneous tissue and is free of hair or blemishes. Allow the skin to dry completely before administering the injection to avoid inactivating the antigen.)
To perform single-puncture intradermal tests (recall antigen tests, tests to detect exposure to disease, such as the Mantoux test, allergy tests):
• Inject each antigen being tested intradermally into the volar aspect of the patient's forearm. Use a separate tuberculin syringe for each antigen.
• Circle each injection site with a pen and label each according to the antigen given.

• Instruct the patient to avoid washing off the circles until the test is completed.

• If a control wheal is required, as in the recall antigen test, inject normal saline solution or test diluent into the other arm, following the same procedure.

• Inspect injection sites for reactivity after 48 and 72 hours.

• Record induration and erythema in millimeters.

• Confirm a negative test at the first concentration of antigen by using a higher concentration.

To perform multipuncture tests, such as the tine test, Aplitest, and Mono-Vacc:

• Always read the enclosed directions. The following steps are general guidelines.

• Remove the protective cap from the unit.

• Hold the patient's forearm with one hand, and stretch taut the cleansed skin area with your fingers. Grasp the unit with your other hand, and firmly press the tines completely into the patient's skin without twisting the unit.

• Hold the device in place for at least 1 second. If you have applied sufficient pressure, you will see four distinct punctures and a circular depression made by the device on the skin. Recap the device and discard it.

• Read tine test and Aplitest results 48 to 72 hours after injection; Mono-Vacc test results, 48 to 96 hours after injection. Record test results.

• The administration phase of the test takes about 5 to 10 minutes for each antigen.

Special precautions

• Store antigens in lyophilized (freeze-dried) form at 39.2° F. (4° C.), protected from light. Reconstitute them shortly before use, and check their expiration dates. If the patient is suspected of hypersensitivity to the antigens, apply them first in low concentrations.

• If the forearms are not free from disease (for example, if the patient has atopic dermatitis), use other sites, such as the back.

• In intradermal injections, after withdrawing the needle, apply gentle pressure to the injection site. Do not rub the site (to avoid irritating underlying tissues, which may affect test results).

• Be sure a wheal appears after you inject the antigen; if none appears, repeat the test.

CLINICAL ALERT: **Observe the patient carefully for signs of anaphylactic shock—urticaria, respiratory distress, and hypotension. If such signs develop, administer epinephrine, as ordered, and notify the physician immediately.**

Schick Test

Although not performed routinely in the United States, the Schick test determines susceptibility or immunity to diphtheria—an acute, highly contagious bacterial infection. In this skin test, 0.1 ml of purified diphtheria toxin dissolved in buffered human serum albumin is injected intradermally into one forearm, and 0.1 ml of purified diphtheria toxoid is injected into the other forearm, as a control. Both sites are examined after 24 and 48 hours, and again 4 to 7 days after injection.

Patients susceptible to diphtheria—those who have slight amounts of or no circulating antitoxin—demonstrate inflammation and induration at the site of toxin injection within 24 hours and a peak reaction within 7 days. This reaction generally has a dark red center and may reach 3 cm in diameter. Conversely, the site of toxoid injection shows no reaction.

In patients immune to diphtheria (those with antitoxin levels between 1/30 and 1/100 unit), neither site shows a reaction.

Patient care checklist
Before the test

☑ Explain or clarify test purpose and procedure.

☑ Tell the patient that it takes about 5 to 10 minutes for each antigen to be administered. Also tell the patient when the test results must be read.

☑ Evaluate patient understanding.

☑ Check the patient's history for hypersensitivity to any of the test antigens; if not listed in his history, ask the patient if he has had a skin test previously and, if so, what his reactions were. If the patient's history reveals no sensitivity or hypersensitivity, it is appropriate to test with intermediate-strength antigens.

After the test

☑ Watch the patient closely for severe local reactions that may occur at the test site, such as pain, blistering, swelling, induration, itching, and ulceration. Scarring or hyperpigmentation may result. Also observe for swelling and tenderness in the lymph nodes at the elbow or axillary region. Check for tachycardia and fever, although these rarely occur. Symptoms generally appear in 15 to 30 minutes.

☑ Tell the patient experiencing hypersensitivity that steroids will control the reaction, but skin lesions may persist for 10 to 14 days. Instruct him to avoid scratching or otherwise disturbing the affected area.

Interfering factors

• Use of antigens that have expired or been exposed to heat and light or to bacterial contamination interferes with accurate testing.

• Poor injection technique—subcutaneous instead of intradermal injection—may produce negative results.

• Inaccurate dilution of antigens or error in reading or timing test results causes inaccurate test results.

• A strong, immediate reaction to the antigen at the site of injection may cause a false-negative delayed reaction.

• Oral contraceptives may cause negative results by inhibiting lymphocyte mitosis.

Tensilon test

Purpose

• To aid in diagnosis of myasthenia gravis
• To aid in differentiation between myasthenic and cholinergic crises
• To monitor oral anticholinesterase therapy.

Normal results

Persons who do not have myasthenia gravis usually develop fasciculations in response to Tensilon. The physician must interpret the responses carefully to distinguish a normal person from one with myasthenia gravis.

Abnormal results
Myasthenia gravis:

Muscle strength should improve promptly following administration of Tensilon. The degree of improvement depends on the muscle group being tested. Improvement usually becomes obvious within 30 seconds; although the maximum benefit lasts only several minutes, lingering effects may persist—up to 2 hours in a patient receiving prednisone, for example.

Myasthenic crisis (exacerbation of the disease requiring anticholinesterase therapy):

Brief improvement in muscle strength should occur after Tensilon administration.

Cholinergic crisis (anticholinesterase overdose):

Tensilon will promptly exaggerate muscle weakness.

The basics

This test involves careful observation of the patient following I.V. administration of Tensilon (edrophonium chloride), a rapid, short-acting anticholinesterase that improves muscle strength by increasing muscular response to nerve impulses. It is especially useful in diagnosing myasthenia gravis, an abnormality of the myoneural junction in which nerve impulses fail to induce normal muscular responses. Patients with myasthenia gravis experience extreme fatigue at the end of the day or after repetitive activity or stress.

Although all patients with myasthenia gravis show improved muscle strength in this test, some respond only slightly, and the test may need to be repeated to confirm diagnosis. This test gives inconsistent results when myasthenia gravis affects only ocular muscles, as in mild or early forms of the disorder. It may produce a positive response in motor neuron disease and in some neuropathies and myopathies. However, the response is usually less dramatic and less consistent than in myasthenia gravis. Results of other procedures, including electromyography, may supplement Tensilon test findings in diagnosing this disease.

Contraindications (because of the systemic adverse effects Tensilon may produce) include the presence of hypotension, bradycardia, apnea, and mechanical obstruction of the intestine or urinary tract.

Procedure

Begin I.V. infusion of 5% dextrose in water or normal saline solution.

For the adult patient suspected of having myasthenia gravis:
• Administer 2 mg of Tensilon initially. (Dosage must be adjusted for an infant or child. See *Tensilon Dosage for Infants and Children*.)
• Before the rest of the dosage is administered, the physician may want to fatigue the muscles by asking the patient to perform various exercises, such as looking up until ptosis develops, counting to 100 until his voice diminishes, or holding his arms above his shoulders until they drop.
• When the muscles have been fatigued, administer the remaining 8 mg

---

Tensilon Dosage For Infants and Children

In infants and children, the dosage of Tensilon is adjusted as follows:
• **Infants:** Administer 0.5 mg I.V.
• **Children up to 75 lbs (34 kg):** Beginning with 1 mg I.V., administer up to 5 mg at the rate of 1 mg every 30 to 45 seconds; or administer 2 mg I.M.
• **Children over 75 lbs (34 kg):** Beginning with 2 mg I.V., administer up to 10 mg at the rate of 1 mg every 30 to 45 seconds; or administer 5 mg I.M.

Response to Tensilon is not affected by method of administration except that I.M. administration delays it for 2 to 10 minutes.

---

of Tensilon over 30 seconds. (Note: Some physicians prefer to begin this test with a placebo injection to evaluate the patient's muscular response more accurately. If so, administer the placebo and observe the patient. This placebo is not necessary when cranial muscles are being tested, since cranial strength cannot be simulated voluntarily.)
• After administration of Tensilon, the patient will be asked to perform repetitive muscular movements, such as opening and closing his eyes and crossing and uncrossing his legs. Assist the physician by closely observing the patient for improved muscle strength.
• If muscle strength does not improve within 3 to 5 minutes, the test may be repeated.

To differentiate between myasthenic crisis and cholinergic crisis:
• Infuse 1 to 2 mg of Tensilon.
• Continually monitor the patient's vital signs after infusion.
• Watch closely for respiratory distress, and be prepared to provide respiratory assistance.
• If muscle strength does not improve, infuse more Tensilon cautiously—1 mg at a time, up to a maximum of 5

mg—and observe the patient for distress.

• Administer neostigmine immediately if the test demonstrates myasthenic crisis; administer atropine for cholinergic crisis.

To evaluate anticholinesterase therapy:

• Infuse 2 mg of Tensilon 1 hour after the patient's last dose of the anticholinesterase.

• Observe the patient carefully for adverse effects and muscular response. (If Tensilon decreases muscle strength in a person with prominent adverse effects, therapy should be reduced. If the test shows no change in muscle strength and only mild adverse effects occur, therapy should remain the same.)

• After administration of Tensilon, keep the I.V. line open at a rate of 20 ml/hour until all of the patient's responses have been evaluated.

• When the test is complete, discontinue the I.V., as ordered, and check the patient's vital signs.

• Check the puncture site for hematoma, excessive bleeding, and swelling.

• The test takes 15 to 30 minutes.

Special precautions

CLINICAL ALERT: **Stay with the patient during the test, and observe him closely for adverse effects. Keep resuscitation equipment handy in case of respiratory failure.**

Patient care checklist

Before the test

☑ Explain or clarify test purpose and procedure.

☑ Do not describe the exact response that will be evaluated, since this knowledge may interfere with the test's objectivity.

☑ Advise the patient that Tensilon may produce some unpleasant adverse effects, but reassure him that someone will be with him at all times and that any reactions will quickly disappear.

☑ Tell the patient that, to ensure accurate results, the test may be repeated several times.

☑ Evaluate patient understanding.

☑ Withhold medications that may interfere with test results, as ordered. If they must be continued, note them on the laboratory slip.

☑ Review the patient history for drug sensitivities and respiratory disease. (Patients with respiratory ailments, such as asthma, should receive atropine during the test to minimize Tensilon's adverse effects.)

☑ If the patient is receiving anticholinesterase therapy, note the time the last dose was received on the requisition slip.

Interfering factors

• In patients receiving prednisone, the effect of Tensilon on muscle strength may be delayed.

• Quinidine and anticholinergics interfere with test results by inhibiting the action of Tensilon.

• Procainamide and muscle relaxants interfere with test results by inhibiting normal muscle responses.

Uroflowmetry

Purpose

• To evaluate lower urinary tract function

• To demonstrate bladder outlet obstruction.

Normal results

Flow rate varies according to the patient's age and sex and the volume of urine voided. Normal values are listed below for minimum volumes needed to obtain adequate recordings.

Age	Minimum volume (ml)	Male (ml/sec)	Female (ml/sec)
4 to 7	100	10	10
8 to 13	100	12	15
14 to 45	200	21	18
46 to 65	200	12	15
66 to 80	200	9	10

Abnormal results
Increased flow rate indicates:
   Reduced urethral resistance, possibly associated with external sphincter dysfunction.
Decreased flow rate indicates:
   Outflow obstruction
   Hypotonia of the detrusor muscle.
(For more information, see *Characteristic Uroflow Curves*.)

The basics
This simple, noninvasive test uses a uroflowmeter to detect and evaluate dysfunctional voiding patterns. The uroflowmeter, contained in a funnel into which the patient voids, measures flow rate (volume of urine voided per second), continuous flow time (time of measurable flow), and intermittent flow (total voiding time, including any interruptions).

Several types of uroflowmeters are available: rotary disk, electromagnetic, spectrophotometric, and gravimetric systems. The gravimetric system, which weighs urine as it is voided and plots the weight against time, is the simplest to use and is widely available.

Procedure
(The test procedure is the same with all types of equipment.)
• A male patient is asked to void while standing; a female patient, while sitting.
• The patient is asked to avoid straining to empty the bladder.
• Cable connections are checked, and the patient is left alone.
• The patient pushes the start button on the commode chair, counts for 5 seconds (1-one-thousand, 2-one-thousand, and so on), and voids.
• When finished, he counts for 5 seconds and pushes the button again.
• The volume of urine voided is then recorded and plotted as a curve over the time of voiding.
• The patient's position and the route of fluid intake (oral or intravenous) are noted.

Characteristic Uroflow Curves

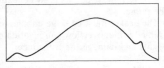

A. Normal curve.

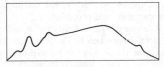

B. Normal peak with hesitancy may result from the patient's embarrassment or advanced age.

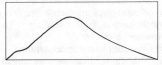

C. High peak flow over short voiding time may indicate incontinence.

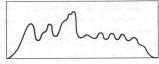

D. Many peaks over normal voiding time indicate abdominal straining and detrusor muscle weakness.

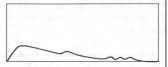

E. Low peak with long voiding time and urethral dribbling indicates obstruction.

• The test takes 10 to 15 minutes.

Special precautions
• The transducer must be level, and the beaker must be centered beneath the funnel.
• The beaker must be large enough to hold all urine; overflow can invalidate results and damage the transducer.

Patient care checklist
Before the test
☑ Explain or clarify test purpose, preparation, and procedure.
☑ Advise the patient not to urinate for several hours before the test, and to increase fluid intake so he will have a full bladder and a strong urge to void.
☑ Instruct the patient to remain still while voiding during the test to help ensure accurate results.
☑ Assure the patient that he will have complete privacy during the test; many people have difficulty voiding in the presence of others.
☑ Evaluate patient understanding.
☑ Withhold medications that may interfere with test results, as ordered.

Interfering factors
• Drugs that affect bladder and sphincter tone, such as urinary spasmolytics and anticholinergics, will alter test results.
• Strong drafts can affect transducer function.
• If the patient moves while seated on the commode chair, flow recording may be inaccurate.
• The presence of toilet tissue in the beaker will invalidate test results.
• If the patient strains to void, test results will be altered.

Vectorcardiography *(VCG)*

Purpose
• To detect ventricular hypertrophy, interventricular conduction disturbances, and myocardial infarction (MI)

• To clarify doubtful EKG results.

Normal results
Three distinct loops (P, QRS, and T) are present, each representing an event in the cardiac cycle. The appearance of the VCG itself may vary with age and sex; the shape of the loops, the spacing of the dashes, and the direction of the arrows have significance in evaluating the heart's electrical activity.

Abnormal results
The VCG may help identify:
    Ventricular hypertrophy
    MI
    Bundle branch blocks
    Myocardial ischemia
    Metabolic disturbances.

The basics
Similar to electrocardiography, vectorcardiography records variations in electrical potential during the cardiac cycle. However, vectorcardiography—unlike electrocardiography—uses two simultaneously recorded lead axes to construct a three-dimensional view of the heart. Vectors, which are composites of electrical potential, possess direction, magnitude, and polarity and are measured along three axes: the X, or horizontal, axis; the Y, or vertical, axis; and the Z, or sagittal, axis. Simultaneous recording of X and Y axes produces the frontal plane; of X and Z axes, the horizontal plane; and of Z and Y axes, the sagittal plane. Since the left atrium and left ventricle dominate the electrical field, most vectors represent forces on the left side of the heart.

In vectorcardiography, electrodes applied to the patient's skin transmit the heart's electrical impulses to a vectorcardiograph. This instrument displays the three vector loops—P, QRS, and T—on its oscilloscope screen, permitting photographic or direct graphic recording of results. These loops represent one complete cardiac cycle and correspond to the P wave, QRS complex, and T wave of the EKG.

Although vectorcardiography requires correlation with patient history, physical examination, and other diagnostic tests, it proves most valuable in evaluating ventricular abnormalities. It is also considered more sensitive than electrocardiography in identifying an MI.

Vectorcardiography is more commonly used in research and teaching than in a clinical setting, but it does prove useful in clarifying questionable EKG results, especially in patients with hypertrophy, bundle branch block, MI, or combinations of these disorders. However, its clinical application is limited because of its high cost. Interpretation of the VCG requires great skill, and definitive standards for normal and abnormal vectors and for lead placement do not exist.

Procedure
• The patient is placed in a supine or sitting position.
• Electrodes, to which conductive jelly has been applied, will be secured to his chest, left leg, back, and nape of the neck or forehead (Frank system). The number and placement of electrodes vary, depending on the system selected.

• The patient is encouraged to relax, breathe quietly, and remain still during the test.
• The VCG machine is turned on, and the desired number of recordings is obtained.
• After completing the recordings, the electrodes and the conductive gel are removed.
• The procedure takes about 15 minutes. Results are usually available in 1 or 2 days.

Patient care checklist
Before the test
☑ Explain or clarify test purpose and procedure.
☑ Reassure the patient that the test, which is similar to electrocardiography, is safe and painless.
☑ Evaluate patient understanding.
☑ Have the patient put on a hospital gown and remove any metallic objects above the waist.

Interfering factors
• Cardioactive drugs, such as antiarrhythmics or digitalis, can alter test results.
• Incorrect placement of electrodes or excessive patient movement during the test can produce inaccurate results.
• In patients with a heavy body build, the QRS loop may simulate right ventricular hypertrophy.

Selected References

Andreoli, Kathleen G., and Fowkes, Virginia K. *Comprehensive Cardiac Care: A Text for Nurses, Physicians, and Other Health Practitioners,* 5th ed. St. Louis: C.V. Mosby Co., 1983.

Babb, J.D., and Leaman, D.M. "Risk of Cardiac Catheterization Today," *Journal of Cardiovascular Medicine* 941-48, October 1980.

Benchimol, Albert O. *Non-Invasive Diagnostic Techniques in Cardiology,* 2nd ed. Baltimore: Williams & Wilkins Co., 1981.

Cardiovascular Disorders. Nurse's Clinical Library. Springhouse, Pa.: Springhouse Corp., 1984.

Clinical Cardiac Electrophysiology: Techniques and Interpretations. Philadelphia: Lea & Febiger, 1979.

Conn, Rex B., ed. *Current Diagnosis,* 7th ed. Philadelphia: W.B. Saunders Co., 1985.

Conover, Mary H. *Understanding Electrocardiography: Physiological and Interpretive Concepts,* 3rd ed. St. Louis: C.V. Mosby Co., 1980.

Diagnostics, 2nd ed. Nurse's Reference Library. Springhouse, Pa.: Springhouse Corp., 1986.

Fischbach, Frances. A Manual of Laboratory Diagnostic Tests, 2nd ed. Philadelphia: J.B. Lippincott Co., 1984.

Fowler, Noble O., ed. Cardiac Diagnosis and Treatment, 3rd ed. Philadelphia: J.B. Lippincott Co., 1980.

Grossman, William, ed. Cardiac Catheterization and Angiography, 2nd ed. Philadelphia: Lea & Febiger, 1980.

Guyton, Arthur C. Textbook of Medical Physiology, 6th ed. Philadelphia: W.B. Saunders Co., 1981.

Harvey, A. McGehee, et al. The Principles and Practice of Medicine, 21st ed. East Norwalk, Conn.: Appleton-Century-Crofts, 1984.

Hermann, Christy S. "Performing Intradermal Skin Tests—The Right Way," Nursing83 13:50-53, October 1983.

Kennedy, Harold L. Ambulatory Electrocardiography: Including Holter Recording Technology. Philadelphia: Lea & Febiger, 1981.

Neurologic Disorders. Nurse's Clinical Library. Springhouse, Pa.: Springhouse Corp., 1984.

Petersdorf, Robert G., and Adams, Raymond D., eds. Harrison's Principles of Internal Medicine, 10th ed. New York: McGraw-Hill Book Co., 1983.

Procedures. Nurse's Reference Library. Springhouse, Pa.: Springhouse Corp., 1985.

Reading EKGs Correctly, 2nd ed. New Nursing Skillbook Series. Springhouse, Pa.: Springhouse Corp., 1984.

Teasley, Deborah. "Don't Let Cardiac Catheterization Strike Fear in Your Patient's Heart," Nursing82 12:52-55, March 1982.

Using Monitors. Nursing Photobook Series. Springhouse, Pa.: Springhouse Corp., 1981.

Vandenbelt, Ronald J., et al. Cardiology—A Clinical Approach. Chicago: Year Book Medical Pubs., 1979.

Visalli, Florence, and Evans, Patricia. "The Swan-Ganz Catheter: A Program for Teaching Safe, Effective Use," Nursing81 11(1):42-47, January 1981.

Wenger, Nanette K., et al. Cardiology for Nurses. New York: McGraw-Hill Book Co., 1980.

Wyngaarden, James, and Smith, Lloyd. Cecil Textbook of Medicine, 16th ed. Philadelphia: W.B. Saunders Co., 1982.

Laboratory Test Values

A

AChR antibodies, serum
negative or ≤ 0.5 nmol/liter

Acid phosphatase, serum
0 to 1.1 Bodansky units/ml
1 to 4 King-Armstrong units/ml
0.13 to 0.63 BLB units/ml

ACTH, plasma
< 120 pg/ml

ACTH, rapid test, plasma
Cortisol rises 7 to 18 mcg/dl
above baseline, 60 minutes
after injection

Activated partial thromboplastin time
25 to 36 seconds

Albumin, peritoneal fluid
50% to 70% of total protein

Albumin, serum
3.3 to 4.5 g/dl

Aldosterone, serum
1 to 21 ng/dl (standing)

Aldosterone, urine
2 to 16 mcg/24 hours

Alkaline phosphatase, peritoneal fluid
Men: > age 18, 90 to 239 units/liter
Women: < age 45, 76 to 196 units/liter; > age 45, 87 to 250 units/liter

Alkaline phosphatase, serum
1.5 to 4 Bodansky units/dl
4 to 13.5 King-Armstrong units/dl
Chemical inhibition method: Men, 90 to 239 units/dl; Women < age 45, 76 to 196 units/liter; Women > age 45, 87 to 250 units/liter

Alpha-fetoprotein, amniotic fluid
≤ 18.5 mcg/ml at 13 or 14 weeks

Alpha-fetoprotein, serum
Nonpregnant women: < 30 ng/ml

Amino acids, urine
50 to 200 mg/24 hours

Ammonia, peritoneal fluid
< 50 mcg/dl

Ammonia, plasma
< 50 mcg/dl

Amniotic fluid
Lecithin/sphingomyelin ratio: > 2
Meconium: Absent
Phosphatidiglycerol: Present

Amylase, peritoneal fluid
138 to 404 amylase units/liter

Amylase, serum
60 to 180 Somogyi units/dl

Amylase, urine
10 to 80 amylase units/hour

Androstenedione
Men: 0.9 to 1.7 ng/ml
Menstruating women: 0.6 to 3 ng/ml
Postmenopausal women: 0.3 to 8 ng/ml

Angiotensin converting enzyme
> age 20: 18 to 67 U/liter

Anion gap
8 to 14 mEq/liter

Antibody screening, serum
Negative

Anti–deoxyribonucleic acid antibodies, serum
< 1 mcg DNA bound/ml

Antidiuretic hormone, serum
1 to 5 pg/ml

Antiglobulin test, direct
Negative

Antimitochondrial antibodies, serum
Negative at 1:5 dilution

Antinuclear antibodies, serum
Negative at ≤ 1:32 titer

Anti–smooth-muscle antibodies, serum
Normal titer < 1:20

Antistreptolysin-O, serum
< 85 Todd units/ml

Antithrombin III
> 50% of normal control values

Antithyroid antibodies, serum
Normal titer < 1:100

Arginine test
Men: hgH increases to > 10 ng/ml
Women: hgH increases to > 15 ng/ml

Arterial blood gases
Pao_2:   75 to 100 mmHg
$Paco_2$:   35 to 45 mmHg
O_2CT: 15% to 23%
O_2 Sat: 94% to 100%
HCO_3^-:   22 to 26 mEq/liter

Arylsulfatase A, urine
Men: 1.4 to 19.3 units/liter
Women: 1.4 to 11 units/liter

(continued)

Laboratory Test Values*(continued)*

Aspergillosis antibody, serum
Normal titer < 1:8

B

B-lymphocyte count
270 to 640/mm³

Bence Jones protein, urine
Negative

Bilirubin, amniotic fluid
Absent at term

Bilirubin, serum
Adult: Direct, < 0.5 mg/dl;
indirect, ≤ 1.1 mg/dl
Neonate: Total, 1 to 12 mg/dl

Bilirubin, urine
Negative

Blastomycosis antibody, serum
Normal titer < 1:8

Bleeding time
Modified template: 2 to 10
minutes
Template: 2 to 8 minutes
Ivy: 1 to 7 minutes
Duke: 1 to 3 minutes

Blood urea nitrogen
8 to 20 mg/dl

C

C-reactive protein, serum
Negative

Calcitonin, plasma
Baseline: Males, ≤ 0.155 ng/ml;
females, ≤ 0.105 ng/ml
Calcium infusion: Males, 0.265
ng/ml; females, 0.120 ng/ml
Pentagastrin infusion: Males,
0.210 ng/ml; females, 0.105
ng/ml

Calcium, serum
4.5 to 5.5 mEq/liter
Atomic absorption: 8.9 to 10.1
mg/dl

Calcium, urine
Men: < 275 mg/24 hours
Women: < 250 mg/24 hours

Capillary fragility
Petechiae:

0 to 10	Score: 1 +
10 to 20	Score: 2 +
20 to 50	Score: 3 +
50	4 +

Carbon dioxide, total, blood
22 to 34 mEq/liter

**Carcinoembryonic antigen,
serum**
< 5 ng/ml

Carotene, serum
48 to 200 mcg/dl

Catecholamines, plasma
Supine: Epinephrine, 0 to 110 pg/
ml; norepinephrine, 70 to 750
pg/ml; dopamine, 0 to 30 pg/ml
Standing: Epinephrine, 0 to 140
pg/ml; norepinephrine, 200 to
1,700 pg/ml; dopamine, 0 to
30 pg/ml

Catecholamines, urine
24-hour specimen: 0 to 135 mcg
Random specimen: 0 to 18 mcg/
dl

Catheterization, pulmonary artery
Right atrial: 1 to 6 mmHg
Systolic right ventricular: 20 to
30 mmHg
End diastolic right ventricular:
< 5 mmHg
Systolic PAP: 20 to 30 mmHg
Diastolic PAP: approximately
10 mmHg
Mean PAP: < 20 mmHg
PAWP: 6 to 12 mmHg
Left atrial: approximately 10
mmHg

Cerebrospinal fluid
Pressure: 50 to 180 mm water
Appearance: Clear, colorless
Gram stain: No organisms

Ceruloplasmin, serum
22.9 to 43.1 mg/dl

Chloride, cerebrospinal fluid
118 to 130 mEq/liter

Chloride, serum
100 to 108 mEq/liter

Chloride, sweat
10 to 35 mEq/liter

Chloride, urine
110 to 250 mEq/24 hours

Cholesterol, total, serum
120 to 330 mg/dl

**Cholinesterase
(pseudocholinesterase)**
8 to 18 units/ml

Chorionic gonadotropin, serum
< 3 mIU/ml

Chorionic gonadotropin, urine
Pregnant Women: First trimester,
≤ 500,000 IU/24 hours;

Laboratory Test Values *(continued)*

Chorionic gonadotropin, urine
(continued)
second trimester, 10,000 to 25,000 IU/24 hours; third trimester, 5,000 to 15,000 IU/24 hours

Clot retraction
50%

Coccidioidomycosis antibody, serum
Normal titer < 1:2

Cold agglutinins, serum
Normal titer < 1:16

Complement, serum
Total: 41 to 90 hemolytic units
CI esterase inhibitor: 16 to 33 mg/dl
C3: Men, 88 to 252 mg/dl; women, 88 to 206 mg/dl
C4: Men, 12 to 72 mg/dl; women, 13 to 75 mg/dl

Complement, synovial fluid
10 mg protein/dl: 3.7 to 33.7 units/ml
20 mg protein/dl: 7.7 to 37.7 units/ml

Copper, urine
15 to 60 mcg/24 hours

Copper reduction test, urine
Negative

Coproporphyrin, urine
Men: 0 to 96 mcg/24 hours
Women: 1 to 57 mcg/24 hours

Cortisol, plasma
Morning: 7 to 28 mcg/dl
Afternoon: 2 to 18 mcg/dl

Cortisol, free, urine
24 to 108 mcg/24 hours

Creatine phosphokinase
Total: Men, 23 to 99 units/liter; women, 15 to 57 units/liter
CPK-BB: None
CPK-MB: 0 to 7 IU/liter
CPK-MM: 5 to 70 IU/liter

Creatine, serum
Men: 0.2 to 0.6 mg/dl
Women: 0.6 to 1 mg/dl

Creatinine, amniotic fluid
> 2 mg/100 ml in mature fetus

Creatinine clearance
Men (age 20): 90 ml/minute/1.73 m²
Women (age 20): 84 ml/minute/1.73 m²

Creatinine, serum
Men: 0.8 to 1.2 mg/dl
Women: 0.6 to 0.9 mg/dl

Creatinine, urine
Men: 1 to 1.9 g/24 hours
Women: 0.8 to 1.7 g/24 hours

Cryoglobulins, serum
Negative

Cryptococcosis antigen, serum
Negative

Cyclic adenosine monophosphate, urine
Parathyroid hormone infusion: 3.6- to 4-μmol increase

D

Delta-aminolevulinic acid, urine
1.5 to 7.5 mg/dl/24 hours

D-xylose absorption
Blood: Children, 730 mg/dl in 1 hour; adults, 25 to 40 mg/dl in 2 hours
Urine: Children, 16% to 33% excreted in 5 hours; adults, > 3.5 g excreted in 5 hours

E

Erythrocyte sedimentation rate
Men: 0 to 10 mm/hour
Women: 0 to 20 mm/hour

Esophageal acidity
pH > 5.0

Estriol, amniotic fluid
16 to 20 weeks: 25.7 ng/ml
Term: < 1,000 ng/ml

Estrogens, serum
Menstruating women: day 1 to 10, 24 to 68 pg/ml; day 11 to 20, 50 to 186 pg/ml; day 21 to 30, 73 to 149 pg/ml
Men: 12 to 34 pg/ml

Estrogens, total urine
Menstruating women: follicular phase, 5 to 25 mcg/24 hours; ovulatory phase, 24 to 100 mcg/24 hours; luteal phase, 12 to 80 mcg/24 hours
Postmenopausal women: < 10 mcg/24 hours
Men: 4 to 25 mcg/24 hours

Euglobulin lysis time
≥ 2 hours

(continued)

Laboratory Test Values *(continued)*

F

Factor II assay
225 to 290 units/ml

Factor V assay
50% to 150% of control

Factor VII assay
65% to 135% of control

Factor VIII assay
55% to 145% of control

Factor IX assay
60% to 140% of control

Factor X assay
45% to 155% of control

Factor XI assay
65% to 135% of control

Factor XII assay
50% to 150% of control

Febrile agglutination, serum
Salmonella *antibody:* < 1:80
Brucellosis *antibody:* < 1:80
Tularemia *antibody:* < 1:40
Rickettsial *antibody:* < 1:40

Ferritin, serum
Men: 20 to 300 ng/ml
Women: 20 to 120 ng/ml

Fibrin split products
Screening assay: < 10 mcg/ml
Quantitative assay: < 3 mcg/ml

Fibrinogen, plasma
195 to 365 mg/dl

Fibrinogen, pleural fluid
Transudate: Absent
Exudate: Present

Fluorescent treponemal absorption, serum
Negative

Folic acid, serum
2 to 14 ng/ml

Follicle-stimulating hormone, serum
Menstruating women: Follicular phase, 5 to 20 mIU/ml; ovulatory phase, 15 to 30 mIU/ml; luteal phase, 5 to 15 mIU//ml
Menopausal women: 5 to 100 mIU/ml
Men: 5 to 20 mIU/ml

Free thyroxine, serum
0.8 to 3.3 ng/dl

Free triiodothyronine
0.2 to 0.6 ng/dl

G

Galactose-1-phosphate uridyl transferase
Qualitative: negative
Quantitative: 18.5 to 28.5 mU/g of hemoglobin

Gamma glutamyl transferase
Men: 6 to 37 units/liter
Women: < age 45, 5 to 27 units/liter; > age 45, 6 to 37 units/liter

Gastric acid stimulation
Men: 18 to 28 mEq/hour
Women: 11 to 21 mEq/hour

Gastric secretion, basal
Men: 1 to 5 mEq/hour
Women: 0.2 to 3.8 mEq/hour

Gastrin, serum
< 300 pg/ml

Gamma globulin, cerebrospinal fluid
3% to 12% of total protein

Globulin, peritoneal fluid
30% to 45% of total protein

Globulin, serum
Alpha$_1$: 0.1 to 0.4 g/dl
Alpha$_2$: 0.5 to 1 g/dl
Beta: 0.7 to 1.2 g/dl
Gamma: 0.5 to 1.6 g/dl

Glucagon, fasting, serum
< 250 pg/ml

Glucose, amniotic fluid
< 45 mg/100 ml

Glucose, cerebrospinal fluid
50 to 80 mg/100 ml

Glucose, peritoneal fluid
70 to 100 mg/dl

Glucose, plasma, fasting
70 to 100 mg/dl

Glucose, plasma, oral tolerance
Peak at 160 to 180 mg/dl, 30 to 60 minutes after challenge dose

Glucose, plasma, 2-hour postprandial
< 145 mg/dl

Glucose, synovial fluid
70 to 100 mg/dl

Glucose, urine
Negative

Glutathione reductase activity index
0.9 to 1.3

Laboratory Test Values *(continued)*

Growth hormone, serum
Men: 0 to 5 ng/ml
Women: 0 to 10 ng/ml
Growth hormone suppression
0 to 3 ng/ml after 30 minutes to 2 hours

H

Haptoglobin, serum
38 to 270 mg/dl
Heinz bodies
Negative
Hematocrit
Men: 42% to 54%
Women: 38% to 46%
Hemoglobin electrophoresis
Hgb A: 95%
Hgb A$_2$: 2% to 3%
Hgb F: > 1%
Hemoglobin, glycosylated
Hgb A$_{1a}$: 1.6% of total RBC Hgb
Hgb A$_{1b}$: 0.8% of total RBC Hgb
Hgb A$_{1c}$: 4% of total RBC Hgb
Total glycosylated Hgb: 5.5% to 9%
Hemoglobin, total
Men: 14 to 18 g/dl
Women: 12 to 16 g/dl
Hemoglobin, urine
Negative
Hemoglobins, unstable
Heat stability: Negative
Isopropanol: Stable
Hemosiderin, urine
Negative
Hepatitis-B surface antigen, serum
Negative
Heterophil agglutination, serum
Normal titer < 1:56
Hexosaminidase A and B, serum
Total: 5 to 12.9 units/liter
(Hex-A is 55% to 76% of total)
Histoplasmosis antibody, serum
Normal titer: < 1:8
Homovanillic acid, urine
< 8 mg/24 hours
Hydroxybutyric dehydrogenase
Serum HBD: 114 to 290 units/ml
LDH/HBD ratio: 1.2 to 1.6:1
17-Hydroxycorticosteroids, urine
Men: 4.5 to 12 mg/24 hours
Women: 2.5 to 10 mg/24 hours
5-Hydroxyindoleacetic acid, urine
< 6 mg/24 hours

I

Immune complex assays, serum
Negative
Immunoglobulins, serum
IgG: 6.4 to 14.3 mg/ml
IgA: 0.3 to 3 mg/ml
IgM: 0.2 to 1.4 mg/ml
Insulin tolerance test
Blood glucose falls to 50% of fasting level 20 to 30 minutes after insulin administration, resulting in a 10- to 20-ng/dl increase over baseline values in both hGh and ACTH. Peak levels occur 60 to 90 minutes after insulin administration.
Inulin clearance, urine
≥ *Age 21:* 90 to 130 ml/minute
Insulin, serum
0 to 25 μU/ml
Iron, serum
Men: 70 to 150 mcg/dl
Women: 80 to 150 mcg/dl
Iron, total binding capacity, serum
Men: 300 to 400 mcg/dl
Women: 300 to 450 mcg/dl
Isocitrate dehydrogenase
1.2 to 7 units/liter

J, K

17-Ketogenic steroids, urine
Men: 4 to 14 mg/24 hours
Women: 2 to 12 mg/24 hours
Ketones, urine
Negative
17-Ketosteroids, urine
Men: 6 to 21 mg/24 hours
Women: 4 to 17 mg/24 hours

L

Lactic acid, blood
0.93 to 1.65 mEq/liter
Lactic dehydrogenase
Total: 48 to 115 IU/liter
LDH$_1$: 18.1% to 29%
LDH$_2$: 29.4% to 37.5%
LDH$_3$: 18.8% to 26%
LDH$_4$: 9.2% to 16.5%
LDH$_5$: 5.3% to 13.4%
Lactose tolerance test, oral
Within 15 to 60 minutes after ingestion of a lactose loading dose, plasma glucose levels
(continued)

Laboratory Test Values *(continued)*

Lactose tolerance test, oral
(continued)
rise more than 20 mg/dl over fasting levels. Stool sample analysis shows normal pH and low glucose content.
Leucine aminopeptidase
< 50 units/liter
Leukoagglutinins
Negative
Lipase
32 to 80 units/liter
Lipids, fecal
< 20% of excreted solids; < 7 g/24 hours
Lipoproteins, serum
HDL-cholesterol: 29 to 77 mg/dl
LDL-cholesterol: 62 to 185 mg/dl
Long-acting thyroid stimulator, serum
Negative
Lupus erythematosus cell preparation
Negative
Luteinizing hormone, plasma
Menstruating women: Follicular phase, 5 to 15 mIU/ml; ovulatory phase, 30 to 60 mIU/ml; luteal phase, 5 to 15 mIU/ml
Postmenopausal women: 50 to 100 mIU/ml
Men: 5 to 20 mIU/ml
Lymphocyte transformation
60% to 90% lymphocytes respond
Lysozyme, urine
< 3 mg/24 hours

M
Magnesium, serum
1.5 to 2.5 mEq/liter
Atomic absorption: 1.7 to 2.1 mg/dl
Magnesium, urine
< 150 mg/24 hours
Manganese, serum
0.4 to 0.85 ng/ml
Melanin, urine
Negative
Myoglobin, serum
30 to 90 ng/ml
Myoglobin, urine
Negative

N
Neonatal thyroid-stimulating hormone
≤ Age 2 days: 25 to 30 gmIU/ml
> Age 2 days: 25 gmIU/ml
5'-Nucleotidase
2 to 17 units/liter

O
Occult blood, fecal
< 2.5 ml/24 hours
Ornithine carbamoyltransferase, serum
0 to 500 Sigma units/ml
Oxalate, urine
≤ 40 mg/24 hours

P
Para-aminohippuric acid excretion, urine
Age 20: 400 to 700 ml/minute (17 ml/minute decrease each decade after age 20)
Parathyroid hormone, serum
20 to 70 μIEq/ml
Pericardial fluid
Amount: 10 to 50 ml
Appearance: Clear, straw-colored
White blood cell count: < 1,000/mm^3
Glucose: approximately whole blood level
Peritoneal fluid
Amount: < 50 ml
Appearance: Clear, straw-colored
Phenylalanine, serum, screening
Negative: < 2 mg/dl
Phenolsulfonphthalein excretion, urine
15 minutes: 25% of dose excreted
30 minutes: 50% to 60% of dose excreted
1 hour: 60% to 79% of dose excreted
2 hours: 70% to 80% of dose excreted
Phosphate, tubular reabsorption, urine and plasma
80% reabsorption
Phosphates, serum
1.8 to 2.6 mEq/liter
Atomic absorption: 2.5 to 4.5 mg/dl

Laboratory Test Values (continued)

Phosphates, urine
< 1,000 mg/24 hours
Phospholipids, plasma
180 to 320 mg/dl
Placental lactogen, serum
Pregnant women: 5 to 27 weeks, < 4.6 mcg/ml; 28 to 31 weeks, 2.4 to 6.1 mcg/ml; 32 to 35 weeks, 3.7 to 7.7 mcg/ml; 36 weeks to term, 5 to 8.6 mcg/ml
Nonpregnant women: < 0.5 mcg/ml
Men: < 0.5 mcg/ml
Plasma plasminogen
2.7 to 4.5 μ/ml (activity units); ≥ 65% (normal control values)
Plasma renin activity
Sodium-depleted, peripheral vein (upright position): Ages 20 to 39, 2.9 to 24 ng/ml/hour; age 40 and over, 2.9 to 10.8 ng/ml/hour
Sodium-replete, peripheral vein (upright position): Ages 20 to 39, 0.1 to 4.3 ng/ml/hour; age 40 and over, 0.1 to 3 ng/ml/hour
Platelet aggregation
3 to 5 minutes
Platelet count
130,000 to 370,000/mm³
Platelet survival
50% tagged platelets disappear within 84 to 116 hours
100% disappear within 8 to 10 days
Pleural fluid
Appearance: Clear (transudate); cloudy, turbulent (exudate)
Specific gravity: < 1.016 (transudate); > 1.016 (exudate)
Porphobilinogen, urine
≤ 1.5 mg/24 hours
Porphyrins, total
16 to 60 mg/dl of packed RBCs
Potassium, serum
3.8 to 5.5 mEq/liter
Pregnanediol, urine
Men: 1.5 mg/24 hours
Women: 0.5 to 1.5 mg/24 hours
Postmenopausal women: 0.2 to 1 mg/24 hours

Pregnanetriol, urine
< 3.5 mg/24 hours
Progesterone, plasma
Menstrual cycle: Follicular phase, < 150 ng/dl; luteal phase, 300 ng/dl; midluteal phase, 2,000 ng/dl
Pregnancy: First trimester, 1,500 to 5,000 ng/dl; second and third trimesters, 8,000 to 20,000 ng/dl
Prolactin, serum
0 to 23 ng/dl
Protein, cerebrospinal fluid
15 to 45 mg/dl
Protein, pleural fluid
Transudate: < 3 g/dl
Exudate: > 3 g/dl
Protein, total, peritoneal fluid
0.3 to 4.1 g/dl
Protein, total, serum
6.6 to 7.9 g/dl
Albumin fraction: 3.3 to 4.5 g/dl
Globulin levels: Alpha₁–globulin, 0.1 to 0.4 g/dl; alpha₂–globulin, 0.5 to 1 g/dl; beta globulin, 0.7 to 1.2 g/dl; gamma globulin, 0.5 to 1.6 g/dl
Protein, total, synovial fluid
10.7 to 21.3 mg/dl
Protein, urine
≤ 150 mg/24 hours
Prothrombin consumption time
20 seconds
Prothrombin time
Men: 9.6 to 11.8 seconds
Women: 9.5 to 11.3 seconds
Protoporphyrins
16 to 60 mg/dl
Pyruvate kinase
Ultraviolet: 2 to 8.8 units/g hemoglobin
Low substrate assay: 0.9 to 3.9 units/g hemoglobin
Pyruvic acid, blood
0.08 to 0.16 mEq/liter

R
Radioallergosorbent test
Negative: < 150% of control
Red blood cell count
Men: 4.5 to 6.2 million/μl venous blood

(continued)

Laboratory Test Values *(continued)*

Red blood cell count *(continued)*
Women: 4.2 to 5.4 million/μl
venous blood
Red blood cell survival time
25 to 35 days
Red blood cells, pleural fluid
Transudate: Few
Exudate: Variable
Red blood cells, urine
0 to 3 per high-power field
Red cell indices
MCV: 84 to 99 μ^3/red cell
MCH: 26 to 32 pg/red cell
MCHC: 30% to 36%
Reticulocyte count
0.5% to 2% of total RBC count
Rheumatoid factor, serum
Negative
Rubella antibodies, serum
Titer of 1:8 or less indicates little
or no immunity

S

Semen
Volume: 1.5 to 5 ml
pH: 7.3 to 7.7
Liquefaction: 30 minutes
Sperm: 60 million to 150 million/
ml
Cervical mucus: ≥ 5 motile
sperm per high-power field
**Serum glutamic-oxaloacetic
transaminase**
8 to 20 units/liter
**Serum glutamic-pyruvic
transaminase**
Men: 10 to 32 units/liter
Women: 9 to 24 units/liter
Sickle cell test
Negative
Sodium, serum
135 to 145 mEq/liter
Sodium, sweat
10 to 30 mEq/liter
Sodium, urine
30 to 280 mEq/24 hours
Sodium chloride, urine
5 to 20 g/24 hours
Sporotrichosis antibody, serum
Normal titers < 1:40
Synovial fluid
Color: Colorless to pale yellow
Clarity: Clear

Synovial fluid *(continued)*
Quantity (in knee): 0.3 to 3.5 ml
Viscosity: 5.7 to 1,160
pH: 7.2 to 7.4
Mucin clot: Good
Pao$_2$: 40 to 60 mm Hg
Paco$_2$: 40 to 60 mm Hg

T

T-lymphocyte count
1,400 to 2,700/mm^3
T$_3$ resin uptake
25% to 35% of T$_3$* binds resin
**Terminal deoxynucleotidyl
transferase, serum**
0 to 10 IU/10^{13} cells
Testosterone, plasma or serum
Men: 30 to 1,200 ng/dl
Women: 30 to 95 ng/dl
Thrombin time, plasma
10 to 15 seconds
**Thyroid-stimulating hormone,
serum**
0 to 15 μIU/ml
Thyroxine, total, serum
5 to 13.5 mcg/dl
**Thyroxine-binding globulin,
serum**
Electrophoresis: From 10 to 26
mcg T$_4$ (binding capacity)/dl to
16 to 24 mcg T$_4$ (binding
capacity)/dl
Radioimmunoassay: 1.3 to 2 ng/dl
Tolbutamide tolerance
Plasma glucose drops to one half
fasting level for 30 minutes,
recovers in 1½ to 3 hours
Transferrin, serum
250 to 390 mcg/dl
Triglycerides, serum
Ages 0 to 29: 10 to 140 mg/dl
Ages 30 to 39: 10 to 150 mg/dl
Ages 40 to 49: 10 to 160 mg/dl
Ages 50 to 59: 10 to 190 mg/dl
Triiodothyronine, serum
90 to 230 ng/dl

U

Urea, urine
Maximal clearance: 64 to 99 ml/
minute
Uric acid, serum
Men: 4.3 to 8 mg/dl
Women: 2.3 to 6 mg/dl

Laboratory Test Values (continued)

Uric acid, synovial fluid
  Men: 2 to 8 mg/dl
  Women: 2 to 6 mg/dl
Uric acid, urine
  250 to 750 mg/24 hours
Urinalysis, routine
  Color: Straw
  Appearance: Clear
  Specific gravity: 1.005 to 1.020
  pH: 4.5 to 8
  Epithelial cells: Few
  Casts: Occasional hyaline casts
  Crystals: Present
Urine hydroxyproline, total
  Adult: 14 to 45 mg/24 hours
Urine osmolality
  Range: 50 to 1,400 mosmol/kg
  Average: 500 to 800 mosmol/kg
Urine potassium
  Excretion: 25 to 125 mEq/24
    hours
  Concentration: < 10 mEq/liter in
    patients with hypokalemia
Urobilinogen, fecal
  50 to 300 mg/24 hours
Urobilinogen, urine
  Men: 0.3 to 2.1 Ehrlich units/2
    hours
  Women: 0.1 to 1.1 Ehrlich units/
    2 hours
Uroporphyrin, urine
  Men: 0 to 42 mcg/24 hours
  Women: 1 to 22 mcg/24 hours
Uroporphyrinogen I synthase
  Men: 7.9 to 14.7 nm/sec/liter
  Women: 8.1 to 16.8 nm/sec/liter

V
Vanillylmandelic acid, urine
  0.7 to 6.8 mg/24 hours
VDRL, cerebrospinal fluid
  Negative
VDRL, serum
  Negative
Vitamin A, serum
  125 to 150 IU/dl
Vitamin B$_1$, urine
  100 to 200 mcg/24 hours
Vitamin B$_6$ (tryptophan), urine
  < 50 mcg/24 hours

Vitamin B$_{12}$, serum
  200 to 1,100 pg/ml
Vitamin C, plasma
  0.2 to 2 mg/dl
Vitamin C, urine
  30 mg/24 hours
Vitamin D$_3$, serum
  10 to 55 ng/ml

W
White blood cell count, blood
  4,100 to 10,900/µl
**White blood cell count,
  cerebrospinal fluid**
  0 to 5/mm^3
**White blood cell count, peritoneal
  fluid**
  < 300/µl
**White blood cell count, pleural
  fluid**
  Transudate: Few
  Exudate: Many (may be purulent)
**White blood cell count, synovial
  fluid**
  0 to 200/µl
White blood cell count, urine
  0 to 4 per high-power field
**White blood cell differential,
  blood**
  Neutrophils: 47.6% to 76.8%
  Lymphocytes: 16.2% to 43%
  Monocytes: 0.6% to 9.6%
  Eosinophils: 0.3% to 7%
  Basophils: 0.3% to 2%
**White blood cell differential,
  synovial fluid**
  Lymphocytes: 0 to 78/µl
  Monocytes: 0 to 71/µl
  Clasmatocytes: 0 to 26/µl
  Polymorphonuclears: 0 to 25/µl
  Other phagocytes: 0 to 21/µl
  Synovial lining cells: 0 to 12/µl
Whole blood clotting time
  5 to 15 minutes

Z
Zinc, serum
  0.75 to 1.4 mcg/ml

International System of Units (SI Units)

Clinical laboratory data is expressed in SI (or metric system) units throughout most of the world. (The abbreviation SI stands for "Système International" in French or "International System" in English.) It was adopted by Canada in 1970. In the U.S., the transition from conventional units to SI units will occur in the near future and will represent a major national change. The metric system is the cornerstone of SI units. This system is actually a simplified system because it uses fewer types of base units than previous measurement systems. There are only 7 base units in SI, and other derived units come from these 7 units.

Base Units of the International System (SI)

Physical quantity	Base unit	SI symbol
length	meter	m
mass	kilogram	kg
time	second	s
amount of substance	mole	mol
thermodynamic temperature	kelvin	K
electric current	ampere	amp
luminous intensity	candela	cd

The important SI unit which affects much laboratory data is the mole. This one unit will (for the most part) be used to measure amounts of substances, instead of the many units used in the conventional system. The mole is the amount of a substance which contains as many atoms or molecules as there are atoms in 0.012 kilogram of carbon-12. This means that equal quantities of different substances, expressed in molar amounts, contain equal numbers of atoms or molecules.

International System of Units *(continued)*

The following chart gives normal (reference) chemistry values for common tests. The SI unit is included as well as the conversion factor for changing to conventional values. For enzyme values, you are instructed to consult your laboratory. We have included approximate SI values. For most constituents, the changes from Mass units (conventional) to SI units, and vice versa, involves the application of a simple factor which is independent of method. However, for enzymes, the factors are dependent on the substrate, technique, and temperature involved. Furthermore, there is still debate regarding the use of the SI unit, "katal," to express enzyme activity. Many countries have merely adopted U/L as the standard form. Conversion from U/L to katal/L always involves the same factor: 0.06 from nkat/L to U/L, or 60 from ukat/L to U/L.

Because of the large variety of enzyme substrates, conversion factors for enzymes have NOT been stated in the following list. Great care should be taken to establish which method has been used and to ensure that results of enzyme determinations are contrasted with appropriate reference ranges quoted by your laboratory.

(continued)

International System of Units *(continued)*

BLOOD CHEMISTRY	NORMAL LABORATORY TEST VALUES		
Constituent	SI Units	Conversion Factor (SI→ Conventional)	Conventional Values
Acid phosphatase Example only: King-Armstrong	2 to 8 U/L 20 to 65 nkat/L	0.561 0.060	1 to 4 King-Armstrong units/ml
Albumin, serum	33 to 45 g/L	10.0	3.3 to 4.5 g/dl
Alkaline phosphatase Example only: King-Armstrong	28 to 100 U/L 9.5 to 1.7 ukat/L	0.14 60.00	4 to 13.5 King-Armstrong units/dl
Amylase CONSULT LABORATORY	approx 0 to 2.2 kat/L		
Arterial blood gases pO_2 pCO_2 pH	10.0 to 13.3 kPa 4.7 to 6.0 kPa 37 to 45 nmol/L	7.5 7.5 Complex	75 to 100 mm Hg 35 to 45 mm Hg 7.35 to 7.42
Bilirubin, serum Adult direct Adult indirect	<8 umol/L ≤18 umol/L	0.0585	<0.5 mg/dl ≤1.1 mg/dl
Blood urea nitrogen	2.9 to 7.1 mmol/L	2.80	8 to 20 mg/dl
Calcium, serum	2.30 to 2.65 mmol/L	2.0 4.0	4.5 to 5.5 mEq/L 8.9 to 10.1 mg/dl
Carbon dioxide, total blood	22 to 34 mmol/L	1.0	22 to 34 mEq/L
Catecholamines, plasma Supine: Epinephrine Norepinephrine Dopamine	0 to 600 pmol/L 0.4 to 4.4 nmol/L 0 to 196 pmol/L	0.183 169.0 0.153	0 to 110 pg/ml 70 to 750 pg/ml 0 to 30 pg/ml
Standing: Epinephrine Norepinephrine Dopamine	0 to 765 pmol/L 1.2 to 10.1 nmol/L 0 to 196 pmol/L	0.183 169.0 0.153	0 to 140 pg/ml 200 to 1,700 pg/ml 0 to 30 pg/ml
Chloride, serum	100 to 108 mmol/L	1.0	100 to 108 mEq/L

International System of Units *(continued)*

BLOOD CHEMISTRY	NORMAL LABORATORY TEST VALUES		
Constituent	SI Units	Conversion Factor (SI→ Conventional)	Conventional Values
Cholesterol, total, serum	3.1 to 8.6 mmol/L	38.7	120 to 330 mg/dl
Creatine phosphokinase CONSULT LABORATORY	Approx 0 to 2.2 ukat/L		
Creatine, serum Males: Females:	15 to 46 umol/L 46 to 76 umol/L	0.0131	0.2 to 0.6 mg/dl 0.6 to 1 mg/dl
Creatinine, serum Males: Females:	71 to 106 umol/L 53 to 80 umol/L	0.0113	0.8 to 1.2 mg/dl 0.6 to 0.9 mg/dl
Free thyroxine	10 to 42 pmol/L	0.0777	0.8 to 3.3 mg/dl
Free triiodothyronine	3.1 to 9.2 pmol/L	0.0651	0.2 to 0.6 ng/dl
Gamma glutamyl transferase CONSULT LABORATORY	Approx 0 to 0.5 ukat/L		
Glucose, fasting, plasma	3.9 to 5.6 mmol/L	18.0	70 to 100 mg/dl
Glucose, plasma, oral tolerance	Peak at 8.9 to 10.0 mmol/L, 30 to 60 minutes after challenge dose	18.0	Peak at 160 to 180 mg/dl, 30 to 60 minutes after challenge dose
Glucose, plasma, 2-hour postprandial	<8.1 mmol/L	18.0	<145 mg/dl
Iron, serum Men: Women:	13 to 27 umol/L 14 to 27 umol/L	5.6	70 to 150 mcg/dl 80 to 150 mcg/dl
Lactic acid, blood	0.93 to 1.65 mmol/L	1.0	0.93 to 1.65 mEq/L

(continued)

International System of Units *(continued)*

BLOOD CHEMISTRY	NORMAL LABORATORY TEST VALUES		
Constituent	**SI Units**	**Conversion Factor (SI→ Conventional)**	**Conventional Values**
Lactic dehydrogenase CONSULT LABORATORY	Approx 0.8 to 2.7 ukat/L		
Lipase CONSULT LABORATORY	Approx 0 to 2.7 ukat/L		
Lipoproteins, serum HDL-cholesterol LDL-cholesterol	0.8 to 2.0 mmol/L 1.6 to 4.8 mmol/L	38.7	29 to 77 mg/dl 62 to 185 mg/dl
Magnesium, serum	0.9 to 1.3 mmol/L	2.0 or 2.4	1.5 to 2.5 mEq/L 1.7 to 2.1 mg/dl
Phosphates, serum	0.8 to 1.5 mmol/L	3.1	2.5 to 4.5 mg/dl
Potassium, serum	3.8 to 5.5 mmol/L	1.0	3.8 to 5.5 mEq/L
Protein, total, serum	66 to 79 g/L	10.0	6.6 to 7.9 g/dl
Serum GOT (aspartate transferase— AST) CONSULT LABORATORY	Approx 0 to 0.6 ukat/L		
Serum GPT (alanine transferase—ALT) CONSULT LABORATORY	Approx 0 to 0.6 ukat/L		
Sodium, serum	135 to 145 mmol/L	1.0	135 to 145 mEq/L
Thyroxine, total, serum	64 to 174 nmol/L	0.0777	5 to 13.5 mcg/dl

International System of Units *(continued)*			

BLOOD CHEMISTRY — NORMAL LABORATORY TEST VALUES

Constituent	SI Units	Conversion Factor (SI→ Conventional)	Conventional Values
Triglycerides, serum			
Ages 0 to 29	0.11 to 1.58 mmol/L	0.0113	10 to 140 mg/dl
Ages 30 to 39	0.11 to 1.69 mmol/L		10 to 150 mg/dl
Ages 40 to 49	0.11 to 1.81 mmol/L		10 to 160 mg/dl
Ages 50 to 59	0.11 to 2.14 mmol/L		10 to 190 mg/dl
Uric acid, serum			
Men:	256 to 476 umol/L	0.0168	4.3 to 8 mg/dl
Women:	137 to 357 umol/L		2.3 to 6 mg/dl

URINE CHEMISTRY — NORMAL LABORATORY TEST VALUES

Constituent	SI Units	Conversion Factor (SI→ Conventional)	Conventional Values
Calcium, urine			
Males:	<6.9 mmol/d	40.0	<275 mg/24 hours
Females:	<6.3 mmol/d		<250 mg/24 hours
Catecholamines, urine			
24-hour specimen	0 to 800 nmol/d (expressed as norepinephrine)	0.169	0 to 135 mcg
Random specimen	0 to 1,065 nmol/L (1.07 umol/L)		0 to 18 mcg/dl
Creatinine, urine			
Men:	9 to 17 mmol/24 hours	0.113	1 to 1.9 g/24 hours
Women:	7 to 15 mmol/24 hours		0.8 to 1.7 g/24 hours

(continued)

International System of Units (continued)

URINE CHEMISTRY	NORMAL LABORATORY TEST VALUES		
Constituent	SI Units	Conversion Factor (SI→ Conventional)	Conventional Values
17-Hydroxycortico-steroids, urine			
Men:	12 to 33 umol/d	0.362	4.5 to 12 mg/24 hours
Women:	7 to 28 umol/d		2.5 to 10 mg/24 hours
17-Ketogenic steroids, urine			
Men:	14 to 49 umol/d	0.288	4 to 14 mg/24 hours
Women:	7 to 42 umol/d (as dehydro-epiandrosterone)		2 to 12 mg/24 hours
17-Ketosteroids			
Men:	21 to 73 umol/d	0.288	6 to 21 mg/24 hours
Women:	14 to 59 umol/d (as dehydro-epiandrosterone)		4 to 17 mg/24 hours
Osmolality			
Range	50 to 1,400 mmol/kg	1.0	
Average	300 to 800 mmol/kg		
Sodium, urine	30 to 280 mmol/d	1.0	30 to 280 mEq/24 hours
Uric acid, urine	1.5 to 4.5 mmol/d	168.0	250 to 750 mg/24 hours
VMA (4-hydroxy-3-methoxy mandelic acid—HMMA)	3.5 to 34 umol/d	0.198	0.7 to 6.8 mg/24 hours

Laboratory Values for Therapeutic Drug Monitoring

In therapeutic monitoring, analytic measurements of blood drug levels are taken serially to determine and maintain dosage at an effective level. Drug monitoring is especially useful when the margin of safety between therapeutic and toxic levels is narrow. Such monitoring is commonly restricted to drugs for which a known correlation exists between blood levels and therapeutic effects. In patients who require these special groups of drugs, blood level monitoring can evaluate the patient's compliance, adequacy of dosage, and current clinical status.

Drug	Peak time	Steady state	Therapeutic level	Toxic level
Antiarrhythmics				
Disopyramide, serum (Norpace)	P.O.: 2 hours	25 to 30 hours	2 to 4.5 mcg/ml	> 9 mcg/ml
Lidocaine, serum (Xylocaine)	I.V.: immediate	5 to 10 hours	2 to 6 mcg/ml	> 7 mcg/ml
Procainamide, serum (Pronestyl)	P.O.: 60 minutes I.V.: 25 to 60 minutes	11 to 20 hours	4 to 8 mcg/ml	> 12 mcg/ml
N-acetyl-procainamide			2 to 8 mcg/ml	> 30 mcg/ml
Propranolol, serum (Inderal)	P.O.: 60 to 90 minutes I.V.: 2 to 4 hours	10 to 30 hours	40 to 85 ng/ml (If patient's condition does not improve with serum level of 100 ng, treatment is unsuccessful.)	> 150 ng/ml (Toxic concentrations vary and require correlation with clinical status.)
Quinidine, serum (Quinaglute, Cardioquin, Quinidex)	P.O.: 1 to 3 hours I.V.: immediate I.M.: 30 to 90 minutes	20 to 35 hours	2.4 to 5 mcg/ml	> 6 mcg/ml
Verapamil, serum (Calan, Isoptin)	P.O.: 1 to 2 hours I.V.: 5 minutes	15 to 35 hours	0.08 to 0.3 mcg/ml	Unknown

(continued)

Laboratory Values for Therapeutic Drug Monitoring *(continued)*

Drug	Peak time	Steady state	Therapeutic level	Toxic level
Antibiotics				
Amikacin, serum (Amikin)	I.M.: 30 minutes to 1 hour I.V.: 15 to 30 minutes	1 to 2 days	8 to 16 mcg/ml	Peak: > 35 mcg/ml Trough: > 8 mcg/ml*
Gentamicin, serum (Garamycin)	I.M.: 30 minutes to 1 hour I.V.: 15 to 30 minutes	1 to 2 days	4 to 10 mcg/ml	Peak: > 12 mcg/ml Trough: > 2 mcg/ml*
Kanamycin, serum (Kantrex)	I.M.: 30 minutes to 1 hour	1 to 2 days	8 to 16 mcg/ml	Peak: > 35 mcg/ml Trough: > 8 mcg/ml*
Netilmicin, serum (Netromycin)	I.M.: 30 minutes to 1 hour I.V.: 15 to 30 minutes	1 to 2 days	0.5 to 10 mcg/ml	Peak: > 16 mcg/ml Trough: > 4 mcg/ml*
Tobramycin, serum (Nebcin)	I.M.: 30 minutes to 1 hour I.V.: 15 to 30 minutes	1 to 2 days	4 to 8 mcg/ml	Peak: > 12 mcg/ml Trough: > 2 mcg/ml*
(*Toxic trough levels may be below therapeutic levels due to the nephrotoxicity of antibiotics.)				
Anticonvulsants				
Carbamazepine, serum (Tegretol)	2 to 6 hours	2 to 4 days	2 to 10 mcg/ml	> 12 mcg/ml (Toxic concentrations vary and require correlation with clinical status.)
Ethosuximide, serum (Zarontin)	1 to 2 hours	8 to 10 days	40 to 80 mcg/ml	> 100 mcg/ml
Phenobarbital, serum (Luminal)	6 to 18 hours	14 to 21 days	20 to 40 mcg/ml	> 55 mcg/ml

Laboratory Values for Therapeutic Drug Monitoring *(continued)*

Drug	Peak time	Steady state	Therapeutic level	Toxic level
Anticonvulsants *(continued)*				
Phenytoin, serum (Dilantin)	4 to 8 hours	5 to 11 days	10 to 20 mcg/ml	> 80 mcg/ml (Toxic concentrations vary and require correlation with clinical status.)
Primidone, serum (Mysoline)	2 to 4 hours	4 to 7 days	7 to 11 mcg/ml	> 12 mcg/ml (Toxic concentrations vary and require correlation with clinical status.)
Bronchodilators				
Aminophylline, serum or Theophylline, serum (Aminodur Dura-tab, Corophyllin	P.O.: 2 to 3 hours I.V.: 15 minutes	15 to 40 hours	10 to 20 mcg/ml	> 20 mcg/ml (Toxic concentrations vary and require correlation with clinical status.)
Cardiac Glycosides				
Digitoxin (Crystodigin)	4 to 12 hours	25 to 35 days	5 to 30 ng/ml	> 35 ng/ml
Digoxin, serum (Lanoxin)	1½ to 5 hours	7 days	0.5 to 2 ng/ml	> 2.5 ng/ml

Laboratory Values in Toxicology

Toxicity determinations may include emergency tests to evaluate the type and amount of legal or illegal drugs taken in accidental or intentional overdoses. Generally, blood or urine is the specimen of choice, but appropriate specimens may include gastric contents or lavage fluid, if the test is performed soon after ingestion.

Drug/Substance	Therapeutic level	Toxic level
Alcohol		
Ethanol, serum		> 0.1% wt/vol (100 mg/dl) (If blood alcohol level is between 0.05% and 0.1% wt/vol (50 to 100 mg/dl), a person is, by law, intoxicated; however, behavior and other circumstances are considered by the court.)
Isopropanol, serum (isopropyl alcohol, rubbing alcohol)		30 mg/dl (Lethal level: 150 mg/dl)
Methanol, serum (antifreeze)		20 mg/dl (Lethal level: 80 mg/dl)
Amphetamines		
Amphetamine, urine	2 to 3 mcg/ml	> 30 mcg/ml
Dextroamphetamine, urine (Dexedrine)	1 to 1.5 mcg/ml	> 15 mcg/ml
Methamphetamine, urine (Desoxyn)	3 to 5 mcg/ml	> 40 mcg/ml
Phenmetrazine, urine (Preludin)	5 to 30 mcg/ml	> 50 mcg/ml
Antidepressants		
Amitriptyline (and metabolite Nortriptylline), serum or plasma (Amitril, Triavil, Elavil)	75 to 200 ng/ml	> 1,000 ng/ml
Desipramine, serum or plasma (Norpramin)	20 to 160 ng/ml	> 1,000 ng/ml

Laboratory Values in Toxicology *(continued)*

Drug/Substance	Therapeutic level	Toxic level
Antidepressants *(continued)*		
Doxepin (and metabolite desmethyldoxepin), serum or plasma (Adapin, Sinequan)	90 to 250 ng/ml	> 1,000 ng/ml
Imipramine (and metabolite desipramine), serum or plasma (Tofranil)	200 ng/ml	> 1,000 ng/ml
Lithium, serum or plasma (Lithobid)	0.9 to 1.4 mEq	1.5 mEq
Nortriptyline, serum or plasma (Aventyl)	75 to 150 ng/ml	> 300 ng/ml
Barbiturates and Hypnotics		
Amobarbital, serum (Amytal)	Unknown	> 50 mcg/ml Lethal: > 50 mcg/ml
Glutethimide, serum (Doriden)	2 to 7 mcg/ml	> 10 mcg/ml
Pentobarbital, serum (Nembutal)	1 to 10 mcg/ml	> 10 mcg/ml Lethal: > 30 mcg/ml
Phenobarbital, serum (Luminal)	15 to 40 mcg/ml	> 60 mcg/ml Lethal: > 80 mcg/ml
Secobarbital, serum (Seconal)	5 to 15 mcg/ml	> 15 mcg/ml Lethal: > 30 mcg/ml
Nonnarcotic Analgesics		
Acetaminophen, serum (Tylenol, Datril)	5 to 20 mcg/ml	After 4 hours: > 120 mcg/ml After 8 hours: > 60 mcg/ml
Salicylates, serum (Aspirin)	2 to 30 mg/100 ml	> 40 mg/100 ml
Phenothiazines		
Chlorpromazine, serum (Thorazine)	< 0.5 mcg/ml	> 1.0 mcg/ml

(continued)

Laboratory Values in Toxicology *(continued)*

Drug/Substance	Therapeutic level	Toxic level
Phenothiazines *(continued)*		
Prochlorperazine, serum (Compazine)	< 0.5 mcg/ml	> 1.0 mcg/ml
Thioridazine, serum (Mellaril)	< 1.25 mcg/ml	> 10 mcg/ml
Trifluoperazine, serum (Stelazine)	< 0.5 mcg/ml	> 1.0 mcg/ml

Drug/Substance	Normal level	Toxic level
Hemoglobin Derivatives		
Carboxyhemoglobin (Results from union of hemoglobin and carbon monoxide)	3% of the total hemoglobin (up to 15% in tobacco smokers)	For acute carbon monoxide toxicity: 20% to 30% of total hemoglobin (Lethal level: 60% to 80%)
Methemoglobin (Results from oxidation of ferrous iron to the ferric form, usually from chemicals and drugs, such as nitrates, nitrites, sulfonamides, aniline, chlorates, or phenacetin, or from primary methemoglobinemia)	< 3% of the total hemoglobin	10% to 70% of total hemoglobin (Lethal level: > 70%)
Sulfhemoglobin (Results from combining hemoglobin with certain drugs, such as phenacetin or sulfonamides)	Undetectable	10 g/dl (Produces cyanosis but few or no toxic symptoms)

Home Tests

With the exception of measuring urine glucose, home testing is relatively new and growing in popularity. Improved technology brings more products, easier test performance, and quicker results.

A representative sample of home tests, with summaries of their procedures, is included in the chart below. Commercial kits provide more detailed instructions for use.

Product	Procedure overview	Comments
Tests for glucose: Currently, there is a definite trend toward testing blood rather than urine for glucose. Testing the blood instead of urine results in improved patient motivation and, thus, better control of diabetes.		
Visidex II® reagent strips, Chemstrip® bG, BetaScan Trendstrips™, Glucostix® reagent strips	A drop of blood from the finger or earlobe is placed on the reagent pads of the test strip. After a specified period, the resulting reagent pad colors are compared to a standardized color chart usually found on the vial label.	For quantitative measurements, the Chemstrip bG can be read by the Accu-Chek™ bG Blood Glucose Monitor; the BetaScan Trendstrips by the Trend Meter; Glucostix reagent strips by the Glucometer II® Blood Glucose Monitor.
Glucometer II® Blood Glucose Monitor	After obtaining a blood sample, placing it on the Glucostix® reagent strip, and blotting as directed, the strip is inserted into the Glucometer II®, which reads the color on the test reagent pads electronically and displays a digital value.	The Glucometer and other similar blood-sugar meters are accurate, economical, and easy to use. These devices need to be calibrated before use.
Clinistix®, Diastix®, Chemstrip®	The reagent pad of the test strip is dipped in urine; excess urine is removed, and, after waiting a specified time, the approximate glucose level is determined by comparing the reagent pad color to a standardized chart on the container.	These tests are specific for glucose but are not as accurate as blood glucose tests. Excess vitamin C can affect test results.
Clinitest®	The Clinitest tablet is added to a test tube containing a specified amount of urine. A heat-producing chemical reaction takes place. Comparison of the resulting color of the test tube liquid with the standardized color chart gives the approximate level of urine glucose.	This test is not as accurate as blood tests.

(continued)

Home Tests *(continued)*

Product	Procedure overview	Comments
Tests for infection: Home testing for infections includes detection of urinary tract infection and of gonorrhea in males.		
V.D. Alert	The male obtains a urethral discharge on a slide and sends it to the specified laboratory. After 48 hours, he phones the lab, using a toll-free number, and identifies himself only by a code number. He is informed whether *Neisseria gonorrhoeae* is present.	This test, which allows complete anonymity, detects gonorrhea but not other sexually transmitted diseases. The patient must contact his physician for treatment if results are positive. The test is not applicable to females.
Microstix-Nitrite®	Three Microstix-Nitrite reagent test strips are used to test first-morning urine specimens on three consecutive mornings. If nitrite is present in urine, the test strip will turn pink.	Nitrate from dietary sources is converted in urine to nitrite by such organisms as *Escherichia coli*. Positive results mean that 100,000 or more nitrate-reducing bacteria are present; these organisms cause about 90% of urinary tract infections. If results are positive, a physician should be contacted as soon as possible.
Tests for occult blood: Tests for fecal occult blood verify that blood is present but do not specify the source. These tests can serve as useful screening tests for colorectal cancer. Over 90% of patients with colorectal cancer could survive 5 or more years with early detection and treatment.		
ColoScreen Self-Test™	A reagent-impregnated pad is dropped into the toilet with feces. The edge will change to orange-red if blood is present. The test must be performed for three successive bowel movements.	This test is based on detection of hemoglobin released from feces. Dietary and medication restrictions include none for fruits and vegetables, but vitamin C and red meats are restricted.
Early Detector™	After a bowel movement, a specimen pad is used to pat the anal area. A developer solution is then sprayed onto the stool specimen. If there is blood present, the area around	Dietary and medication restrictions include items such as vitamin C, fruits, vegetables, and red meat for 2 days prior to and during the test.

Home Tests *(continued)*

Product	Procedure overview	Comments
Tests for occult blood *(continued)*		
Early Detector™ *(continued)*	*the specimen will turn blue. The test must be performed for three successive bowel movements.*	
Hemoccult® Home Test	Two small fecal specimens from three consecutive bowel movements are applied to prepared slides. Any trace or shade of blue may mean that there is blood present.	This test uses paper that has been treated with guaiac, a chemical that is sensitive to blood in the stool. Dietary and medication restrictions include items such as vitamin C, iron preparations, aspirin, red meat, turnips, and melons for 2 days prior to and during the test.

Tests for ovulation: These tests are based on detecting the surge of luteinizing hormone (LH) that normally appears shortly before ovulation. Their purpose is to help maximize the chances of conception. The tests use a plastic dipstick coated with monoclonal antibodies specific for LH.

OvuSTICK™ Self-Test; First Response™ Ovulation Predictor Test; Ovutime™ Ovulation Predictor Test	Urine is tested daily for a specified number of days in the menstrual cycle. For each test, a dipstick coated with monoclonal antibodies specific for LH is inserted into the urine sample. The dipstick turns blue during the LH surge, indicating that ovulation will occur shortly.	Each product specifies testing time and indicates when ovulation is likely to occur.

Tests for pregnancy. All home pregnancy tests are based on the ability to detect human chorionic gonadotropin (hCG) in urine. This hormone is produced by the human placenta and secreted in urine. Since the hormone is not normally found in nonpregnant women, its presence usually indicates pregnancy. Newer tests use monoclonal antibody technology and are performed more easily.

First Response™ Pregnancy Test	A dipstick is used to test the urine sample. If, after following all steps, a blue liquid is observed in the vial, this indicates that hCG is present and pregnancy is probable.	Earliest possible detection: First day of missed period. Testing time: 20 minutes. This test uses monoclonal antibody technology.

(continued)

Home Tests *(continued)*

Product	Procedure overview	Comments
Tests for pregnancy *(continued)*		
Advance®	*A plastic "Colorstick" is dipped in urine; if, after following all steps, a blue color appears on the rounded end of the dipstick, this indicates the presence of hCG in urine and probable pregnancy.*	*Earliest possible detection: 3 days after the last missed period. Testing time: 30 minutes. This test uses monoclonal antibody technology.*
Fact™	*A dark ring reflected in the mirror under the test tube containing urine indicates hCG is present and pregnancy is probable.*	*Earliest possible detection: 3 days after the last missed period. Testing time: 45 minutes.*

INDEX